D1395280

Dietary Supplements

Dietary Supplements

THIRD EDITION

Pamela Mason

BSc, MSc, PhD, MRPharmS
Pharmacist and Registered Nutritionist Writer and Consultant
Grosmont, Monmouthshire, UK

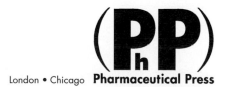

London • Chicago **Pharmaceutical Press**

Published by the Pharmaceutical Press

An imprint of RPS Publishing

1 Lambeth High Street, London SE1 7JN, UK
100 South Atkinson Road, Suite 200, Grayslake, IL 60030–7820, USA

© Pharmaceutical Press 2007

(**PP**) is a trade mark of RPS Publishing

RPS Publishing is the publishing organisation of the Royal
Pharmaceutical Society of Great Britain

First edition published by Blackwell Science Ltd 1995
Reprinted 1998
Second edition 2001
Third edition 2007

Typeset by Techbooks, New Delhi, India
Printed in Great Britain by Cromwell Press, Trowbridge, Wiltshire

ISBN 978 0 85369 653 7

Contents

Preface

SINCE THE SECOND EDITON of this book was published five years ago, the UK and worldwide market for food supplements has continued to grow. Vitamins and minerals – in multiple-ingredient products and as single ingredients – remain very popular. Indeed, multivitamins and minerals have the largest share of the market in most countries.

However, since the last edition, there has been an enormous growth in interest in other supplements, such as carotenoids, glucosamine, isoflavones, omega-3 fatty acids and probiotics, substances that were hardly known to the general public until very recently. Technological advances are increasingly making it possible to include such ingredients in both dietary supplements and foods, hence the blurring of boundaries between 'supplements', 'functional foods' and the 'nutraceutical' ingredients that go into them. As the range of substances identified in foods, and knowledge of their potential benefits in disease, continues to grow, it is likely that many more such substances will be included in food supplements in the future.

The amount of information about food supplements has grown exponentially during the last few years, most of it appearing on the Internet and fully accessible to the public. Added to which is the huge variety of food supplements on the shelves of pharmacies, health food shops, supermarkets and on the Internet. Finding an evidence-based path through the maze of information and products is an enormous challenge for the health professional, and it is very confusing for the potential buyer who wants to know 'what really works'.

Few health professionals, including pharmacists, nurses, doctors or dieticians, have an in-depth knowledge of dietary supplements, yet the public expects them to be able to answer questions on these products. Although there is an abundance of spurious information, there is, alongside this, a growing evidence base for dietary supplements. A large number of peer-reviewed, high-quality trials, systematic reviews and meta-analyses have been published since the second edition of this book, offering health professionals a better evidence base from which to offer information to the public.

There are still, of course, many uncertainties, and the inevitable 'more research needed' will continue to apply to many dietary supplements for some time to come. However, this should not prevent health professionals from giving evidence-based information where it exists and being honest enough to say 'research has not yet provided the answers' where appropriate.

So, what has changed in the third edition of *Dietary Supplements*? The answer to this lies mainly in the depth of information provided in the monographs, which has arisen entirely because of the growth in the research base. Ten new monographs have also been added. Another significant change is the inclusion of maximum safe upper levels for vitamins and minerals, which have been published in the UK since the second edition. The regulatory framework for dietary supplements has also changed in the UK, in that the European Union Food Supplements Directive has now come into force. Although this has meant limited change to the book, the labelling and marketing of supplements is likely to change in the near future.

The easy-to-use encyclopaedic format continues to be retained and it is my intention that this book is primarily a reference source, which I hope will continue to be useful to many colleagues around the world.

Pamela Mason
January 2007

About the author

PAMELA MASON is a pharmacist and registered nutritionist working as a writer and consultant based in Grosmont, Monmouthshire. She qualified as a pharmacist at Manchester University and worked as a community pharmacist for several years before studying at King's College London, where she completed an MSc and PhD in nutrition. Her interest in food supplements began as a result of her studies in nutrition and her experience in community pharmacy, where she was often asked questions about these products. She is the author of three other books, several open learning programmes and over 300 articles. She teaches nutrition to pharmacists at both undergraduate and postgraduate level and gives conference presentations about supplements both in the UK and abroad.

Introduction

There is now considerable interest in dietary supplements, and increasing numbers of people are using them. In the National Diet and Nutrition Survey of British adults aged 19–64 years, 40% were taking supplements.[1] In the UK, sales of dietary supplements in 2005 were approximately £326 million in 'bricks and mortar' shops (excluding health food shops).[2] Sales of some of the different types of supplements (2005 figures) are shown in Table 1.

Table 1 Sales of different types of supplements in the UK (2005)

Type of supplement	Sales(£ million)
Fish oils	116
Multivitamins	72
Single vitamins	35
Evening primrose oil and other GLA products	13
Garlic	7
Other	83
Total	326

GLA = gamma-linolenic acid.

Individuals buy supplements for many different reasons, which may include the following:

- As an insurance policy, to supplement what an individual may consider to be a poor diet (e.g. no time or inclination to eat regular meals).
- To improve overall health and fitness.
- To prolong vitality and delay the onset of age-associated problems.
- As a tonic or 'pick-me-up' when feeling run-down or after illness.
- For symptoms of stress.
- Recommended by an alternative health practitioner or health professional.
- Pregnancy.
- Slimming.
- Smoking.
- To improve performance and body-building in sports and athletics.
- To prevent or treat various signs and symptoms (e.g. colds, cardiovascular disease, cancer, poor sight, skin problems, arthritis, premenstrual syndrome, etc.).

While there is a great deal of information about these substances – increasingly so on the Internet – not all of it is reliable. Indeed, there are probably few areas associated with health care where such confusion exists. This confusion extends to health professionals as well as the general public. Because dietary supplements are not considered to be drugs, pharmacists are often unfamiliar with them and, because they are not foods (in the sense of being part of a normal diet), dieticians are understandably wary of recommending them. Doctors typically receive little nutritional education and may not have the knowledge or the time to give informed advice.

In addition, supplements are a topic about which there is a great deal of disagreement even between nutrition experts. Some say they are largely unnecessary because a balanced diet provides all the required vitamins and minerals, others say that supplements make a worthwhile contribution to a healthy diet, while increasingly, some experts say that optimal health cannot easily be achieved in some areas without them.

Given the growth in sales of dietary supplements, it is appropriate to ask what evidence there is that they work. Are there rigorous trials to show that these products work? Until the early 1990s, there were relatively few well-conducted trials involving vitamins and minerals, and fewer still on substances such as garlic, fish oils, ginseng, and so on. Evidence was largely limited to anecdotal reports and single case studies. The argument often used to be made that controlled trials could not be conducted with supplements, because they often contain a range of natural ingredients whose effects are difficult to separate. However, such arguments are often misguided, and an increasing body of evidence is now emerging from double-blind randomised controlled trials, and also from systematic reviews and meta-analyses. Some of these suggest that some supplements (e.g. folic acid, fish oils) are effective in some groups of the population in certain circumstances. However, for other supplements (e.g. royal jelly), there is little evidence of benefit.

What are dietary supplements?

Definition

Various definitions for dietary supplements exist worldwide. In the UK, the definition developed by the Proprietary Association of Great Britain (PAGB), British Herbal Manufacturers' Association (BHMA) and the Health Food Manufacturers' Association (HFMA) is that they are:

> foods in unit dosage form, e.g. tablets, capsules and elixirs, taken to supplement the diet. Most are products containing nutrients normally present in foods which are used by the body to develop cells, bone, muscle etc, to replace co-enzymes depleted by infection and illness, and generally to maintain good health.

In addition to vitamins and minerals, this definition also covers ingredients such as garlic, fish oils, evening primrose oil and ginseng, which can be taken to supplement dietary intake or for their suggested health benefits.

For the purposes of the European Union (EU) Directive on food supplements the term 'food supplements' means:

> foodstuffs the purpose of which is to supplement the normal diet and which are concentrated sources of nutrients or other substances with a nutritional or physiological effect, alone or in combination, marketed in dose form, namely forms such as capsules, pastilles, tablets, pills and other similar forms, sachets of powder, ampoules of liquids, drop dispensing bottles, and other similar forms of liquids and powders designed to be taken in measured small unit quantities.

In the USA, the Dietary Supplement Health Education Act (DSHEA) 1994 defines a dietary supplement as:

> a product (other than tobacco) that is intended to supplement the diet which bears or contains one or more of the following dietary ingredients: a vitamin, a mineral, a herb or other botanical, an amino acid, a dietary substance for use by man to supplement the diet by increasing the total daily intake, or a concentrate, metabolite, constituent, extract or combinations of these ingredients. It is intended for ingestion in pill, capsule, tablet or liquid form, is not represented for use as a conventional food or as the sole item of a meal or diet and is labelled as a dietary supplement.

This definition, like that in the UK, also expands the meaning of dietary supplements beyond essential nutrients, to include such substances as ginseng, garlic, psyllium, other plant ingredients, enzymes, fish oils and mixtures of these. The EU definition does not currently include substances apart from vitamins and minerals, but other substances may be included in the future.

One of the key points in these definitions is that dietary supplements are products consumed in unit quantities in addition to normal food intake. This differentiates supplements from other foods, such as fortified foods and functional foods, to which nutrients are added. However, a major difference in the US definition is the explicit inclusion of 'herbs or other botanicals' in the list of dietary ingredients.

In the UK, herbal products are currently marketed under a variety of arrangements – either as fully licensed medicines, under the

Traditional Herbal Medicines Product (THMP) Directive, 'medicines exempt from licensing' under section 12 of the 1968 Medicines Act, or as cosmetics or foods, so they do not fall entirely in the food supplements category.

Enteral feeds (e.g. Complan and Ensure) and slimming aids are also classified as dietary supplements by nutritionists and dieticians, but for the purposes of this book, these products will be ignored.

Classification

Dietary supplements fall into several categories in relation to ingredients. These are:

1 Vitamins and minerals
  • Multivitamins and minerals. These normally contain around 100% of the Recommended Daily Allowance (RDA) for vitamins, with varying amounts of minerals and trace elements.
  • Single vitamins and minerals. These may contain very large amounts, and when levels exceed ten times the RDA, they are often termed 'megadoses'.
  • Combinations of vitamins and minerals. These may be marketed for specific population groups, e.g. athletes, children, pregnant women, slimmers, teenagers, vegetarians, etc.
  • Combinations of vitamins and minerals with other substances, such as evening primrose oil and ginseng.
2 'Unofficial' vitamins and minerals, for which a requirement and a deficiency disorder in humans has not, so far, been recognised, e.g. boron, choline, inositol, silicon.
3 Natural oils containing fatty acids for which there is some evidence of beneficial effects, e.g. evening primrose oil and fish oils.
4 Natural substances containing 'herbal' ingredients with recognised pharmacological actions but whose composition and effects have not been fully defined, e.g. echinacea, garlic, ginkgo biloba and ginseng.
5 Natural substances whose composition and effects are not well defined but which are marketed for their 'health giving properties', e.g. *chlorella*, royal jelly and spirulina.

6 Enzymes with known physiological effects, but of doubtful efficacy when taken by mouth, e.g. superoxide dismutase.
7 Amino acids or amino acid derivatives, e.g. N-acetyl cysteine, S-adenosyl methionine.

Uses of supplements

There are two main approaches to the use of supplements. They can be used to:

• treat or prevent nutritional deficiency; and to
• reduce the risk of non-deficiency disease and promote optimal health.

When vitamins were first discovered during the early years of the 20th century, their only indication was for the prevention and treatment of deficiency disease such as scurvy, beri-beri, pellagra, etc. This led to the development of dietary standards such as RDAs and, more recently, to the Dietary Reference Values (DRVs).[3] These values were based on amounts of nutrients required to prevent deficiency, and even though subject to various limitations, they are still the best measure of dietary adequacy.

After the Second World War, it was thought that nutritional deficiencies had largely disappeared and scientific interest in vitamins and minerals waned. However, with the increase in various chronic diseases such as cardiovascular disease and cancer, vitamins became an area of growing interest again, and it was suggested that supplements might help to reduce the risk of such disease. At the start of the 21st century, there is growing concern among the public to improve quality of life and supplements are increasingly used to promote so-called optimum health.

Despite the idea that nutritional deficiency had disappeared, recent UK national diet and nutrition surveys have shown that there is no room for complacency. Although average dietary intakes may appear adequate, some groups of the surveyed populations are clearly at risk of marginal deficiencies.

The National Diet and Nutrition Survey in pre-school children[4] showed that 8% of the surveyed youngsters aged 1½ to 4½ were anaemic, a further 12% were mildly iron-deficient and 15% had a poor intake of zinc. Vitamin A deficiency was present in 8%, vitamin B_2 deficiency in 23% and vitamin C deficiency in 3%.

A similar nutritional survey of older children[5] again showed average nutrient intakes were largely fine, but anaemia was present in 1.5% of boys and 5% of girls, with respective totals of 13% and 27% having low serum ferritin – an indication of iron deficiency. In addition, zinc was found to be low in the diets of 10% of boys and 20% of girls. Also of concern were calcium intakes, which were below the Lower Reference Nutrient Intake (LRNI) in 6% of boys and 12% of girls. For magnesium, the respective figures were 12% and 27% and for vitamin A, 10% and 11%. Furthermore, some of the surveyed youngsters also appeared to have poor status for vitamin B_{12}, vitamin C, vitamin D, folate, riboflavin and thiamine.

The National Diet and Nutrition Survey of people aged 65 years and over[6] showed that there were nutritional problems in some individuals. Up to 38% of the survey population was deficient in vitamin D, up to 38% were deficient in vitamin C, up to 18% in folate, up to 15% in vitamin B_{12} and up to 30% in iron. Of the free-living individuals, 11% of men and 9% of women were anaemic.

The most recent National Diet and Nutrition Survey involving British adults aged 19–64 years[1] found that mean intakes of all nutrients in men are $\geq$ 100% of the RNI. For women, mean intakes of iron, magnesium and copper were below the RNI. However, mean intakes fail to show the proportion of people that do not achieve the RNI. For example, for women, mean magnesium intake was 85% of the RNI, but 74% in this survey failed to achieve the RNI. Mean intakes also fail to show that intakes in some age groups are particularly poor. For example, iron intake in women overall was 82% of the RNI while in 19–24-year-old women it was 60% of the RNI. Overall, 91% of women failed to achieve the RNI for iron while 41% of women aged 19 to 34 had intakes of iron below the LRNI. For magnesium and copper, intake overall in women is 85% and 86% of the RNI, respectively, but for women aged 19–24 years it was 76% of the RNI for both minerals. Indeed, men and women aged 19–24 had significantly poorer intakes of all vitamins and minerals than those aged 50–64, with mineral and trace element intakes in the women aged 19–24 years a particular cause for concern.

Although good diet is the most appropriate route to achieving improved nutrition in these population groups, there is no evidence to suggest that risk of deficiency is a thing of the past.

Various groups of the population could be at risk of nutrient deficiency and could benefit from supplementation. These include:

- People in a particular demographic category, e.g. infants and children, adolescents, women during pregnancy and lactation and throughout the reproductive period, the elderly and ethnic minorities.
- People whose nutritional status may be compromised by lifestyle (enforced or voluntary), e.g. smokers, alcoholics, drug addicts, slimmers, strict vegetarians (i.e. vegans), food faddists, individuals on low incomes and athletes.
- People whose nutritional status may be compromised by surgery and/or disease, e.g. malabsorption syndromes, hepato-biliary disorders, severe burns and wounds and inborn errors of metabolism.
- People whose nutritional status may be compromised by long-term drug administration (e.g. anticonvulsants may increase the requirement for vitamin D).

Increasingly, people are taking supplements for reasons other than prevention of deficiency and at amounts higher than the RDA. Moreover, evidence is increasing that, at least for some nutrients (e.g. folic acid, vitamin D), there may be benefits in achieving higher intakes than the RDA.

However, while there is agreement about the beneficial effects of nutrients in the prevention of deficiency disease and the amounts required to achieve such effects, there is controversy about amounts required for reduction in risk of chronic disease and so-called 'optimum health'. Some would argue that higher amounts are required and that basing requirements for nutrients only on the prevention of deficiency disease is inadequate. But what other end points should be used is open to debate; longevity, increased resistance to cancer and coronary heart disease, improved athletic performance, etc. Higher levels of intake cannot always easily be obtained from diet alone, and supplementation is required. However, excessive intake of some nutrients can lead to toxicity, and it is with this in mind that several committees worldwide have established safe upper limits for supplement intake.

Legal status

The UK

In the UK, the majority of dietary supplements are classified legally as foods, and sold under food law. There are just a few exceptions (e.g. Abidec, Pregaday, Epogam, Efamast, Maxepa and some generic vitamin and mineral preparations), which are licensed medicines. Unlike medicines, most supplements are not, therefore, subject to the controls of the Medicines Act (1968). Because supplements classed as foods do not require product licences, they do not have to go through such rigorous clinical trials, and are therefore much cheaper to put on the market than medicines.

Dietary supplements are not controlled by quite the same strict conditions of dosage, labelling, purity criteria and levels of ingredients as medicines. The retail supply of those vitamins that have product licences (i.e. medicines) are subject to limitations which depend on their strength and maximum daily dose, as shown in Table 2.

Dietary supplements containing levels of vitamins in excess of those in prescription-only medicines are available to the public. However, in recognition of the fact that consumers are increasingly using high-dose products, the Food Standards Agency (FSA) Expert Group on Vitamins and Minerals (EVM) has published safe levels of intake for vitamins and minerals.[6] (See Appendix 3.)

Claims that can be made for supplements are currently regulated by food law, but will also be regulated at European level, possibly from 2007 (see below). Advertising of dietary supplements is regulated by various advertising codes for both the broadcast media (TV and

Table 2 Limitations on the sale or supply of licensed medicines containing certain vitamins

Vitamin	Legal status
Vitamin A	Up to 2250 µg (7500 units) GSL
	Over 2250 µg (7500 units) POM
Vitamin D	Up to 10 µg (400 units) GSL
	Over 10 µg (400 units) P
Cyanocobalamin	Up to 10 µg GSL
	Over 10 µg P
Folic acid	Up to 200 µg GSL
	200–500 µg P
	Over 500 µg POM

GSL = subject to control under the Medicines (General Sales List) Order, 1977.

POM = subject to control under the Medicines (Prescriptions Only) Order, 1977.

P = Pharmacy only products.

radio advertising standards codes) and the non-broadcast media. These codes are policed by the Advertising Standards Authority (ASA), an independent body set up by the advertising industry.

Europe

Across the countries of the European Union (EU), the diversity of regulation for food supplements has been wide, with several approaches to regulating vitamin and mineral supplements such that one product of the same strength (e.g. vitamin C 1000 mg) can be a food in one country but a medicine in another.

However, the regulatory environment in Europe is changing rapidly. The European Commission has adopted Directive 2002/46/EC, which lays down specific rules for vitamins and minerals used as ingredients for food supplements (see http://europa.eu.int). All food supplements containing vitamins or minerals as well as other ingredients should conform to the specific rules for vitamins and minerals laid down in the Directive. The Directive was implemented in the UK in August 2005.

The Directive includes a 'positive list' of vitamins and minerals permitted in food supplements (Annex 1), and a second list identifying the chemical substances that can be used in their manufacture (Annex 2). Only vitamins and minerals in the forms listed may be used in the manufacture of food supplements. However, until 31 December 2009, Member States may allow the use of vitamins and minerals not listed in Annex 1 or in forms not listed in Annex 2 provided that:

- the substance was an ingredient in a food supplement marketed in the EC before 12 July 2002;
- the European Food Safety Authority (EFSA) has not given an unfavourable opinion in respect of the use of the substance, or its use in that form, in the manufacture of food supplements, on the basis of a dossier supporting use of the substance that had to be submitted to the Commission by the Member State not later than 12 July 2005.

Dossiers have been submitted for around 300 substances (see http://europa.eu.int). These are principally salts of minerals and trace elements, such as salts of boron, calcium, chromium, cobalt, copper, iron, magnesium, manganese, molybdenum, potassium, selenium, vanadium and zinc. However, some vitamin ingredients also appear on the list of submitted dossiers.

Specific rules concerning nutrients, other than vitamins and minerals, or other substances with a nutritional or physiological effect used as ingredients of food supplements (e.g. fatty acids, amino acids, fibre, and herbal ingredients) will be laid down at a later stage. A proposal on the advisability of establishing specific rules on other nutritional substances is expected by mid-2007.

The Directive will also establish maximum permitted levels of vitamins and minerals for food supplements. These will take into account upper safe levels of vitamins and minerals established by scientific risk assessment based on generally accepted scientific data, intake of vitamins and minerals from other dietary sources and the varying degrees of sensitivity of different consumer groups. Figures for upper levels of vitamins and minerals unlikely to have adverse effects have been published by official groups such as the EU Scientific Committee on Food (SCF), the UK Expert Vitamin and

Mineral Group and the US National Academy of Sciences (see Appendix 3).

The Directive also pays attention to advertising, presentation, purity criteria and labelling of content and dosage. Labels on dietary supplements express their nutrient content in terms of RDAs. EU RDAs are based on the requirements of men and are said to apply to average adults. They take no account of differences in nutritional requirements according to age, sex and other factors, and are therefore simple approximations used for labels only.

Labelling should not imply that a varied and adequate diet cannot provide sufficient quantities of nutrients. In addition, 'medicinal' claims relating to the prevention, treatment or cure of disease in the labelling, advertising or promotion of food supplements are prohibited.

Health claims will be regulated by the proposed Health and Nutrition Claims Regulation, which is expected to be adopted before the end of 2006 and be applied six months later, by the middle of 2007. Health claims such as 'calcium is good for your bones' may be used on a label so long as they are proven to apply to the food supplement in question. Within 3 years of the Regulation entering force, the Commission is to draw up a list of well-established health claims to be used on labels, and Member States will be asked to submit a list of claims already approved at national level. New health claims submitted for the list after this period or any disease risk reduction claims such as 'calcium helps reduce the risk of osteoporosis' or 'X reduces cholesterol', will have to be assessed by the European Food Safety Agency (EFSA) and be approved by the Commission. In the UK, the work of the Joint Health Claims Initiative (see http://www.jhci.org.uk) has helped to inform health claims regulation at European level.

This EC Regulation will also apply to trademarks. Within 15 years of the Regulation entering into force, existing brand names suggesting health benefits (such as promises of weight loss) that do not meet the requirements of the Regulation must be phased out and removed from the market. However, certain generic descriptors such as 'digestives' may apply for derogation from this rule (see http://ec.europa.eu/comm./food/labellingnutri-tion/claims/index_en.htm).

The USA

In the USA, the Food and Drug Administration (FDA) regulates dietary supplements according to the Dietary Supplement Health and Education Act (DSHEA) 1994. Under this law, supplements are regulated in a similar manner to food products, while prohibiting their regulation as medicines or food additives. This Act includes a framework for safety, guidelines for third-party literature provided at the point of sale, guidance on good manufacturing practice (GMP) and labelling standards. Under DSHEA, manufacturers are responsible for marketing safe and properly labelled products, but the FDA bears the burden of proving that a product is unsafe or improperly labelled. However, the FDA has insufficient resources for doing this, and there is concern that not all supplements are marketed according to best standards of practice.

DSHEA regulates the labelling of supplements and the claims that can be made. This includes permissible statements describing the link between a nutrient and a deficiency or between a nutrient and its effect on the body's structure or function, or its effect on well-being. Examples include 'promotes relaxation' or 'builds strong bones'. But to make these claims, the supplement label must also carry the disclaimer: 'This statement has not been validated by the Food and Drug Administration. This product is not intended to diagnose, treat, cure or prevent any disease.'

Under the US Nutrition Labelling and Education Act of 1990, a number of specific health claims are also permitted. These describe the link between a specific nutrient and the reduction in risk of a particular disease or condition and they are based on significant scientific agreement. Claims applicable to dietary supplements include those in relation to calcium and osteoporosis, folic acid and neural tube defects, soluble fibre (from oat bran and psyllium seed) and coronary heart disease and soya and coronary heart disease.

International

Global standards for vitamin and mineral supplements have also been developed and adopted at an international level by the Codex Alimentarius Commission. The Codex Alimentarius Commission or Codex was created by two UN organisations (the Food and Agricultural Organization and the World Health Organization) and its main purpose is to protect consumer health and ensure fair practice in international trade in food through the development of food standards, codes of practice, guidelines and other recommendations.

The Codex guidelines on vitamin and mineral supplements are voluntary and apply to supplements that contain vitamins and/or minerals that are regulated as foods. The guidelines address the composition of vitamin and mineral supplements, including the safety, purity and bioavailability of the sources of vitamins and minerals. They do not specify upper limits for vitamins and minerals in supplements, but provide criteria for establishing maximum amounts of vitamins and minerals per daily portion of supplement consumed, as recommended by the manufacturer. The criteria specify that maximum amounts should be established by scientific risk assessment based on generally accepted scientific data and taking into consideration, as appropriate, the varying degrees of sensitivity of different population groups. The guidelines also address the packaging and labelling of vitamin and mineral supplements.

Law enforcement

In the UK, enforcement of food law, including health claims, is the responsibility of the local authorities' trading standards officers. The local authority associations are in turn coordinated by LACORS (Local Authorities Co-ordinators of Regulatory Services). LACORS (formerly LACOTS) is responsible for improving the quality of trading standards and food enforcement by promoting coordination, consistency and good regulation.

Other EU countries have various arrangements for enforcing the law, while in the USA it is the responsibility of the FDA.

Patient/client counselling

The following questions may be used by health professionals before making any recommendations about supplement use:

1 Who is the supplement for? The individual buying the product may not be the consumer; requirements for vitamins and minerals vary according to age and sex.
2 Why do you think you need a supplement? The individual may have misconceptions about the need for and benefits of supplements that should be addressed.
3 What are your symptoms (if any) and how long have you had them? The individual could have a serious underlying disorder that should be referred for appropriate diagnosis and treatment.
4 What do you eat? A simple dietary assessment should be undertaken to give some indication as to whether vitamin and mineral deficiency is likely.
5 Is your diet restricted in any way? Slimming, vegetarianism or religious conviction could increase the risk of nutritional deficiency.
6 Do you take any prescription or over-the-counter medicines? This information can be used to assess possible drug–nutrient interactions.
7 Do you take other supplements? If so, which ones? This information can be used to assess potential overdosage of supplements which could be toxic.
8 Do you suffer from any chronic illness, e.g. diabetes, epilepsy, Crohn's disease? Nutrient requirements in patients with chronic disease may be greater than in healthy individuals.
9 Are you pregnant or breast-feeding? Nutrient requirements may be increased.
10 Do you take part in sports or other regular physical activity?
11 Do you smoke? Requirements for some vitamins (e.g. vitamin C) may be increased.
12 How much alcohol do you drink? Excessive alcohol consumption may lead to deficiency of the B vitamins.

Guidelines for supplement use

The following guidelines may be useful in making recommendations:

- Compare labels with dietary standards (usually RDAs).
- In the absence of an indication for a specific nutrient, a balanced multivitamin/mineral product is normally preferable to one that contains one or two specific nutrients.
- Use a product that provides approximately 100% of the RDA for as wide a range of vitamins and minerals as possible.
- Avoid preparations containing unrecognised nutrients or nutrients in minute amounts; this increases the cost, but not the value.
- Avoid preparations that claim to be natural, organic or high potency; this increases the cost and, in the case of high-potency products, the risk of toxicity.
- Distinguish between credible claims and unsubstantiated claims.
- If there is uncertainty about product quality, check with the companies concerned. Ask about quality assurance. For example, is the final product analysed to guarantee the contents in the bottle match the label declarations? Are tests for disintegration, dissolution or other tests for bioavailability conducted?

Role of the health professional

When asked about supplements, health professionals should emphasise the importance of consuming a diet based on healthy eating guidelines. This is a diet rich in starchy, fibrous carbohydrates, including fruit and vegetables, and low in fat, sugar and salt. Dietary supplements do not convert a poor diet into a good one.

Health professionals should be aware of dietary standards and good food sources for nutrients. They should be able to assess an individual's risk of nutrient deficiency and need for further referral, by asking questions to detect cultural, physical, environmental and social conditions which may predispose to inadequate intakes.

There is a need to be aware of the potential for adverse effects with supplements. Thus, when a client or patient presents with any symptoms, questions should be asked about the use of dietary supplements. Individuals will not always volunteer this information without prompting because they believe that supplements are 'natural' and therefore safe.

Health professionals should make their clients aware of the existence of badly worded claims and adverts and of the dangers of supplement misuse.

Pharmacists have a particular responsibility, simply because they sell these products. When supplying any supplement with perceived health benefits, pharmacists must be careful to avoid giving their professional authority to a product that may lack any health or therapeutic benefit and has risks associated with its use. In accordance with the Code of Ethics of the Royal Pharmaceutical Society of Great Britain, this may involve not stocking or selling the product. Pharmacists must not give the impression that any dietary supplement is efficacious when there is no evidence for such efficacy.

However, providing a product is not harmful for a particular individual, the freedom to use it should be respected. What is important is that consumers are able to make informed and intelligent choices about the products they buy.

References

1 Henderson L, Irving K, Gregory J (Office for National Statistics), with Bates CJ, Prentice A, Parks J (Medical Resource Council, Human Nutrition Research), and Swan G, Farron M (Food Standards Agency) The National Diet and Nutrition Survey: adults aged 19 to 64 years. Volume 3. *Vitamin and mineral intake and urinary analysis*. London: HMSO, 2003.
2 Figures from Information Resources Inc. (IRI) provided by the Proprietary Association of Great Britain (PAGB).
3 Department of Health. *Dietary Reference Values for Food Energy and Nutrients for the United Kingdom*. Report on Health and Social Subjects No 41. London: HMSO, 1991.
4 *The National Diet and Nutrition Survey: children aged $1\frac{1}{2}$ to $4\frac{1}{2}$ years*. London: HMSO, 1995.
5 *The National Diet and Nutrition Survey: young people aged 4 to 18 years*. London: HMSO, 2000.
6 *The National Diet and Nutrition Survey. People aged 65 years and over*. Report of the diet and nutrition survey. London: HMSO, 1998.
7 European Commission. Scientific Committee on Food (SCF). Tolerable Upper Intake Levels for Vitamins and Minerals. http://ec.europa.eu/comm./food/fs/sc/scf/out80_en.htm (accessed 12 November 2006).

How to use this book

This book covers 82 commonly available dietary supplements, including vitamins, minerals, trace elements and other substances, such as garlic, ginseng and fish oils. For ease of reference, they are arranged in alphabetical order and give information, where appropriate, under the following standard headings.

Description

States the type of substance; e.g. a vitamin, mineral, fatty acid, amino acid, enzyme, plant extract, etc.

Nomenclature

Lists names and alternative names in current usage.

Units

Includes alternative units and conversion factors.

Constituents

Lists active ingredients in supplements that are not pure vitamins or minerals (e.g. evening primrose oil contains gamma-linolenic acid).

Human requirements

Lists for different ages and sex (where established):

- UK Dietary Reference Values and safe upper levels;

- US Recommended Dietary Allowances (RDAs) and Tolerable Upper Intake Levels (ULs);
- World Health Organization (WHO) Reference Nutrient Intakes;
- European Union Recommended Dietary Allowances (RDAs).

Definitions

The UK

Dietary reference values (DRVs) were established in 1991 to replace recommended daily amounts (RDAs).

- EAR: Estimated Average Requirement. An assessment of the average requirement for energy or protein for a vitamin or mineral. About half the population will need more than the EAR, and half less.
- LRNI: Lower Reference Nutrient Intake. The amount of protein, vitamin or mineral considered to be sufficient for the few people in a group who have low needs. Most people will need more than the LRNI and if people consistently consume less they may be at risk of deficiency of that nutrient.
- RNI: Reference Nutrient Intake. The amount of protein, vitamin or mineral sufficient for almost every individual. This level of intake is much higher than many people need.
- Safe Intake: A term used to indicate intake or range of intakes of a nutrient for which there is not enough information to estimate RNI, EAR or LRNI. It is considered to be adequate for almost everyone's needs but not large enough to cause undesirable effects.
- DRV: Dietary Reference Value. A term used to cover LRNI, EAR, RNI and safe intake.

The USA

The US Institute of Medicine and the Food and Nutrition Board have established a set of reference values to replace the previous RDAs. The Dietary Reference Intakes encompass EARs, RDAs, AI (adequate intakes) and Tolerable Upper Intake Levels (UIs). RDAs and AIs are set at levels that should decrease the risk of developing a nutritional deficiency disease.

- RDA: Recommended Dietary Allowance. The average amount of energy or a nutrient recommended to cover the needs of groups of healthy people.
- Safe Intake and Adequate Daily Dietary Intakes: These are given for some vitamins and minerals where there is less information on which to base allowances, and figures are provided in the form of ranges.
- Tolerable Upper Intake Levels: Defined by the Food and Nutrition Board of the US National Academy of Sciences as the highest total level of a nutrient (diet plus supplements) which could be consumed safely on a daily basis, that is unlikely to cause adverse health effects to almost all individuals in the general population. As intakes rise above the UL, the risk of adverse effects increases. The UL describes long-term intakes, so an isolated dose above the UL need not necessarily cause adverse effects. The UL defines safety limits and is not a recommended intake for most people most of the time.

Europe

RDA: Recommended Dietary Allowance. Provides sufficient for most individuals. The EU RDA is used on dietary supplement labels.

The following points should be noted in relation to dietary standards:

- Dietary standards are intended to assess the diets of populations, not of individuals. Thus, both the RDA and the UK Reference Nutrient Intake (RNI) are set at two standard deviations above the average population requirement and are intended to cover the needs of 95% of the population. So, if an individual is typically consuming the RDA or the RNI for a particular nutrient, it can be assumed that his or her diet provides adequate amounts (or more than adequate amounts) of that nutrient to prevent deficiency. If intake is regularly below the RNI, it cannot necessarily be assumed that the diet is inadequate, because the person may have a lower requirement for that nutrient. However, if an individual is consistently consuming less than the Lower Reference Nutrient Intake (LRNI) for a nutrient, it can be assumed that the diet is deficient in that nutrient. Nevertheless, individuals differ in the amounts of nutrients they need and the quantities they absorb and utilise, and although the dietary standards are the best figures currently available, they were never intended to assess the adequacy of individual diets.
- Dietary standards are estimates, which are assessed from a variety of epidemiological, biochemical and nutritional data, including:
  - The intake of a nutrient required to prevent or cure clinical signs of deficiency.
  - The intake of a nutrient required to maintain balance (i.e. intake − output = zero).
  - The intake of a nutrient required to maintain a given blood level, tissue concentration or degree of enzyme saturation.
  - The intake of a nutrient in the diet of a healthy population.
- Dietary standards apply only to healthy people but not to those with disease whose nutrient needs may be very different. Requirements may be increased in patients with disorders of the gastrointestinal tract, liver and kidney, and in those with inborn errors of metabolism, cancer, severe infections, wounds, burns and following surgery. Drug administration may also alter nutrient requirements.

Dietary intake

States amounts of nutrients provided by the average adult diet in the UK.[1]

Action

Describes the role of the substance in maintaining physiological function and identifies pharmacological actions where appropriate.

Dietary sources

Lists significant food sources based on average portion sizes. In addition, a food may be described as an *excellent* or *good* source of a nutrient. This does not describe any food as 'excellent' or 'good' overall. It defines only the amount of the nutrient (per portion or serving) in relation to the Reference Nutrient Intake (RNI) of the nutrient for the average adult male.

Thus, an excellent source provides 30% or more of the RNI; a good source provides 15–30% of the RNI.

Where no RNI has been set for a particular nutrient, *excellent* and *good* are numerically defined.

Metabolism

Discusses absorption, transport, distribution and excretion.

Bioavailability

Includes the effects of cooking, processing, storage methods, and substances in food which may alter bioavailability.

Deficiency

Lists signs and symptoms of deficiency.

Uses

Discusses potential indications for use with the level of evidence. Evidence for use of supplements is obtained from several types of studies:

- Epidemiological studies. These are population-based studies and early evidence for the potential value of a nutrient usually comes from epidemiological research. For example, the idea that antioxidant supplements could reduce the risk of cancer came from studies in populations that high intake of fruit and vegetables was associated with a low risk of cancer.
- *In vitro* (laboratory) studies and animal studies. Data from these studies can be used to support evidence, but is not enough on its own. Although both types of study allow for good control of variables such as nutrients and more aggressive intervention, each suffers from uncertainties of extrapolating any observed effects to human.

- Observational studies. These may be prospective and retrospective and include, in decreasing order of persuasiveness, cohort studies, case-control studies and uncontrolled studies. In prospective studies, subjects are recruited and observed prior to the occurrence of the outcome. In retrospective studies, investigators review the records of subjects and interview subjects after the outcome has occurred. Retrospective studies are more vulnerable to recall bias and measurement error but less likely to suffer from the subject selection bias that can occur in prospective studies. In all observational studies, the investigator has no control of the intervention.

- Intervention studies. The investigator controls whether subjects receive an intervention or not. The randomised controlled trial (RCT) is the gold standard. Intervention trials with supplements differ from those for drugs. Unlike studies with drugs, those with foods and nutrients may have additional confounders secondary to the intervention itself. For example, results from intervention studies with antioxidant supplements (e.g. vitamins A, C and E) in the prevention of cancer are inconsistent, even though epidemiological studies have consistently shown that diets high in these nutrients are associated with reduced cancer risk. This could be because such diets contain a range of other substances apart from those in the tested supplements and the antioxidants are merely acting as markers for a type of diet that is protective. Moreover, chronic disease, such as cancer and coronary heart disease, develops over many years and to investigate the effect of a supplement on disease risk therefore requires a prolonged study period (e.g. 20–30 years) as well as a huge number of subjects, and this makes such studies difficult and expensive to conduct. However, without such trials, evidence for efficacy of many supplements will remain sparse.

- Systematic reviews and meta-analyses. These may include RCTs only or they may also include observational studies. Decisions on the part of reviewers to include or leave out certain types of studies can lead to differing conclusions from the analysis.

Precautions/contraindications

Lists diseases and conditions in which the substance should be avoided or used with caution.

Pregnancy and breast-feeding

Comments on safety or potential toxicity during pregnancy and lactation.

Adverse effects

Describes the risks that may accompany excessive intake, and signs and symptoms of toxicity.

Interactions

Lists drugs and other nutrients that may interact with the supplement. This includes drugs that affect vitamin and mineral status and supplements that influence drug metabolism.

Dose

Gives usual recommended dosage (if established).

References

1   Henderson L, Irving K, Gregory J (Office for National Statistics), with Bates CJ, Prentice A, Parks J (Medical Resource Council, Human Nutrition Research), and Swan G, Farron M (Food Standards Agency) *The National Diet and Nutrition Survey: adults aged 19 to 64 years. Volume 3. Vitamin and mineral intake and urinary analysis.* London: HMSO, 2003.

Abbreviations

ACE — angiotensin-converting enzyme
ADP — adenosine 5'-diphosphate
ARMD — age-related macular degeneration
ATP — adenosine triphosphate
BCAAs — branched-chain amino acids
BMD — bone mineral density
CHD — coronary heart disease
CHF — congestive heart failure
CNS — central nervous system
COPD — chronic obstructive pulmonary disease
CVD — cardiovascular disease
DNA — deoxyribonucleic acid
DRI — Dietary Reference Intake
DRV — Dietary Reference Value
EAR — Estimated Average Requirement

HDL — high-density lipoprotein
HIV — human immunodeficiency virus
HRT — hormone replacement therapy
IBS — irritable bowel syndrome
LDL — low-density lipoprotein
NSAID — non-steroidal anti-inflammatory drug
PMS — premenstrual syndrome
PUFAs — polyunsaturated fatty acids
RCT — randomised controlled trial
RDA — Recommended Daily Allowance
RNA — ribonucleic acid
RNI — Reference Nutrient Intake
SLE — systemic lupus erythematosus
VLDL — very-low-density lipoprotein

Aloe vera

Description

Aloe vera is the mucilaginous substance obtained from the central parenchymatous tissues of the large blade-like leaves of *Aloe vera*. It should not be confused with aloes, which is obtained by evaporating water from the bitter yellow juice that is drained from the leaf.

Constituents

Aloe vera contains polysaccharides, tannins, sterols, saponins, vitamins, minerals, cholesterol, gamma-linolenic acid and arachidonic acid. Unlike aloes, aloe vera does not contain anthraquinone compounds and does not therefore exert a laxative action.

Action

Used externally, aloe vera acts as a moisturiser and reduces inflammation. Internally, it may act as an anti-inflammatory, hypoglycaemic and hyperlipidaemic agent. It also has anti-platelet activity.

Possible uses

Topical

Topical aloe vera has been investigated for its effects on wound healing and psoriasis, while oral aloe vera has been investigated in patients with diabetes mellitus and hyperlipidaemia.

A review in 1987 concluded that topical application of aloe vera gel reduces acute inflammation, promotes wound healing, reduces pain and exerts an antipruritic effect.[1] A further review in 1999[2] stated that research had continued to confirm these benefits.

A double-blind, placebo-controlled study of 60 people with psoriasis of mean duration 8.5 years found that applying aloe vera to skin lesions three times a day for 8 months led to significant improvement in 83% of aloe vera patients but in only 6% of those who used placebo.[3]

In rabbits, aloe vera cream was found to be better than placebo and as effective as oral pentoxifylline in improving tissue survival after frostbite.[4]

In a study of 27 patients, aloe vera gel healed burns faster than Vaseline gauze,[5] and in rats enhanced wound healing in second-degree burns.[6]

However, a recent Cochrane review identified a single trial of aloe vera supplementation that suggested delayed wound healing with aloe vera, but the reviewers concluded that the results of the trial were not easily interpretable.[7]

Systemic

A recent systematic review of 10 studies[8] showed that oral aloe vera might be useful as an adjunct for lowering blood glucose concentrations in diabetes and for reducing blood lipid levels in hyperlipidaemia.

There is some evidence that the anti-inflammatory actions of aloe vera might have therapeutic potential in inflammatory bowel disease. An *in vitro* study found that aloe vera gel had a dose-dependent inhibitory effect on the production of reactive oxygen metabolites and eicosanoids in human colorectal mucosa.[9]

A randomised controlled study in 44 patients with ulcerative colitis found that aloe vera gel 100 ml four times weekly produced a clinical response more often than placebo, reducing histological disease activity. The researchers recommended that further evaluation of aloe vera in inflammatory bowel disease is needed.[10]

Conclusion

A huge number of *in vitro* and animal studies have examined aloe vera over the past 30 years. However, there have been few studies in humans, and these have been poorly controlled.

Topical aloe vera may be helpful in psoriasis, but whether it is useful for wound healing is unclear. There is some – albeit limited – evidence that oral aloe vera may be useful for lowering blood glucose in diabetes, reducing blood lipids in hyperlipidaemia and it may have therapeutic potential in inflammatory bowel disease.

Precautions/contraindications

None established, although the potential hypoglycaemic effect means that it should be used with caution in patients with diabetes mellitus. Preliminary research in rats has suggested that aloe vera has a hypoglycaemic effect.[11]

Pregnancy and breast-feeding

No problems have been reported, but there have not been sufficient studies to guarantee the safety of aloe vera in pregnancy and breast-feeding.

Adverse effects

None reported apart from occasional allergic reactions. However, there are no long-term studies investigating the safety of aloe vera.

Interactions

Aloe vera has antiplatelet activity and could theoretically interact with drugs with antiplatelet effects. A case study in one individual found a potential interaction between aloe vera and sevoflurane, in which the woman lost 5 L of blood during surgery.[12]

Dose

Aloe vera is available in the form of creams, gels, tablets, capsules and juice. The International Aloe Science Council operates a voluntary approval scheme that gives an official seal ('IASC – certified') on products containing certified raw ingredients processed according to standard guidelines.

Used internally, there is no established dose. Product manufacturers suggest $\frac{1}{2}$ to $\frac{3}{4}$ cup of juice or 1 to 2 capsules three times a day. The juice in the product should ideally contain at least 98% aloe vera and no aloin.

Used externally, aloe vera should be applied liberally as needed. The product should contain at least 20% aloe vera.

References

1 Heggers JP, Kucukcelebi A, Listengarten B, *et al*. Beneficial effects of aloe in wound healing in an excisional wound model. *J Altern Complement Med* 1996; 2: 271–277.

2 Reynolds T. Aloe vera leaf gel: a review update. *J Ethnopharmacol* 1999; 68: 3–37.

3 Syed TA, Ahmad SA, Holt AH, *et al*. Management of psoriasis with aloe vera extract in a hydrophilic cream: a placebo controlled double blind study. *Trop Med Int Health* 1996; 1: 505–509.

4 Miller MB. Treatment of experimental frostbite with pentoxifylline and aloe vera cream. *Arch Otolaryngol Head Neck Surg* 1995; 121: 678–680.

5 Visuthikosol V, Chowchuen B, Sukwanarat Y, *et al*. Effect of aloe vera gel to healing of burn wound: a clinical and histological study. *J Med Assoc Thai* 1995; 78: 403–409.

6 Somboonwong J, Thanamittramanee S, Jariyapongshul A, Patumraj S. Therapeutic effects of aloe vera on cutaneous microcirculation and wound healing in second degree burn model in rats. *J Med Assoc Thai* 2000; 83: 417–425.

7 Vermeulen H, Ubbink D, Goossens A, *et al*. Dressings and topical agents for surgical wounds healing by secondary intention. Cochrane database, issue 2, 2004. London: Macmillan.

8 Vogler BK, Ernst E. Aloe vera: a systematic review of its clinical effectiveness. *Br J Clin Pract* 1999; 49: 823–828.

9 Langmead L, Makins RJ, Rampton DS. Anti-inflammatory effects of aloe vera gel in human colorectal mucosa *in vitro*. *Aliment Pharmacol Ther* 2004; 19: 521–527.

10 Langmead L, Feakins RM, Goldthorpe S, *et al.* Randomized, double-blind, placebo-controlled trial of oral aloe vera gel for active ulcerative colitis. *Aliment Pharmacol Ther* 2004; 19: 739–747.

11 Rajasekaran S, Sivagnanam K, Ravi K, Subramanian S. Hypoglycaemic effect of aloe vera gel on streptozotocin-induced diabetes in experimental rats. *J Med Food* 2004; 7: 61–66.

12 Lee A, Chui PT, Aun CS, *et al.* Possible interaction between sevoflurane and aloe vera. *Ann Pharmacother* 2004; 38: 1651–1654.

Alpha-lipoic acid

Description

Alpha-lipoic acid is a naturally-occurring sulphur-containing cofactor. It is synthesised in humans.

Nomenclature

Alternative names include alpha-lipoate, thioctic acid, lipoic acid, 2-dithiolane-3-pentatonic acid, and 1,2-dithiolane-3-valeric acid.

Action

Alpha-lipoic acid functions as a potent antioxidant and as a cofactor for various enzymes (e.g. pyruvate dehydrogenase and alpha-ketoglutarate dehydrogenase) in energy-producing metabolic reactions of the Krebs cycle.

In addition, it appears to improve recycling of other antioxidant compounds, including vitamins C and E,[1] coenzyme Q[2] and glutathione.[3] It may also protect against arsenic,[4] cadmium,[5] lead[6] and mercury[7] poisoning.

Dietary sources

Alpha-lipoic acid is present in foods such as spinach, meat (especially liver) and brewer's yeast, but it is difficult to obtain amounts used in clinical studies (i.e. possibly therapeutic amounts) from food.

Metabolism

Alpha-lipoic acid is both fat-soluble and water-soluble, and this facilitates its diffusion into lipophilic and hydrophilic environments. It is metabolised to dihydrolipoic acid (DHLA), which also demonstrates antioxidant properties.

Possible uses

As a dietary supplement, alpha-lipoic acid is claimed to improve glucose metabolism and insulin sensitivity in diabetes, and to reduce replication of the human immunodeficiency virus (HIV). It has been investigated for possible use in patients with diabetes mellitus, glaucoma, HIV, hypertension and Alzheimer's disease.

Diabetes mellitus

Alpha-lipoic acid has long been of interest as a potential therapeutic agent in diabetes, including both the microvascular and neuropathic pathologies. This stems from alpha-lipoic acid's metabolic role and also because diabetes results in chronic oxidative stress. Alpha-lipoic acid appears to increase muscle cell glucose uptake and increase insulin sensitivity in individuals with type 2 diabetes mellitus. *In vitro*, alpha-lipoic acid has been found to stimulate glucose uptake by muscle cells in a manner similar to insulin.[8]

In an uncontrolled study, patients with type 2 diabetes given 1000 mg lipoic acid intravenously experienced a 50% improvement in insulin-stimulated glucose uptake.[9] In a further uncontrolled pilot study,[10] 20 patients with type 2 diabetes were given 500 mg lipoic acid intravenously for 10 days. Glucose uptake increased by an average of 30%, but there were no changes in either fasting blood glucose or insulin levels.

In a study involving 10 lean and 10 obese patients with type 2 diabetes,[11] alpha-lipoic acid improved glucose effectiveness and prevented hyperglycaemia-induced increases in serum lactate and pyruvate. In the lean diabetic patients, but not the obese patients, alpha-lipoic acid resulted in improved insulin sensitivity and lower fasting glucose.

In a placebo-controlled, multicentre pilot study,[12] 74 patients with type 2 diabetes were randomised to receive alpha-lipoic acid 600 mg once, twice or three times a day, or placebo. When compared to placebo, significantly more patients had an increase in insulin-stimulated glucose disposal. As there was no dose effect, all three treatment groups were combined into one active group and compared with placebo. The increase in insulin-stimulated glucose disposal was then statistically significant, suggesting that oral administration of alpha-lipoic acid can improve insulin sensitivity in patients with type 2 diabetes.

Diabetic neuropathy

Alpha-lipoic acid has been used extensively in Germany for the treatment of diabetic neuropathy. An *in vitro* study showed that lipoic acid reduced lipid peroxidation of nerve tissue.[13] A study in rats with diabetes induced by streptozotocin showed that alpha-lipoic acid reversed the reduction in glucose uptake that occurs in diabetes, and that this change was associated with an improvement in peripheral nerve function.[14]

In a randomised, double-blind, placebo-controlled multicentre trial, 73 patients with non-insulin-dependent diabetes mellitus were assigned to receive oral alpha-lipoic acid 800 mg daily or placebo for 4 months. Of the total, 17 patients dropped out of the study, but the results suggested that alpha-lipoic acid might slightly improve cardiac autonomic neuropathy (assessed by measures of heart rate variability) in non-insulin-dependent diabetic patients.[15]

In a randomised, placebo-controlled study involving 24 patients with type 2 diabetes,[16] oral treatment with 600 mg alpha-lipoic acid three times a day for 3 weeks appeared to reduce the chief symptoms of diabetic neuropathy. A further placebo-controlled, randomised, double-blind trial showed that oral alpha-lipoic acid 600 mg once or twice a day appeared to have a beneficial effect on nerve conduction in patients with both type 1 and type 2 diabetes.[17]

A review[18] of the evidence of the effect of alpha-lipoic acid in the treatment of diabetic neuropathy concluded that short-term treatment with oral or intravenous alpha-lipoic acid appears to reduce the chief symptoms of diabetic neuropathy, but this needs to be confirmed by larger studies.

A meta-analysis of four trials of alpha-lipoic acid involving 1258 patients found a benefit of 16–25% (compared with placebo) in signs and symptoms of neuropathy (e.g. ankle reflexes, pain, burning, numbness, pin-prick and touch-pressure sensation) after 3 weeks of treatment. This is supported by three more recent trials, which have also shown favourable results with alpha-lipoic acid in diabetic neuropathy.[19] Three non-blinded trials (one in Korea and two in Bulgaria) tested alpha-lipoic acid in a dose of 600 mg daily. In the Korean study, total symptom score was significantly reduced at 8 weeks, as were individual symptom scores for pain, burning sensation, paraesthesia and numbness.[20] In one of the Bulgarian trials, there was a significant improvement in several aspects of autonomic function, including postural blood pressure change and overall cardiovascular autonomic neuropathy score.[21] In the second Bulgarian study, alpha-lipoic acid was found to be effective in peripheral and autonomic diabetic neuropathy and also diabetic mononeuropathy of the cranial nerves, leading to full recovery of the patients.[22]

Glaucoma

In a study involving 75 patients with open-angle glaucoma,[23] alpha-lipoic acid was administered in a dose of either 75 mg daily for 2 months or 150 mg daily for 1 month. Improvements in biochemical parameters and visual function were found, particularly in the group receiving 150 mg lipoic acid.

Human immunodeficiency virus

Alpha-lipoic acid blocks activation of NF-kappa B, which is required for HIV virus transcription, and has also been noted to improve antioxidant status, T-helper lymphocytes, and the

T-helper/suppressor cell ratio in HIV-infected T-cells.[24] However, it is not known whether supplementation would improve survival in individuals who are HIV-positive.

Miscellaneous

Results of preliminary studies suggest that alpha-lipoic acid may lower blood pressure,[25] improve the symptoms of burning mouth syndrome[26] and improve T-cell functions *in vitro* in advanced stage cancer patients.[27] Alpha-lipoic acid has also been investigated for a potential role in dementia, but there is only very limited evidence available.[28,29] Alpha-lipoic acid has been investigated for an effect in conditions such as cancer cachexia, liver disease, ischaemia reperfusion injury, photoageing of the skin and cataract. However, there is no convincing data as yet from human randomised controlled trial (RCT) data.

Conclusion

There is evidence that alpha-lipoic acid might have a role in patients with diabetes mellitus in improving glucose utilisation, insulin sensitivity and diabetic neuropathy. Very limited evidence also exists that alpha-lipoic acid may be helpful in glaucoma, dementia, hypertension and slow replication of HIV and cancer cells, but evidence of benefit in all these conditions, including diabetes, is too limited to make recommendations for supplementation.

Precautions/contraindications

Alpha-lipoic acid should be used with caution in patients predisposed to hypoglycaemia, including patients taking antidiabetic agents.

Pregnancy and breast-feeding

No problems have been reported, but there have not been sufficient studies to guarantee the safety of alpha-lipoic acid in pregnancy and breast-feeding.

Adverse effects

None reported, apart from occasional skin rashes. Studies investigating the effect of alpha-lipoic acid have suggested that it is a safe supplement at reasonable doses. However, there are no long-term studies assessing the safety of alpha-lipoic acid.

Interactions

Drugs

Oral hypoglycaemics and insulin: Theoretically, alpha-lipoic acid could enhance the effects of these drugs.

Dose

Alpha-lipoic acid is available in the form of tablets and capsules.

The dose is not established. Studies have used 300–600 mg daily. Dietary supplements provide 50–300 mg daily.

References

1 Scholich H, Murphy ME, Sies H. Antioxidant activity of dihydrolipoate against microsomal lipid peroxidation and its dependence on α-tocopherol. *Biochem Biophys Acta* 1989; 1001: 256–261.
2 Kagan V, Serbinova E, Packer L. Antioxidant effects of ubiquinones in microsomes and mitochondria are mediated by tocopherol recycling. *Biochem Biophys Res Comm* 1990; 169: 851–857.
3 Busse E, Zimmer G, Schopohl B, *et al.* Influence of alpha-lipoic acid on intracellular glutathione in vitro and in vivo. *Arzneimittelforschung* 1992; 42: 829–831.
4 Grunert RR. The effect of DL-α-lipoic acid on heavy metal intoxication in mice and dogs. *Arch Biochem Biophys* 1960; 86: 190–194.
5 Muller L, Menzel H. Studies on the effect of lipoate and dihydrolipoate in the alteration of cadmium toxicity in isolated hepatocytes. *Biochem Biophys Acta* 1990; 1052: 386–391.
6 Gurer H, Ozgunes H, Oztezcan S, Ercal N. Antioxidant role of alpha-lipoic acid in lead toxicity. *Free Radic Biol Med* 1999; 27: 75–81.
7 Keith RL, Setiarahardjo I, Fernando Q, *et al.* Utilization of renal slices to evaluate the efficacy of chelating agents for removing mercury from the kidney. *Toxicology* 1997; 116: 67–75.
8 Estrada DE, Ewart HS, Tsakiridis T, *et al.* Stimulation of glucose uptake by the natural coenzyme

alpha-lipoic acid/thioctic acid: participation of elements of the insulin signaling pathway. *Diabetes* 1996; 45: 1798–1804.

9 Jacob S, Henricksen EJ, Schiemann AL, *et al.* Enhancement of glucose disposal in patients with type 2 diabetes by alpha-lipoic acid. *Arzneimittelforschung* 1995; 45: 872–874.

10 Jacob S, Henricksen EJ, Tritschler HJ, *et al.* Improvement of insulin-stimulated glucose disposal in type 2 diabetes after repeated parenteral administration of thioctic acid. *Exp Clin Endocrinol Diabetes* 1996; 104: 284–288.

11 Konrad T, Vicini P, Kusterer K, *et al.* Alpha-lipoic acid treatment decreases serum lactate and pyruvate concentrations and improves glucose effectiveness in lean and obese patients with type 2 diabetes. *Diabetes Care* 1999; 22: 280–287.

12 Jacob S, Ruus P, Hermann R, *et al.* Oral administration of RAC-alpha-lipoic acid modulates insulin sensitivity in patients with type 2 diabetes mellitus: a placebo-controlled pilot trial. *Free Radic Biol Med* 1999; 27: 309–314.

13 Nickander KK, McPhee BR, Low PA, *et al.* Alpha-lipoic acid: antioxidant potency against lipid peroxidation of neural tissues in vitro and implications for diabetic neuropathy. *Free Radic Biol Med* 1996; 21: 631–639.

14 Kishi Y, Schmeizer JD, Yao JK, *et al.* Alpha-lipoic acid: effect of glucose uptake, sorbitol pathway, and energy metabolism in experimental diabetic neuropathy. *Diabetes* 1999; 48: 2045–2051.

15 Ziegler D, Schatz H, Conrad F, *et al.* Effects of treatment with the antioxidant alpha-lipoic acid on cardiac autonomic neuropathy in NIDDM patients. A 4-month randomized controlled multicenter trial (DEKAN Study). Deutsche Kardiale Autonome Neuropathie. *Diabetes Care* 1997; 20: 369–373.

16 Ruhnau KJ, Meissner HP, Finn JR. Effects of a 3-week oral treatment with the antioxidant thioctic acid (alpha-lipoic acid) in symptomatic diabetic polyneuropathy. *Diabet Med* 1999; 16: 1040–1043.

17 Reljanovic M, Reichel G, Rett K, *et al.* Treatment of diabetic polyneuropathy with the antioxidant thioctic acid (alpha-lipoic acid): a two year multicenter randomized double-blind placebo-controlled trial (ALADIN II). Alpha-lipoic acid in diabetic neuropathy. *Free Radic Res* 1999; 31: 171–179.

18 Ziegler D, Reljanovic M, Mehnert H. Alpha-lipoic acid in the treatment of diabetic polyneuropathy in Germany: current evidence from clinical trials. *Exp Clin Endocrinol Diabetes* 1999; 107: 421–430.

19 Ziegler D, Nowak H, Kempler P, *et al.* Treatment of symptomatic diabetic polyneuropathy with the antioxidant alpha-lipoic acid: a meta-analysis. *Diabet Med* 2004; 21: 114–121.

20 Hahm JR, Kim BJ, Kim KW. Clinical experience with thioctacid (thioctic acid) in the treatment of distal symmetric polyneuropathy in Korean diabetic patients. *J Diabetes Complications* 2004; 18: 79–85.

21 Tankova T, Koev D, Dakovska L. Alpha-lipoic acid in the treatment of autonomic diabetic neuropathy (controlled, randomized, open-label study). *Rom J Intern Med* 2004; 42: 457–464.

22 Tankova T, Cherninkova S, Koev D. Treatment for diabetic mononeuropathy with alpha-lipoic acid. *Int J Clin Pract* 2005; 59: 645–650.

23 Filina AA, Davydova NG, Endrikhovskii SN, *et al.* Lipoic acid as a means of metabolic therapy of open-angle glaucoma. *Vestn Oftalmol* 1995; 111: 6–8.

24 Baur A, Harrer T, Peukert M, *et al.* Alpha-lipoic acid is an effective inhibitor of human immunodeficiency virus (HIV-1) replication. *Klin Wochenschr* 1991; 69: 722–724.

25 Vasdev S, Ford CA, Parai S, *et al.* Dietary alpha-lipoic acid supplementation lowers blood pressure in spontaneously hypertensive rats. *J Hypertens* 2000; 18: 567–573.

26 Zakrzewska JM, Forssell H, Glenny AM. Interventions for the treatment of burning mouth syndrome. Cochrane database, issue 1, 2005. London: Macmillan.

27 Mantovani G, Maccio A, Melis G, *et al.* Restoration of functional defects in peripheral blood mononuclear cells isolated from cancer patients by thiol antioxidants alpha-lipoic acid and N-acetyl cysteine. *Int J Cancer* 2000; 86: 842–847.

28 Savitha S, Sivarajan K, Havipriya D, *et al.* Efficacy of levo carnitine and alpha-lipoic acid in ameliorating the decline in mitochondrial enzymes during aging. *Clin Nutr* 2005; 24: 794–800.

29 Sauer J, Tabet N, Howard R. Alpha-lipoic acid for dementia. Cochrane database, issue 1, 2004. London: Macmillan.

Antioxidants

Description

Various antioxidant systems have evolved to offer protection against free radicals and prevent damage to vital biological structures such as lipid membranes, proteins and DNA. Antioxidant capacity is a concept used to describe the overall ability of tissues to inhibit processes mediated by free radicals.[1] It is dependent on the concentrations of individual antioxidants and the activity of protective enzymes. The most common and important antioxidant defences are shown in Table 1.

The antioxidant vitamins can be divided into those that are water-soluble and exist in aqueous solution – primarily vitamin C – and those that are fat-soluble and exist in membranes or lipoproteins – primarily vitamin E. Lipid membranes are particularly vulnerable to oxidative breakdown by free radicals. Vitamin E protects cell membranes from destruction by undergoing preferential oxidation and destruction. Carotenoids, such as beta-carotene, which are found in most dark green, red or yellow fruits and vegetables and some quinones, such as ubiquinone (coenzyme Q) also appear to have antioxidant properties. Flavonoids and other phenols and polyphenols found in foods such as green tea, red wine, olive oil, grapes and many other fruits are also antioxidants. All these substances can act as free radical scavengers and can react directly with free radicals.

Some trace elements act as essential components of antioxidant enzymes – copper, magnesium or zinc for superoxide dismutase and selenium for glutathione peroxidase.

Supplements that are marketed as having antioxidant activity include:

- vitamin A (usually as beta-carotene), vitamins C and E (ACE vitamins, often with selenium)
- alpha-lipoic acid (see Alpha-lipoic acid)
- carnitine (see Carnitine)
- carotenoids (see Carotenoids)
- coenzyme Q (see Coenzyme Q)
- green tea (see Green tea extract)
- zinc (see Zinc).

Action

Antioxidants are believed to protect against certain diseases by preventing the deleterious effects of processes mediated by free radicals in cell membranes and by reducing the susceptibility of tissues to oxidative stress.

Free radicals

Each orbital surrounding the nucleus of an atom is occupied by a pair of electrons. If an orbital in the outer shell of a molecule loses an electron, the molecule becomes a free radical. As a result of the unpaired electron, the molecule becomes unstable and, therefore, highly reactive. The free radical may then react with any other nearby molecule, also converting that molecule to a free radical which can then initiate another reaction. Some free radicals are capable of severely damaging cells.

Theoretically, a single free radical can ultimately cause an endless number of reactions. This chain reaction is terminated either by the free radical's reaction with another free radical, resulting in the formation of a covalently bound molecule, or by the free radical's reaction with an antioxidant, an antioxidant enzyme, or both. Fortunately, many enzyme systems have

---

Table 1   Antioxidant defences

- **Intracellular antioxidants**
  Enzymes
    catalase
    glutathione peroxidase
    superoxide dismutase
- **Extracellular antioxidants**
  Vitamin C
  Sulphydryl groups
- **Membrane antioxidants**
  Carotenoids
  Ubiquinone
  Vitamin E
- **Substances essential for synthesis of antioxidant enzymes**
  Copper
  Manganese
  Selenium
  Zinc

---

evolved to provide protection from free radical production.

Because antioxidant defences are not completely efficient, increased free radical formation in the body is likely to increase damage. The term 'oxidative stress' is often used to refer to this effect. If mild oxidative stress occurs, tissues often respond by increasing their antioxidant defences. However, severe oxidative stress can cause cell injury and cell death.

There is growing evidence that free-radical damage is involved in the development of many diseases, such as atherosclerosis, cancer, Parkinson's disease and other neurodegenerative disorders, inflammatory bowel disease and lung disease.

Possible uses

Epidemiological evidence suggests that low plasma levels of antioxidant nutrients and low dietary intakes are related to an increased risk of diseases such as coronary heart disease (CHD) and cancer. There is also increasing evidence that these diseases can be prevented or delayed to some extent by dietary changes, in particular by increased consumption of fruits and vegetables. Several substances in fruit and vegetables (e.g. beta-carotene, vitamin C and vitamin E) may act to diminish oxidative damage *in vivo* and, because endogenous antioxidant defences are not completely effective, dietary antioxidants may be important in diminishing the cumulative effects of oxidative damage in the human body.

A question of particular interest is whether supplementation of adequately nourished subjects with antioxidant nutrients will reduce the incidence of such diseases. The few intervention trials of antioxidants reported so far have shown little evidence for the value of supplements. Some have shown harmful effects.

Cardiovascular disease

Epidemiological studies

Experimental studies suggest an inverse association between CHD mortality and vitamins C, E and beta-carotene, and argue strongly in favour of a protective role of antioxidants in the development of atherosclerosis.

In a cross-cultural study of middle-aged men representing 16 European populations,[1] differences in mortality from ischaemic heart disease were primarily attributable to plasma levels of vitamin E. Twelve of the 16 populations had similar blood cholesterol levels and blood pressure but differed greatly in tocopherol levels and heart disease death rates. For vitamin E, mean plasma levels lower than 25 µmol/L were associated with a high risk of CHD, whereas plasma levels above this value were associated with a higher risk of the disease. In the case of vitamin C, mean plasma levels less than 22.7 µmol/L were found in those regions that had a moderate to high risk of CHD, whereas plasma levels in excess of this level tended to be found in those areas at low risk.

In a large case-control study in Scotland,[2] 6000 men aged 35–54 were studied for a possible association between antioxidant status and risk of angina pectoris. Highly significant correlations between low plasma concentrations of beta-carotene, vitamin C, vitamin E and risk of angina were found.

The Health Professionals Study,[3] a large prospective investigation that looked at 39 910

US male health professionals aged 40–75, showed that men who took more than 100 units of vitamin E daily for over 2 years had a 37% reduction in risk of heart disease. The Nurses' Health Study,[4] in which 87 245 female nurses aged 34–59 took part, showed that women who took more than 200 units of vitamin E daily for more than 2 years had a 41% reduction in risk of CHD.

Intervention trials

The first intervention trial published was a study of 333 male physicians aged between 40 and 84 with angina pectoris and/or coronary revascularisation, which showed that 50 mg of beta-carotene on alternate days resulted in a 44% reduction in major coronary events.[5]

However, another study[6] tested aspirin, vitamin E and beta-carotene in the prevention of cardiovascular disease (CVD) and cancer in 39 876 women aged 45 and older. Among those randomly assigned to receive 50 mg beta-carotene or a placebo every other day, there were no statistically significant differences in incidence of CVD, cancer or overall death rate after a median of 2 years of treatment and 2 years of follow-up.

In a study of 1862 smoking men aged 50 to 59 [participants in the Finnish Alpha-Tocopherol, Beta-Carotene Cancer Prevention (ATBC) Study][7] who were followed for a median of 5.3 years, dietary supplements of alpha-tocopherol (50 mg a day), beta-carotene (20 mg a day), both, or a placebo were given. There were significantly more deaths from CHD among those who took beta-carotene supplements, and a non-significant trend towards more deaths in the vitamin E group. This same study also found that neither alpha-tocopherol nor beta-carotene had a preventive effect for large abdominal aortic aneurysm.[8] During the 6-year post-trial follow-up in the ATBC study, beta-carotene increased the post-trial risk of first-ever non-fatal myocardial infarction, suggesting that these supplements should not be used in the prevention of CVD among male smokers.[9]

Another large trial involving 20 536 UK adults aged 40–80 with coronary disease, other occlusive arterial disease or diabetes, randomly allocated participants to receive antioxidant vitamin supplementation (600 mg vitamin E, 250 mg vitamin C and 20 mg beta-carotene daily) or matching placebo over 5 years. There were no significant differences in all-cause mortality, or in deaths due to vascular or non-vascular causes. Nor were there any significant differences in the number of participants having non-fatal myocardial infarction or coronary death, non-fatal or fatal stroke, or coronary or non-coronary revascularisation. For the first occurrence of these major vascular events, there were no material differences overall and no significant differences in cancer incidence and hospitalisation for any other non-vascular disease.[10]

A double-blind clinical trial[11] found that taking high doses of vitamin C (500 mg twice a day) and E (700 units twice a day) and beta-carotene (30 000 units twice a day) did not reduce the risk of arteries re-clogging after balloon coronary angioplasty. The patients took probucol, probucol plus three antioxidants, the antioxidants alone or placebo. All patients also received aspirin. After 6 months the rates of repeated angioplasty were 11% in the probucol group, 16.2% in the combined treatment group, 24.4% in the multivitamin group and 26.6% in the placebo group.

A trial in post-menopausal women with coronary disease found that supplementation with vitamin E 400 units twice daily and vitamin C 500 mg twice daily did not retard atherosclerosis and provided no cardiovascular benefit.[12] Results from the SU.VI.MAX trial also suggested that a combination of antioxidants (120 mg vitamin C, 30 mg vitamin E, 6 mg beta-carotene, 100 μg selenium, 20 mg zinc) over an average of 7.2 years had no beneficial effects on carotid atherosclerosis and arterial stiffness[13] or risk of hypertension[14] in healthy patients. A further trial in 520 smoking and non-smoking men and post-menopausal women (all of whom had serum cholesterol > 5 mmol/L) found that supplementation with combination vitamin E and slow-release vitamin C slows down atherosclerotic progression.[15]

More recent trials have shown some beneficial effect of antioxidant supplements on certain aspects of CVD. A Polish trial involving 800 patients with acute myocardial infarction found that supplementation with vitamin C 1200 mg daily and vitamin E 600 mg daily over 30 days had a positive influence on primary end points (i.e. in-hospital cardiac mortality, non-fatal new myocardial infarction) and concluded that a larger study is warranted to generate further evidence for this particular regimen.[16]

An RCT involving 100 patients with asymptomatic or mildly symptomatic moderate aortic stenosis found that supplementation with vitamin E (400 units) and vitamin C (1000 mg) daily had modest anti-inflammatory effect, although the clinical relevance requires further clarification.[17] A 15-day clinical trial in patients with early-stage untreated type 2 diabetes mellitus or impaired glucose tolerance found that supplementation with N-acetyl cysteine 600 mg daily, vitamin E 300 mg daily and vitamin C 250 mg daily reversed unfavourable oxidative changes occurring after a moderate fat meal and may therefore have decreased oxidative stress.[18] A further trial involving 48 acute ischaemic stroke patients (evaluated within 12 h of symptom onset) found that compared with placebo alpha-tocopherol 800 units daily and vitamin C 500 mg daily over 14 days increased antioxidant capacity, reduced lipid peroxidation products and may have an anti-inflammatory effect.[19]

There is some evidence that folate status could have an influence on the response to antioxidant supplementation in patients at cardiovascular risk. One study found that folate deficiency may amplify the effect of other risk factors such as elevated homocysteine or variant methylene tetrahydrofolate reductase (MTHFR) genotype, as well as influencing the ability of antioxidant supplementation to protect against genetic damage.[20] A reduction in systolic blood pressure has been observed in young healthy men supplemented with both folic acid (10 mg daily) and antioxidants (vitamin C 100 mg, vitamin E 800 mg).[21] However, in a further study involving patients in the immediate aftermath of stroke, supplementation with antioxidant vitamins (vitamin E 800 units and vitamin C 500 mg daily), or B group vitamins (5 mg folic acid, 5 mg vitamin B_2, 50 mg vitamin B_6, 0.4 mg vitamin B_{12}), both vitamins together or no supplements found that supplementation with antioxidant vitamins with or without B-group vitamins enhances antioxidant capacity, mitigates oxidative damage and may have an anti-inflammatory effect immediately post-infarct in stroke.[22]

The effect of antioxidant supplementation in CVD has been evaluated in systematic reviews and meta-analyses. One systematic review assessed whether antioxidants in food or supplements can offer primary prevention against myocardial infarction or stroke.[23] Eight RCTs were included, six of which tested supplements of beta-carotene, four tested alpha-tocopherol and two ascorbic acid. None of the RCTs showed any benefit of antioxidant supplementation on CVD. In one study there was a significantly increased risk for fatal or non-fatal intracerebral and subarachnoid haemorrhage in participants taking alpha-tocopherol. The reviewers concluded that from these RCTs (which had limitations) antioxidants as food supplements had no beneficial effects in the primary prevention of myocardial infarction and stroke and cannot be recommended for such purposes.

A meta-analysis that looked at the effect of antioxidant vitamins on long-term cardiovascular outcomes included 12 RCTs, of which seven examined vitamin E and eight beta-carotene.[24] Over all the studies there was no statistically significant difference between vitamin E and control for all-cause mortality, cardiovascular mortality or cerebrovascular accident. Beta-carotene was associated with a slight statistically significant increase in all-cause mortality and cardiovascular death compared with control. The authors concluded that the routine use of vitamin E cannot be recommended and that the use of supplements containing beta-carotene should be actively discouraged.

The US Agency for Healthcare Research and Quality (AHRQ) commissioned an extensive report on the efficacy and safety of antioxidant supplements (vitamins C, E and coenzyme Q_{10}) for the prevention and treatment of CVD.[25] From a review and analysis of the 144 clinical trials the authors identified, the following conclusions were reached. Firstly, the evidence does not suggest a benefit of supplements containing vitamin E or vitamin C (either alone or in combination) on either CVD or all-cause mortality, but there was no suggestion of harm. Secondly, there was no consistent support for a beneficial effect on fatal or non-fatal myocardial infarction or upon plasma lipid levels. Evidence on coenzyme Q_{10} was judged to be insufficient to reach conclusions on its effects in CVD.

A pooled analysis of nine cohort studies evaluated the relationship between the intake of antioxidant vitamins and CHD risk. Dietary intake of antioxidants was only weakly related to CHD risk. However, subjects with a higher supplemental vitamin C intake had a lower CHD incidence, while supplemental vitamin E intake was not significantly associated with CHD risk.[26]

In 2004, the American Heart Association Council on Nutrition, Physical Activity and Metabolism concluded that antioxidant supplements have little or no proven value for preventing or treating CVD.[27]

Cancer

Epidemiological studies

There is now good evidence linking high intake of fruit and vegetables with lower incidence of certain cancers, and it is presumed that the protective nutrients are some or all of the antioxidant nutrients.

In a study of 25 802 volunteers in Washington County, Maryland,[28] prediagnostic blood samples from 436 cancer cases at nine cancer sites were compared with 765 matched control cases. Serum beta-carotene levels showed a strong protective association with lung cancer, suggestive protective associations with melanoma and bladder cancer, and a suggestive but non-protective association with lung cancer. Serum vitamin E levels showed a protective association with lung cancer, but none of the other cancer sites studied showed impressive associations. Low levels of serum lycopene (a carotenoid occurring in ripe fruits) were strongly associated with pancreatic cancer and less strongly associated with cancer of the bladder and rectum.

The Basel study from Switzerland[29] demonstrated that patients who had died from all cancers, including cancer of the bronchus and stomach, had statistically lower mean carotene levels compared with a matched group of healthy survivors.

In a Finnish study,[30] individuals with low serum levels of vitamin E had about a 1.5-fold risk of cancer compared with those with a higher serum level of vitamin E. The strength of the association between serum vitamin E level and cancer risk varied for different cancer sites and was strongest for some gastrointestinal cancers and for the combined group of cancers unrelated to smoking.

Intervention trials

An intervention trial in Linxian, China,[31] provided some of the earliest clinical data on the effects of specific vitamin–mineral supplementation on cancer incidence and disease-specific mortality. Linxian County has one of the world's highest rates of oesophageal and gastric cancers. Combined daily doses of 15 mg beta-carotene, 30 mg vitamin E and 50 µg selenium taken over 5 years were associated with a 13% reduction in deaths from cancer, and an overall reduction in mortality of 9%. These results, although impressive, might have been achieved because the population studied had low intakes and were deficient in the nutrients investigated. A similar study is required in a well-nourished population.

Not all studies have shown positive results. The ATBC Study in Finland[32] found no reduction in the incidence of lung cancer among male smokers after 5 to 8 years of dietary supplementation with vitamin E or beta-carotene; incidence of lung cancer increased by 18% and overall death rate by 8% in the group receiving beta-carotene. However, these results should be considered in the context of the population studied – the subjects had smoked an average of 20 cigarettes a day for 36 years. Most studies with antioxidants suggest that their protective properties are associated with the early stages of cancer and it is likely that this intervention took place too late in the carcinogenic process. In addition, the study could have employed too low a dose (50 mg vitamin E and/or 20 mg beta-carotene were used) or was of too short a duration. The excess risks of beta-carotene on lung cancer were no longer evident 46 years after the intervention had ended.[33] More recent data from this study suggest no association between dietary vitamin C or E, alpha- or gamma-tocopherol, alpha- or beta-carotene, lycopene or lutein and risk for colorectal cancer.[34] No overall preventive effect of long-term supplementation with alpha-tocopherol or beta-carotene on gastric cancer was found.[35]

Another trial,[36] which tested a combination of beta-carotene and vitamin A, was terminated after 4 years because it appeared that those taking the supplements and who also smoked had a 28% higher incidence of lung cancer and a 17% higher death rate.

In the Nurses' Health Study,[37] large intakes of vitamin C or E did not protect women from breast cancer. In contrast, there was a significant inverse association of vitamin A intake with risk of this disease. The authors concluded, however, that vitamin A supplements are unlikely to influence the risk of breast cancer among women whose dietary intake of this vitamin is already adequate.

In the Polyp Prevention Study,[38] there was no evidence that supplements of either beta-carotene or vitamins C and E reduced the incidence of colorectal adenomas. Compared with placebo, alpha-tocopherol supplementation increased the occurrence of second primary cancers in head and neck patients.[39]

A further study found that low-dose antioxidant supplementation (over 7.5 years) lowered total cancer incidence and all-cause mortality in men, but not in women. The authors suggested that the effectiveness of supplementation in men may have been because of their lower baseline status of certain antioxidants, especially beta-carotene.[40] In a further study, supplemental beta-carotene intake at a dose of at least 2000 µg daily was associated with a decreased risk of prostate cancer in men with low dietary beta-carotene intake. Among current and recent smokers, increasing dose (>400 units daily) and duration (> 10 years) of supplemental vitamin E use was also associated with reduced prostate cancer risk.[41]

AHRQ commissioned a report to investigate the effectiveness of vitamin E, vitamin C and coenzyme Q_{10} in the prevention and treatment of cancer.[42] They found no evidence to support the beneficial effects of vitamin E and/or vitamin C in the prevention of new tumours, the development of colonic polyps or in the treatment of patients with advanced cancer.[42] A systematic review and meta-analysis found no evidence that antioxidant supplements (beta-carotene, vitamin A, C and E) can prevent gastrointestinal cancers, but rather that they seemed to increase overall mortality. There was evidence from four of the included trials that selenium has a beneficial effect on the incidence of gastrointestinal cancer. However, good clinical trials are needed to confirm this benefit.[43]

Cataract

Antioxidants are also being investigated for a possible protective effect in cataract. Low vitamin C intakes have been associated with increased risk of cataract.[44] Increased levels of supplementary vitamins C and E correlated with a 50% reduction in the risk of cataracts,[45] while the Nurses' Health Study[46] found that dietary carotenoids, although not necessarily beta-carotene, and long-term vitamin C supplementation may reduce the risk of cataracts.

The Age-Related Eye Disease Study (AREDS), an 11-centre trial, evaluated the effect of a high-dose antioxidant supplement (vitamin C 500 mg, vitamin E 400 units, beta-carotene 15 mg) on the development and progression of age-related lens opacities and visual acuity loss. Of 4757 participants enrolled, 4629 who were aged from 55 to 80 had at least one natural lens present and were followed up for an average of 6.3 years. No statistically significant effect of the antioxidant formulation was seen on the development or progression of age-related lens opacities or visual acuity loss.[47]

A further trial – the Roche European American Cataract Trial (REACT) – randomised 445 patients with age-related cataract (in English and American outpatient settings) to a mixture of oral antioxidant micronutrients (beta-carotene 18 mg daily, vitamin C 750 mg daily and vitamin E 600 mg daily) or placebo and followed for 2–4 years. After 2 years of treatment, there was a small positive treatment effect in the US group and after 3 years a positive effect was apparent in both the US and UK groups. The positive effect in the US group was even more positive after 3 years, but the benefit in the UK group did not reach statistical significance.[48]

Age-related macular degeneration (ARMD)

Research is being conducted to determine whether taking supplements or consuming foods rich in antioxidants can protect against age-related macular degeneration (ARMD), a disease in which the central portion of the retina deteriorates so that only peripheral vision remains. A study following 3654 individuals aged 49 or older found no statistically significant association between ARMD and dietary intake of either carotene, zinc or vitamins A or C, either from diet, supplements or both.[49] An earlier study involving 156 subjects with ARMD showed that neither serum alpha-tocopherol nor beta-carotene was significantly associated with age-related maculopathy.[50]

In 29 000 smoking males aged 50 to 69 randomly assigned to alpha-tocopherol (50 mg a day), beta-carotene (20 mg a day), placebo or both, no beneficial effect of supplementation on the occurrence of ARMD was found.[51] However in a study involving 21 120 male physicians,[52] those who used vitamin E supplements or multivitamins had a possible but non-significant reduced risk of ARMD, but the authors concluded that large reductions in the risk of ARMD were unlikely.

A Cochrane review[53] (which included one study) concluded in 2000 that there was no evidence to date that people without ARMD should take antioxidant vitamin and mineral supplements to prevent or delay the onset of the disease.

The AREDS (see above) also evaluated the effect of antioxidants with the addition of zinc (80 mg daily) and copper (2 mg daily) on ARMD. All patients had best eye visual acuity of 20/32 or better in at least one eye. They had category 2, 3 or 4 disease, meaning that they had small to intermediate drusen. The main outcome was progression to advanced macular degeneration. Antioxidants combined with zinc were associated with lower rates of development of advanced ARMD and loss of visual acuity. Both zinc and antioxidants plus zinc significantly reduced the odds of developing advanced ARMD in the higher-risk group. In conclusion this trial showed that the combination of antioxidants plus zinc was worth while in people with extant macular degeneration to prevent or slow further development to the advanced form.[54] This study did not show this supplement had benefits at other stages of ARMD.

A recent Dutch cohort study involving 4170 participants aged 55 or older in a suburb of Rotterdam found that dietary intake of both vitamin E and zinc was inversely associated with incident ARMD. An above median intake of beta-carotene, vitamin C, vitamin E and zinc was associated with a 35% reduced risk of ARMD.[55]

A Cochrane review including eight trials concluded that evidence for the effectiveness of antioxidant vitamin and mineral supplementation in halting progression of ARMD comes mainly from the AREDS. However, it also concluded that the generalisability of these findings to other populations is unknown and further large trials are required.[56]

Pre-eclampsia

Antioxidants have also been evaluated for possible prevention of pre-eclampsia, with mixed results.[57–59] A Cochrane review of seven (mostly poor quality) trials found that antioxidant supplementation seems to reduce the risk of pre-eclampsia, with a reduction in risk of having a small-for-dates baby associated with antioxidants, although there is an increase in the risk of pre-term birth. Several large trials are ongoing and the results of these are needed before antioxidants can be recommended for clinical practice.[60]

Physical exercise

Intense physical exercise has been associated with an increase in free radical production and an increase in oxidative stress. Antioxidant supplements have been evaluated for an effect on exercise stress. Supplementation has been associated with a decrease in oxidative stress markers in basketball players,[61] an increase in antioxidant enzymes in athletes,[62] enhancement in neutrophil oxidative burst in trained runners,[63] prevention of decreases in serum iron in endurance athletes,[64] prevention of exercise-induced lipid peroxidation in ultra-marathon runners,[65] but not prevention of muscle damage in response to an ultra-marathon run.[66]

Miscellaneous

Antioxidant supplements have been investigated for a wide range of other conditions. Current research interests include asthma, lung function and critical illness in hospital. However, good clinical trials have not yet been conducted in these areas.

Adverse effects

Antioxidants are considered to be largely safe in low doses. However, routine use of combinations of antioxidants exceeding the Recommended Daily Allowance (RDA) should not be recommended for long-term use. One study has found that antioxidants (vitamins E and C, beta-carotene and selenium) could block the favourable effects of statins combined with

> ### Conclusion
> Biochemical evidence suggests that oxidative stress caused by accumulation of free radicals is involved in the pathogenesis of several diseases. Appropriate levels of antioxidant nutrients might therefore be expected to delay or prevent these diseases. Several epidemiological studies have found lower serum levels of antioxidant nutrients in patients with CVD, cancer and cataract, but there is no good evidence that supplements of antioxidant nutrients prevent CVD or cancer. Evidence suggests that some may cause harm and increase mortality. Further intervention trials are needed. In the meantime, the best advice to give is to eat plenty of fruit and vegetables (five or more servings a day). An antioxidant combination has been found to delay progression of ARMD.

niacin (a drug combination used in the USA). This interaction could have implications for the management of CVD.[67]

Interactions

None reported.

References

1 Gey KF, Puska P, Jordan P, Moser UK. Inverse correlation between plasma vitamin E and mortality from ischaemic heart disease in cross-cultural epidemiology. *Am J Clin Nutr* 1991; 53: 326S–346S.
2 Riemersma RA, Wood DA, MacIntyre CCA, *et al*. Risk of angina pectoris and plasma concentrations of vitamins A, C and E and carotene. *Lancet* 1991; 337: 1–5.
3 Rimm EB, Stampfer MJ, Ascherio A, *et al*. Vitamin E consumption and the risk of coronary heart disease in men. *N Engl J Med* 1993; 328: 1450–1456.
4 Stampfer MJ, Hennekens CH, Manson JE, *et al*. Vitamin E consumption and the risk of coronary heart disease in women. *N Engl J Med* 1993; 328: 1444–1449.
5 Gaziano JM, Manson JE, Ridker PM, *et al*. Beta-carotene therapy for chronic stable angina. *Circulation* 1990; 82 (Suppl. III): 201 (abstract 0796).
6 Rapola JM, Virtamo J, Ripatti S, *et al*. Randomised trial of alpha-tocopherol and beta-carotene supplements on incidence of major coronary events in men with previous myocardial infarction. *Lancet* 1997; 349: 1715–1720.
7 Hennekens CH, Buring JE, Manson JE, *et al*. Lack of effect of long term supplementation with beta-carotene on the incidence of malignant neoplasms and cardiovascular disease. *N Engl J Med* 1996; 334: 1145–1149.
8 Tornwall ME, Virtamo J, Haukka JK, *et al*. Alpha-tocopherol (vitamin E) and beta-carotene supplementation does not affect the risk for large abdominal aortic aneurysm in a controlled trial. *Atherosclerosis* 2001; 157: 167–173.
9 Tornwall ME, Virtamo J, Korhonen PA, *et al*. Effect of alpha-tocopherol and beta-carotene supplementation on coronary heart disease during the 6-year post-trial follow-up in the ATBC study. *Eur Heart J* 2004; 25: 1171–1178.
10 Heart Protection Study Collaborative Group. MRC/BHF Heart Protection Study of antioxidant vitamin supplementation in 20,536 high-risk individuals: a randomised placebo-controlled trial. *Lancet* 2002; 360: 23–33.

11 Tardif JC. Probucol and multivitamins in the prevention of restenosis after coronary angioplasty. *N Engl J Med* 1997; 337: 365–372.

12 Waters DD, Alderman EL, Hsia J, *et al*. Effects of hormone replacement therapy and antioxidant vitamin supplements on coronary atherosclerosis in postmenopasal women. *JAMA* 2002; 288: 2432–2440.

13 Zureik M, Galan P, Bertrais S, *et al*. Effects of long-term daily low-dose supplementation with anti-oxidant vitamins and minerals on structure and function of large arteries. *Arterioscler Thromb Vasc Biol* 2004; 24: 1485–1491.

14 Czernichow S, Bertrais S, Blacher J, *et al*. Effect of supplementation with antioxidants upon long-term risk of hypertension in the SU.VI.MAX study: association with plasma antioxidant levels. *J Hypertens* 2005; 23: 2013–18.

15 Salonen RM, Nyyssonen K, Kaikkonene J, *et al*. Six-year effect of combined vitamin C and E supplementation on atherosclerotic progression: the Antioxidant Supplementation in Atherosclerotic Prevention (ASAP) Study. *Circulation* 2003; 107: 947–953.

16 Jaxa-Chamiec T, Bednarz B, Drozdowska D, *et al*. Antioxidant effects of combined vitamins C and E in acute myocardial infarction. The randomized, double-blind, placebo controlled, multicenter pilot Myocardial Infarction and VITamins (MIVIT) trial. *Kardiol Pol* 2005; 62: 344–50.

17 Tahir M, Foley B, Pate G, *et al*. Impact of vitamin E and C supplementation on serum adhesion molecules in chronic degenerative aortic stenosis: a randomized controlled trial. *Am Heart J* 2005; 150: 302–306.

18 Signorelli NS, Torrisi B, Pulvirenti D, *et al*. Effects of antioxidant supplementation on postprandial oxidative stress and endothelial dysfunction: a single-blind, 15-day clinical trial in patients with untreated type 2 diabetes, subjects with impaired glucose tolerance, and healthy controls. *Clin Ther* 2005; 27: 1764–1773.

19 Ullegaddi R, Powers HJ, Gariballa SE. Antioxidant supplementation enhances antioxidant capacity and mitigates oxidative damage following acute ischemic stroke. *Eur J Clin Nutr* 2005; 59: 1367–1373.

20 Smolkova B, Dusinska M, Raslova K, *et al*. Folate levels determine effect of antioxidant supplementation on micronuclei in subjects with cardiovascular risk. *Mutagenesis* 2004; 19: 469–476.

21 Schutte AE, Huisman HW, Oosthuizen W, *et al*. Cardiovascular effects of oral supplementation of vitamin C, E and folic acid in young healthy males. *Int J Vitam Nutr Res* 2004; 74: 285–293.

22 Ullegaddi R, Powers HJ, Gariballa SE. Antioxidant supplementation with or without B-group vitamins after acute ischaemic stroke: a randomised controlled trial. *J Parenter Enteral Nutr* 2006; 30: 108–114.

23 Asplund K. Antioxidant vitamins in the prevention of cardiovascular disease: a systematic review. *J Intern Med* 2002; 251: 372–392.

24 Vivekananthan DP, Penn MS, Sapp SK, *et al*. Use of antioxidant vitamins for the prevention of cardiovascular disease: meta-analysis of randomized trials. *Lancet* 2003; 361: 2017–2023.

25 Agency for Healthcare Research and Quality. *Effect of Supplemental Antioxidants Vitamin C, Vitamin E, and Coenzyme Q$_{10}$ for the Prevention and Treatment of Cardiovascular Disease*. Evidence Report/Technology Assessment: Number 83. AHRQ Publication Number 03-E042. Available from http://www.ahrq.gov/clinic/epcsums/antioxsum.htm (accessed 6 November 2006). Rockville, MD: AHRQ, June 2003.

26 Knekt P, Ritz J, Pereira MA, *et al*. Antioxidant vitamins and coronary heart disease risk: a pooled analysis of 9 cohorts. *Am J Clin Nutr* 2004; 80: 1508–1520.

27 Kris-Etherton PM, Lichtenstein AH, Howard BV, *et al*. Antioxidant vitamin supplements and cardiovascular disease. *Circulation* 2004; 110: 637–641.

28 Comstock GW, Helzlsouer KJ, Bush T. Prediagnostic serum levels of carotenoids and vitamin E as related to subsequent cancer in Washington County, Maryland. *Am J Clin Nutr* 1991; 53: 260S–264S.

29 Stahelin HB, Gey KF, Eichholzer M, Ludin E. Beta-carotene and cancer prevention: the Basel study. *Am J Clin Nutr* 1991; 53: 265S–269S.

30 Knekt P, Aromaa A, Maatela J, *et al*. Vitamin E and cancer prevention. *Am J Clin Nutr* 1991; 53: 283S–286S.

31 Blot WJ, Li JY, Taylor PR. Nutrition intervention trials in Linxian, China: supplementation with specific vitamin/mineral combinations, cancer incidence, and disease-specific mortality in the general population. *J Natl Cancer Inst* 1993; 85: 1483–1492.

32 The Alpha-Tocopherol, Beta-Carotene Cancer Prevention Study Group. The effect of vitamin E and beta carotene on the incidence of lung cancer in male smokers. *N Engl J Med* 1994; 330: 1029–1035.

33 Virtamo J, Pietinen P, Huttunen JK, *et al*. Incidence of cancer and mortality following alpha-tocopherol and beta-carotene supplementation: a postintervention follow-up. *JAMA* 2003; 290: 476–485.

34 Malila N, Virtamo J, Virtanen M, *et al*. Dietary and serum alpha-tocopherol, beta-carotene and retinol, and risk for colorectal cancer in male smokers. *Eur J Clin Nutr* 2002; 56: 615–621.

35 Malila N, Taylor PR, Virtanen MJ, *et al*. Effects of alpha-tocopherol and beta-carotene supplementation on gastric cancer incidence in male smokers (ATBC Study, Finland). *Cancer Causes Control* 2002; 13: 617–623.

36 Omenn GS, Goodman GE, Thornquist MD, *et al.* Effects of a combination of betacarotene and vitamin A on lung cancer and cardiovascular disease. *N Engl J Med* 1996; 334: 1150–1155.

37 Hunter DJ, Manson JE, Colditz GA, *et al.* A prospective study of vitamins C, E and A and the risk of breast cancer. *N Engl J Med* 1993; 329: 234–240.

38 Greenberg ER, Baron JA, Tosteson TD, *et al.* A clinical trial of antioxidant vitamins to prevent colorectal adenoma. *N Engl J Med* 1994; 331: 141–147.

39 Bairati I, Meyer F, Gelinas M, *et al.* A randomized trial of antioxidant vitamins to prevent second primary cancers in head and neck cancer patients. *J Natl Cancer Inst* 2003; 97: 468–470.

40 Hercberg S, Galan P, Preziosi P, *et al.* The SU.VI.MAX Study: a randomized, placebo-controlled trial of the health effects of antioxidant vitamins and minerals. *Arch Intern Med* 2004; 164: 2335–2342.

41 Kirsch VA, Hayes RB, Mayne ST, *et al.* Supplemental vitamin E, beta-carotene, and vitamin C intakes and prostate cancer risk. *J Natl Cancer Inst* 2006; 98: 245–254.

42 Agency for Healthcare Research and Quality. *Effect of the Supplemental Use of Antioxidants Vitamin C, Vitamin E, and Coenzyme Q_{10} for the Prevention and Treatment of Cancer.* Evidence Report/Technology Assessment: Number 75. AHRQ Publications Number 04-E002. Available from http://www.ahrq.gov/clinic/epcsums/aoxcansum.htm (accessed 6 November 2006). Rockville, MD: AHRQ, October 2003.

43 Bjelakovic G, Nikolova D, Simonetti RG, Gluud C. Antioxidant supplements for prevention of gastrointestinal cancers: a systematic review and meta-analysis. *Lancet* 2004; 364: 1219–1228.

44 Jacques PF, Chylack LT. Epidemiologic evidence of a role for the antioxidant vitamins and carotenoids in cancer prevention. *Am J Clin Nutr* 1991; 53: 352S–355S.

45 Robertson J McD, Donner AP, Trevithick JR. A possible role for vitamins C and E in cataract prevention. *Am J Clin Nutr* 1991; 53: 346S–351S.

46 Hankinson SE, Stampfer MJ, Seddon JM, *et al.* Nutrient intake and cataract extraction in women: a prospective study. *BMJ* 1992; 305: 335–339.

47 Age-Related Eye Disease Study Research Group. A randomized, placebo-controlled, clinical trial of high-dose supplementation with vitamins C and E and beta-carotene for age-related cataract and vision loss: AREDS report no. 9. *Arch Ophthalmol* 2001; 119: 1439–1452.

48 Chylack LT Jr, Brown NP, Bron A, *et al.* The Roche American Cataract Trial (REACT): a randomised clinical trial to investigate the efficacy of an oral antioxidant micronutrient mixture to slow progression of age-related cataract. *Ophthalmic Epidemiol* 2002; 9: 49–80.

49 Smith W, Mitchell P, Webb K, Leeder SR. Dietary antioxidants and age-related maculopathy: The Blue Mountains Study. *Ophthalmology* 1999; 106: 761–767.

50 Smith W, Mitchell P, Rochester C, *et al.* Serum betacarotene, alpha tocopherol and age-related maculopathy: the Blue Mountain study. *Am J Ophthalmol* 1997; 124: 839–840.

51 Teikari JM, Laatikainen L, Virtamo J, *et al.* Six-year supplementation with alpha-tocopherol and beta-carotene and age-related maculopathy. *Acta Ophthalmol Scand* 1998; 76: 224–229.

52 Christen WG, Ajani UA, Glynn RG, *et al.* Prospective cohort study of antioxidant vitamin supplement use and the risk of age-related maculopathy. *Am J Epidemiol* 1999; 149: 476–484.

53 Evans JR, Henshaw K. Antioxidant vitamin and mineral supplementation for preventing age related macular degeneration. Cochrane database, issue 2, 2006. London: Macmillan.

54 Age-Related Eye Disease Study Research Group. A randomized, placebo-controlled, clinical trial of high-dose supplementation with vitamins C and E, beta-carotene and zinc for age-related cataract and vision loss: AREDS report no. 8. *Arch Ophthalmol* 2001; 119: 1417–1436.

55 van Leeuwen R, Boekhoorn S, Vingerling JR, *et al.* Dietary intake of antioxidants and risk of age-related macular degeneration. *JAMA* 2005; 294: 3101–3107.

56 Evans JR. Antioxidant vitamin and mineral supplements for slowing the progression of age-related macular degeneration. Cochrane database, issue 2, 2006. London: Macmillan.

57 Beazley D, Ahokas R, Livingston J, *et al.* Vitamin C and E supplementation in women at high risk for preeclampsia: a double-blind, placebo-controlled trial. *Am J Obstet Gynecol* 2005; 192: 520–521.

58 Rumbold AR, Crowther CA, Haslam RR, *et al.* Vitamins C and E and the risks of preeclampsia and perinatal complications. *N Engl J Med* 2006; 27: 354: 1796–1806.

59 Poston L, Briley AL, Seed PT, *et al.* Vitamin C and vitamin E in pregnant women at risk for preeclampsia (VIP) trial: randomised placebo-controlled trial. *Lancet* 2006; 367: 1145–1154.

60 Rumbold A, Duley L, Crowther C, Haslam R. Antioxidants for preventing preeclampsia. Cochrane database, issue 4, 2005. London: Macmillan.

61 Schroder H, Navarro E, Mora J, *et al.* Effects of alpha-tocopherol, beta-carotene and ascorbic acid on oxidative, hormonal and enzymatic exercise stress markers in habitual training activity of professional basketball players. *Eur J Clin Nutr* 2001; 40: 178–184.

62 Tauler P, Aguilo A, Fuentespina E, *et al*. Diet supplementation with vitamin E, vitamin C and beta-carotene cocktail enhances basal neutrophil antioxidant enzymes in athletes. *Pflugers Arch* 2002; 443: 791–797.

63 Robson PJ, Bouic PJ, Myburgh KH. Antioxidant supplementation enhances neutrophil oxidative burst in trained runners following prolonged exercise. *Int J Sport Nutr Exerc Metab* 2003; 13: 369–381.

64 Aguilo A, Tauler P, Fuentespina E, *et al*. Antioxidant diet supplementation influences blood iron status in endurance athletes. *Int J Sport Nutr Exerc Metab* 2004; 14: 147–160.

65 Mastaloudis A, Morrow JD, Hopkins DW, *et al*. Antioxidant supplementation prevents exercise-induced lipid peroxidation, but not inflammation, in ultramarathon runners. *Free Radic Biol Med* 2004; 36: 1329–1341.

66 Mastaloudis A, Traver MG, Carstensen K, Widrick JJ. Antioxidants did not prevent muscle damage in response to an ultramarathon run. *Med Sci Sports Exerc* 2006; 38: 72–80.

67 Cheung MC, Zhao XQ, Chait A. Antioxidant supplements block the response of HDL to simvastatin-niacin therapy in patients with coronary artery disease and low HDL. *Arterioscler Thromb Vasc Biol* 2001; 21: 1320–1326.

Bee pollen

Description

Bee pollen consists of flower pollen and nectar from male seed flowers. It is collected by the worker honey bee, mixed with secretions from the bee such as saliva, which contains digestive enzymes, and is then carried back to the beehive on the hind legs of the bee. The pollen is harvested at the entrance to the beehive as bees travel through the wire mesh brushing their legs against a collecting vessel. Commercial quantities of pollen can also be collected directly from the flowers.

Constituents

Bee pollen consists of protein, carbohydrates, minerals, and essential fatty acids such as alpha-linolenic acid and linoleic acids. It also contains small amounts of B vitamins, vitamin C, flavonoids and various amino acids, hormones, enzymes and coenzymes. In nutritional terms the amounts of vitamins and minerals are too small to be significant.

Action

Bee pollen may have antioxidant and anti-inflammatory activity.

Possible uses

Bee pollen has been claimed to be useful for improving prostatitis and benign prostatic hypertrophy, although all the studies conducted so far have been uncontrolled and none published in English. Bee pollen has also been claimed to be beneficial in reducing the risk of atherosclerosis, hypertension and varicose veins, but there are no clinical studies to support these claims.

Two double-blind, placebo-controlled trials in humans have investigated the effects of bee pollen in cross-country runners,[1] and in elderly patients with memory deterioration.[2] However, there were no improvements in running speed or memory function in these two studies.

Precautions/contraindications

Bee pollen is contraindicated in people with a known history of atopy or allergy to pollen or plant products because of the risk of hypersensitivity.

Pregnancy and breast-feeding

No problems have been reported, but there have not been sufficient studies to guarantee the safety of bee pollen in pregnancy and breast-feeding.

Adverse effects

Bee pollen may cause allergic reactions, including nausea, vomiting and anaphylaxis. One 19-year-old man with asthma had a fatal reaction to bee pollen.[3] Anecdotally, bee pollen has been shown to promote hyperglycaemia in diabetes.

Interactions

None reported.

Dose

Bee pollen is available in the form of capsules and powder.

The dose is not established. Product manufacturers tend to recommend doses of

500–1500 mg daily from capsules or ½–1 tea-spoon of the powder.

References

1 Steben RE, Boudreaux P. The effects of pollen and protein extracts on selected blood factors and performance of athletes. *J Sports Med Phys Fitness* 1978; 18: 221–226.

2 Iversen T, Fiigaard KM, Schriver P, *et al.* The effects of NaO Li Su on memory functions and blood chemistry in elderly people. *J Ethnopharmacol* 1997; 56: 109–116.

3 Prichard M, Turner KJ. Acute hypersensitivity to ingested processed pollen. *Aust NZ J Med* 1985; 15: 346–347.

Betaine

Description

Betaine is a cofactor in various methylation reactions.

Action

Betaine works with choline, vitamin B_{12}, and also S-adenosyl methionine (SAMe), a derivative of the amino acid methionine, from which homocysteine is synthesised. It reduces homocysteine levels by remethylating homocysteine to produce methionine.

Possible uses

As a supplement, betaine is available in the form of the hydrochloride and as such contains 23% hydrochloric acid. It has been used as a digestive aid to treat people with achlorhydria and to reduce high levels of homocysteine. Whether it can reduce near normal levels of homocysteine is open to question.

Betaine has been reported to play a role in reducing plasma homocysteine levels, which may reduce the risk of heart disease. A study in 15 healthy men and women aged 18–35 years showed that betaine 6 g daily for 3 weeks reduced plasma homocysteine concentration after 2 weeks by 0.9 μmol/L and after 3 weeks by 0.6 μmol/L.[1] However, the extent of the decrease was much smaller than that in patients with homocystinuria[2] and appears to be smaller than that established by interventions with folic acid.[3] An RCT in 42 obese subjects[4] found that betaine supplementation (6 g daily for 12 weeks) decreased plasma homocysteine concentration by 8.76 ± 1.63 μmol/L at the start of the study and 7.93 ± 1.52 μmol/L at the end of the study.

However, there is insufficient evidence to recommend betaine supplements for the prevention of CHD.

Precautions/contraindications

Betaine should be avoided in patients with peptic ulcer.

Pregnancy and breast-feeding

No problems have been reported, but there have not been sufficient studies to guarantee the safety of betaine in pregnancy and breast-feeding.

Adverse effects

Betaine may cause gastrointestinal irritation.

Interactions

None reported.

Dose

Betaine is available in the form of tablets and capsules.

The dose is not established. Dietary supplements provide 250–500 mg in each dose.

References

1 Brouwer IA, Verhoef P, Urgert R. Betaine supplementation and plasma homocysteine in healthy volunteers. *Arch Intern Med* 2000; 160: 911.
2 Wilcken DE, Wilcken B, Dudman NP, Tyrell PA. Homocystinuria: the effects of betaine in the

treatment of patients not responsive to pyridoxine. *N Engl J Med* 1983; 309: 448–453.

3 Homocysteine Lowering Trialists' Collaboration. Lowering blood homocysteine with folic acid based supplements: meta-analysis of randomised trials. *BMJ* 1998; 316: 894–898.

4 Schwab U, Torronen A, Toppinen L, *et al*. Betaine supplementation decreases plasma homocysteine concentrations but does not affect body weight, body composition, or resting energy expenditure in human subjects. *Am J Clin Nutr* 2002; 76: 961–967.

Biotin

Description

Biotin is a water-soluble vitamin and a member of the vitamin B complex.

Nomenclature

Biotin was formerly known as vitamin H or coenzyme R.

Human requirements

See Table 1 for Dietary Reference Values for biotin.

Dietary intake

In the UK, the average dietary intake in adult women is 28 µg daily and in adult men is 39 µg daily. Biotin is also produced by colonic bacteria, but the effect of this on biotin requirements is not known.

Action

Biotin functions as an integral part of the enzymes that transport carboxyl units and fix carbon dioxide. Biotin enzymes are important in carbohydrate and lipid metabolism, and are involved in gluconeogenesis, fatty acid synthesis, propionate metabolism and the catabolism of amino acids.

Dietary sources

Biotin is ubiquitous in the diet. The richest sources of biotin are liver, kidney, eggs, soya beans and peanuts. Meat, wholegrain cereals, wholemeal bread, milk and cheese are also good sources. Green vegetables contain very little biotin.

Table 1 Dietary Reference Values for biotin (µg/day)

Age	UK safe intake	UK EVM	USA AI	FAO/WHO RNI
EU RDA = 150 µg				
Males and females				
0–6 months			5	5
7–12 months			6	6
1–3 years			8	8
4–6 years			–	12
4–8 years			12	–
7–9 years			–	20
9–13 years			20	–
10–18 years			–	25
14–18 years			25	–
19–50 years			30	45
51+ years			30	45
11–50+ years	10–20	970	–	–
Pregnancy			30	30
Lactation			35	35

AI = adequate intake
EVM = likely safe daily intake from supplements alone.
TUL = Tolerable Upper Intake Level (not determined for biotin).

Metabolism

Absorption

Biotin is absorbed rapidly from the gastro-intestinal tract by facilitated transport (at low concentrations) and by passive diffusion (at high concentrations). Absorption is greater in the jejunum than the ileum and minimal in the colon.

Distribution
Biotin is bound to plasma proteins.

Elimination
Excess biotin is excreted largely unchanged in the urine. It also appears in breast milk.

Deficiency

Biotin deficiency is a risk only in those patients on prolonged parenteral nutrition (who will automatically be given multivitamin supplements). Deficiency has been induced by the ingestion of large amounts of raw egg white, which contain the biotin-binding protein, avidin, to a diet low in biotin.[1] Marginal biotin deficiency may also occur in pregnancy.[2]

Symptoms of biotin deficiency include anorexia, nausea, vomiting, dry scaly dermatitis, glossitis, loss of taste, somnolence, panic and an increase in serum cholesterol and bile pigments.

Possible uses

Biotin has been claimed to be of value in the treatment of brittle finger nails, acne, seborrhoeic dermatitis, hair fragility and alopecia, but such claims need further confirmation by controlled clinical trials.

A trial of biotin (2.5 mg four times daily) in women with brittle nails found a 25% increase in nail thickness, as assessed by electron microscopy.[3]

Biotin deficiency has been associated with sudden infant death syndrome (SIDS). In one study, the median biotin levels in the livers of infants who died from SIDS were significantly lower than those of infants who died from explicable causes.[4] However, evidence that biotin deficiency is an important contributory factor in SIDS is circumstantial and there is no unequivocal proof. There is no requirement for biotin supplements in newborn or young infants. Supplements should *not* be sold to parents for this purpose.

Precautions/contraindications
No problems have been reported.

Pregnancy and breast-feeding
No problems have been reported.

Adverse effects
None reported.

Interactions
Drugs
Anticonvulsants (carbamazepine, phenobarbitone, phenytoin and primidone): requirements for biotin may be increased.

Dose

Biotin is available in the form of tablets and capsules. However, it is available mainly in multivitamin preparations.

The dose is not established. Dietary supplements provide 100–300 µg daily.

Upper safety levels

The UK Expert Group on Vitamins and Minerals (EVM) has identified a likely safe total daily intake of biotin from supplements alone of 970 µg.

References

1   Baugh CM, Malone JW, Butterworth Jr, CE. Human biotin deficiency. A case history of biotin deficiency induced by raw egg consumption in a cirrhotic patient. *Am J Clin Nutr* 1968; 1: 173–182.
2   Mock DM, Quirk JG, Mock NI. Marginal biotin deficiency during normal pregnancy. *Am J Clin Nutr* 2002; 5: 295–299.
3   Colombo VE, Gerber F, Bronhofer M, *et al*. Treatment of brittle fingernails and onychoschizia with biotin: scanning electron microscopy. *J Am Acad Dermatol* 1990; 23: 1127–1132.
4   Heard GS, Hood RL, Johnson AR. Hepatic biotin and sudden infant death syndrome. *Med J Aust* 1983; 2: 305–306.

Boron

Description

Boron is an ultratrace mineral.

Human requirements

Boron is essential in plants and some animals, and evidence of essentiality is accumulating in humans; however requirements have not so far been defined. The Food Standards Agency Expert Vitamins and Minerals (EVM) group set a safe upper level from supplements alone of 5.9 mg daily.

Dietary intake

Most UK diets appear to provide about 2 mg daily.

Action

Boron appears to be important in calcium metabolism, and can affect the composition, structure and strength of bone. It may also influence the metabolism of calcium, copper, magnesium, phosphorus, potassium and vitamin D. In addition, boron affects the activity of certain enzymes. It also affects brain function; boron deprivation appears to depress mental alertness.

Dietary sources

Foods of plant origin, especially non-citrus fruits, leafy vegetables and nuts, are rich sources of boron, but there is little in meat, fish and poultry. Beer, wine and cider contain significant amounts.

Metabolism

Absorption

Dietary boron is rapidly absorbed. The mechanism of absorption from the gastrointestinal tract has not been elucidated.

Distribution

Boron is distributed throughout the body tissues; the highest concentrations are found in the bone, teeth, fingernails, spleen and thyroid.

Elimination

Boron is excreted mainly in the urine.

Deficiency

No precise signs and symptoms of boron deficiency have been defined.

Possible uses

Boron has been claimed to prevent osteoporosis and to both prevent and relieve the symptoms of osteoarthritis, as well as to improve memory.

Bone

In a study of 12 post-menopausal women,[1] boron supplementation (3 mg daily) reduced urinary excretions of calcium and magnesium, and elevated serum concentrations of oestradiol and ionised calcium.

A further study[2] has provided evidence that boron can both enhance and mimic some effects of oestrogen ingestion in post-menopausal women. In women receiving oestrogen therapy, an increase in boron intake increased serum oestradiol concentrations to higher levels than when boron intake was low. However, there is no evidence that boron supplements can relieve the symptoms of the menopause. The effects seen in this study did not occur in men or in women not receiving oestrogen therapy. However, another study[3] in men found that supplementation with boron (10 mg a day) significantly increased oestradiol concentrations, and there was also a trend for plasma testosterone to increase. These findings support the contention that, if oestrogen is beneficial to calcium metabolism, then boron might also be beneficial.

However, another study[4] in post-menopausal women showed that 3 mg boron daily had no effect on bone mineral absorption and excretion, plasma sex steroid levels and urinary excretion of pyridinium crosslink markers of bone turnover. Moreover, in this study a low-boron diet appeared to induce hyperabsorption of calcium because positive calcium balances were found in combination with elevated urinary calcium excretion. The authors concluded that this phenomenon may have inhibited or obscured any effect of boron supplementation.

Arthritis

Boron has been claimed to relieve the symptoms of arthritis, but evidence is very weak. Epidemiological studies suggest that incidence of arthritis is higher in areas of the world where boron intake is low, and subjects with arthritis have been found to have lower bone boron concentrations.[5] One double-blind controlled (but not randomised) trial in 20 patients with osteoarthritis found that boron (6 mg daily) improved symptoms in five out of 10 subjects in the treated group, and one out of 10 subjects in the placebo group. However, statistical analysis was not performed because of the small number of subjects.[6]

Brain function

Three placebo-controlled, double-blind randomised trials in 28 healthy adults showed that low dietary boron (0.25 mg/2000 kcals) was associated with poorer performance of a variety of cognitive and psychomotor tasks and

also depression of mental alertness than higher intake (3.25 mg/2000 kcals).[7]

> **Conclusion**
> There is preliminary evidence that boron has beneficial effects on calcium metabolism in post-menopausal women by preventing calcium loss and bone demineralisation, but no evidence that it can prevent or be of benefit in treating osteoarthritis. There is some evidence that diets low in boron impair cognitive function.

Precautions/contraindications

No problems have been reported.

Pregnancy and breast-feeding

No problems have been reported, but there have not been sufficient studies to guarantee the safety of boron in pregnancy and breast-feeding. However, supplements are probably best avoided because of possible changes in oestrogen metabolism.

Adverse effects

Boron is relatively non-toxic when administered orally at doses contained in food supplements. High oral doses (> 100 mg daily) are associated with disturbances in appetite and digestion, nausea, vomiting, diarrhoea, dermatitis and lethargy.

Toxicity has occurred, especially in children, from the application of boron-containing dusting powders and lotions (in the form of borax or boric acid) to areas of broken skin and mucous membranes. Such preparations are no longer recommended.

Interactions

Nutrients

Riboflavin: large doses of boron may increase excretion of riboflavin.

Magnesium: boron supplementation may reduce urinary magnesium excretion and increase serum magnesium concentrations.

Dose

Boron is available in the form of tablets and capsules.

The dose is not established. Dietary supplements provide, on average, 3 mg per daily dose.

Upper safety levels

The UK Expert Group on Vitamins and Minerals (EVM) has identified a safe total intake of boron for adults from supplements alone of 5.9 mg daily.

The US Tolerable Upper Intake Level (UL) for boron, the highest total amount from diet and supplements unlikely to pose no risk for most people, is 20 mg daily for adults; 17 mg daily for youngsters aged 14–18; 11 mg daily for youngsters aged 9–13; 6 mg daily for children aged 4–8; and 3 mg daily for children aged 1–3.

References

1 Nielsen FH, Hunt CD, Mullen LM, Hunt JR. Effect of dietary boron on mineral, estrogen and testosterone metabolism in postmenopausal women. *FASEB J* 1987; 1: 394–397.

2 Nielsen FH, Mullen LM, Gallagher SK. Effect of boron depletion and repletion on blood indicators of calcium status in humans fed a magnesium-low diet. *J Trace Elem Exp Med* 1990; 3: 45–54.

3 Naghii MR, Samman S. The effect of boron supplementation on its urinary excretion and selected cardiovascular risk factors in healthy male subjects. *Biol Trace Elem Res* 1997; 56: 273–286.

4 Beattie JH, Peace HS. The influence of a low-boron diet and boron supplementation on bone, major mineral and sex steroid metabolism in postmenopausal women. *Br J Nutr* 1993; 69: 871–884.

5 Newnham RE. Essentiality of boron for healthy bones and joints. *Environ Health Perspect* 1994; 102 (Suppl. 7): 83–85.

6 Travers RL, Rennie GC, Newnham RE. Boron and arthritis: the results of a double-blind, pilot study. *J Nutr Med* 1990; 1: 127–132.

7 Penland JG. Dietary boron, brain function, and cognitive performance. *Environ Health Perspect* 1994; 102 (Suppl. 7): 65–72.

Branched-chain amino acids

Description

Branched-chain amino acids (BCAAs) are a group of essential amino acids. They are all found in the muscle, accounting for one-third of all amino acids in muscle protein.

Constituents

L-leucine, L-isoleucine, L-valine.

Action

As with all amino acids, the primary function of BCAAs is as precursors for the synthesis of proteins. In addition, they may be broken down if necessary to serve as an energy source. They may be used directly by skeletal muscle, as opposed to other amino acids which require prior gluconeogenesis in the liver to produce a useful energy source. Muscle tissue appears to demonstrate an increased need for these amino acids during times of intense physical exercise, and there is some evidence that serum BCAA levels fall during exercise.

In addition, because BCAAs are not readily degraded by the liver, they circulate in the blood and compete with the amino acid tryptophan for uptake into the brain. Tryptophan is a precursor of serotonin (5-hydroxytryptamine), which may produce symptoms of fatigue. It appears that exercise increases the ratio of free tryptophan:BCAA, thus raising serotonin levels in the brain. Some researchers think that supplementation with BCAAs will reduce this ratio and raise serum levels of BCAAs, so improving mental and physical performance.

Possible uses

Exercise performance

Researchers have been interested in the potential role of BCAAs in exercise and whether they can improve performance.

A placebo-controlled (not blinded) study involving 193 experienced runners given 16 g BCAAs or placebo showed that running performance was improved in the slow runners but not the fast runners with BCAAs. A second part of the study showed that 7.5 g BCAAs improved mental performance during exercise compared with placebo, but the study has been criticised for lack of dietary control and poor choice of performance measures.[1]

Another placebo-controlled, but in this case double-blind, study in 16 subjects, participating in a 21-day trek at a mean altitude of 3255 m found that supplementation with BCAAs (11.52 g) improved indices of muscle loss and concluded that BCAAs could prevent muscle loss during chronic hypoxia of high altitude.[2]

In a double-blind, placebo-controlled study, 10 endurance-trained male athletes were studied during cycle exercise while ingesting in random order drinks containing sucrose, sucrose plus tryptophan, sucrose plus BCAAs (6 g) or sucrose plus BCAAs (18 g). There were no differences between the treatment groups in time to exhaustion, suggesting that BCAAs did not improve exercise performance. However, BCAAs reduced brain tryptophan uptake and significantly increased plasma ammonia levels compared to the control group.[3]

In a double-blind, placebo-controlled, randomised, crossover study, nine well-trained male cyclists performed three laboratory trials consisting of 100 km cycling after ingesting either glucose, glucose plus BCAA, or placebo. Neither the glucose nor the BCAAs enhanced performance in these cyclists.[4]

In a further study of seven well-trained male cyclists, perceived exhaustion was 7% lower and ratings of mental fatigue were 15% lower than when they were given placebo, but there was no difference in physical performance. However, the ratio of tryptophan:BCAA, which increased during exercise, remained unchanged or decreased when BCAAs were ingested.[5]

In a double-blind, placebo-controlled trial, six women and seven women participated in a cycle trial in the heat. Cycle time to exhaustion increased with BCAAs, indicating that BCAA supplementation prolongs moderate exercise performance in the heat.[6]

In a further double-blind, placebo-controlled trial, eight subjects performed three exercise trials and were given either carbohydrate drinks, carbohydrate plus BCAAs (7 g) or placebo 1 hour before and then during exercise. Subjects ran longer with both carbohydrate and carbohydrate plus BCAAs, but there were no differences between the carbohydrate and carbohydrate and BCAA groups, indicating that BCAAs are of no added benefit in exercise.[7]

Other studies have suggested that BCAAs could prevent or decrease the net rate of protein degradation seen in heavy exercise,[8,9] while others have not.[10] One study indicated that BCAAs might have a sparing effect on muscle glycogen degradation during exercise.[11] There is also some evidence that BCAAs can alter mood and cognitive performance during exercise.[12]

Miscellaneous

BCAAs can activate glutamate dehydrogenase, an enzyme deficient in amyotrophic lateral sclerosis (ALS). In one double-blind, randomised, placebo-controlled trial of BCAA, supplements helped maintenance of muscle strength and continued ability to walk in such patients.[13] However, a larger study was ended early when BCAAs not only failed to cause benefit, but also led to excess mortality.[14] BCAAs have also been investigated for potential value in anorexia and cachexia. A review concluded that they could exert significant anti-anorectic and anti-

cachectic effects and that their supplementation may represent a viable intervention for patients suffering from chronic disease such as cancer, chronic renal failure and liver cirrhosis and for patients at risk of muscle wasting due to age, immobility or bed rest.[15]

> ### Conclusion
> Evidence from well-controlled trials shows no benefit of BCAAs in exercise performance. Benefit has been shown mainly in poorly controlled trials.

Precautions/contraindications

No problems have been reported, but BCAAs should probably not be used in hepatic and renal impairment without medical supervision. However, BCAAs are used occasionally in patients with these conditions but in a medical setting.

Pregnancy and breast-feeding

No problems have been reported, but there have not been sufficient studies to guarantee the safety of BCAAs in pregnancy and breast-feeding.

Adverse effects

None reported, but there are no long-term studies assessing the safety of BCAAs. Large doses of BCAAs (> 20 g) may increase plasma ammonia levels and may impair water absorption, causing gastrointestinal discomfort.

Interactions

None reported. BCAAs compete with aromatic amino acids (e.g. phenylalanine, tyrosine, tryptophan) for transport into the brain.

Dose

BCAAs are available in tablet and powder form.

The dose is not established. Dietary supplements provide 7–20 g per dose.

References

1 Blomstrand E, Hassmen P, Ekblom B, *et al.* Administration of branched-chain amino acids during sustained exercise – effects on performance and plasma concentrations of some amino acids. *Eur J Appl Physiol Occup Physiol* 1991; 63: 83–88.

2 Schena F, Guerrini F, Tregnaghi P, Kayser B. Branched-chain amino acid supplementation during trekking at high altitude. The effects on loss of body mass, body composition and muscle power. *Eur J Appl Physiol Occup Physiol* 1992; 65: 394–398.

3 Van Hall G, Raaymakers J, Saris W, *et al.* Ingestion of branched chain amino acids and tryptophan during sustained exercise in man: failure to affect performance. *J Physiol* 1995; 486: 789–794.

4 Madsen K, MacLean DA, Kiens B, *et al.* Effects of glucose, glucose plus branched chain amino acids or placebo on bike performance over 100 km. *J Appl Physiol* 1996; 81: 2644–2650.

5 Blomstrand E, Hassmen P, Ek S, *et al.* Influence of ingesting a solution of branched chain amino acids on perceived exertion during exercise. *Acta Physiol Scand* 1997; 159: 41–49.

6 Mittleman KD, Ricci MR, Bailey SP. Branched-chain amino acids prolong exercise during heat stress in men and women. *Med Sci Sports Exerc* 1998; 30: 83–91.

7 Davis JM, Welsh RS, De Volve KL, Alderson NA. Effects of branched-chain amino acids and carbohydrate on fatigue during intermittent, high intensity running. *Int J Sports Med* 1999; 20: 309–314.

8 Blomstrand E, Newsholme EA. Effect of branched-chain amino acid supplementation on the exercise induced change in aromatic amino acid concentration in human muscle. *Acta Physiol Scand* 1992; 146: 293–298.

9 MacLean DA, Graham TE, Saltin B. Branched-chain amino acids augment ammonia metabolism while attenuating protein breakdown during exercise. *Am J Physiol* 1994; 267: E1010–E1022.

10 Blomstrand E, Andersson S, Hassmen P, *et al.* Effect of branched-chain amino acid and carbohydrate supplementation on the exercise-induced change in plasma and muscle concentration of amino acids in human subjects. *Acta Physiol Scand* 1995; 153: 87–96.

11 Blomstrand E, Ek S, Newsholme EA. Influence of ingesting a solution of branched-chain amino acids on plasma and muscle concentrations of amino acids during prolonged submaximal exercise. *Nutrition* 1996; 12: 485–490.

12 Hassmen P, Blomstrand E, Ekblom B, Newsholme EA. Branched chain amino acid supplementation during 30-km competitive run: mood and cognitive performance. *Nutrition* 1994; 10: 405–410.

13 Plaitakis A, Smith J, Mandeli J, Yahr MD. Pilot trial of branched-chain amino acids in amyotrophic lateral sclerosis. *Lancet* 1988; 1: 1015–1018.

14 The Italian ALS Study Group. Branched-chain amino acids and amyotrophic lateral sclerosis: a treatment failure? *Neurology* 1993; 43: 2466–2470.

15 Laviano A, Muscaritoli M, Cascino A, *et al.* Branched-chain amino acids: the best compromise to achieve anabolism? *Curr Opin Clin Nutr Metab Care* 2005; 8: 408–414.

Brewer's yeast

Description

Brewer's yeast is *Saccharomyces cerevisiae*.

Constituents

The average nutrient composition of dried brewer's yeast is shown in Table 1.

Possible uses

Brewer's yeast is a useful source of B vitamins and several minerals (see Table 1).

Brewer's yeast has been used to treat diarrhoea caused by *Clostridium difficile*.[1] A review concluded that it appears successful in many cases, but it is unclear whether it acts as a probiotic or as a source of B vitamins.[2] Because brewer's yeast contains chromium it has been claimed to help in the control of blood glucose levels. It is also claimed to prevent hypercholesterolaemia. However, there is insufficient evidence for these claims.

> **Conclusion**
> Brewer's yeast has a suggested value in controlling blood glucose levels, preventing hypercholesterolaemia and controlling diarrhoea caused by *Clostridium difficile*. Little evidence is available to support its efficacy in all but the last of these conditions.

Precautions/contraindications

Brewer's yeast should be avoided by patients taking monoamine oxidase inhibitors (see Interactions). It is also best avoided by patients with gout; this is because of high concentrations

Table 1 Average nutrient composition of dried brewer's yeast

Nutrient	Per teaspoon 8 g	% RNI[1] (approx.)
Vitamin A	Trace	–
Thiamine (mg)	1.2	133
Riboflavin (mg)	0.4	33
Niacin (mg)	2.0	14
Vitamin B$_6$ (mg)	0.2	16
Folic acid (µg)	320	160
Pantothenic acid (mg)	0.9	–
Biotin (µg)	16	–
Vitamin C	Trace	–
Calcium (mg)	6	0.9
Magnesium (mg)	18	6
Potassium (mg)	160	4.5
Phosphorus (mg)	103	19
Iron (mg)	1.6	13
Zinc (mg)	0.6	7
Copper (mg)	0.4	33
Chromium (µg)		
Selenium (µg)		

[1] Reference Nutrient Intake for men aged 19–50 years.

Note: Brewer's yeast tablets contain approximately 300 mg brewer's yeast per tablet; extra B vitamins are often added.

of nucleic acids, which may lead to purine formation.

Pregnancy and breast-feeding

No problems have been reported.

Adverse effects

None reported except flatulence.

Interactions

Drugs

Monoamine oxidase inhibitors: may provoke hypertensive crisis.

Dose

Brewer's yeast is available in the form of tablets and powder.

The dose is not established.

References

1   Schellenberg D, Bonington A, Champion CM, *et al*. Treatment of *Clostridium difficile* diarrhoea with brewer's yeast. *Lancet* 1994; 343: 171.
2   Sargent G, Wickens H. Brewers' yeast in C *difficile infection*: probiotic or B group vitamins? *Pharm J* 2004; 273: 230–231.

Bromelain

Description

Bromelain is the name for the protease enzymes extracted from the stem and fruit of fresh pineapple. The commercial supplement is usually obtained only from the stem of the pineapple, which contains a higher concentration of the enzymes than the fruit.

Constituents

Bromelains are sulphydryl proteolytic enzymes, including several proteases. In addition, bromelain also contains small amounts of non-proteolytic enzymes (including acid phosphatase, peroxidase and cellulase), polypeptide protease inhibitors and organically bound calcium.

Action

Bromelain is an anti-inflammatory agent and is thought to act through direct or indirect effects on inflammatory mediators. It inhibits the enzyme thromboxane synthetase, which converts prostaglandin H_2 into pro-inflammatory prostaglandins and thromboxanes. Bromelain also stimulates the breakdown of fibrin, which stimulates pro-inflammatory prostaglandins responsible for fluid retention and clot formation. It also appears to promote the conversion of plasminogen to plasmin, causing an increase in fibrinolysis.

Possible uses

Various claims are made for the value of bromelain supplementation, but much of the research underpinning these claims was carried out in the 1960s and 1970s, and there are very few well-controlled human studies.

Bromelain has been associated with improvement in symptoms of sinusitis, acceleration of wound healing, potentiation of antibiotic action, healing of gastric ulcers, treatment of inflammation and soft tissue injuries, reduction in severity of angina, reduction in sputum production in patients with chronic bronchitis and pneumonia and decrease in symptoms of thrombophlebitis.[1]

Sinusitis

Two double-blind, placebo-controlled studies showed that bromelain 160 mg (400 000 units) could reduce some symptoms of sinusitis.[2,3] However, headache was not improved in either study.

Musculoskeletal injuries

In a double-blind, placebo controlled trial,[4] 146 boxers with bruises to the face and haematomas to the eyes, lips, ears, arms and chest received either 160 mg bromelain daily or placebo for 14 days. At day 4, 78% of the bromelain-treated group were completely cured of their bruises compared with 15% of the placebo group. However, this result was not tested for statistical significance. A randomised, double-blind trial in 40 subjects with muscle soreness as a result of exercise compared the outcomes with ingestion of either ibuprofen or bromelain. There was no difference between treatments.[5]

Arthritis

There is preliminary clinical evidence that the anti-inflammatory and analgesic properties of bromelain help to reduce symptoms of osteo- and rheumatoid arthritis. In a controlled trial involving 77 subjects suffering from mild knee pain, ingestion of bromelain (200 and 400 mg) resulted in improvements in total symptoms, stiffness and physical function in a dose-dependent manner. The authors concluded that double-blind, placebo-controlled studies are now warranted to confirm these results.[6]

Surgical procedures
Bromelain has been reported in at least two studies[7,8] to reduce the degree and duration of swelling and oral pain with oral surgery. However, one study was not controlled and the other had no statistical analysis.

Antibacterial
Bromelain could be useful as an anti-diarrhoeal agent. In an *in vitro* study,[9] bromelain was shown to prevent intestinal fluid secretion mediated by *Escherichia coli* and *Vibrio cholerae*, and in other studies[10,11] to protect piglets from diarrhoea. However, there are no human studies to date.

Cardiovascular disease
Bromelain has been reported to reduce the severity of angina,[12] and several *in vitro* studies[13,14] have demonstrated that bromelain reduces platelet aggregation.

Ulcerative colitis
A letter from two US consultants[15] stated that two patients with ulcerative colitis achieved complete clinical and endoscopic remission after initiation of therapy with bromelain.

Cystitis
One double-blind study in humans revealed that bromelain was effective in treating non-infectious cystitis.[16]

Conclusion

Many claims have been made for bromelain, based largely on studies conducted in the 1960s and 1970s. Many of the published trials are uncontrolled human studies or animal or *in vitro* studies, and well-controlled clinical trials are required to establish the role of bromelain as a potential supplement.

Precautions/contraindications
No problems have been reported, but based on the potential pharmacological activity of bromelain, i.e. that it may inhibit platelet aggregation, bromelain should be used with caution in patients with a history of bleeding or haemostatic disorders.

Pregnancy and breast-feeding
No problems have been reported, but there have been insufficient studies to guarantee the safety of bromelain in pregnancy and breast-feeding.

Adverse effects
None reported, but there are no long-term studies assessing the safety of bromelain.

Interactions
Drugs
None reported, but theoretically, bleeding tendency may be increased with anticoagulants, aspirin and antiplatelet drugs.

Dose
Bromelain is available in the form of tablets, capsules and powders. A variety of designations have been used to indicate the activity of bromelain. These include rorer units (ru), gelatine-dissolving units (gdu) and milk clotting units (mcu). One gram of bromelain standardised to 2000 mcu would be approximately equal to 1 gram with 1200 gdu of activity or 8 g with 100 000 ru activity.[1]

The dose is not established. Dietary supplements provide 125–500 mg in a dose.

References
1   Anonymous. Bromelain. *Altern Med Rev* 1998; 3: 302–308.
2   Ryan RE. A double-blind clinical evaluation of bromelains in the treatment of acute sinusitis. *Headache* 1967; 7: 13–17.
3   Seltzer AP. Adjunctive use of bromelains in sinusitis: a controlled study. *Eye Ear Nose Throat Mon* 1967; 46: 1281–1288.

4 Blonstein JL. Control of swelling in boxing injuries. *Practitioner* 1960; 185: 78.

5 Stone MB, Merrick MA, Ingersoll CD, Edwards JE. Preliminary comparison of bromelain and ibuprofen for delayed onset muscle soreness management. *Clin J Sports Med* 2002; 12: 373–378.

6 Walker AF, Bundy R, Hicks SM, Middleton RW. Bromelain reduces mild acute knee pain and improves well-being in a dose-dependent fashion in an open study of otherwise healthy adults. *Phytomedicine* 2002; 9: 681–686.

7 Tassman GC, Zafran JN, Zayon GM. Evaluation of a plant proteolytic enzyme for the control of inflammation and pain. *J Dent Med* 1964; 19: 73–77.

8 Tassman GC, Zafran JN, Zayon GM. A double blind crossover study of a plant proteolytic enzyme in oral surgery. *J Dent Med* 1965; 20: 51–54.

9 Mynott TL, Guandalini S, Raimondi F, *et al*. Bromelain prevents secretion caused by *Vibrio cholerae* and *Escherichia coli* enterotoxins in rabbit ileum in vitro. *Gastroenterology* 1997; 113: 175–184.

10 Mynott TL, Luke RKJ, Chandler DS. Oral administration of protease inhibits enterotoxigenic *Escherichia coli* (ETEC) activity in piglet small intestine. *Gut* 1996; 38: 28–32.

11 Chandler DS, Mynott TL. Bromelain protects piglets from diarrhoea caused by oral challenge with K88-positive enterotoxigenic *Escherichia coli*. *Gut* 1998; 43: 196–202.

12 Nieper HA. Effect of bromelain on coronary heart disease and angina pectoris. *Acta Med Empirica* 1978; 5: 274–278.

13 Heinicke RM, Van der Wal M, Yokoyama MM. Effect of bromelain (Ananase) on human platelet aggregation. *Experientia* 1972; 28: 844–845.

14 Metzig C, Grabowska E, Eckert K, *et al*. Bromelain proteases reduce human platelet aggregation in vitro, adhesion to bovine endothelial cells, and thrombus formation in rat vessels in vivo. *In Vivo* 1999; 13: 7–12.

15 Kane S, Goldberg MJ. Use of bromelain for mild ulcerative colitis (letter). *Ann Intern Med* 2000; 132: 680.

16 Lotti T, Mirone V, Imbimbo C, *et al*. Controlled clinical studies of nimesulide in the treatment of urogenital inflammation. *Drugs* 1993; 46 (Suppl. 1): 144–146.

Calcium

Description

Calcium is an essential mineral.

Human requirements

Dietary Reference Values for calcium are shown in Table 1.

Dietary intake

In the UK, the average diet provides: for men, 1007 mg daily; women, 774 mg daily.

Action

Calcium has a structural role in bones and teeth. Some 99% of calcium is found in the skeleton. Bone density increases during the first three decades of life, reaching its peak about the age of 30. After this age, bone density declines, and the decline increases more rapidly in women after the menopause. However, bone density also declines in older men. Calcium is also essential for cellular structure, blood clotting, muscle contraction, nerve transmission, enzyme activation and hormone function.

Dietary sources

Dietary sources of calcium are shown in Table 2.

Metabolism

Absorption

Calcium is absorbed in the duodenum, jejunum and ileum by an active saturable process that involves vitamin D. At high intakes, some calcium is absorbed by passive diffusion (independent of vitamin D). It can also be absorbed from the colon.

Distribution

More than 99% of the body's calcium is stored in the bones and teeth. The physiologically active form of calcium is the ionised form (in the blood). Blood calcium levels are controlled homeostatically by parathyroid hormone, calcitonin and vitamin D and a range of other hormones.

Elimination

Excretion of calcium occurs in the urine, although a large amount is reabsorbed in the kidney tubules, the amount excreted varying with the quantity of calcium absorbed and the degree of bone loss. Elimination of unabsorbed and endogenously secreted calcium occurs in the faeces. Calcium is also lost in the sweat and is excreted in breast milk.

Bioavailability

Bioavailability is dependent to some extent on vitamin D status. Absorption is reduced by phytates (present in bran and high-fibre cereals), but high-fibre diets at currently recommended levels of intake do not significantly affect calcium absorption in the long term. Absorption is reduced by oxalic acid (present in cauliflower, spinach and rhubarb). High sodium intake may reduce calcium retention.

The efficiency of absorption is increased during periods of high physiological requirement (e.g. in childhood, adolescence,

Table 1   Dietary Reference Values for calcium (mg/day)

Age	UK			EVM	USA		WHO RNI
						EU RDA = 800 mg	
	LNRI	EAR	RNI		AI	TUL	RNI
0–6 months	240	400	525		210	–	300[2]
7–12 months	240	400	525		270	–	400
1–3 years	200	275	350		500	2500	500
4–6 years	275	350	450		–	–	600
4–8 years	–	–	–		800	2500	–
7–10 years	325	425	550		800	–	700[a]
9–18 years	–	–	–		1300	2500	–
Males							
11–14 years	450	750	1000		–	–	1300[b]
15–18 years	450	750	1000		–	–	1300
19–24 years	400	525	700	1500	–	2500	1000
25–50 years	400	525	700	1500	1000	2500	1000
50+ years	400	525	700	1500	1200	2500	1000[3]
Females							
11–14 years	480	625	800		–	–	1300[b]
15–18 years	480	625	800		–	–	1300
19–50 years	400	525	700	1500	1000	2500	1000
50+ years	400	525	700	1500	1200	2500	1300
Pregnancy	*	*	*		1000[1]	2500	1200[4]
Lactation		+550			1000[1]	2500	1000

* No increment.
[a] 7–9 years.   [b] 10–14 years.
[1] ≤18 years, 1300 mg.   [2] 400 mg for cows' milk feed.   [3] 1300 mg for men > 65 years.   [4] third trimester.
AI = Adequate Intake.
EVM = Likely safe daily intake from supplements alone.
TUL = Tolerable Upper Intake Level from diet and supplements.
Note: The National Osteoporosis Society has produced separate guidelines for recommended daily calcium intake as follows: 7–12 years, 800 mg; 13–19 years, 1000 mg; men 20–45 years, 1000 mg; men >45 years, 1500 mg; women 20–45 years, 1000 mg; women >45 years, 1500 mg; women > 45 years (using HRT), 1000 mg; pregnant and breast-feeding women, 1200 mg; pregnant and breast-feeding teenagers, 1500 mg.

pregnancy and breast-feeding) and impaired in the elderly.

Deficiency

Simple calcium deficiency is not a recognised clinical disorder. However, low dietary intake during adolescence and young adulthood may reduce peak bone mass and bone mineral content and increase the risk of osteoporosis in later life.

However, requirements may be increased and/or and supplements may be necessary in:

- children, adolescents, pre- and post-menopausal women
- pregnant and breast-feeding women
- vegans and others who avoid milk and milk products; and
- those with lactose intolerance (because of avoidance of milk and milk products).

Table 2   Dietary sources of calcium

Food portion	Calcium content (mg)
Cereal products	
Bread, brown, 2 slices	70
white, 2 slices	70
wholemeal, 2 slices	35
1 chapati	20
Milk and dairy products	
½ pint (280 ml) milk, whole,	**350**
semi-skimmed or skimmed	
½ pint (280 ml) soya milk	50
1 pot yoghurt, plain (150 g)	300
fruit (150 g)	250
Cheese, Brie (50 g)	270
Camembert (50 g)	175
Cheddar (50 g)	**360**
Cheddar, reduced fat (50 g)	**420**
Cottage cheese (100 g)	73
Cream cheese (30 g)	35
Edam (50 g)	**350**
Feta (50 g)	*180*
Fromage frais (100 g)	85
White cheese (50 g)	*280*
1 egg, size 2 (60 g)	35
Fish	
Pilchards, canned (105 g)	*105*
Prawns (80 g)	*120*
Salmon, canned (115 g)	100
Sardines, canned (70 g)	**350**
Shrimps (80 g)	100
Whitebait (100 g)	**860**
Vegetables	
Broccoli (100 g)	40
Spinach (100 g)	*150*
Spring greens (100 g)	75
1 small can baked beans (200 g)	106
Dahl, chickpea (150 g)	100
Lentils, kidney beans or chick	40–70
peas (105 g)	40–70
Soya beans, cooked (100 g)	85
Tofu (60 g)	*300*
Fruit	
1 large orange	70
Nuts	
20 almonds	50
1 tablespoon sesame seeds (20 g)	*140*
Tahini paste on 1 slice bread (10 g)	70
Milk chocolate (100 g)	*240*

Excellent sources (**bold**); good source (*italics*).

Possible uses

The role of calcium has been investigated in a number of conditions, including osteoporosis, hypertension, colon cancer, obesity, menstrual symptoms and pre-eclampsia.

Osteoporosis

Calcium supplements may have a role in the prevention of osteoporosis. Most of the available evidence has been obtained from studies looking at three different population groups (i.e. children and adolescents, pre-menopausal women and post-menopausal women).

Children and adolescents

Adequate intake of calcium is important throughout life, but seems to be particularly important during skeletal growth and development of peak bone mass.[1, 2] There are also data to show that high intake of milk and dairy produce increases bone mineralisation and bone growth in adolescence – effects that may not be due entirely to the high calcium content of milk.[3,4] In addition to other minerals, such as magnesium, phosphorus and zinc (which are themselves important for bone health), milk also provides energy and protein, both of which may stimulate bone growth through their influence on insulin growth factor 1 (IGF-1).

Several controlled intervention studies[5–8] using calcium supplements in children and adolescents have shown that calcium intakes above the current British Reference Nutrient Intake are effective in increasing bone mineral accretion, particularly in those youngsters with habitually low calcium intakes. However, another study has demonstrated that calcium supplementation (500 mg daily) has only a modest effect on bone mineral density (BMD) in girls aged 12–14, and this effect was independent of habitual calcium intake.[9]

Whether any benefits are sustained if calcium intake is reduced is not clear. However, a follow-up study of a trial in which 1000 mg calcium was given to adolescent girls for 1 year has shown that increased bone mineral accretion may be sustained for a period of 3.5 years after supplementation has been discontinued.[10] A further RCT has demonstrated that calcium supplementation given from childhood to young adulthood significantly improved bone accretion during the pubertal growth spurt with a diminishing effect thereafter.[11]

A Cochrane review,[12] including 19 trials, has assessed the effectiveness of calcium supplementation for improving BMD in children. There was no effect of calcium supplementation on femoral neck or lumbar spine BMD. There was a small effect on total body bone mineral content and upper limb BMD, but only the effect in the upper limb persisted after supplementation stopped. This effect is unlikely to result in a clinically significant reduction in fracture risk and the review concluded that the results do not support the use of calcium supplementation in healthy children as a public health intervention.

Pre-menopausal women

In pre-menopausal women, results from studies examining the relationship between dietary calcium intake and bone mass and also those from calcium supplementation studies are contradictory. Some show a positive effect of calcium[13,14] on BMD, but others do not.[15–17]

Post-menopausal women

After the menopause, bone loss occurs at an increasing rate, and while calcium may help to slow the loss, it does not prevent it. Moreover, the influence of calcium at this stage of life seems to vary with the length of time that has passed since the menopause. Most studies fail to show a relationship between calcium intake, from either food or supplements, and bone loss during the 5 years immediately following the menopause. The rapid loss of oestrogen causes a very high rate of bone resorption, which increases serum calcium concentrations and inhibits intestinal absorption of calcium.[18]

In one study,[19] women who had undergone the menopause within the last 5 years had rapid bone loss that was not affected by a calcium supplement of 500 mg a day. However, one RCT in women over 45 showed that calcium and vitamin D supplementation during a 30-month period showed a positive effect on BMD in both peri- and post-menopausal subjects.[20]

In women who were more than 6 years after the menopause (and had a calcium intake of <400 mg a day), the same supplement significantly reduced bone loss. Another study in women 10 years after the menopause[21] showed that a calcium supplement of 1000 mg a day had a benefit on both total and site-specific bone mass even though their habitual calcium intake was satisfactory, and that this effect of supplementation could last for 4 years and result in fewer fractures.[22]

Using fracture rather than bone loss as the end point, some recent studies have demonstrated a benefit of calcium given with vitamin D in older people. A French study (Decalyos I),[23] showed considerable reduction in fracture rates in a large group of elderly people (mean age 84 ± 6) who were living in a nursing home and given 1200 mg calcium with 800 units of vitamin D. Protection became apparent after 6–12 months, and after 3 years the probability of hip fractures was reduced by 29%.

In a more recent study,[24] also in elderly people, similar results were obtained from calcium supplementation alone, but the subjects were vitamin D replete. Researchers in the USA[25] looked at the effects of 500 mg of calcium plus 700 units of vitamin D for 3 years in 176 men and 213 women aged 65 or older who were living at home. The supplemented group had a reduced incidence of non-vertebral fracture and lower bone loss in the femoral neck and the total body than the non-supplemented group.

A further study conducted by the French group (Decalyos II) has confirmed the results of Decalyos I and found that calcium (1200 mg) plus vitamin D (800 units) reduces both hip bone loss and the risk of hip fracture in elderly institutionalised women.[26] Analysis of the Decalyos data showed that this supplementation strategy is cost-saving.[27]

A recent meta-analysis has confirmed that calcium supplementation slows bone loss in post-menopausal women with a trend towards a reduction in vertebral fractures.[28]

A trial involving 36 282 post-menopausal women aged 50–79 randomised participants to receive 1000 mg of elemental calcium with 400 units of vitamin D_3 daily or placebo. There was a small but significant 1% improvement in hip bone density for those taking calcium combined with vitamin D compared with those taking placebo. There was also a 12% reduction in hip fracture, but this was non-significant. However, women who consistently took the full supplement dose experienced a 29% decrease in hip fracture. Women older than 60 had a significant 21% reduction in hip fracture. The supplements had no significant effect on spine or total fractures and were associated with an increased risk of kidney stones.[29]

A 5-year, double-blind, placebo-controlled study involving 1460 women over the age of 70 found that 1200 mg calcium daily is effective in preventing fracture in those who are compliant, but as a public health intervention in the ambulatory elderly population is ineffective because of poor long-term compliance.[30]

Corticosteroid-induced osteoporosis

Steroids cause bone loss and it has been suggested that patients on steroids should receive preventive treatment (e.g. calcium, vitamin D, bisphosphonates, oestrogens). A Cochrane meta-analysis of five trials involving 274 patients found a clinically and statistically significant prevention of bone loss at the lumbar spine and forearm with vitamin D and calcium in corticosteroid treated patients. The authors recommended that because of low toxicity and low cost, all patients being started on corticosteroids should receive prophylactic therapy with calcium and vitamin D.[31]

Hypertension

Epidemiological studies[32,33] support an inverse relationship between the amount of calcium in the diet and blood pressure. However, based on multivariate analyses, the absolute contribution of calcium is very small. Some clinical intervention studies have reported reduction in blood pressure in normotensive and hypertensive subjects[34–36] or no effect.[37] A meta-analysis of 33 RCTs concluded that calcium (800–2000 mg daily) may lead to a small reduction in systolic blood pressure.[38] Another meta-analysis of 22 randomised clinical trials showed that calcium supplements (500–1000 mg daily) produced a significant decrease in systolic but not diastolic blood pressure, but the authors concluded that the effect was too small to support the use of calcium supplementation in hypertension.[39] Calcium may be most effective in patients

with hypertension who are Afro-Caribbean[40] or who are responsive to manipulation of dietary sodium.[41]

A Cochrane review of 13 RCTs found that calcium supplementation was associated with a statistically significant reduction in systolic blood pressure (mean difference: –2.5 mmHg; 95% CI, –4.5 to –0.6) but not diastolic blood pressure (mean difference: –0.8 mmHg; 95% CI, 2.1 to 0.4). The review concluded that evidence in favour of causal association between calcium supplementation and blood pressure reduction is weak and that longer duration, better quality studies are needed.[42]

Cancer

Calcium supplementation may reduce the occurrence of colorectal cancer, but study results are inconsistent. High calcium intake (1200–1400 mg daily) has been linked with reduced colon cancer risk in epidemiological studies, and high dietary and supplemental calcium have been associated with reduced recurrence of adenomatous polyps,[43–45] and reduced colorectal cancer risk.[46] Other studies have shown no significant effects of calcium supplementation on colorectal cell proliferation in subjects at high risk for colorectal cancer.[47,48] There is also evidence that vitamin D acts with calcium in reducing risk of colorectal adenomal recurrence.[49] A pooled analysis of 10 cohort studies found that higher consumption of calcium is associated with lower risk of colorectal cancer.[50]

Evidence from the Calcium Polyp Prevention Study, which involved patients with recent colorectal adenoma, showed that calcium (1200 mg daily) may have a more pronounced antineoplastic effect on advanced colorectal lesions than on other types of polyps.[51] In the Polyp Prevention Trial, calcium and vitamin D intake was inversely associated with recurrence of adenomatous polyps in the large bowel.[52] A recent Cochrane review concluded that evidence from two RCTs suggests that calcium supplementation might contribute to a moderate degree to the prevention of colorectal adenomatous polyps, but that this does not constitute sufficient evidence to recommend the general use of calcium supplements to prevent colorectal cancer.[53] A systematic review and meta-analysis of three trials also suggested that calcium supplementation prevents recurrent colorectal adenomas.[54]

Calcium has been associated with increased risk of prostate cancer. In the Physician's Health Study, men consuming >600 mg calcium a day from dairy products had a 32% higher risk of prostate cancer compared with men consuming <150 mg daily.[55] However, in a recent RCT involving 672 men, calcium 1200 mg daily was not associated with increased prostate cancer risk.[56] A meta-analysis of 12 studies found that high intake of dairy products and calcium may be associated with an increased risk of prostate cancer, although the effect appeared to be small.[57]

Menstrual symptoms

Calcium supplementation (1200 mg daily for three menstrual cycles) was effective in reducing premenstrual but not menstrual pain in a prospective, randomised, double-blind, placebo-controlled trial.[58] In another trial, when given with manganese, calcium (1336 mg daily) reduced menstrual pain and undesirable behavioural symptoms.[59] A further trial showed that calcium (1000 mg daily) reduced both premenstrual and menstrual symptom scores, and there was a significant effect of calcium on menstrual pain.[60]

Pre-eclampsia

Use of calcium supplements during pregnancy may reduce the risk of pre-eclampsia. An analysis of clinical trials that examined the effects of calcium intake on pre-eclampsia and pregnancy outcomes in 2500 women found that those who consumed 1500–2000 mg of calcium a day were 70% less likely to suffer from hypertension in pregnancy.[61] However, a large study involving 4589 healthy first-time mothers found that calcium supplementation (2000 mg daily) had no effect on the incidence of hypertension, protein excretion or complications of childbirth.[62]

A Cochrane systematic review of pregnancy-induced hypertension identified nine placebo-controlled RCTs. Calcium significantly reduced the relative risk of hypertension, especially in women at high risk of hypertension and with low dietary calcium.[63]

Obesity

Dietary calcium plays a pivotal role in the regulation of energy metabolism. High-calcium diets reduce adipose tissue accretion and weight gain during periods of overconsumption and increase fat breakdown to preserve thermogenesis during energy restriction, thereby accelerating weight loss.[64] A review analysing data from six observational studies and three controlled trials has shown that high calcium intakes are associated with lower weight gain at mid-life.[65] An RCT looking at the effect of calcium supplementation (1000 mg daily) in 100 women found no significant differences between body weight or fat mass changes between the placebo and calcium-supplemented groups. However, there was a trend to increased loss of body weight in the calcium group, which the authors suggested to be consistent with a small effect.[66]

> ### Conclusion
> There is evidence that calcium supplementation can improve bone density in adolescents. Calcium may also help to reduce the decline in bone density in post-menopausal women, particularly when given in conjunction with vitamin D. However, there is less evidence that calcium supplementation attenuates the reduction in bone density around the time of the menopause. Calcium supplementation may lower blood pressure, but the effect is too small to recommend its use in hypertension. Evidence linking calcium to colon cancer and prostate cancer is conflicting. There is preliminary evidence that calcium supplementation may help symptoms of premenstrual syndrome (PMS), particularly pain, and may also reduce the risk of pre-eclampsia. Evidence of the value of calcium supplements in obesity is limited.

Precautions/contraindications

Calcium supplements should be avoided in conditions associated with hypercalcaemia and hypercalcuria, and in renal impairment (chronic). They should be used with caution and with medical supervision in hypertension because blood pressure control may be altered.

Traditionally, a low-calcium diet was advised in patients with or at risk of kidney stones. Recent studies have suggested that the risk of kidney stones is not increased by calcium.[67–70] In two studies, however, supplemental calcium was positively associated with risk.[29,71]

A recent review on developments in stone prevention states: 'Calcium should not be restricted. There is clear evidence from clinical and experimental studies that a normal or high calcium supply is appropriate in calcium stone disease. Only in absorptive hypercalcuria calcium restriction remains beneficial in combination with thiazide and citrate therapy.'[72]

Pregnancy and breast-feeding

No problems have been reported. Calcium supplements may be required during pregnancy and breast-feeding. Some studies have shown that the use of calcium supplements in pregnancy may lower the risk of pre-eclampsia, while another has not (see above).

Adverse effects

Reported adverse effects with supplements include nausea, constipation and flatulence (usually mild). Calcium metabolism is under such tight control that accumulation in blood or tissues from excessive intakes is almost unknown; accumulation is usually due to failure of control mechanisms. Toxic effects and hypercalcaemia are unlikely with oral doses of < 2000 mg daily. However, in young children, calcium supplements should be used under medical supervision because of a risk of bowel perforation.

Interactions

Drugs

Alcohol: excessive alcohol intake may reduce calcium absorption.
Aluminium-containing antacids: may reduce calcium absorption.
Anticonvulsants: may reduce serum calcium levels.

Bisphosphonates: calcium may reduce absorption of etidronate; give 2 h apart.
Cardiac glycosides: concurrent use with parenteral calcium preparations may increase risk of cardiac arrhythmias (ECG monitoring recommended).
Corticosteroids: may reduce serum calcium levels.
Laxatives: prolonged use of laxatives may reduce calcium absorption.
Loop diuretics: increased excretion of calcium.
4-Quinolones: may reduce absorption of 4-quinolones; give 2 h apart.
Tamoxifen: calcium supplements may increase the risk of hypercalcaemia (a rare side-effect of tamoxifen therapy); calcium supplements are best avoided.
Tetracyclines: may reduce absorption of tetracyclines; give 2 h apart.
Thiazide diuretics: may reduce calcium excretion.

Nutrients

Fluoride: may reduce absorption of fluoride and vice versa; give 2 h apart.
Iron: calcium carbonate or calcium phosphate may reduce absorption of iron; give 2 h apart (absorption of iron in multiple formulations containing iron and calcium is not significantly altered).
Vitamin D: increased absorption of calcium and increased risk of hypercalcaemia; may be advantageous in some individuals.
Zinc: may reduce absorption of zinc.

Dose

Calcium is available in the form of tablets and capsules. A review of 35 US calcium supplements showed that four brands contained lower levels of calcium than claimed on the label. However, none of the products failed testing for exceeding contamination levels for lead and other heavy metals.[73] Another survey showed that calcium supplements may contain lead,[74] but levels were not high enough to cause concern.[75]

The dose for potential prevention of osteoporosis is 1000–1200 mg (as elemental

Table 3 Calcium content of commonly used calcium salts

Calcium salt	Calcium(mg/g)	Calcium(%)
Calcium amino acid chelate	180	18
Calcium carbonate	400	40
Calcium chloride	272	27.2
Calcium glubionate	65	6.5
Calcium gluconate	90	9
Calcium lactate	130	13
Calcium lactate gluconate	129	13
Calcium orotate	210	21
Calcium phosphate (dibasic)	230	23

Note: Calcium lactate and gluconate are more efficiently absorbed than calcium carbonate (particularly in patients with achlorhydria).

calcium) daily with 800 units of cholecalciferol. Patients who may require supplementation include: those aged 65 and over who are confined to their homes and care institutes; post-menopausal women below the age of 65, where lifestyle modification is unsustainable; secondary prevention of osteoporotic fractures in post-menopausal women (this is covered by the 2005 NICE guideline[76]); prevention of osteoporotic fractures in patients taking glucocorticoids.

Note: doses are given in terms of elemental calcium. Patients should be advised that calcium supplements are not identical; they provide different amounts of elemental calcium. The calcium content of various calcium salts commonly used in supplements is shown in Table 3.

Upper safety levels

The UK Expert Group on Vitamins and Minerals (EVM) has identified a likely safe total intake of calcium for adults from supplements alone of 1500 mg daily.

The US Tolerable Upper Intake Level (UL) for calcium, the highest total amount from diet and supplements unlikely to pose no risk for most people, is 2500 mg daily for adults and children from the age of 12 months.

References

1 Matkovik V. Calcium metabolism and calcium requirements during skeletal modelling and consolidation of bone mass. *Am J Clin Nutr* 1991; 54(Suppl.): 245S–259S.
2 Recker RR, Davies MK, Hinders SM, *et al*. Bone gain in young adult women. *JAMA* 1992; 268: 2403–2408.
3 Chan GM, Hoffman K, McMurry M. Effects of dairy produce on bone and body composition in pubertal girls. *J Pediatr* 1995; 126: 551–556.
4 Cadogan J, Eastell R, Jones M, Barker ME. A study of bone growth in adolescents: the effect of an 18-month, milk-based dietary intervention. *BMJ* 1997; 315: 1255–1260.
5 Johnston CC, Miller JZ, Slemenda CW, *et al*. Calcium supplementation and increases in bone mineral density in children. *N Engl J Med* 1992; 327: 82–87.
6 Lloyd T, Andon MB, Rollings N, *et al*. Calcium supplementation and bone mineral density in adolescent girls. *JAMA* 1993; 270: 841–844.
7 Lee WTK, Leung SSF, Leung DMT, *et al*. A randomised double-blind controlled calcium supplementation trial and bone and height acquisition in children. *Br J Nutr* 1995; 74: 125–139.
8 Rozen GS, Rennert G, Dodiuk-Gad RP, *et al*. Calcium supplementation provides an extended window of opportunity for bone mass accretion after menarche. *Am J Clin Nutr* 2003; 78: 993–998.
9 Molgaard C, Thomsen BL, Michaelsen KF. Effect of habitual dietary calcium intake on calcium supplementation in 12–14 year old girls. *Am J Clin Nutr* 2004; 80: 1422–1427.
10 Dodiuk-Gad RP, Rozen GS, Rennert G, *et al*. Sustained effect of short-term calcium supplementation on bone mass in adolescent girls with low calcium intake. *Am J Clin Nutr* 2005; 81: 168–174.
11 Matkovic V, Goel PK, Badenhop-Stevens NE. Calcium supplementation and bone mineral density in females from childhood to young adulthood: a randomized controlled trial. *Am J Clin Nutr* 2005; 81: 175–188.
12 Winzenberg TM, Shaw K, Fryer J, Jones G. Calcium supplementation for improving bone mineral density in children. Cochrane database, issue 2, 2006. London: Macmillan.
13 Ramsdale SJ, Bassy EJ, Pye DJ. Dietary calcium intake relates to bone mineral density in pre-menopausal women. *Br J Nutr* 1994; 71: 77–84.

14 Rico H, Revilla M, Villa LF, *et al.* Longitudinal study of the effect of calcium pidolate on bone mass in eugonadal women. *Calcif Tissue Int* 1994; 54: 47–80.

15 Valimaki MJ, Karkkainen M, Lamberg-Allardt C, *et al.* Exercise, smoking and calcium intake during adolescence and early adulthood as determinants of peak bone mass. *BMJ* 1994; 309: 230–235.

16 New SA, Bolton-Smith C, Grubb DA, Reid DM. Nutritional influences on bone mineral density: a cross sectional study in premenopausal women. *Am J Clin Nutr* 1997; 65: 1831–1839.

17 Earnshaw SA, Worley A, Hosking DJ. Current diet does not relate to bone mineral density after the menopause. The Nottingham Early Postmenopausal Intervention Cohort (EPIC) Study Group. *Br J Nutr* 1997; 78: 65–72.

18 Chiu KM. Efficacy of calcium supplements on bone mass in postmenopausal women. *J Gerontol A Biol Med Sci* 1999; 54: M275–280.

19 Dawson-Hughes B, Dallal GE, Krall EA, *et al.* A controlled trial of the effect of calcium supplementation on bone density in post-menopausal women. *N Engl J Med* 1990; 323: 878–883.

20 Di Daniele N, Carbonelli MG, Candeloro N, *et al.* Effect of supplementation of calcium and vitamin D on bone density and bone mineral content in peri- and post-menopause women; a double-blind, randomized controlled trial. *Pharmacol Res* 2004; 50: 637–641.

21 Reid IR, Ames RW, Evans MC, *et al.* Effect of calcium supplementation on bone loss in postmenopausal women. *N Engl J Med* 1993; 328; 460–464.

22 Reid IR, Ames RW, Evans MC, *et al.* Long term effects of calcium supplementation on bone loss and fractures in postmenopausal women: a randomised controlled trial. *Am J Med* 1995; 98: 331–335.

23 Chapuy MC, Arlot ME, Duboeuf F, *et al.* Vitamin D and calcium to prevent hip fractures in elderly women. *N Engl J Med* 1992; 327: 1637–1642.

24 Chevalley T, Rizzoli R, Nydegger V, *et al.* The effects of calcium supplements on femoral bone mineral density and vertebral fracture rate in vitamin D-replete elderly patients. *Osteoporosis Int* 1994; 4: 245–252.

25 Dawson-Hughes B, Harris SS, Krall EA, Dallal GE. Effect of calcium and vitamin D supplementation on bone density in men and women 65 years of age or older. *N Engl J Med* 1997; 337: 670–676.

26 Chapuy MC, Pamphile R, Paris E, *et al.* Combined calcium and vitamin D3 supplementation in elderly women: confirmation of reversal of secondary hyperparathyroidism and hip fracture risk: the Decalyos II study. *Osteoporosis Int* 2002; 13: 257–264.

27 Lilliu H, Pamphile R, Chapuy MC, *et al.* Calcium-vitamin D3 supplementation is cost-effective in hip fractures prevention. *Maturitas* 2003; 44; 299–305.

28 Shea B, Wells G, Cranney A, *et al.* Calcium supplementation on bone loss in postmenopausal women. Cochrane database, issue 1, 2004. London: Macmillan.

29 Jackson RD, LaCroix AZ, Gass M, *et al.* Calcium plus vitamin D supplementation and the risk of fractures. *N Engl J Med* 2006; 354: 669–683.

30 Prince RL, Devine A, Dhaliwal SS, Dick IM. Effects of bone supplementation on clinical fracture and bone structure. *Arch Intern Med* 2006; 166: 869–875.

31 Homik JJEH, Cranney A, Shea BJ, *et al.* Calcium and vitamin D for corticosteroid-induced osteoporosis. Cochrane database, issue 2, 1998. London: Macmillan.

32 Iso H, Terao A, Kitamura A. Calcium intake and blood pressure in seven Japanese populations. *Am J Epidemiol* 1991; 133: 776–783.

33 McCarron DA, Morris CD. The calcium deficiency hypothesis of hypertension. *Ann Intern Med* 1987; 107: 919–922.

34 Grobbee DE, Hofman A. Effect of calcium supplementation on diastolic blood pressure in young people with mild hypertension. *Lancet* 1986; 2: 703–707.

35 McCarron DA, Lipkin M, Rivlin RS, Heaney RP. Dietary calcium and chronic diseases. *Med Hypotheses* 1990; 31: 265–273.

36 Kawano Y, Yoshimi H, Matsuoka H, *et al.* Calcium supplementation in patients with essential hypertension: assessment by office, home and ambulatory blood pressure. *J Hypertens* 1998; 16: 1693–1699.

37 Galloe AM, Graudal N, Moller J, *et al.* Effect of oral calcium supplementation on blood pressure in patients with hypertension: a randomised, double-blind, placebo-controlled, crossover study. *J Hum Hypertens* 1993; 7: 43–45.

38 Bucher HC, Cook RJ, Guyatt GH, *et al.* Effects of dietary calcium supplementation on blood pressure – a meta-analysis of randomized controlled trials. *JAMA* 1996; 275: 1016–1022.

39 Allender PS, Cutler JA, Follman D, *et al.* Dietary calcium and blood pressure: a meta-analysis of randomized controlled trials. *Ann Intern Med* 1996; 124: 825–831.

40 Zemel MB. Dietary calcium, calcitrophic hormones, and hypertension. *Nutr Metab Cardiovasc Dis* 1994; 4: 224–228.

41 Weinberger MH, Wagner UL, Fineberg NS, *et al.* The blood pressure effects of calcium supplementation in humans of known sodium responsiveness. *Am J Hypertens* 1993; 6: 799–805.

42 Dickinson HO, Nicolson DJ, Cook JV, et al. Calcium supplementation for the management of primary hypertension in adults. Cochrane database, issue 2, 2006. London: Macmillan.

43 Hofstad B, Almendigen K, Vatn M, et al. Growth and recurrence of colorectal polyps: a double-blind 3-year intervention with calcium and antioxidants. *Digestion* 1998; 59: 148–156.

44 Hyman J, Baron JA, Dain BJ, et al. Dietary and supplemental calcium and the recurrence of colorectal adenomas. *Cancer Epidemiol Biomarkers Prev* 1998; 7: 291–295.

45 Bonithon-Kopp C, Kronborg Ole, Giacosa A, et al. Calcium and fibre supplementation in prevention of colorectal adenoma recurrence: randomised intervantion trial. *Lancet* 2000; 356: 1300–1306.

46 Terry P, Baron JA, Bergkvist L, et al. Dietary calcium and vitamin D intake and risk of colorectal cancer: a prospective cohort in women. *Nutr Cancer* 2002; 43: 39–46.

47 Baron JA, Tosteson TD, Wargovich MJ, et al. Calcium supplementation and rectal mucosal proliferation: a randomized controlled trial. *J Natl Cancer Inst* 1995; 87: 1303–1307.

48 Weisberger UM, Boeing H, Owen RW, et al. Effect of long-term placebo controlled calcium supplementation on sigmoidal cell proliferation in patients with sporadic adenomatous polyps. *Gut* 1996; 38: 396–402.

49 Grau MV, Baron JA, Sandler RS, et al. Vitamin D, calcium supplementation, and colorectal adenoma: results of a randomized trial. *J Natl Cancer Inst* 2003; 95: 1765–1771.

50 Cho E, Smith-Warner SA, Spiegelman D, et al. Dairy foods, calcium, and colorectal cancer: a pooled analysis of 10 cohort studies. *J Natl Cancer Inst* 2004; 96: 1015–1022.

51 Wallace K, Baron JA, Cole BF, et al. Effect of calcium supplementation on the risk of large bowel polyps. *J Natl Cancer Inst* 2004; 96: 921–925.

52 Hartman TJ, Albert PS, Snyder K, et al. The association of calcium and vitamin D with risk of colorectal adenomas. *J Nutr* 2005; 135: 252–259.

53 Weingarten MA, Zalmanovici A, Yaphe J. Dietary calcium supplementation for preventing colorectal cancer and adenomatous polyps. Cochrane database, issue 2, 2005. London: Macmillan.

54 Shaukat A, Scouras N, Schunemann HJ. Role of supplemental calcium in the recurrence of colorectal adenomas: a meta-analysis of randomized controlled trials. *Am J Gastroenterol* 2005; 100: 395–396.

55 Chan JM, Stampfer MJ, Ma J, et al. Dairy products, calcium and prostate cancer risk in the Physician's Health Study. *Am J Clin Nutr* 2001; 74: 549–554.

56 Baron JA, Beach M, Wallace K, et al. Risk of prostate cancer in a randomized clinical trial of calcium supplementation. *Cancer Epidemiol Biomarkers Prev* 2005; 14: 586–589.

57 Gao X, LaValley MP, Tucker KL. Prospective studies of dairy product and calcium intakes and prostate cancer risk: a meta-analysis. *J Natl Cancer Inst* 2005; 97; 1768–1777.

58 Thys-Jacobs S, Starkey P, Bernstein D, et al. Calcium carbonate and the premenstrual syndrome: effects on premenstrual and menstrual symptoms (Premenstrual Syndrome Study Group), *Am J Obstet Gynecol* 1998; 179: 444–452.

59 Penland JG, Johnson PE. Dietary calcium and manganese effects on menstrual cycle symptoms. *Am J Obstet Gynecol* 1993; 168: 1417–1423.

60 Thys-Jacobs S, Ceccarelli S, Bierman A, et al. Calcium supplementation in premenstrual syndrome: a randomized crossover trial. *J Gen Intern Med* 1989; 4: 183–189.

61 Herrara JA, Arevala Herrara M, Herrara S, et al. Prevention of preeclampsia by linoleic acid and calcium supplementation: a randomized controlled trial. *Obstet Gynecol* 1998; 91: 585–590.

62 Bucher HC, Guyatt GH, Cook RJ, et al. Effect of calcium supplementation on pregnancy induced hypertension and preeclampsia: a meta-analysis of randomized controlled trials. *JAMA* 1996; 275: 1113–1117.

63 Atallah AN, Hofmeyr GJ, Duley L. Calcium supplementation during pregnancy for preventing hypertensive disorders and related problems. Cochrane database, issue 3, 2000. London: Macmillan.

64 Zemel MB. Regulation of adiposity and obesity risk by dietary calcium: mechanisms and implications. *J Am Coll Nutr* 2002; 21: S146–S151.

65 Heaney RP, Davies KM, Barger-Lux MJ. Calcium and weight: clinical studies. *J Am Coll Nutr* 2002; 21: S152–S155.

66 Shapses SA, Heshka S, Heymsfield SB. Effect of calcium supplementation on weight and fat loss in women. *J Clin Endocrinol Metab* 2004; 89: 632–637.

67 Taylor EN, Stampfer MJ, Curhan GC. Dietary factors and the risk of incident kidney stones in men: new insights after 14 years of follow-up. *J Am Soc Nephrol* 2004; 15: 3225–3232.

68 Curhan GC. A prospective study of dietary calcium and other nutrients and the risk of symptomatic kidney stones. *N Engl J Med* 1993; 328: 833–838.

69 Borghi L, Schianchi T, Meschi T, et al. Comparison of two diets for the prevention of recurrent stones in idiopathic hypercalcuria. *N Engl J Med* 2002; 36: 77–84.

70 Sowers MR, Jannausch M, Wood C, et al. Prevalence of renal stones in a population-based study with

dietary calcium, oxalate and medication exposures. *Am J Epidemiol* 1998; 147: 914–920.

71 Curhan GC, Willett WC, Speizer FE, *et al*. Comparison of dietary calcium with supplemental calcium and other nutrients as factors affecting the risk of kidney stones in women. *Am Intern Med* 1997; 126: 497–504.

72 Straub M, Hautmann RE. Developments in stone prevention. *Curr Opin Urol* 2005; 15: 119.

73 Consumerlab. Product review. Calcium. http://www.consumerlab.com (accessed 10 November 2006).

74 Ross EA, Szabo NJ, Tebbett IR. Lead content of calcium supplements. *JAMA* 2000; 284: 1425–1429.

75 Heaney R. Lead in calcium supplements. Cause for alarm or celebration? *JAMA* 2000; 284: 1263–1270.

76 National Institute for Health and Clinical Excellence. Osteoporosis-secondary prevention. The clinical effectiveness and cost effectiveness of technologies for the secondary prevention of osteoporotic fractures in postmenopausal women. NICE, January 2005.

Carnitine

Description

Carnitine is an amino acid derivative.

Nomenclature

Carnitine is sometimes known as vitamin B_T; it is not an officially recognised vitamin.

Constituents

Carnitine exists as two distinct isomers, L-carnitine (naturally occurring carnitine) and D-carnitine (synthetic carnitine). Dietary supplements contain L-carnitine or a DL-carnitine mixture.

Human requirements

No proof of a dietary need exists. Carnitine is synthesised in sufficient quantities to meet human requirements.

Dietary intake

The average omnivorous diet is estimated to provide 100–300 mg of carnitine daily.

Dietary sources

Meat and dairy products are the best sources. Fruit, vegetables and cereals are poor sources of carnitine. Carnitine is added to infant milk formulae.

Action

Carnitine has the following physiological functions:

- Regulation of long-chain fatty acid transport across cell membranes.
- Facilitation of beta-oxidation of long-chain fatty acids and ketoacids.
- Transportation of acyl CoA compounds.

Metabolism

Dietary carnitine is absorbed rapidly from the intestine by both passive and active transport mechanisms. Carnitine is synthesised in the liver, brain and kidney from the essential amino acids, lysine and methionine.

Deficiency

Primary carnitine deficiency is caused by impairment in the membrane transport of carnitine. Symptoms may include: chronic muscle weakness (due to muscle carnitine deficiency); recurrent episodes of coma and hypoglycaemia (usually in infants and children); encephalopathy; and cardiomyopathy.

Secondary carnitine deficiency occurs in several inherited disorders of metabolism (especially organic acidurias and disorders of beta-oxidation).

Despite the fact that plant foods are poor sources of carnitine, there is no evidence that vegetarians are deficient in carnitine. Endogenous synthesis prevents deficiencies.

Possible uses

Carnitine supplementation has been investigated for its potential benefit in CVD, exercise performance, chronic fatigue syndrome and Alzheimer's disease.

Cardiovascular disease

Carnitine may be beneficial in patients with ischaemic heart disease, but only those who have low serum carnitine levels.

Orally administered L-carnitine (2 g daily) has been shown to improve symptoms of angina,[1] and to reduce anginal attacks and glyceryl trinitrate consumption.[2] In a dose of 900 mg daily for 12 weeks, it has also been shown to improve exercise tolerance in patients with stable angina.[3]

Carnitine supplementation (4 g daily) has also been reported to improve heart rate, arterial pressures, angina and lipid patterns in a controlled study of patients who had experienced a recent myocardial infarction.[4] Yet another study showed that L-carnitine (1 g twice daily for 45 days) may be beneficial in congestive heart failure (CHF), by reducing heart rate, dyspnoea and oedema, and increasing diuresis. Supplementation also allowed for a reduction in daily digoxin dose.[5]

Another study has provided some evidence that L-carnitine (2 g twice a day for 3 weeks) increases walking distance in patients with intermittent claudication.[6]

Hyperlipidaemias

Preliminary studies have shown that L-carnitine may reduce blood cholesterol levels. Oral administration of L-carnitine (3–4 g daily) significantly reduced serum levels of total cholesterol or triglyceride or both, and increased those of high-density lipoprotein (HDL) cholesterol.[7–9]

Exercise performance

There is a potential for carnitine to improve athletic performance by increasing lipid utilisation and conserving glycogen supplies in the muscles.

An increase in maximal aerobic power was observed in subjects who received L-carnitine 2 g daily[10] and 4 g daily.[11,12] Other studies have shown no effect of supplemental carnitine on muscle carnitine.[13,14]

Double-blind placebo-controlled trials have shown no benefit of oral carnitine 2 g,[15] 3 g[16] or 4 g[17] on exercise performance in healthy subjects.

Chronic fatigue syndrome

Patients with chronic fatigue syndrome have been reported to have low carnitine levels. One crossover (not blinded) parallel design study randomised 30 patients with chronic fatigue syndrome to either 3 g L-carnitine or 100 mg amantadine.[18] At the end of the 2-month study, the carnitine group experienced clinical improvement in 12 out of the 18 studied parameters. However, no statistical comparison between carnitine and amantadine was conducted.

Alzheimer's disease

Preliminary evidence from two double-blind, placebo-controlled trials[19,20] suggests that carnitine supplementation could reduce the deterioration in some symptoms of Alzheimer's disease. A meta-analysis of 21 double-blind RCTs of acetyl-L-carnitine (ALC) versus placebo in the treatment of mild cognitive impairment and mild Alzheimer's disease concluded that ALC improved mild cognitive impairment or prevented deterioration, and was well tolerated.[21] More recent evidence from a Cochrane review of 16 trials suggests evidence of benefit for acetyl-L-carnitine on clinical global impression and on the Mini Mental State Examination (MMSE – test for Alzheimer's disease), but there is no evidence using objective assessments in any other area of outcome. In many cases the trial methodologies were poor with vague descriptions of dementia. The Cochrane review concluded that at present there is no evidence to recommend the use of acetyl-L-carnitine in clinical practice.[22]

Miscellaneous

There is some evidence that carnitine improves insulin resistance in type II diabetes.[23] ALC is also a promising treatment for symptoms, particularly pain, of diabetic neuropathy.[24,25] It may support treatment for epilepsy[26] and complement antiretroviral therapy in patients with HIV,[27,28] but studies have not assessed the effect of carnitine on morbidity and mortality from AIDS.

Conclusion

Preliminary evidence suggests that carnitine supplementation may be of benefit in several cardiovascular disorders, such as angina, hyperlipidaemia, myocardial infarction, CHF and intermittent claudication. Evidence also exists that carnitine may be beneficial in Alzheimer's disease, chronic fatigue syndrome and diabetic neuropathy. While these results are clearly of interest, further evidence is required before the role of carnitine, if any, in the management of these conditions can be defined. Despite a theoretical rationale, there is as yet no good evidence that carnitine supplementation improves exercise performance.

Precautions/contraindications

The administration of the D-isomer (including a DL-mixture, contained in some supplements) may interfere with the normal function of the L-isomer and should not be used. Only the L-isomer has been used in studies.

Pregnancy and breast-feeding

No problems have been reported, but there have not been sufficient studies to guarantee the safety of carnitine in pregnancy and breast-feeding.

Adverse effects

Serious toxicity has not been reported. Nausea, vomiting and diarrhoea may occur with high doses. The risk of toxicity is greater with the D-isomer than with L-carnitine (see Precautions/contraindications); myasthenia has been reported with ingestion of DL-carnitine.

Interactions

Drugs

Anticonvulsants: increased excretion of carnitine.
Pivampicillin: increased excretion of carnitine.

Pivmecillinam: increased excretion of carnitine.

Dose

L-carnitine supplements are available in the form of tablets and capsules.

The dose is not established. In studies, doses of 1–6 g L-carnitine daily have been used.

References

1   Cherchi A, Lai C, Angelino F, Trucco G, Caponnetto S. Effects of L-carnitine in exercise tolerance in chronic stable angina: a multicenter, double-blind, randomized placebo controlled crossover study. *Int J Clin Pharmacol Ther Toxicol* 1985; 23: 569–572.
2   Garyza G, Amico RM. Comparative study on the activity of racemic and laevorotatory carnitine in stable angina pectoris. *Int J Tissue React* 1980; 2: 175–180.
3   Kamikawa T, Suzuki Y, Kobayashi A, *et al*. Effects of L-carnitine on exercise tolerance in patients with stable angina pectoris. *Jpn Heart J* 1984; 25: 587–597.
4   Davini P, Bigalli A, Lamanna F, *et al*. Controlled study on L-carnitine therapeutic efficacy in post-infarction. *Drugs Exp Clin Res* 1992; 18: 355–365.
5   Ghidini O, Azzurro M, Vita G, *et al*. Evaluation of the therapeutic efficacy of L-carnitine in congestive heart failure. *Int J Clin Pharmacol Ther Toxicol* 1988; 26: 217–220.
6   Brevetti G, Chiariello M, Ferulano G, *et al*. Increases in walking distance in patients with peripheral vascular disease treated with L-carnitine: a double-blind, cross-over study. *Circulation* 1988; 77: 767–773.
7   Pola P, Savi L, Grilli M, *et al*. Carnitine in the therapy of dyslipidemic patients. *Curr Ther Res* 1979; 27: 208–216.
8   Pola P, Tondi P, Dal Lago A, *et al*. Statistical evaluation of long-term L-carnitine therapy in hyperlipoproteinaemias. *Drugs Exp Clin Res* 1983; 12: 925–935.
9   Rossi CS, Silprandi N. Effect of carnitine on serum HDL-cholesterol: report of two cases. *Johns Hopkins Med J* 1982; 150: 51–54.
10 Swart I, Rossouw J, Loots J, *et al*. The effect of L-carnitine supplementation on plasma carnitine levels and various parameters of male marathon athletes. *Nutr Res* 1997; 17: 405–414.
11 Angelini C, Vergani L, Costa L, *et al*. Clinical study of efficacy of L-carnitine and metabolic observations in exercise physiology. In: Borum D, ed. *Clinical*

Aspects of Human Carnitine Deficiency. New York: Pergamon Press, 1986: 36–42.

12 Marconi C, Sassi G, Carpinelli A, Cerretelli P. Effects of L-carnitine loading on the aerobic and aerobic performance of endurance athletes. *Eur J Appl Physiol* 1985; 54: 131–135.

13 Barnett C, Costill D, Vukovitch M, *et al*. Effect of L-carnitine supplementation on muscle and blood carnitine content and lactate accumulation during high-intensity spring cycling. *Int J Sport Nutr* 1994; 4: 280–288.

14 Vukovitch M, Costill D, Fink W, *et al*. Carnitine supplementation: effect on muscle carnitine and glycogen content during exercise. *Med Sci Sports Exerc* 1994; 26: 1122–1129.

15 Colombani P, Wenk C, Kunz I, *et al*. Effects of L-carnitine supplementation on physical performance and energy metabolism of endurance trained athletes: a double-blind crossover field study. *Eur J Appl Physiol* 1996; 73: 434–439.

16 Trappe SW, Costill DL, Goodpaster P, *et al*. The effects of L-carnitine on performance during interval swimming. *Int J Sports Med* 1994; 15: 181–185.

17 Giamberardino MA, Dragani L, Valente R, *et al*. Effects of prolonged L-carnitine administration on delayed muscle pain and CK release after eccentric effort. *Int J Sports Med* 1996; 17: 320–324.

18 Pliophys A, Pliophys S. Amantadine and L-carnitine treatment of chronic fatigue syndrome. *Neuropsychobiology* 1997; 35: 16–23.

19 Sano M, Bell K, Cote L, *et al*. Double-blind parallel design pilot study of acetyl levocarnitine in patients with Alzheimer's disease. *Arch Neurol* 1992; 49: 1137–1141.

20 Spagnoli A, Lucca U, Menasce G, *et al*. Long term acetyl-L-carnitine treatment in Alzheimer's disease. *Neurology* 1991; 41: 1726–1732.

21 Montgomery SA, Thal LJ, Amrein R. Meta-analysis of double blind randomized controlled clinical trials of acetyl-L-carnitine versus placebo in the treatment of mild cognitive impairment and mild Alzheimer's disease. *Int Clin Psychopharmacol* 2003; 18: 61–71.

22 Hudson S, Tabet N. Acetyl-L-carnitine for dementia. Cochrane database, issue 2, 2003. London: Macmillan.

23 Mingrone G, Greco AV, Capristo E. L-carnitine improves glucose disposal in type 2 diabetic patients. *J Am Coll Nutr* 1999; 18: 77–82.

24 De Grandis D, Minardi C. Acetyl-L-carnitine in the treatment of diabetic neuropathy. A long-term, randomised, double-blind, placebo-controlled study. *Drugs R D* 2002; 3: 223–231.

25 Sima AA, Calvani M, Mehra M, *et al*. Acetyl-L-carnitine improves pain, nerve regeneration, and vibratory perception in patients with chronic diabetic neuropathy: an analysis of two randomized placebo-controlled trials. *Diabetes Care* 2005; 1: 89–94.

26 Shuper A, Gutman A, Mimoumi M. Intractable epilepsy. *Lancet* 1999; 353: 1238.

27 Moretti S, Alesse E, Di Marzio L. Effect of L-carnitine on human immunodeficiency virus-1 infection-associated apoptosis: a pilot study. *Blood* 1998; 91: 3817–3824.

28 De Simone C, Tzantzoglou S, Famularo G. High dose L-carnitine improves immunologic and metabolic parameters in AIDS patients. *Immunopharmacol Immunotoxicol* 1993; 15: 1–12.

Carotenoids

Description

Carotenoids are natural pigments found in plants, including fruit and vegetables, giving them their bright colour. About 600 carotenoids have been identified, of which about six appear to be used in significant ways by the blood or other tissues. About 50 have pro-vitamin A activity, and of these, all-*trans* beta-carotene is the most active on a weight basis and makes the most important quantitative contribution to human nutrition. Beta-carotene is fat soluble. Apart from beta-carotene, other significant carotenoids (according to research conducted so far) are alpha-carotene, astaxanthin, cryptoxanthin, lycopene, lutein and zeaxanthin.

Units

The bioavailability of those carotenoids with pro-vitamin A activity (e.g. alpha-carotene, beta-carotene, cryptoxanthin) is less than that of retinol (preformed vitamin A).

The absorption and utilisation of carotenoids varies, but the generally accepted relationship in the UK is that 1 µg retinol is equivalent to 6 µg beta-carotene or 12 µg of other pro-vitamin A carotenoids. (Other carotenoids with pro-vitamin A activity are not converted to vitamin to the same extent as is beta-carotene.) However, the bioactivity of carotenoids in foods is now known to be less than was previously thought and there is much debate about the conversion factors. The US Food and Nutrition Board revised its conversion factors in 2001 such that 1 µg retinol is equivalent to 12 µg beta-carotene or 24 µg of other provitamin A carotenoids.

The amount of beta-carotene in dietary supplements may be expressed in terms of micrograms or International Units. One unit of beta-carotene is defined as the activity of 0.6 µg beta-carotene. Thus:

- 1 unit beta-carotene = 0.6 µg beta-carotene; and
- 1 µg beta-carotene = 1.67 units beta-carotene.

Human requirements

There is currently no UK Dietary Reference Value for beta-carotene (or any other carotenoids). This is because, until recently, its only role has been considered to be as a precursor of vitamin A. Some authorities are starting to make recommendations for beta-carotene, e.g. 6 mg daily (Finland); 4 mg daily (France); 2 mg daily (Germany).

Dietary intake

In the UK, the average adult diet provides 2.28 mg (beta-carotene) daily.

Action

Carotenoids have the following functions. They:

- quench singlet oxygen and prevent the formation of free radicals. *Note*: natural beta-carotene (*cis* form) acts as an antioxidant, while the synthetic (*trans*) form has been suggested to be pro-oxidant;[1]
- react with or scavenge free radicals directly and thus act as an antioxidant;
- enhance some aspects of immune function; and
- act as precursors for vitamin A (e.g. alpha-carotene, beta-carotene, cryptoxanthin).

51

Table 1   Carotenoid composition of typical fruits and vegetables (μg/100 g portion)

Food	Alpha-carotene	Beta-carotene	Beta-cryptoxanthin	Lutein + zeaxanthin	Lycopene
Apricots, dried	0	17 600	0	0	864
Beet greens	3	2 560	0	7 700	0
Broccoli, boiled	0	1 042	0	2 226	0
Brussels sprouts, boiled	0	465	0	1 290	0
Cantaloupe melon	27	1 595	0	40	0
Carrots, cooked	3700	9 800	0	260	0
Grapefruit, pink	5	603	12	13	1 462
Kale, cooked	0	6 202	0	15798	0
Lettuce, cos	0	1 272	0	2 635	0
Mandarin orange	14	71	485	243	0
Mango, raw	17	445	11	–	–
Mango, canned, drained	–	13 120	1 550	–	–
Orange juice	2	4	15	36	0
Oranges	16	51	122	187	0
Papaya	0	276	761	75	0
Pasta with tomato sauce	0	127	0	0	3 162
Peppers, red, raw	59	2 379	2 205	–	–
Pizza, with tomato sauce	0	170	0	20	2 071
Spinach, cooked	0	5 242	0	7 043	0
Sweetcorn, canned	33	30	0	884	0
Sweet potato, cooked	0	9 488	0	0	0
Tomato soup, canned	0	235	0	90	10 920
Tomato, raw	0	520	0	100	3 100

Data from USDA-NCC Carotenoid Database for US Foods, 1998.

Dietary sources

Carotenoids are found in a wide variety of fruits and vegetables, although they may not be the ones commonly consumed. Alpha-carotene is found in palm oil, maize, carrots and pumpkin. Lycopene is concentrated in red fruits, such as tomatoes (particularly cooked and pureed tomatoes), guava, watermelon, apricots, peaches and red grapefruit. Lutein and zeaxanthin are found in dark green vegetables, red pepper and pumpkin. Cryptoxanthin is present in mangoes, oranges and peaches. The carotenoid content of various fruits and vegetables is shown in Table 1.

Metabolism

Although there are a huge number of carotenoids, most research has been conducted on beta-carotene, and less is known about the others, particularly in terms of metabolism. Hence, only the metabolism of beta-carotene is described here.

Absorption

Beta-carotene consists of two molecules of vitamin A, which are hydrolysed in the gastro-intestinal tract. It is absorbed into the mucosal cells of the small intestine and converted to retinol. The efficiency of absorption is usually 20–50%, but can be as low as 10% when intake is high. The conversion of beta-carotene to retinol is regulated by the vitamin A stores of the individual and by the amount ingested; conversion efficiency varies from 2:1 at low intakes to 12:1 at higher intakes. On average, 25% of absorbed beta-carotene appears to remain intact and 75% is converted to retinol.

Distribution

Intact beta-carotene is transported in very-low-density lipoprotein (VLDL) or low-density lipoprotein (LDL) cholesterol. Blood levels, unlike those of retinol, are not maintained constant but vary roughly in proportion to the amounts ingested. Increased blood levels (hypercarotenaemia) are sometimes associated (as a secondary condition) with hypothyroidism, diabetes mellitus, and hepatic and renal disease. Hypercarotenaemia can also be caused by a rare genetic inability to convert beta-carotene to vitamin A.

All carotenoids are deposited in the liver to a less extent than is vitamin A. Most are stored in the adipose tissue, epidermal and dermal layers of the skin and the adrenals; there are high levels in the corpus luteum and in colostrum.

Elimination

Beta-carotene is eliminated mainly in the faeces.

Bioavailability

Beta-carotene is not very stable, and potency is lost if it is exposed to oxygen. Mild cooking processes can improve bioavailability, e.g. absorption from raw carrot can be as low as 1%, but this figure increases dramatically when carrots are subject to short periods of boiling. However, overcooking reduces bioavailability. Significant losses can also occur during frying, freezing and canning.

Deficiency

No specific symptoms have been defined.

Possible uses

Carotenoids are being investigated in a variety of conditions, particularly cancer, CVD and cataract.

Beta-carotene

Cancer

Epidemiological studies More than 50 epidemiological studies have demonstrated that a high intake of foods rich in carotenoids (i.e. fruit and vegetables) and high serum levels of beta-carotene are associated with reduced risk of certain cancers, especially lung cancer, but also cancers of the cervix, endometrium, breast, oesophagus, mouth and stomach.[2]

Fruit and vegetables contain several types of carotenoids in addition to beta-carotene, and it is incorrect to assume that beta-carotene is responsible for all the preventive effects of fruit and vegetables. For example, increased alpha-carotene intakes from diet have been associated with a reduced risk of lung cancer,[3,4] with suggestive inverse associations for other carotenoids also.

However, serum analysis has also shown an association between low serum beta-carotene levels and increased cancer risk, possibly indicating a more specific link. Intervention studies published so far have provided very little evidence for a beneficial effect of beta-carotene supplementation on cancer risk; indeed, some have indicated that there may be an increased risk.

Intervention trials A 12-year US study involving 22 071 male physicians randomly allocated to 50 mg beta-carotene every other day or placebo did not demonstrate any statistically significant benefit or harm from supplementation. In the beta-carotene group, 1273 subjects developed malignant neoplasms compared with 1293 in the placebo group. No serious adverse effects were noted in the study.[5]

In a double-blind, placebo-controlled Finnish intervention trial, known as the Alpha-Tocopherol, Beta-Carotene Prevention (ATBC) Study,[6] 29 000 male smokers were randomised to receive beta-carotene 20 mg daily, alpha-tocopherol 50 mg daily, both beta-carotene and alpha-tocopherol, or placebo. Lung cancer incidence increased in all the groups receiving beta-carotene, but the effect was stronger in those who smoked heavily, a finding consistent with the CARET study (see below). However, lung cancer incidence was not correlated with serum beta-carotene, suggesting that this was not a direct effect of beta-carotene.[7] There was also no significant effect on incidence or mortality of cancer of the pancreas,[8] nor on the incidence of colorectal adenomas.[9]

Another US study (the beta-carotene and retinol efficacy trial – CARET) in 4060 subjects with substantial work-related exposure to asbestos and also 14 254 heavy smokers, showed that beta-carotene 30 mg with vitamin A 25 000 units increased the risk of lung cancer compared with placebo. Mortality was also 17% higher. As a consequence, this trial was stopped prematurely.[10]

These unexpected results were reviewed extensively and numerous possible explanations were proposed. One possible explanation for the negative results of the human beta-carotene intervention trials is that the positive effects of beta-carotene shown in case-control studies were instead the results of other nutrients that co-vary with carotenoids and carotenoids are only one of several factors in fruits and vegetables that must be consumed together to be effective. Carotenoids could also be a marker for a generally healthy lifestyle that includes a diet low in fat and high in fruits and vegetables.[11]

Another hypothesis is that a large dose of beta-carotene, such as was used in these trials, is metabolised differently than a smaller dietary dose, resulting in adverse effects. The idea was tested experimentally in a model of smoke-exposed, beta-carotene-treated ferrets. In the lungs of these animals, retinoid oxidative enzymes were elevated and retinoid levels were reduced.[12] This was found, in part, to be the result of enhanced oxidative excentric cleaving of beta-carotene to produce various beta-carotene metabolites (e.g. beta-apo-carotenals). However, when alpha-tocopherol and ascorbic acid were added to beta-carotene in ferrets exposed to cigarette smoke, the production of beta-apo-carotenals was inhibited, while the production of retinoids was increased. When either alpha-tocopherol or vitamin C alone was added, the production of retinoids was not affected, suggesting that alpha-tocopherol and ascorbic acid may act synergistically in preventing the enhanced oxidative cleavage of beta-carotene induced by smoking exposure.[13] A more recent study in a ferret lung cancer model indicates that combined antioxidative supplementation could be a useful chemopreventive strategy against

lung carcinogenesis through maintaining tissue retinoid levels and inhibiting cell proliferation and other potentially carcinogenesis pathways in the lung.[14]

In patients with documented cervical dysplasia given either beta-carotene 30 mg or placebo for 9 months, complete remission occurred in 23% of the supplemented group and 47% of the placebo group, showing that beta-carotene had no beneficial effect on resolution of cervical dysplasia.[15] However, in another study there was an inverse relationship between breast cancer and beta-carotene intake in pre-menopausal women.[16]

In a further study, beta-carotene was neither beneficial nor harmful in reducing the risk of developing skin cancer. A total of 1621 subjects aged 20 to 69 were randomised into four groups – beta-carotene and sunscreen, sunscreen and placebo, beta-carotene and no sunscreen, and no sunscreen and placebo. Sunscreen was applied daily to all exposed areas of the head, neck, arms and hands, with re-application after swimming or increased perspiration. No dosing details were given for beta-carotene. At the end of the study, there were no statistically significant differences in development of basal or squamous cell carcinoma between the beta-carotene and placebo groups.[17] A lack of effect of beta-carotene supplementation in non-melanoma skin cancer was observed among men with low baseline plasma beta-carotene.[18]

More recent trials continue to show mixed results with beta-carotene alone. One RCT in 264 patients who had been treated for a recent early-stage squamous cell carcinoma of the oral cavity, pharynx or larynx found that beta-carotene 50 mg daily had no significant effect on second cancers of the head and neck (RR 0.69; 5% CI, 0.39 to 1.25) or lung cancer (RR 1.44; 5% CI, 0.62 to 3.39) and total mortality was not affected. However, in this study the point estimates suggested a possible decrease in second head and neck cancer risk but a possible increase in lung cancer risk.[19] In a further trial involving patients treated for head and neck cancer, beta-carotene (75 mg daily) had no significant effect on the incidence of second primary tumours, but there was a statistically non-significant 40% reduction in the risk of death among subjects assigned to beta-carotene and no increase in death from CVD.[20] In patients with early-stage head and neck cancer, supplemental beta-carotene did not have pro-oxidant effects in either smokers or non-smokers.[21]

Beta-carotene has been shown in one RCT to be protective of colorectal adenoma recurrence among subjects who neither smoked cigarettes nor drank alcohol. A total of 864 subjects who had had an adenoma removed and were polyp-free were randomised to receive beta-carotene (25 mg) and/or vitamins C and E in combination (1000 mg and 400 mg, respectively) or placebo. They were followed at 1 and 4 years for adenoma recurrence. Among subjects who did not smoke or drink, beta-carotene was associated with a marked decrease in risk of one or more recurrent adenomas (RR 0.56, 95% CI, 0.35 to 0.89), but beta-carotene supplementation conferred a modest increase in the risk of recurrence in those who smoked or drank. For people who smoked and drank more than one alcoholic drink a day, beta-carotene doubled the risk of adenoma recurrence, suggesting that both alcohol and smoking modify the effect of beta-carotene supplementation on the risk of colorectal adenoma recurrence.[22] Vitamin A and alpha-carotene have also been found to protect against recurrence of adenomatous polyps in non-smokers and non-drinkers.[23]

Cardiovascular disease

Diets rich in fruit and vegetables are generally associated with a lower risk of CVD, but evidence for a direct protective effect of beta-carotene was reported from the US Physicians' Health Study.[23] In an analysis of a subgroup of volunteers who had previously had stable angina or coronary revascularisation, 50 mg beta-carotene on alternate days reduced subsequent coronary events by 50% compared with placebo.

However, in a large placebo-controlled trial involving men between 50 and 69 who smoked five or more cigarettes a day, supplementation with beta-carotene was not helpful in angina pectoris and may have slightly increased the incidence of the condition.[24] In this study, 5602 patients received beta-carotene 20 mg daily,

5570 patients received alpha-tocopherol 50 mg daily, 5548 patients received alpha-tocopherol 50 mg and beta-carotene 20 mg daily, and 5549 received placebo. Follow-up continued for a maximum of 7 years. Patients taking vitamin E alone or in combination with beta-carotene showed a minor decrease in angina pectoris, but beta-carotene alone was associated with a slight increase in angina incidence.

Incidence of myocardial infarction was not reduced by beta-carotene supplementation (50 mg daily) in US male physicians.[25] Beta-carotene was not effective in the treatment of increased serum triglycerides or cholesterol levels,[26] and was not shown to reduce the risk of stroke.[27]

A meta-analysis that looked at the effect of antioxidant vitamins on long-term cardiovascular outcomes included 12 RCTs, of which eight involved beta-carotene.[28] Beta-carotene was associated with a slight statistically significant increase in all-cause mortality and cardiovascular death compared with the control. The authors concluded that the use of supplements containing beta-carotene should be actively discouraged.

Cataract

Beta-carotene may protect against cataract formation. In a retrospective study,[29] the group with the lowest serum beta-carotene levels had over five times the risk of developing cataract as the group with the highest serum levels. Two RCTs have evaluated the influence of beta-carotene supplements in age-related cataract. In the US Physicians' Health Study, 22 071 men aged 40–84 were randomly assigned to receive either beta-carotene 50 mg on alternate days or placebo for 12 years. There was no difference between the beta-carotene and placebo groups in the overall incidence of cataract, relative risk or cataract extraction. In smokers, however, beta-carotene appeared to attenuate excess risk of cataract by about 25%.[30] In the Women's Health Study, 39 867 female health professionals aged 45 or older were randomised to receive beta-carotene 50 mg on alternate days, vitamin E and aspirin for the prevention of cancer and CVD. The beta-carotene arm was terminated early and the main outcome measures were visually significant cataract and cataract extraction. However, 2 years of beta-carotene treatment had no large beneficial (or harmful) effect on the development of cataract.[31]

Diabetes

Serum beta-carotene levels may be reduced in diabetic patients, and one case-control study has shown a negative correlation between beta-carotene and glycaemic control.[32] However, in the US Physicians' Health Study, beta-carotene supplementation (50 mg daily) was ineffective in reducing the risk of developing type 2 diabetes.[33]

Immune function

Data on beta-carotene's influence on the immune system are conflicting. One study showed that supplementation (beta-carotene 15 mg daily for 26 days) resulted in a significant increase in the proportion of monocytes involved in initiating immune responses.[34] However, in other studies, T-cell immunity was unaffected by beta-carotene supplementation.[35]

Lutein

Lutein is a carotenoid found in high concentrations in the eye, where it filters out blue light, and it may have a protective role in the visual apparatus and its vascular supply. There is evidence that lutein may help to prevent ARMD[36] and cataracts.[37] Supplements may also help to improve visual function in patients with retinal degeneration.[38]

A study in Miami tested the effects of 30 mg of lutein on eye pigment in two people for a period of 140 days. The results showed that 20–40 days after starting the lutein supplement, the density of the pigment in the subject's eyes started to increase. The amount of blue light reaching the photoreceptors, Bruch's membrane and the retinal pigment epithelium (vulnerable eye tissues affected in macular degeneration) was reduced by 30–40%.[39] Another carotenoid, lycopene, appears to confer protection against oxidative changes in the epithelial cells of the lens.[40]

Dietary intake of lutein and its isomer zeaxanthin may reduce the risk of developing both cataract and macular degeneration.[41] In the US Nurses' Health Study, those in the highest quintile for consumption of lutein and zeaxanthin had a 22% reduced risk of cataract extraction compared with those in the lowest quintile.[42] In the US Physicians' Health Study, those in the highest quintile for lutein and zeaxanthin intake had a 19% reduction in risk for cataract extraction when smoking, age, and other risk factors were controlled for.[43] Other carotenoids (alpha-carotene, beta-carotene, beta-cryptoxanthin, lycopene) were not associated with a reduced risk of cataract.

Similarly, in the US Beaver Dam Eye Study, lutein and zeaxanthin were the only carotenoids of those examined associated with reduction in cataracts – in this case, nuclear cataracts. People in the highest quintile of lutein intake in the distant past were half as likely to have an incidence of cataract as those in the lowest quintile.[37] As part of the same study, 252 subjects were followed over a 5-year period. Only a trend towards an inverse relationship between serum lutein and cryptoxanthin and risk of cataract development was noted.[44]

In a UK cross-sectional survey, the risk of posterior subscapular cataract was lowest in those with higher plasma concentrations of lutein and the risk of cortical cataract was lowest in people with the highest plasma concentrations of lycopene. However, the risk of nuclear cataract was lowest in people with the highest plasma concentrations of alpha- or beta-carotene.[45]

In the first published intervention trial involving lutein, 17 patients with age-related cataracts were randomised in a double-blind study involving dietary supplementation with lutein 15 mg, alpha-tocopherol 100 mg or placebo three times a week for up to 2 years. Visual performance (visual acuity and glare sensitivity) improved in the lutein group but not with alpha-tocopherol or placebo.[46]

The second trial was a 21-month randomised, double-masked, placebo-controlled trial that involved 90 patients with atrophic ARMD. One group of patients received lutein 10 mg daily, another group received lutein 10 mg with antioxidants and vitamins and minerals while the third group received a placebo. Visual function (as measured by macular pigment optical density, Snellen equivalent visual acuity and contrast sensitivity) improved with both lutein alone and lutein together with the other nutrients compared with placebo.[47] The authors concluded that lutein or lutein together with antioxidant vitamins was not a cure for ARMD but could reverse various symptoms of the condition and improve visual function.

Lycopene

Lycopene is a carotenoid pigment that functions as a free radical scavenger and antioxidant. Supplementation has been reported to protect against macular degeneration,[48] atherosclerosis,[49] and cancer, especially prostate cancer.[50,51]

Intervention trials have begun to evaluate the effects of lycopene supplements in prostate cancer. In a pilot trial, 26 men with newly diagnosed, clinically localised prostate cancer were randomised to receive 15 mg of lycopene twice daily or no supplementation for 3 weeks before radical prostatectomy. The results suggested that lycopene supplementation may reduce the growth of prostate cancer, but the authors emphasised that no firm conclusions could be reached because of the small sample size.[52]

The same research group conducted a further pilot trial involving the use of a tomato extract containing 30 mg lycopene each day in 26 men – again for 3 weeks before radical prostatectomy. After intervention, subjects in the intervention group had smaller tumours, less involvement of extra-prostatic tissue with cancer and less diffuse involvement of the prostate by high-grade prostatic intraepithelial neoplasia. Mean prostate-specific antigen (PSA) was lower in the intervention group than the placebo group. The authors concluded that this pilot study suggests that lycopene may have beneficial effects in prostate cancer, although large trials are warranted to investigate the potential preventive and/or therapeutic role of lycopene in the disease.[53]

In another trial, 54 men with prostate cancer were assigned to receive orchidectomy alone or orchidectomy plus lycopene (2 mg twice daily). At 6 months there was a significant reduction in PSA in both treatment arms, but this was more marked in the lycopene group. This change was more consistent after 2 years. Adding lycopene to orchidectomy produced a more reliable and consistent reduction in PSA, shrinking the primary tumour, diminishing secondary tumours, providing better relief from bone pain and lower urinary tract symptoms and improving survival compared with orchidectomy alone.[54] A further trial using a supplement containing lycopene, isoflavones, silymarin and antioxidants found that this supplement delayed PSA progression after potentially curative treatment (radical prostatectomy).[55]

A meta-analysis of 11 case-control studies and 10 cohort studies or nested case-control studies involving tomato, tomato products or lycopene concluded that tomato products may play a role in the prevention of prostate cancer, but the effect is small.[56]

Conclusion

Diets rich in carotenoids are protective against various conditions, particularly cancer and CVD. However, evidence that beta-carotene supplements are beneficial for this purpose is lacking. Other carotenoids, such as lycopene and lutein, are now being studied. Preliminary evidence suggests that lutein may be protective in cataract and macular degeneration, while lycopene may be protective against macular degeneration and prostate cancer.

Precautions/contraindications

No serious problems have been reported. Supplements should be avoided by people with known hypersensitivity to carotenoids.

Pregnancy and breast-feeding

No problems have been reported.

Adverse effects

Unlike retinol, carotenoids are generally non-toxic. Even when ingested in large amounts, they are not known to cause birth defects or to cause hypervitaminosis A, primarily because efficiency of absorption decreases rapidly as the dose increases and because conversion to vitamin A is not sufficiently rapid to induce toxicity.

Intake of >30 mg daily (either from commercial supplements or tomato or carrot juice) may lead to hypercarotenaemia, which is characterised by a yellowish coloration of the skin (including the palms of the hands and soles of the feet), and a very high concentration of carotenoids in the plasma. This is harmless and reversible and gradually disappears when excessive intake of carotenoids is corrected.

Hypercarotenaemia is clearly differentiated from jaundice by the appearance of the whites of the eyes (yellow in hypercarotenaemia but not in jaundice).

Diarrhoea, dizziness and arthralgia may occur occasionally with carotene supplements. Allergic reactions (hay fever and facial swelling), amenorrhoea and leucopenia have been reported rarely.

According to FAO/WHO, intakes up to 5 mg beta-carotene/kg body weight are acceptable.

The only serious toxic manifestation of carotenoid intake is canthaxanthin retinopathy, which can develop in patients with erythropoietic protoporphyria and related disorders who are treated with large daily doses (50–100 mg) of canthaxanthin (a derivative of beta-carotene) for long periods.

Interactions

None specifically established (see also Vitamin A).

Dose

Beta-carotene, lutein, lycopene and mixed carotenoids are available in the form of tablets and capsules.

Beta-carotene as a single supplement should not be recommended.

References

1 Levin G, Yeshurun M, Mockady S. In vitro antiperoxidative effect of 9-*cis* beta-carotene compared with that of the all-*trans* isomer. *J Nutr Cancer* 1997; 27: 293–297.

2 Gaby SK, Singh VN. Betacarotene. In: Gaby SK, Bendich A, Singh VN, Machlin LJ, eds. *Vitamin Intake and Health. A Scientific Review*. New York: Marcel Dekker, 1991: 89–106.

3 Michaud DS, Feskanich D, Rimm EB, *et al*. Intake of specific carotenoids and risk of lung cancer in 2 prospective US cohorts. *Am J Clin Nutr* 2000; 72: 990–997.

4 Knekt P, Jarvinen R, Tempo, *et al*. Role of various carotenoids in lung cancer prevention. *J Natl Cancer Inst* 1999; 91: 182–184.

5 Hennekens CH, Buring JE, Manson JE, *et al*. Lack of effect of long-term supplementation with beta-carotene on the incidence of malignant neoplasms and cardiovascular disease. *N Engl J Med* 1996; 334: 1145–1149.

6 The Alpha-Tocopherol, Beta-Carotene Cancer Prevention Study Group. The effect of vitamin E and beta carotene on the incidence of lung cancer in male smokers. *N Engl J Med* 1994; 330: 1029–1035.

7 Albanes E, Heinonen OP, Taylor PR, *et al*. Alpha-tocopherol and beta-carotene supplements and lung cancer incidence in the alpha-tocopherol, beta-carotene cancer prevention study: effects of base-line characteristics and study compliance. *J Natl Cancer Inst* 1996; 88: 1560–1570.

8 Rautalahti MT, Virtamo JRK, Taylor PR, *et al*. The effects of supplementation with alpha-tocopherol and beta-carotene on the incidence and mortality of carcinoma of the pancreas in a randomised, controlled trial. *Cancer* 1999; 86: 37–42.

9 Maliula N, Virtamo J, Virtanen M, *et al*. The effect of alpha-tocopherol and β-carotene supplementation on colorectal adenomas in middle-aged male smokers. *Cancer Epidemiol Biomarkers Prev* 1999; 8: 489–493.

10 Omenn GS, Goodman GE, Thornquist MD, *et al*. Effects of a combination of betacarotene and vitamin A on lung cancer and cardiovascular disease. *N Engl J Med* 1996; 334: 1150–1155.

11 Mayne ST. Antioxidant nutrients and chronic disease: use of biomarkers of exposure and oxidative stress status in epidemiologic research. *J Nutr* 2003; 33 (Suppl.): S933–940.

12 Liu C, Russell RM, Wang XD. Exposing ferrets to cigarette smoke and a pharmacological dose of β-carotene supplementation enhance in vitro retinoic acid catabolism in lungs via induction of cytochrome P450 enzymes. *J Nutr* 2003; 133: 173–179.

13 Liu C, Russell RM, Wang XD. Alpha-tocopherol and ascorbic acid decrease the production of beta-apo-carotenals and increase the formation of retinoids from β-carotene in the lung tissues of cigarette smoke-exposed ferrets in vitro. *J Nutr* 2004; 134: 426–430.

14 Kim Y, Chongviriyaphan N, Liu C, *et al*. Combined antioxidant (beta-carotene, alpha-tocopherol and ascorbic acid) supplementation increases the levels of lung retinoic acid and inhibits the activation of mitogen-activated protein kinase in the ferret lung cancer model. *Carcinogenesis* 2006; 27: 1410–1419.

15 Romney SL, Ho GYF, Palan PR, *et al*. Effects of betacarotene and other factors on outcome of cervical dysplasia and human papillomavirus infection. *Gynecol Oncol* 1997; 65: 483–492.

16 Bohlke K, Spiegelman D, Trichopoulou A, *et al*. Vitamins A, C and E and the risk of breast cancer: results from a case control study in Greece. *Br J Cancer* 1999; 79: 23–29.

17 Green A, Williams G, Neale R, *et al*. Daily sunscreen application and betacarotene supplementation in prevention of basal cell and squamous cell carcinomas of the skin. *Lancet* 1999; 354: 723–729.

18 Schaumberg DA, Frieling UM, Rifai N, Cook N. No effect of beta-carotene supplementation on risk of nonmelanoma skin cancer among men with low baseline plasma beta-carotene. *Cancer Epidemiol Biomarkers Prev* 2004; 6: 1079–1080.

19 Mayne ST, Cartmel B, Baum M, *et al*. Randomized trial of supplemental beta-carotene to prevent second head and neck cancer. *Cancer Res* 2001; 61: 1457–1463.

20 Toma S, Bonelli L, Sartoris A, *et al*. Beta-carotene supplementation in patients radically treated for stage I–II head and neck cancer: results of a randomized trial. *Oncol Rep* 2003; 10: 1895–1901.

21 Mayne ST, Walter M, Cartmel B, *et al*. Supplemental bete-carotene, smoking, and urinary F2-isoprostane excretion in patients with prior early stage head and neck cancer. *Nutr Cancer* 2004; 49: 1–6.

22 Baron JA, Cole BF, Mott L, *et al*. Neoplastic and antineoplastic effects of beta-carotene on colorectal adenoma recurrence: results of a randomized trial. *J Natl Cancer Inst* 2003; 95: 717–722.

23 Steck-Stott S, Forman MR, Sowell A, *et al*. Carotenoids, vitamin A and risk of adenomatous polyp recurrence in the polyp prevention trial. *Int J Cancer* 2004; 112: 295–305.

24 Gaziano JM, Manson JE, Ridker PM, *et al*. Beta-carotene supplementation for chronic stable angina. *Circulation* 1990; 82 (Suppl. III): 201 (abstract 0796).

25 Rapola JM, Virtamo J, Haukka JK, *et al*. Effect of vitamin E and betacarotene on the incidence of angina pectoris: a randomized, double-blind, controlled trial. *JAMA* 1996; 275: 693–698.

26 Redlich C, Chung J, Cullen M, *et al*. Effect of long-term betacarotene and vitamin A on serum cholesterol and triglycerides among participants in the carotene and retinol efficacy trial (CARET). *Atherosclerosis* 1999; 145: 425–432.

27 Ascherio A, Rimm E, Hernan MA, *et al*. Relation of consumption of vitamin E, vitamin C and carotenoids to risk for stroke among men in the United States. *Ann Intern Med* 1999; 130: 963–970.

28 Vivekananthan DP, Penn MS, Sapp SK, *et al*. Use of antioxidant vitamins for the prevention of cardiovascular disease: meta-analysis of randomized trials. *Lancet* 2003; 361: 2017–2023.

29 Jacques PF, Hartz SC, Chylack LT, *et al*. Nutritional status in persons with and without senile cataract: blood vitamin and mineral levels. *Am J Clin Nutr* 1988; 48: 152–158.

30 Christen WG, Manson JE, Glynn RJ, *et al*. A randomized trial of beta carotene and age-related cataract in US physicians. *Arch Ophthalmol* 2003; 121: 372–378.

31 Christen W, Glynn R, Sperduto R, *et al*. Age-related cataract in a randomized trial of beta-carotene in women. *Ophthalmic Epidemiol* 2004; 11: 401–412.

32 Abahusain MA, Wright J, Dickerson JWT, *et al*. Retinol, alpha-tocopherol and carotenoids in diabetes. *Eur J Clin Nutr* 1999; 53: 630–635.

33 Liu S, Ajanu U, Chae C, *et al*. Long-term β-carotene supplementation and risk of type 2 diabetes mellitus. *JAMA* 1999; 282: 1073–1075.

34 Hughes DA, Wright AJA, Finglas PM, *et al*. The effect of beta-carotene supplementation on the immune function of blood monocytes from healthy male non-smokers. *J Lab Clin Med* 1997; 129: 309–317.

35 Santos MS, Leka LS, Ribaya-Mercado D, *et al*. Short and long-term beta-carotene supplementation do not influence T cell-mediated immunity in healthy elderly persons. *Am J Clin Nutr* 1997; 66: 917–924.

36 Hammond BR Jr, Johnson EJ, Russell RM, *et al*. Dietary modification of human macular pigment density. *Invest Ophthalmol Vis Sci* 1997; 38: 1795–1801.

37 Lyle BJ, Mares-Perlman JA, Klein BE, *et al*. Antioxidant intake and risk of incident age related nuclear cataracts in the Beaver Dam Eye Study. *Am J Epidemiol* 1999; 149: 801–809.

38 Dagnelie G, Zorge IS, McDonald TM. Lutein improves visual function in some patients with retinal degeneration: a pilot study via the Internet. *Optometry* 2000; 7: 147–164.

39 Landrum JT, Bone RA, Joa H, *et al*. A one year study of the macular pigment: the effect of 140 days of a lutein supplement. *Exp Eye Res* 1997; 65: 57–62.

40 Mohanty I, Joshi S, Trivedi D, *et al*. Lycopene prevents sugar-induced morphological changes and modulates antioxidant status of human lens epithelial cells. *Br J Nutr* 2002; 88: 347–354.

41 Mares-Perlman JA, Millen AE, Ficek TL, Hankinson SE. The body of evidence to support a protective role

for lutein and zeaxanthin in delaying chronic disease. *J Nutr* 2002; 132 (Suppl.): S518–524.

42 Chasan-Taber L, Willett WC, Seddon JM, *et al*. A prospective study of carotenoid and vitamin A status and risk of cataract extraction in US women. *Am J Clin Nutr* 1999; 70: 509–516.

43 Brown L, Rimm EB, Seddon JM, *et al*. A prospective study of carotenoid extraction in US men. *Am J Clin Nutr* 1999; 70: 517–524.

44 Lyle BJ, Mares-Perlman JA, Klein BE, *et al*. Serum carotenoids and tocopherols and incidence of age-related nuclear cataract. *Am J Clin Nutr* 1999; 69: 272–277.

45 Gale CR, Hall NF, Phillips DIW, Martyn C. Plasma antioxidant vitamins and carotenoids and age-related cataract. *Ophthalmology* 2001; 108: 1992–1998.

46 Olmedilla B, Granado F, Blanco I, Vaquero M. Lutein, but not alpha-tocopherol, supplementation improves visual function in patients with age-related cataracts: a 2-y double-blind, placebo-controlled pilot study. *Nutrition* 2003; 19: 21–4.

47 Richer S, Stiles W, Statuke L, *et al*. Double-masked, placebo-controlled, randomized trial of lutein antioxidant supplementation in the intervention of atrophic age-related macular degeneration: the Veterans LAST study (Lutein Antioxidant Supplementation Trial). *Optometry* 2004; 75: 216–230.

48 Mares-Perlman JA, Brady WE, Klein R, *et al*. Serum antioxidants and age related macular degeneration in a population-based case-control study. *Arch Ophthalmol* 1995; 113: 1518–1523.

49 Agarwal S, Rao AV. Tomato lycopene and low density lipoprotein oxidation: a human dietary intervention study. *Lipids* 1998; 33: 981–984.

50 Giovanucci E. Tomatoes, tomato-based products, lycopene and cancer. Review of the epidemiologic literature. *J Natl Cancer Inst* 1999; 91: 317–331.

51 Gann PH, Ma J, Giovannucci E, *et al*. Lower prostate cancer risk in men with elevated plasma lycopene levels: results of a prospective analysis. *Cancer Res* 1999; 59: 1225–1230.

52 Kucuk O, Sarkar FH, Sakr W, *et al*. Phase II randomized clinical trial of lycopene supplementation before radical prostatectomy. *Cancer Epidemiol Biomarkers Prev* 2001; 8: 861–868.

53 Kucuk O, Sarkar FH, Djuric Z, *et al*. Effects of lycopene supplementation in patients with localized prostate cancer. *Exp Biol Med* 2002; 227: 881–885.

54 Ansari MS, Gupta NP. A comparison of lycopene and orchidectomy vs orchidectomy alone in the management of advanced prostate cancer. *BJU Int* 2003; 92: 375–378.

55 Schroder FH, Roobol MJ, Boeve ER, *et al*. Randomized, double-blind, placebo-controlled crossover study in men with prostate cancer and rising PSA: effectiveness of a dietary supplement. *Eur Urol* 2005; 48: 922–930.

56 Etminan M, Takkouche B, Caamano-Isorna F. The role of tomato products and lycopene in the prevention of prostate cancer: a meta-analysis of observational studies. *Cancer Epidemiol Biomarkers Prev* 2004; 3: 340–345.

Chitosan

Description

Chitosan is a fibre extracted from chitin, which is a structural component of crustacean shells, crabs, shrimps and lobsters. Chitin is de-acetylated to produce chitosan.

Constituents

Chitosan is a polysaccharide containing numerous acetyl groups.

Action

Chitosan binds fat molecules as a result of its ionic nature. When taken orally, chitosan has been reported to be able to bind 8–10 times its own weight in fat from food that has been consumed. This prevents fat from being absorbed and the body then has to burn stored fat, which may lead to reductions in body fat and body weight.

Possible uses

Weight loss

In mice treated with chitosan and given a high-fat diet, chitosan prevented the increase in body weight, hyperlipidaemia and fatty liver normally induced by such a diet.[1]

In a randomised, placebo-controlled, double-blind study, 34 overweight human volunteers were given four capsules of chitosan or placebo for 28 consecutive days. Subjects maintained their normal diet and documented their food intake. After 4 weeks of treatment, body mass index, serum cholesterol, triglycerides, vitamin A, D and E and beta-carotene were not significantly different in the two groups. The results

suggest that chitosan in the dose given had no effect on body weight in overweight subjects. No serious adverse effects were reported.[2]

In another placebo-controlled, double-blind study, 51 healthy obese women were given chitosan 1200 mg twice a day for 8 weeks. No reductions in weight were observed in any treatment group. LDL cholesterol fell to a greater extent in the chitosan group than the placebo group, but there was no significant change in HDL cholesterol and triglycerides were slightly increased.[3]

A 24-week randomised, double-blind, placebo-controlled trial involving 250 obese women found that the chitosan group lost more weight than the placebo group but the effects were very small.[4] A systematic review of 14 RCTs involving a total of 1071 participants found that weight loss in high-quality studies was less than in lower quality studies. The review concluded that the effect of chitosan on body weight is minimal and unlikely to be of clinical significance.[5]

Chitosan reduced blood glucose and cholesterol in an animal model of lean-type non-insulin-dependent diabetes mellitus with hypoinsulinaemia,[6] but had no effect in an animal model of obese-type NIDDM with hyperinsulinaemia.[7] The authors concluded that chitosan could be a useful treatment for lean-type NIDDM with hypoinsulinaemia.[6] Two recent double-blind RCTs in humans investigating the effect of chitosan on plasma cholesterol have shown conflicting results. One was a Japanese study involving 90 women with mild to moderate hypercholesterolaemia, which found that chitosan significantly reduced cholesterol although the effect was small.[8] The second was a Finnish study in 130 men and women

61

with moderately increased plasma cholesterol, which found that chitosan had no effect on the concentrations of plasma lipids or glucose.[9]

Conclusion

Chitosan is promoted for weight loss, but there have been few trials, and results have been conflicting. Any effect of chitosan on body weight is likely to be very small. Chitosan has also been investigated for an effect on plasma cholesterol, but the effects are likely to be very small, if any.

Precautions/contraindications

Chitosan should be avoided in patients with gastrointestinal malabsorption conditions.

Pregnancy and breast-feeding

No problems have been reported, but weight loss should not be attempted during pregnancy.

Adverse effects

There are no long-term studies assessing the safety of chitosan. However, chitosan may reduce the absorption of fat-soluble vitamins (A, D, E and K). This has been shown in animals,[7] but not in humans.[2,3]

Interactions

None reported.

Dose

Chitosan is available in the form of tablets and capsules.

The dose is not established. Dietary supplements provide 1500–3000 mg per daily dose.

References

1 Han LK, Kimura Y, Okuda H. Reduction in fat storage during chitin-chitosan treatment in mice fed a high-fat diet. *Int J Obes Relat Metab Disord* 1999; 23: 174–179.
2 Pittler MH, Abbott NC, Harkness EF, Ernst E. Randomized, double-blind trial of chitosan for body weight reduction. *Eur J Clin Nutr* 1999; 53: 379–381.
3 Wuolijoki E, Hirvela T, Ylitalo P. Decrease in serum LDL cholesterol with microcrystalline chitosan. *Methods Find Exp Clin Pharmacol* 1999; 21: 357–361.
4 Mhurchu CN, Poppitt SD, McGill AT, *et al.* The effect of the dietary supplement, chitosan, on body weight: a randomised controlled trial in 250 overweight and obese adults. *Int J Obes Relat Metab Disord* 2004; 28: 1149–1156.
5 Mhurchu CN, Dunshea-Mooij C, Bennett D, Rodgers A. Effect of chitosan on weight loss in overweight and obese individuals: a systematic review of randomized controlled trials. *Obes Rev* 2005; 6: 3–4.
6 Miura T, Usami M, Tsuura Y, *et al.* Hypoglycemic and hypolipidemic effect of chitosan in normal and neonatal streptozotocin-induced diabetic mice. *Biol Pharm Bull* 1995; 18: 1623–1625.
7 Deuchi K, Kanauchi O, Shizukuishi M, *et al.* Continuous and massive intake of chitosan affects soluble vitamin status in rats fed on a high fat diet. *Biosci Biotech Biochem* 1995; 59: 1211–1216.
8 Bokura H, Kobayashi S. Chitosan decreases total cholesterol in women: a randomized, double-blind, placebo-controlled trial. *Eur J Clin Nutr* 2003; 57: 721–725.
9 Metso S, Ylitalo R, Nikkila M, *et al.* The effect of long-term microcrystalline chitosan therapy on plasma lipids and glucose concentrations in subjects with increased plasma total cholesterol: a randomised placebo-controlled double-blind crossover trial in healthy men and women. *Eur J Clin Pharmacol* 2003; 59: 741–746.

Chlorella

Description

Chlorella is a single-celled freshwater alga.

Constituents

Chlorella is rich in chlorophyll. Manufacturers claim that it is a source of amino acids, nucleic acids, fatty acids, vitamins and minerals. However, content varies with conditions of growing, harvesting and processing. *Chlorella* is claimed to contain a unique substance called Chlorella Growth Factor. The claimed nutrient content of *Chlorella* is shown in Table 1.

Action

Chlorella may have antitumour and antiviral activities, and may also be able to stimulate the immune system, but these effects have not been clarified in human studies.

Possible uses

Chlorella is promoted as a tonic for general health maintenance; it is a useful source of some nutrients (e.g. beta-carotene, riboflavine, vitamin B_{12}, iron and zinc; see Constituents).

In addition, *Chlorella* is claimed to be useful in: accelerating the healing of wounds and ulcers; improving digestion and bowel function; stimulating growth and repair of tissues; slowing down ageing; strengthening the immune system; improving the condition of the hair, skin, teeth and nails; treating colds and respiratory infections; and removing poisonous substances from the body. These claims are based largely on anecdote; *Chlorella* has no proven efficacy for these conditions.

Table 1 Claimed[1] nutrient content of *Chlorella*

Nutrient	per 100 g	per typical dose(3 g)	% RNI[2]
Protein (g)	66	2	–
Fat (g)	9	0.3	–
Carbohydrate (g)	11	0.3	–
Vitamin A (μg) (as beta-carotene)	5500	165	28
Thiamine (mg)	2.0	0.06	8
Riboflavin (mg)	7.0	0.2	24
Niacin (mg)	30	0.9	6
Vitamin B_6 (mg)	1.5	0.05	4
Vitamin B_{12} (μg)	134	4	270
Folic acid (μg)	25	0.75	0.4
Pantothenic acid (mg)	3.0	0.09	–
Biotin (μg)	190	6	–
Vitamin C (mg)	60	1.8	5
Vitamin E (mg)	17	0.5	–
Choline (mg)	270	8.1	–
Inositol (mg)	190	5.7	–
Calcium (mg)	500	15	2
Magnesium (mg)	300	9	3
Potassium (mg)	700	21	0.6
Phosphorus (mg)	1200	36	6.5
Iron (mg)	260	8	80
Zinc (mg)	70	2	26
Copper (μg)	80	2.4	0.2
Iodine (μg)	600	18	13

[1] Reported on a product label.
[2] Reference Nutrient Intake for men aged 19–50 years.

Preliminary evidence from an uncontrolled study in 20 patients over a period of 2 months showed that *Chlorella* supplementation may help relieve the symptoms of fibromyalgia.[1] However, the authors concluded that a larger, more comprehensive double-blind, placebo-controlled trial in these patients is warranted.

Other preliminary evidence suggests that *Chlorella* could help patients with brain tumours to better tolerate chemotherapy and radiotherapy. However, there appears to be no effect on tumour progression or survival.[2]

> **Conclusion**
> There is insufficient reliable information to recommend the use of *Chlorella* for any indication.

Precautions/contraindications

No problems have been reported.

Pregnancy and breast-feeding

No problems have been reported.

Adverse effects

None reported, but *Chlorella* may provoke allergic reactions.

Interactions

None reported, but *Chlorella* may contain significant amounts of vitamin K. This could inhibit the activity of warfarin and other anti-coagulants.

Dose

Chlorella is available in the form of tablets, capsules, liquid extracts and powder.

The dose is not established. Dietary supplements provide 500–3000 mg of the intact organism per daily dose.

References

1 Merchant RE, Carmack CA, Wise CM. Nutritional supplementation with *Chlorella pyredinosa* for patients with fibromyalgia syndrome: a pilot study. *Phytother Res* 2000; 14: 167–173.
2 Merchant RE, Rice CD, Young HF. Dietary *Chlorella pyredinosa* for patients with malignant glioma: effects on immunocompetence, quality of life and survival. *Phytother Res* 1990; 4: 220–231.

Choline

Description

Choline is associated with the vitamin B complex; it is not an officially recognised vitamin. Choline is a component of phosphatidylcholine and an active constituent of dietary lecithin, but the two substances are not synonymous.

Human requirements

Choline is an essential nutrient for several mammalian organisms, but there is no agreement over its essentiality as a vitamin for humans. However, the US Food and Nutrition Board of the National Institute of Medicine has established a Dietary Reference Intake for adults of 550 mg a day for men and 425 mg a day for women, with lower amounts for children, together with an upper intake level of 3.5 g daily for adults over 18 years.

Dietary intake

Estimated dietary intake in the UK is 250–500 mg daily. Choline can also be synthesised in the body from phosphatidylethanolamine.

Action

Choline serves as a source of labile methyl groups for transmethylation reactions. It functions as a component of other molecules such as the neurotransmitter acetylcholine, phosphatidylcholine (lecithin) and sphingomyelin, structural constituents of cell membranes and plasma lipoproteins, platelet activating factor and plasmalogen (a phospholipid found in highest concentrations in cardiac muscle membranes).

Lecithin and sphingomyelin participate in signal transduction,[1] an essential process for cell growth, regulation and function. Animal studies suggest that choline or lecithin deficiency may interfere with this critical process and that alterations in signal transduction may lead to abnormalities such as cancer and Alzheimer's disease.

Dietary sources

Choline is widely distributed in foods (mainly in the form of lecithin). The richest sources of choline are brewer's yeast, egg yolk, liver, wheatgerm, soya beans, kidney and brain. Oats, peanuts, beans and cauliflower contain significant amounts.

Metabolism

Absorption
Some choline is absorbed intact, probably by a carrier-mediated mechanism; some is metabolised by the gastrointestinal flora to trimethylamine (which produces a fishy odour).

Distribution
Choline is stored in the brain, kidney and liver, primarily as phosphatidylcholine (lecithin) and sphingomyelin.

Elimination
Elimination of choline occurs mainly via the urine.

Deficiency

Dietary choline deficiency occurs in animals, and abnormal liver function, liver cirrhosis and fatty liver may be associated with choline deficiency in humans. Observations in patients on total parenteral nutrition (TPN) have shown a choline-deficient diet to result in fatty infiltration of the liver, hepatocellular damage and liver dysfunction.[2,3]

Possible uses

As a precursor of acetylcholine, it has been suggested that choline could increase the concentration of acetylcholine in the brain. It has been suggested, therefore, that choline could be beneficial in patients with disease related to impaired cholinergic transmission (e.g. tardive dyskinesia, Huntington's chorea, Alzheimer's disease, Gilles de la Tourette, mania, memory impairment and ataxia). However, experimental evidence suggests that oral choline has no effect on choline metabolites in the brain.[4]

Comparison of studies involving choline is often complicated by lack of standardisation of doses used. However, clinical trials with tardive dyskinesia patients using choline have met with some success.[4–7]

Choline has also been suggested to improve performance in athletes. This idea arose because of findings that plasma choline concentrations were reduced in trained runners[8] and athletes[9] after sporting events. However, a double-blind crossover study in 20 cyclists showed that choline supplementation did not delay fatigue during brief or prolonged exercise.[10]

Claims have been made for the value of choline in the prevention of CVD, including angina, atherosclerosis, hypertension, stroke and thrombosis. However, scientific evidence for these claims from RCTs is lacking. Interest has recently focused on the potential for choline (as a precursor of betaine) to reduce plasma homocysteine. One crossover study showed that phosphatidylcholine supplementation (2.6 g choline daily for 2 weeks) lowers fasting as well as post-methionine-loading plasma homocysteine concentrations in healthy men with mildly elevated homocysteine concentrations.[11] Choline (in conjunction with carnitine) supplementation has also been shown to lower lipid peroxidation and promote conservation of antioxidants (e.g. retinol and alpha-tocopherol) in women.[12]

Choline has also been claimed to prevent and/or treat Alzheimer's disease, senile dementia and memory loss. A Cochrane review of 14 studies found some evidence that cytidine-diphosphocholine (CDP-choline) has a positive effect on memory and behaviour at least in the short to medium term, but evidence is limited by the quality of the studies.[13]

> ### Conclusion
> Research on choline supplementation is limited and studies are generally very poorly controlled. The limited research shows that choline does not appear to improve athletic performance. Very preliminary evidence suggests choline might be beneficial in poor memory and tardive dyskinesia, but evidence is not sufficient to recommend supplementation.

Precautions/contraindications

No problems have been reported.

Pregnancy and breast-feeding

No problems have been reported.

Adverse effects

Fishy odour; more severe symptoms relate to excessive cholinergic transmission (doses of 10 g daily or more) and include diarrhoea, nausea, dizziness, sweating, salivation, depression and a longer P-R interval in electrocardiograms.

Interactions

None established.

Dose

Choline is available in the form of tablets and capsules.

The dose is not established. Dietary supplements generally provide 250–500 mg per dose (choline chloride provides 80% choline and choline tartrate 50% choline).

References

1 Canty DJ, Zeisel SH. Lecithin and choline in human health and disease. *Nutr Rev* 1994; 52: 327–339.

2 Sheard NF, Tayek JA, Bistrian BR, Blackburn GL, Zeisel SH. Plasma choline concentration in humans fed parenterally. *Am J Clin Nutr* 1986; 43: 219–224.

3 Zeisel SH, DaCosta KA, Franklin PD. Choline, an essential nutrient for humans. *FASEB J* 1991; 5: 2093–2098.

4 Davis KL, Berger PA, Hollister LE. Choline for tardive dyskinesia. *N Engl J Med* 1975; 293: 152–153.

5 Gelenberg AJ, Doller-Wojcik JC, Growdon JH. Choline and lecithin in the treatment of tardive dyskinesia: preliminary results from a pilot study. *Am J Psychiatr* 1979; 136: 772–776.

6 Growdon JH, Hirsch MJ, Wurtman RJ, Wiener W. Oral choline administration to patients with tardive dyskinesia. *N Engl J Med* 1977; 297: 524–527.

7 Tamminga CA, Smith RC, Erickson SE, *et al.* Cholinergic influences in tardive dyskinesia. *Am J Psychiatr* 1977; 134: 769–774.

8 Conlay LA, Saboujian LA, Wurtman RJ. Exercise and neuromodulators: choline and acetylcholine in marathon runners. *Int J Sports Med* 1992; 13: S141–142.

9 Von Allworden HN, Horn S, Kahl J, *et al.* The influence of lecithin on plasma choline concentrations in triathletes and adolescent runners during exercise. *Eur J Appl Physiol* 1993; 67: 87–91.

10 Spector SA, Jackman MR, Sabounjian LA, *et al.* Effect of choline supplementation on fatigue in trained cyclists. *Med Sci Sports Exerc* 1995; 27: 668–673.

11 Olthof MR, Brink EJ, Katan MB, Verhoef P. Choline supplemented as phosphatidylcholine decreases fasting and postmethionine-loading plasma homocysteine concentrations in healthy men. *Am J Clin Nutr* 2005; 82: 111–117.

12 Sachan DS, Hongu N, Johnsen M. Decreasing oxidative stress with choline and carnitine in women. *J Am Coll Nutr* 2005; 24: 172–176.

13 Fioravanti M, Yanagi M. Cytidinediphosphocholine (CDP-choline) for cognitive and behavioural disturbances associated with chronic cerebral disorders in the elderly. Cochrane database, issue 2, 2005. London: Macmillan.

Chondroitin

Description

Chondroitin is a natural physiological compound that is synthesised endogenously and secreted by the chondrocytes. It is found in joint cartilage and connective tissue (including vessel walls).

Constituents

Chondroitin is a mixture of high molecular weight glycosaminoglycans and disaccharide polymers composed of equimolar amounts of D-glucuronic acid, D-acetylgalactosamine and sulphates in 10–30 disaccharide units. (Glycosaminoglycans are the substances in which collagen fibres are embedded in cartilage.)

Action

Chondroitin absorbs water, adding to the thickness and elasticity of cartilage and its ability to absorb and distribute compressive forces. It also appears to control the formation of new cartilage matrix, by stimulating chondrocyte metabolism and synthesis of collagen and proteoglycan. Chondroitin also inhibits degradative enzymes (elastase and hyaluronidase), which break down cartilage matrix and synovial fluid, contributing to cartilage destruction and loss of joint function.

Possible uses

Osteoarthritis

Chondroitin is claimed to be useful as a dietary supplement in combination with glucosamine in osteoarthritis and related disorders. Preliminary evidence suggests that chondroitin reduces the pain of osteoarthritis in the knee compared with placebo.

In a multicentre, randomised, double-blind, controlled study, involving 127 patients with osteoarthritis of the knee, 40 were treated with chondroitin sulphate oral gel 1200 mg daily, capsules 1200 mg daily or placebo for 3 months. Chondroitin (both formulations) significantly improved subjective symptoms, including joint mobility.[1]

In a randomised, double-blind, placebo-controlled study, 80 patients with knee osteoarthritis participated in a 6-month study and received either 2×400 mg chondroitin capsules twice a day or placebo. Symptoms of joint pain and time to perform a 20-metre walk were significantly reduced in the treated group, and there was a non-significant trend for the placebo group to use more paracetamol.[2]

A 1-year, randomised, double-blind, controlled pilot study included 42 patients with symptomatic knee osteoarthritis. Patients were treated orally with 800 mg chondroitin sulphate or placebo. Chondroitin sulphate was well tolerated and significantly reduced pain and increased overall mobility. In addition, bone and joint metabolism stabilised in the treated patients, but not in those on placebo.[3]

A meta-analysis that included seven trials of 372 patients taking chondroitin found that over 120 or more days, chondroitin was significantly superior to placebo with respect to the Lesquesne index and pain rating on a visual analogue scale (VAS). Pooling the data confirmed these results, and showed at least 50% improvement in the treated versus the placebo patients. The authors concluded that further investigations using larger cohorts of patients for longer time periods were needed to prove the usefulness of chondroitin as a symptom-modifying agent in osteoarthritis.[4]

A randomised, double-blind, double-dummy study compared the efficacy of chondroitin with diclofenac in 146 patients with knee osteoarthritis. During the first month, patients received either 3×50 mg diclofenac tablets daily plus 3×400 mg placebo sachets, or 3×400 mg chondroitin sachets daily plus 3×50 mg placebo tablets. From months two to three, the diclofenac patients were given placebo sachets alone, and the chondroitin patients were given chondroitin sachets. Both groups were treated with placebo sachets from months four to six. The diclofenac group showed prompt pain reduction, which disappeared after the end of treatment. In the chondroitin group, the therapeutic response appeared later, but lasted for up to 3 months after the end of treatment.[5]

Chondroitin sulphate 1 g daily was investigated in a prospective, double-blind, placebo-controlled, multicentre clinical study in patients with femetotibial osteoarthritis. Treatment continued for 3 months and there was a 3-month post-treatment period. There was a trend towards efficacy, with good tolerability after 3 months' treatment, and persistent efficacy 1 month post-treatment.[6]

Conclusion

Chondroitin appears to offer some pain relief in osteoarthritis. However, studies conducted so far have involved small numbers of subjects and have been short. Further research is required to establish the place of chondroitin as a supplement for osteoarthritis.

Precautions/contraindications

No problems have been reported.

Pregnancy and breast-feeding

No problems have been reported but there have not been sufficient studies to guarantee the safety of chondroitin in pregnancy and breast-feeding. Chondroitin is probably best avoided.

Adverse effects

There are no known serious side-effects. However, there are no long term studies assessing the safety of chondroitin. Rarely, gastrointestinal effects and headache have been reported. However, studies in animals have found significantly decreased haematocrit, haemoglobin, white blood cells and platelet count, and the risk of internal bleeding has been suggested.[7] However, there are no reports of bleeding as a result of chondroitin use in humans.

Interactions

Drugs

Anticoagulants: Theoretically, chondroitin could potentiate the effects of anticoagulants.

Dose

Chondroitin is available in the form of capsules, typically containing 250–750 mg, often in combination with glucosamine. A review of two US products containing chondroitin showed that both had lower chondroitin levels than declared on the labels; this was also found for six out of 13 glucosamine and chondroitin combination products, all due to low chondroitin levels.[8]

The dose is not established. Manufacturers tend to recommend 400–1200 mg daily.

References

1 Bourgeois P, Chales G, Dehais J, *et al*. Efficacy and tolerability of chondroitin sulfate 1200 mg/day vs chondroitin 3 x 400 mg/day vs placebo. *Osteoarthritis Cartilage* 1998; 6 (Suppl. A): 5–30.

2 Bucsi L, Poor G. Efficacy and tolerability of oral chondroitin sulfate as a symptomatic slow-acting drug for osteoarthritis (SYASDOA) in the treatment of knee osteoarthritis. *Osteoarthritis Cartilage* 1998; 6 (Suppl. A): 1–6.

3 Uebelhart D, Thonar EJ, Delmad PD, *et al*. Effects of oral chondroitin sulfate on the progression of knee osteoarthritis: a pilot study. *Osteoarthritis Cartilage* 1998; 6 (Suppl. A): 9–46.

4 Leeb BF, Schweitzer H, Montag K, Smolen JS. A meta-analysis of chondroitin sulfate in the treatment of osteoarthritis. *J Rheumatol* 2000; 7: 205–211.

5 Morreale P, Manopulo R, Galati M. Comparison of anti-inflammatory efficacy of chondroitin sulfate

and diclofenac sodium in patients with knee osteo-arthritis. *J Rheumatol* 1996; 3: 1385–1391.

6   Mazieres B, Combe B, Phan Van A, *et al*. Chondroitin sulphate in osteoarthritis of the knee: a prospective, double-blind, placebo-controlled multicenter clinical study. *J Rheumatol* 2001; 28: 173–181.

7   McNamara PS, Barr SC, Erb HN, *et al*. Hematologic, hemostatic and biochemical effects in dogs receiving an oral chondroprotective agent for thirty days. *Am J Vet Res* 1996; 57: 1390–1394.

8   Consumerlab. Product review. Glucosamine and chondroitin. http://www.consumerlab.com (accessed 12 November 2006).

Chromium

Description

Chromium is an essential trace mineral.

Human requirements

In the UK, no Reference Nutrient Intake or Estimated Average Requirement has been set. A safe and adequate intake is, for adults, 50–400 µg daily; for children and adolescents, 0.1–1.0 µg/kg daily.

In the USA, the Adequate Intake (AI) for men (19–50 years) is 35 µg daily and for women (19–50 years) is 25 µg daily. For those aged over 51, the AI is 30 µg daily for men and 20 µg daily for women.

Dietary intake

In the UK, the average adult diet provides 13.6–47.7 µg daily.

Action

Chromium functions as an organic complex known as glucose tolerance factor (GTF), which is thought to be a complex of chromium, nicotinic acid and amino acids. It potentiates the action of insulin and thus influences carbohydrate, fat and protein metabolism. Chromium also appears to influence nucleic acid synthesis and to play a role in gene expression.

Dietary sources

Wholegrain cereals (including bran cereals), brewer's yeast, broccoli, processed meats and spices are the best sources. Dairy products and most fruits and vegetables are poor sources.

Metabolism

Absorption

Chromium is poorly absorbed (0.5–2% of intake); absorption occurs in the small intestine by mechanisms that have not been clearly elucidated, but which appear to involve processes other than simple diffusion.

Distribution

Chromium is transported in the serum or plasma bound to transferrin and albumin. It is widely distributed in the tissues.

Elimination

Absorbed chromium is excreted mainly by the kidneys, with small amounts lost in hair, sweat and bile.

Bioavailability

Absorption of chromium is increased by oxalate and by iron deficiency, and reduced by phytate. Diets high in simple sugars (glucose, fructose, sucrose) increase urinary chromium losses. Absorption is also increased in patients with diabetes mellitus, and depressed in the elderly. Stress and increased physical activity appear to increase urinary losses.

Deficiency

Gross chromium deficiency is rarely seen in humans, but signs and symptoms of marginal deficiency include: impaired glucose intolerance, fasting hyperglycaemia, raised circulating insulin levels, glycosuria, decreased insulin binding, reduced number of insulin receptors, elevated serum cholesterol, elevated serum triglycerides, and central and peripheral neuropathy.

Possible uses

Because of its effects on insulin, chromium has been investigated for a potential role in diabetes mellitus, and it has also been promoted for body building in athletes. It has also been investigated for a potential role in cholesterol lowering and reducing the risk of CVD.

Diabetes mellitus

Chromium deficiency may result in insulin resistance,[1] although other researchers have concluded that low-chromium diets have no effect on either insulin or blood glucose.[2] Chromium supplementation may improve glycaemic control in some patients with type 1 and 2 diabetes and gestational diabetes, but relatively high doses (e.g. 1000 µg daily) may be needed. Serum lipid fractions may also be reduced by chromium in patients with diabetes.

Chromium picolinate (200 µg three times a day) reduced glycosylated haemoglobin in a woman with type 1 diabetes mellitus, and the patient also reported improved blood glucose values.[3] Chromium picolinate (200 µg daily) increased insulin sensitivity in patients with type 1 and type 2 diabetes, allowing for a reduction in dose of insulin or hypoglycaemic drugs without compromising glucose control.[4] Steroid-induced diabetes was improved after supplementation with chromium 200 µg three times a day, and chromium 200 µg daily was sufficient to maintain normal blood glucose thereafter.[5]

In a double-blind, placebo-controlled trial, 180 patients with type 2 diabetes were randomised to receive 250 µg chromium twice a day, 100 µg chromium twice a day, or placebo. After 2 months, glycosylated haemoglobin levels were significantly lower in the high-dose chromium group and after 4 months were lower in both chromium groups compared with placebo. Fasting and 2-hour insulin levels were significantly lower in both chromium groups at 2 and 4 months, but significantly lower

glucose values and lower plasma cholesterol were found only in the high-dose chromium group.[6]

In a prospective, double-blind, placebo-controlled, crossover study in 28 subjects with type 2 diabetes, serum triglycerides were significantly reduced by chromium (200 µg daily for 2 months).[7] However, there was no change in fasting glucose, or plasma LDL or HDL levels.

In a double-blind, placebo-controlled, crossover study, 78 patients with type 2 diabetes in Saudi Arabia received in random order brewer's yeast (23 µg chromium) and 200 µg chromium from chromium chloride for 4 weeks each. Mean HDL cholesterol and serum and urinary chromium were all raised by chromium intake. After each chromium phase, mean drug dosage tended to decrease, but was not significant except in the case of glibenclamide. There was no change in dietary intakes or body mass index. Overall, brewer's yeast was associated with better chromium retention and more positive effects than chromium chloride.[8]

Supplementation of nicotinic acid together with chromium may increase its effectiveness. In a study involving 16 healthy elderly volunteers, neither chromium 200 µg daily nor nicotinic acid 100 mg daily affected fasting glucose or glucose tolerance. However, chromium administered with nicotinic acid resulted in a 15% decrease in the area under the glucose curve and a 7% decrease in fasting glucose.[9]

A systematic review and meta-analysis of 15 RCTs involving 618 participants, of whom 193 had type 2 diabetes and 425 were in good health or had impaired glucose tolerance, showed that there was no effect of chromium on glucose or insulin concentrations in non-diabetic subjects and the data for people with diabetes were inconclusive. Only one of the studies in the meta-analysis, involving 155 subjects in China, showed that chromium reduced glucose and insulin concentrations and HbA1c.[10]

Further studies have investigated other potential effects of chromium in patients with diabetes. Chromium supplementation has been found to minimise increased oxidative stress in type 2 diabetes mellitus patients with high HbA1c levels.[11] Chromium supplementation (400 or 800 µg) improved glucose tolerance in 10 out of 13 subjects in a randomised crossover study.[12] Short-term chromium supplementation (1000 µg) has also been found to shorten QTc interval in patients with type 2 diabetes mellitus.[13]

A US review concluded that there is little evidence that chromium has any value in glucose metabolism in those without type 2 diabetes, or on weight loss. The review also suggested that it may have a value in type 2 diabetes but this is still to be established. Another conclusion was that there is some evidence that chromium added to total parenteral nutrition (TPN) solutions may reduce the risk of hyperglycaemia in patients receiving this therapy.[14]

Obesity

In some controlled human studies, chromium has been reported to reduce body fat[15,16] and increase fat-free mass,[17] but to have no effect in others.[18] A meta-analysis of 10 trials found that chromium picolinate had a favourable effect on body weight. However, sensitivity analysis suggested that this effect is largely dependent on the results of a single trial. The authors concluded that the effect of chromium is likely to be small and its clinical relevance debatable.[19]

Body-building

Chromium supplements are claimed to influence body composition during body-building programmes, although there is little evidence for this. In a study involving 36 men on a weight-training programme, chromium supplementation had no effect on strength, fat-free mass or muscle mass.[20] Chromium picolinate (200 µg a day) did not alter body fat, lean body mass and skin-fold thickness in untrained young men on an exercise programme.[21] Neither body composition nor strength changed as a result of chromium picolinate supplementation (200 µg daily) in football players during a 9-week training programme.[22] Young women on a weight-training programme taking chromium picolinate (200 µg daily for 12 weeks) gained significantly more weight than those taking

a placebo, and there was a non-significant increase in lean body mass.[23] However, there were no effects on body composition or strength in the young men on the same programme. In moderately obese women placed on an exercise programme, 12 weeks of chromium supplementation (400 µg daily) did not significantly affect body composition, resting metabolic rate, plasma glucose, serum insulin, plasma glucagons, serum C-peptide and serum lipid concentrations.[24]

Cardiovascular disease

Chromium supplements have been claimed to reduce serum cholesterol levels, and there is some evidence for this.

Two placebo-controlled trials, one in 76 men on beta-blockers (a double-blind study),[25] the other in 76 patients with atherosclerosis (not blinded),[26] showed a significant increase in serum HDL cholesterol with chromium (300 µg daily in the first study, 200 µg daily in the second). In a double-blind, placebo-controlled, crossover study in 28 healthy subjects,[27] chromium supplementation (200 µg daily) resulted in a statistically significant reduction in total and LDL cholesterol. HDL was not raised significantly, although apolipoprotein A-1 (the principal protein in A-1) was increased.

Depression

Patients with depression may respond to chromium. In a double-blind RCT, 113 adults with atypical depression, most of whom were obese, were randomised to receive 600 µg of elemental chromium or placebo. Chromium produced an improvement in carbohydrate craving and appetite increase and diurnal variation in feelings. The results suggested that the main benefit of chromium was in depressed patients with high carbohydrate craving. The authors concluded that further research is needed in depressed patients specifically selected for symptoms of increased appetite and carbohydrate craving.[28]

Conclusion

Preliminary evidence suggests that chromium may improve insulin resistance and glucose control in diabetes, although not all studies have reached this conclusion. Preliminary evidence also suggests that chromium may improve serum lipid levels. However, there is no good evidence that chromium reduces body weight or body fat. Despite claims made for chromium in sports, there is no evidence that it has body-building effects in athletes. Preliminary evidence suggests that chromium may be helpful in depression with carbohydrate craving.

Precautions/contraindications

Chromium supplements containing yeast should be avoided by patients taking monoamine oxidase inhibitors. Patients with diabetes mellitus should not take chromium supplements unless medically supervised (chromium may potentiate insulin).

Pregnancy and breast-feeding

No problems reported at normal intakes.

Adverse effects

Oral chromium, particularly trivalent chromium (the usual form in supplements), is relatively non-toxic and unlikely to induce adverse effects. However, in 2003, the report of the Expert Group on Vitamins and Minerals (EVM) noted that there was some evidence suggesting that chromium picolinate might be genotoxic (i.e. it could damage DNA). In the light of this, the Food Standards Agency advised that consumers who wished to take chromium supplements should use other types of supplements until specialist advice had been received from the Committee on Mutagenicity (COM). The COM reviewed the evidence and recommended more research. On the basis of this research the COM concluded that the balance of evidence suggested that chromium picolinate was not genotoxic.

Industrial exposure to high amounts of chromate dust is associated with an increased incidence of lung cancer and may cause allergic dermatitis and skin ulcers. The hexavalent form (not found in food or supplements) can cause renal and hepatic necrosis.

Interactions

Drugs

Insulin: may reduce insulin requirements in diabetes mellitus (monitor blood glucose).
Oral hypoglycaemics: may potentiate effects of oral hypoglycaemics.

Dose

Chromium is available in the form of chromium picolinate, chromium nicotinic acid, chromium chloride or as an organic complex in brewer's yeast. It is available in tablet and capsule form and is present in multivitamin/mineral preparations.

The dose is not established. Studies have been conducted with 200–500 µg elemental chromium daily. Dietary supplements provide, on average, 200 µg in a daily dose.

References

1   Mertz W. Chromium in human nutrition: a review. *J Nutr* 1993; 123: 626–633.
2   Anderson RA. Nutritional factors influencing the glucose/insulin system: chromium. *J Am Coll Nutr* 1997; 16: 404–410.
3   Fox GN, Sabovic Z. Chromium picolinate supplementation for diabetes mellitus. *J Fam Pract* 1998; 46: 83–86.
4   Ravina A, Slezak L, Rubal A. Clinical use of the trace element chromium(III) in the treatment of diabetes mellitus. *J Trace Elem Exper Med* 1995; 8: 183–190.
5   Ravina A, Slezak L, Mirsky N. Reversal of corticosteroid-induced diabetes mellitus with supplemental chromium. *Diabet Med* 1999; 16: 164–167.
6   Anderson RA, Cheng N, Bryden NA. Elevated intakes of supplemental chromium improve glucose and insulin variables in individuals with type 2 diabetes. *Diabetes* 1997; 46: 1786–1791.

7 Lee NA, Reasner CA. Beneficial effect of chromium supplementation on serum triglyceride levels in NIDDM. *Diabetes Care* 1994; 17: 1449–1452.

8 Bahijiri SM, Mira SA, Mufti AM, *et al.* The effects of inorganic chromium and brewer's yeast supplementation on glucose tolerance, serum lipids, and drug dosage in individuals with type 2 diabetes. *Saudi Med J* 2000; 21: 831–837.

9 Urberg M, Zemel MB. Evidence for synergism between chromium and nicotinic acid in the control of glucose tolerance in elderly humans. *Metabolism* 1987; 36: 896–899.

10 Althuis MD, Jordan NE, Ludington EA, Wittes JT. Glucose and insulin responses to dietary chromium supplements: a meta-analysis. *Am J Clin Nutr* 2002; 76: 148–155.

11 Cheng HH, Lai MH, Hou WC, Huang CL. Antioxidant effects of chromium supplementation with type 2 diabetes mellitus and euglycemic subjects. *J Agric Food Chem* 2004; 52: 1385–1389.

12 Frauchiger MT, Wenk C, Colombani PC. Effects of acute chromium supplementation on postprandial metabolism in healthy young men. *J Am Coll Nutr* 2004; 23: 351–357.

13 Vrtovec M, Vrtovec B, Briski A, *et al.* Chromium supplementation shortens QTc interval duration in patients with type 2 diabetes mellitus. *Am Heart J* 2005; 149: 632–636.

14 Anonymous. Chromium supplements. *Med Lett Drugs Ther* 2006; 48: 7–8.

15 Kaats GR, Blum K, Fisher JA. Effects of chromium picolinate supplementation on body composition: a randomized, double-masked, placebo-controlled study. *Curr Ther Res* 1996; 57: 747–756.

16 Kaats GR, Blum K, Pullin D. A randomized double-masked, placebo-controlled study of the effects of chromium picolinate supplementation on body composition: a replication and extension of a previous study. *Curr Ther Res* 1998; 59: 379–388.

17 Cefalu WT, Bell-Farrow AD, Wang ZQ. The effect of chromium supplementation on carbohydrate metabolism and body fat distribution. *Diabetes* 1997; 46 (Suppl. 1): 55A.

18 Trent LK, Thieding-Cancel D. Effects of chromium picolinate on body composition. *J Sports Med Phys Fitness* 1995; 35: 273–280.

19 Lukaski HC, Bolonchuk WW, Siders WA. Chromium supplementation and resistance training: effects on body composition, strength and trace element status of men. *Am J Clin Nutr* 1982; 35: 661–667.

20 Pittler MH, Stevinson C, Ernst E. Chromium picolinate for reducing body weight: meta-analysis of randomized trials. *Int J Obes Relat Metab Disord* 2003; 27: 522–529.

21 Hallmark MA, Reynolds TH, DeSouza TA. Effects of chromium and resistive training on muscle strength and body composition. *Med Sci Sports Exerc* 1996; 28: 139–144.

22 Clancy SP, Clarkson PM, DeCheke ME. Effects of chromium picolinate supplementation on body composition, strength and urinary chromium loss in football players. *Int J Sports Nutr* 1994; 4: 142–153.

23 Hasten DL, Rome EP, Franks BD. Effects of chromium picolinate on beginning weight training students. *Int J Sports Nutr* 1992; 2: 343–350.

24 Roeback JR, Hla KM, Chambless LE, *et al.* Effects of chromium supplementation on serum high density lipoprotein cholesterol in men taking beta-blockers. A randomized, controlled trial. *Ann Intern Med* 1991; 115: 917–924.

25 Volpe SL, Huang HW, Larpadisorn K, Lesser II. Effect of chromium supplementation and exercise on body composition, resting metabolic rate and selected biochemical parameters in moderately obese women following an exercise program. *J Am Coll Nutr* 2001; 20: 293–306.

26 Abraham AS, Brooks BA, Eylath U. The effect of chromium supplementation on serum glucose and lipids in patients with and without non-insulin dependent diabetes. *Metabolism* 1992; 41: 768–771.

27 Press RI, Geller J, Evans GW. The effect of chromium picolinate on serum cholesterol and apolipoprotein fractions in human subjects. *West J Med* 1990; 152: 41–45.

28 Docherty JP, Sack DA, Roffman M, *et al.* A double-blind, placebo-controlled exploratory trial of chromium picolinate in atypical depression: effect on carbohydrate craving. *J Psychiatr Pract* 2005; 11: 302–14.

Coenzyme Q

Description

Coenzyme Q is a naturally-occurring enzyme cofactor found in the mitochondria of the body cells.

Nomenclature

Several types of coenzyme Q have been identified and numbered from zero upwards. The variety found in human tissue is coenzyme Q_{10} (ubiquinone) and so is the term used here.

Action

Coenzyme Q_{10} has the following functions:

- It is involved in electron transport and supports the synthesis of adenosine triphosphate (ATP) in the mitochondrial membrane.
- It plays a vital role in intracellular energy production.
- It is a fat-soluble antioxidant that helps to stabilise cell membranes, preserving cellular integrity and function. It also helps to regenerate vitamin E to its antioxidant form.
- It is essential for normal myocardial function.
- It has immunostimulant activity.
- It may be obtained from the diet or a food supplement, but it is also produced endogenously.

Dietary sources

Meat and fatty fish products are the most concentrated sources, although smaller quantities are found in wholegrain cereals, soya beans, nuts and vegetables, particularly spinach and broccoli. The relative importance of endogenous synthesis and dietary intake to coenzyme Q_{10} status has not been established. Coenzyme Q_{10} is also found in a number of food supplements, either as the sole active ingredient or in combination with vitamins and/or minerals, especially magnesium.

Metabolism

Absorption of coenzyme Q_{10} from the diet or a supplement occurs in the small intestine and is influenced by the presence of food and drink. It is better absorbed in the presence of a fatty meal. After absorption, it is transported to the liver where it is incorporated into lipoproteins and bound principally to VLDL and LDL cholesterol. It is then concentrated in the tissues. One study found that coenzyme Q_{10} from both foods and supplements significantly raised serum concentrations.[1]

Coenzyme Q_{10} is produced endogenously from tyrosine within all cells of the body, but specifically in the heart, liver, kidney and pancreas, where it plays an indispensable role in intracellular energy production. Several cofactors are involved in its synthesis, including riboflavin, pyridoxine, folic acid, vitamin B_{12}, niacin, pantothenic acid and vitamin C. The ability to synthesise coenzyme Q_{10} decreases as people get older. The concentration of coenzyme Q_{10} in human tissue appears to be related to age, peaking at age 20 and declining after that.[2]

Deficiency

Because coenzyme Q_{10} is not an essential nutrient in the same way as a vitamin or mineral, no Dietary Reference Values or RDAs have been established. However, there is increasing speculation based on serum and/or biopsy samples that certain signs and symptoms are associated with a lack of coenzyme Q_{10}.

Deficiency has been linked to:

- CHF[3]
- ischaemic heart disease[4]
- cardiomyopathy[5]
- hypertension[4]
- use of HMG-CoA reductase inhibitors[6]
- hyperthyroidism[7]
- breast cancer.[8]

Whether the observed lack of coenzyme Q_{10} in these conditions is a true deficiency that contributes to the development of the disease or is caused by the disease itself is unclear. In heart failure, those with the most advanced disease have lower coenzyme Q_{10} levels than those with less advanced disease.[9] Low serum coenzyme Q_{10} levels are also associated with a significant risk of heart failure or increased mortality.[10]

Deficiency may occur as a result of:

- Inadequate intake or production, particularly if requirements are increased because of disease.
- Inadequate production caused by older age or by deficiencies of nutrients required for its synthesis.
- Genetic or acquired defects in synthesis or metabolism.
- Interactions with medicines. Beta-blockers, clonidine, gemfibrozil, hydralazine, hydrochlorothiazide, methyldopa, statins and tricyclic antidepressants may reduce levels of coenzyme Q_{10}.

Possible uses

Cardiovascular disease

The potential role of coenzyme Q_{10} in CVD has been studied over more than 30 years. Studies increasingly look at its role in specific cardiovascular conditions but an open study in 424 patients published in 1994 indicated that coenzyme Q_{10} supplementation may have benefits in cardiac function in patients with a range of cardiovascular disorders, including ischaemic cardiomyopathy, dilated cardiomyopathy, primary diastolic dysfunction, hypertension, valvular heart disease and mitral valve prolapse.[11]

Congestive heart failure

There is substantive evidence suggesting a role for coenzyme Q_{10} in CHF. Oxidative stress is believed to play a role in the aetiology of CHF. It has been suggested that low coenzyme Q_{10} levels found in patients with CHF contribute to the disease while supplementation with preparations that include coenzyme Q_{10} may produce an improvement.[3]

A double-blind, placebo-controlled study investigated 322 patients with CHF who were randomly assigned to receive 2 mg coenzyme Q_{10}/kg daily or a placebo for 1 year. The number of episodes of pulmonary oedema or cardiac asthma was significantly fewer in the intervention group than the placebo group. The supplemented patients also had fewer hospitalisations.[12] A meta-analysis of eight clinical trials of coenzyme Q_{10} in patients with CHF found that supplemental treatment of CHF was significant, with significant improvement in stroke volume, ejection fraction, cardiac output, cardiac index and diastolic volume index.[13]

Not all clinical trials have produced positive results. In a double-blind, placebo-controlled, crossover study, 30 patients with chronic left ventricular dysfunction were randomised to receive coenzyme Q_{10} or a placebo for 3 months each. Plasma levels of coenzyme Q_{10} increased to more than twice baseline values, but there were no significant differences between treatments in left ventricular ejection fraction, cardiac volumes, haemodynamic indices or quality of life measures.[14] In another RCT, 55 patients with CHF were randomly assigned to receive 200 mg coenzyme Q_{10} or a placebo daily for 6 months. Patients receiving the supplement had higher serum concentrations of coenzyme Q_{10}, but there were no differences in cardiac performance, peak oxygen consumption and exercise duration between the treated group and the placebo group.[15]

Angina

Coenzyme Q_{10} levels tend to be low in patients with ischaemic heart disease and several clinical trials have been conducted in patients with angina. Overall, coenzyme Q_{10} appears to delay onset of angina and increases patients' stamina on a treadmill. In one RCT, 144 patients with acute myocardial infarction were given 120 mg coenzyme Q_{10} or a placebo daily for 28 days, starting within 3 days of the heart attack. There was a significant improvement in angina pectoris, total arrhythmias and poor left ventricular function in the intervention group. Total cardiac events, including cardiac deaths and non-fatal infarction were also significantly lower in the supplemented group than the placebo group.[16]

Hypertension
Coenzyme Q_{10} has been investigated for hypertension both as a stand-alone treatment and as an adjunct to conventional anti-hypertensive medication. In one randomised double-blind study involving 83 patients, an oral dose of 60 mg taken twice a day over 12 weeks was found to produce a mean reduction in systolic blood pressure of 17.8 ± 7.3 mmHg.[17] Another double-blind study in 59 patients with hypertension found that adding 120 mg coenzyme Q_{10} daily to existing anti-hypertensive medication causes an additional reduction in systolic and diastolic blood pressure after 8 weeks' treatment.[18]

Cardiac surgery
Studies have looked at the use of coenzyme Q_{10} supplements before cardiac surgery. Oral supplementation with coenzyme Q_{10} for 2 weeks before cardiac surgery has been shown to improve post-operative heart function and shorten hospital stays.[19] However, supplementation with 600 mg coenzyme Q_{10} 12 h before surgery did not improve myocardial protection in patients undergoing coronary revascularisation.[20]

Exercise performance
Coenzyme Q_{10} is essential in energy metabolism and has therefore been investigated for athletic performance. Controlled trials using doses of 60–150 mg daily over 28 days to 8 weeks have generally shown no improvements in physical performance. However, in one double-blind crossover trial, there were positive results on both objective and subjective parameters of physical performance. In this study, 94% of athletes felt that coenzyme Q_{10} improved their performance and recovery times compared with 33% taking a placebo.[21]

Parkinson's disease
Studies suggest that oxidative damage, inflammation and mitochondrial impairment may play a role in the aetiology of Parkinson's disease.[22] In a multicentre, randomised, placebo-controlled, double-blind study comparing three different doses of coenzyme Q_{10} (300, 600, and 1200 mg) in 80 patients with early Parkinson's disease, significant improvements were reported after 9 months in the group taking 1200 mg daily.[23]

Huntington's chorea
A randomised double-blind study involving 347 patients with early Huntington's chorea showed that a dose of coenzyme Q_{10} 600 mg daily taken over 30 months produced a trend towards slow decline and beneficial improvements in some parameters. However, changes were not significant.[24]

Cancer
Observational studies of women diagnosed with breast cancer have reported reduced blood coenzyme Q_{10} concentrations. There have also been several case reports of remissions or partial remissions in patients with tumours. However, there are no controlled studies to show the effectiveness of coenzyme Q_{10} in cancer.

Migraine
An open trial investigated the effects of coenzyme Q_{10} 150 mg daily for 3 months in 32 individuals with a history of migraine. Coenzyme Q_{10} was associated with a significant reduction in both the frequency of attacks and the number of days with migraine.[25]

Conclusion

Results from preliminary studies with coenzyme Q_{10} suggest that it may help improve symptoms of CHF, and may help to protect against myocardial infarction. Studies in angina and hypertension are inconclusive. Studies conducted so far do not justify the use of coenzyme Q_{10} in cancer, athletes and sports people and AIDS, though some of the preliminary research justifies more rigorous trials to investigate potential benefits. Preliminary evidence from the use of coenzyme Q_{10} in Parkinson's disease is promising. However, there is insufficient evidence to make definite recommendations for coenzyme Q_{10} as a dietary supplement.

Pregnancy and breast-feeding

Safety in pregnancy has not been established.

Adverse effects

Coenzyme Q_{10} seems to be safe and relatively well tolerated in doses of 10–200 mg daily. There are occasional reports of gastrointestinal discomfort, dizziness and skin rash, but these tend to occur with doses > 200 mg daily.

Interactions

Drugs

Statins: Simvastatin, pravastatin and lovastatin reduce endogenous synthesis of coenzyme Q_{10}.[6] The mechanism of action of statins is inhibition of HMG-CoA reductase. Inhibition of this enzyme appears to inhibit the intrinsic biosynthesis of coenzyme Q_{10} at the same time. This reduces coenzyme Q_{10} concentrations, so constituting a new risk for CVD. Supplementation may increase levels without adversely affecting drug efficacy.

Warfarin: Case reports suggest that coenzyme Q_{10} may decrease international normalised ratio (INR) in patients previously stabilised on anticoagulants. However, a double-blind crossover study in 24 patients on long-term warfarin found that oral coenzyme Q_{10} 100 mg daily had no significant effect on INR or warfarin levels.[26] In patients on warfarin, high doses of coenzyme Q_{10} should be used with caution.

Coenzyme Q_{10} should not be used to treat cardiovascular disorders without medical supervision.

Dose

Coenzyme Q_{10} is sold in capsules and tablets in strengths of 10–150 mg. Doses used in studies investigating CVD and prevention of migraine have ranged from 100 to 150 mg daily. However, higher doses have been used in angina (150–600 mg daily) and Parkinson's disease (up to 1200 mg daily). Doses used to prepare for heart surgery have varied between 30 and 100 mg daily for 1–2 weeks before surgery and a month afterwards.

People who wish to try coenzyme Q_{10} for cardiovascular conditions or migraine prevention should be advised it may take 10–12 weeks to have an effect. However all patients with cardiovascular conditions should take medical advice before taking coenzyme Q_{10}.

References

1 Weber C, Bysted A, Holmer G. Coenzyme Q_{10} in the diet – daily intake and relative bioavailability. *Mol Aspects Med* 1997; 18: S251–S254.
2 Kalen A, Appelkvist EL, Dallner G. Age-related changes in the lipid composition of rat and human tissue. *Lipids* 1989; 24: 579–584.
3 Sole MJ, Jeejeebhoy KN. Conditioned nutritional requirements: therapeutic relevance to heart failure. *Herz* 2002; 27: 174–178.
4 Karlsson J, Diamant B, Folkers K, Lund B. Muscle fibre types, ubiquinone content and exercise capacity in hypertension and effort angina. *Ann Med* 1991; 23: 339–344.
5 Mortensen SA, Vadhanavikit S, Muratsu K, Folkers K. Coenzyme Q_{10}: clinical benefits with biochemical correlates suggesting a scientific breakthrough in the management of chronic heart failure. *Int J Tissue React* 1990; 12: 155–162.
6 Overvard K, Diamant B, Holm L, *et al.* Coenzyme Q_{10} in health and disease. *Eur J Clin Nutr* 1999; 53: 764–770.
7 Bianchi G, Solaroli E, Zaccheroni V, *et al.* Oxidative stress and antioxidant metabolites in patients with

hyperthyroidism: effect of treatment. *Horm Metab Res* 1999; 31: 620–624.

8   Folkers K, Osterborg A, Nylander M, *et al*. Activities of vitamin Q_{10} in animal models and a serious deficiency in patients with cancer. *Biochem Biophys Res Commun* 1997; 234: 296–299.

9   Mortensen SA. Perspectives on therapy of cardiovascular diseases with coenzyme Q (ubiquinone). *Clin Investig* 1993; 71: S116–S123.

10   Jameson S. Statistical data support prediction of death within 6 months on low levels of coenzyme Q_{10} and other entities. *Clin Investig* 1993; 71: S137–S139.

11   Langsjoen H, Langsjoen P, Langsjoen P, *et al*. Usefulness of coenzyme Q_{10} in clinical cardiology: a long term study. *Mol Aspects Med* 1994; 15 (Suppl.): S165–S175.

12   Morisco C, Trimarco B, Condorelli M. Effect of coenzyme Q_{10} therapy in patients with congestive heart failure: a long term multicenter randomized study. *Clin Investig* 1993; 71: S134–S136.

13   Soja AM, Mortensen SA. Treatment of congestive heart failure with coenzyme Q_{10} illustrated by meta-analyses of clinical trials. *Mol Aspects Med* 1997; 18: S159–S168.

14   Watson PS, Scalia GM, Galbraith A, *et al*. Lack of effect of coenzyme Q on left ventricular function in patients with congestive heart failure. *J Am Coll Cardiol* 1999; 33: 1549–1552.

15   Khatta M, Alexander BS, Krichten CM, *et al*. The effect of coenzyme Q_{10} with congestive heart failure. *Ann Intern Med* 2000; 132: 636–640.

16   Singh RB, Wander GS, Rastogi A, *et al*. Randomized, double-blind, placebo-controlled trial of coenzyme Q_{10} in patients with acute myocardial infarction. *Cardiovasc Drugs Ther* 1998; 12: 347–353.

17   Burke BE, Neuenschwander R, Olson RD. Randomized, double-blind, placebo-controlled trial of coenzyme Q_{10} in isolated systolic hypertension. *South Med J* 2001; 94: 1112–1117.

18   Singh RB, Niaz MA, Rastogi SS, *et al*. Effect of hydrosoluble coenzyme Q_{10} on blood pressures and insulin resistance in hypertensive patients with coronary artery disease. *J Hum Hypertens* 1999; 13: 203–208.

19   Rosenfeldt FL, Pepe S, Linnane A, *et al*. The effects of ageing on the response to cardiac surgery: protective strategies for the ageing myocardium. *Biogerontology* 2002; 3: 37–40.

20   Taggart DP, Jenkins M, Hooper J, *et al*. Effects of short term supplementation with coenzyme Q_{10} on myocardial protection during cardiac operations. *Ann Thorac Surg* 1996; 61: 829–833.

21   Ylikoski T, Piirainen J, Hanninen O, Penttinen J. The effect of coenzyme Q_{10} on the exercise performance of cross-country skiers. *Mol Aspects Med* 1997; 18: S283–S290.

22   Ebadi M, Govitrapong P, Sharma S, *et al*. Ubiquinone (coenzyme Q_{10}) and mitochondria in oxidative stress in Parkinson's disease. *Biol Signals Recept* 2001; 10: 224–253.

23   Shults CW, Oakes D, Kieburtz K, *et al*. Effects of coenzyme Q_{10} in early Parkinson disease: evidence of slowing of the functional decline. *Arch Neurol* 2002; 59: 1541–1550.

24   Huntington's Study Group. A randomized, placebo-controlled trial of coenzyme Q_{10} and remacemide in Huntington's disease. *Neurology* 2001; 57: 397–404.

25   Rozen TD, Oshinsky ML, Gebeline CA, *et al*. Open label trial of coenzyme Q_{10} as a migraine preventive. *Cephalgia* 2002; 22: 137–141.

26   Engelson J, Nielson JD, Hansen KF. Effect of coenzyme Q_{10} and ginkgo biloba on warfarin dosage in patients on long-term warfarin treatment. A randomized, double-blind, placebo-controlled crossover trial. *Ugeskr Laeger* 2003; 165: 1868–1871.

Conjugated linoleic acid

Description

Conjugated linoleic acid (CLA) is a naturally occurring polyunsaturated fatty acid. Nine different isomers of CLA have been identified, and their double bonds are conjugated at carbons 9 and 11 or 10 and 12 in the *cis* and *trans* configuration. CLA is found in low concentrations in blood and tissues, although the body does not synthesise CLA endogenously. CLA is readily absorbed from food and supplements.

Dietary sources

CLA is present in small quantities in many foods, especially beef and dairy produce. Cooking has been shown to increase the CLA content of meat. Changes in the way beef and dairy animals have been reared in the last decades have reduced the amount of CLA in the diet.

Action

CLA is essential for the delivery of dietary fat into cells. It transports glucose into cells, and helps glucose to be used to provide energy and build muscle rather than being converted to fat. It is this effect that lies behind the claims that CLA is useful for promoting weight loss. CLA is also an antioxidant and enhances the immune system.

Possible uses

CLA is being marketed for loss of body weight, and is also being investigated for prevention of cancer.

Body weight and energy expenditure

CLA is being promoted for control of body weight, and early evidence from animal studies was promising. In mice, CLA has been shown to reduce fat accumulation and increase protein accumulation without any change in food intake,[1] to reduce energy intake, increase metabolism and reduce body fat,[2] to reduce body fat and increase lean body mass without affecting body weight,[3] and to reduce body fat and increase energy expenditure.[4]

Human clinical data are now appearing in the literature, but with somewhat conflicting results. A 12-week randomised double-blind study including 60 overweight or obese volunteers given various doses of CLA from 1.7 to 6.8 g daily found that CLA was associated with a significantly higher reduction in body fat mass than placebo. The reduction in body fat was significant for the groups taking 3.4 and 6.8 g CLA.[5] A 4-week double-blind RCT in 25 obese men aged 39–64 with metabolic disorder found that CLA 4.2 g daily was associated with a significant reduction in abdominal fat but with no concomitant effects on overall obesity and other cardiovascular risk factors.[6]

A Dutch RCT in 54 men and women involved subjects being put on a very low-calorie diet (2.1 MJ/day) for 3 weeks, followed by 13 weeks on either low- or high-dose CLA (1.8 or 3.6 g daily) or placebo. Weight regain after the low-calorie diet was not significantly different between the active and placebo groups, but subjects on CLA did gain a significantly greater proportion of that weight as fat-free mass (4.6% vs 3.4%). The effect was similar for the low- and high-dose CLA.[7] As part of this study, appetite and food intake was also measured. Appetite (hunger, satiety and fullness) was favourably, dose-dependently affected by consumption of both 1.8 and 3.6 g CLA daily. However, this did not affect energy intake at breakfast and did not improve body weight maintenance.[8]

A 12-month study investigated the effect of CLA in 180 healthy overweight adults. Body fat mass was significantly reduced in the CLA groups.[9] As part of the same study, 134 of the participants were included in an open study for a further 12 months to evaluate the safety of CLA and assess its effect on body composition. The extended study found that CLA 3.4 g daily decreases body fat mass and may help maintain initial reductions in body fat mass and weight in the long term. The supplement was well tolerated.[10]

CLA has also been investigated in people who are exercising. A human study showed that 5.6–7.2 g of CLA daily produced non-significant gains in muscle size and strength in experienced and inexperienced training men.[11] A double-blind 12-week RCT in 20 healthy people with body mass index <25 who did standardised exercise in a gym for 90 min three times weekly found that CLA 1.8 g daily reduced body fat but not body weight.[12] A further study investigated the effect of CLA 6 g daily in 23 resistance-trained subjects. Results showed some statistical trends, but CLA did not significantly affect changes in total body mass, percentage body fat, bone mass or fat-free mass, indicating that CLA does not appear to possess significant ergogenic value for experienced resistance-trained athletes.[13]

There is some evidence that a specific isomer of CLA may be the bioactive component in relation to weight change. A US study in 21 adults with type 2 diabetes found that a CLA mixture of predominantly two isomers (c911t and t10c12) resulted in an increase in plasma CLA that was inversely correlated with body weight and serum leptin levels. However, these significant correlations were only seen with the t10c12-CLA.[14]

Atherosclerosis

Animal research suggests an effect of CLA supplementation on preventing atherosclerosis,[15,16] but one study has shown that CLA does not produce beneficial lipid profiles.[17] One human study in 17 healthy female volunteers found that CLA 3.9 g daily for 2 months did not alter blood cholesterol or lipoprotein levels.[18] In the same study, there were no effects of CLA on blood coagulation and platelet function.[19] Another human RCT in 51 normolipidaemic patients found that an isomeric blend of CLA significantly reduced plasma triglycerides and VLDL cholesterol concentrations.[20]

Insulin sensitivity

Based on preliminary work in animals,[21] there has been some hope that CLA could improve insulin resistance. An 8-week Canadian RCT in 16 normal weight, healthy young adults living a sedentary lifestyle found that an isomeric blend of CLA 4 g daily significantly improved insulin sensitivity by 27% compared with the control group. Insulin sensitivity improved in six out of 10 of the treated group while two deteriorated and two had no change.[22]

An Irish RCT in 32 overweight diabetic subjects found the opposite. Treatment consisted of 8 weeks of either placebo or an isomeric blend of CLA (3 g daily). CLA produced a 6.3% significant increase in fasting glucose concentration and a reduction in insulin sensitivity.[23] Two further studies from the same research group found that both of the common CLA isomers have a negative effect on insulin resistance in obese non-diabetics.[24,25]

Cancer

Preliminary evidence from *in vitro* work and animals suggests that CLA may reduce the risk of cancer,[26–28] but other studies have not confirmed this.[29] Linoleic acid itself has been shown to promote tumorigenesis in some studies.

Miscellaneous

Based on findings in experimental animals and cells in culture that CLA can positively influence calcium and bone metabolism, research is now being conducted in humans. However, one double-blind RCT in 60 healthy adult men aged 39–64 found that CLA 3 g daily for 6 weeks had no significant effect on markers of bone formation or bone resorption or on serum or urinary calcium levels.[30]

CLA has also been investigated for effects on immune function. One study in humans found that CLA supplementation results in a dose-dependent reduction in mitogen-induced T-lymphocyte activation,[31] while a further study showed that CLA had a minimal effect on the markers of human immune function.[32]

> ### Conclusion
> Studies in animals suggest that CLA reduces body fat and increases lean body mass. Human clinical data are conflicting, with only limited evidence that CLA can influence lean body mass. CLA may also increase insulin resistance and overweight people are likely to be those with insulin resistance. Animal studies suggest that CLA may have beneficial effects on atherosclerosis, bone metabolism and immune function, but preliminary human studies have not demonstrated such beneficial effects.

Precautions/contraindications

Until more is known, caution should be exercised in the use of CLA supplements because of potential problems with insulin resistance. Although this is not proven, people likely to use CLA will be overweight and most likely to suffer from insulin resistance.

Pregnancy and breast-feeding

No problems have been reported, but there have not been sufficient studies to guarantee the safety of CLA in pregnancy and breast-feeding.

Adverse effects

No known toxicity or side-effects, apart from one report of gastrointestinal side-effects. However, there are no long-term studies assessing the safety of CLA.

Interactions

None reported.

Dose

CLA is produced for supplements from sunflower oil and is available in the form of capsules.

The dose is not established. Animal research has used large doses, equivalent to several grams a day for humans. However, dietary supplements tend to provide a dose of 1–4 g daily.

References

1 DeLany JP, Blohm F, Truett AA, *et al.* Conjugated linoleic acid rapidly reduces body fat content in mice without affecting energy intake. *Am J Physiol* 1999; 276 (part 2): R1172–1179.

2 West DB, DeLany JP, Camet PM, *et al.* Effects of conjugated linoleic acid on body fat and energy metabolism in the mouse. *Am J Physiol* 1998 (part 2); 275: R667–672.

3 Park Y, Allbright KJ, Liu W, *et al.* Effect of conjugated linoleic acid on body composition in mice. *Lipids* 1997; 32: 853–858.

4 West DB, Blohm FY, Truett AA, DeLany JP. Conjugated linoleic acid persistently increases total energy expenditure in AKR/J mice without uncoupling protein gene expression. *J Nutr* 2000; 130: 2471–2477.

5 Blankson H, Stakkestad JA, Fagertun H, *et al.* Conjugated linoleic acid reduces body fat mass in overweight and obese humans. *J Nutr* 2000; 130: 2943–2948.

6 Riserus U, Berglund L, Vessby B. Conjugated linoleic acid reduced abdominal adipose tissue in obese middle-aged men with signs of the metabolic syndrome: a randomised controlled trial. *Int J Obes Relat Metab Disord* 2001; 25: 1129–1135.

7 Kamphuis MM, Lejeune MP, Saris WH, Westerterp-Plantenga MS. The effect of conjugated linoleic acid supplementation after weight loss on body weight regain, body composition and resting metabolic rate in overweight subjects. *Int J Obes Relat Metab Disord* 2003; 27: 840–847.

8 Kamphuis MM, Lejeune MP, Saris WH, Westerterp-Plantenga MS. Effect of conjugated linoleic acid supplementation after weight loss on appetite and food intake in overweight subjects. *Eur J Clin Nutr* 2003; 57: 1268–1274.

9 Gaullier JM, Halse J, Hoye K, *et al.* Conjugated linoleic acid supplementation for 1 y reduces body fat mass in healthy overweight humans. *Am J Clin Nutr* 2004; 79: 1118–1125.

10 Gaullier JM, Halse J, Hoyce K, *et al.* Supplementation with conjugated linoleic acid for 24 months

is well tolerated by and reduces body fat mass in healthy, overweight humans. *J Nutr* 2005; 135: 778–784.

11 Ferreira M, Krieder R, Wilson M. Effects of CLA supplementation during resistance training on body muscle and strength. *J Strength Cond Res* 1998; 11: 280.

12 Thom E, Wadstein J, Gudmundsen O. Conjugated linoleic acid reduces body fat in healthy exercising humans. *J Int Med Res* 2001; 29: 392–396.

13 Kreider RB, Ferreira MP, Greenwood M, *et al.* Effects of conjugated linoleic acid supplementation during resistance training on body composition, bone density, strength and selected haematological markers. *J Strength Cond Res* 2002; 16: 325–334.

14 Belury MA, Mahon A, Banni S. The conjugated linoleic acid (CLA) isomer, t10c12-CLA, is inversely associated with changes in body weight and serum leptin in subjects with type 2 diabetes mellitus. *J Nutr* 2003; 133: S257S–S260.

15 Lee KN, Kritchevsky D, Pariza MW. Conjugated linoleic acid and atherosclerosis in rabbits. *Atherosclerosis* 1994; 108: 19–25.

16 Nicolosi RJ, Rogers EJ, Kritchevsky D, *et al.* Dietary conjugated linoleic acid reduces plasma lipoproteins and early aortic atherosclerosis in hypercholesterolemic hamsters. *Artery* 1997; 22: 266–277.

17 Kritchevsky D, Tepper SA, Wright S, *et al.* Influence of conjugated linoleic acid (CLA) on establishment and progression of atherosclerosis in rabbits. *J Am Coll Nutr* 2000; 19: S472S–S477.

18 Benito P, Nelson GJ, Kelley DS, *et al.* The effect of conjugated linoleic acid on plasma lipoproteins and tissue fatty acid composition in humans. *Lipids* 2001; 36: 229–236.

19 Benito P, Nelson GJ, Kelley DS, *et al.* The effect of conjugated linoleic acid on platelet function, platelet fatty acid composition and blood coagulation in humans. *Lipids* 2001; 36: 221–227.

20 Noone EJ, Roche HM, Nugent AP, Gibney MJ. The effect of dietary suppelementation using isomeric blends of conjugated linoleic acid on lipid metabolism in healthy human subjects. *Br J Nutr* 2002; 88: 243–251.

21 Houseknecht KL, Vanden Heuvel JP, Moya-Camarena SY, *et al.* Dietary conjugated linoleic acid normalises impaired glucose tolerance in the Zucker diabetic fatty fa/fa rat. *Biochem Biophys Res Commun* 1998; 244: 678–682.

22 Eyjolfson V, Spriet LL, Dyck DJ. Conjugated linoleic acid improves insulin sensitivity in young, sedentary humans. *Med Sci Sports Exerc* 2004; 36: 814–820.

23 Moloney F, Yeow TP, Mullen A, *et al.* Conjugated linoleic acid supplementation, insulin sensitivity, and lipoprotein metabolism in patients with type 2 diabetes mellitus. *Am J Clin Nutr* 2004; 80: 887–895.

24 Riserus U, Vessby B, Amlov J, Basu S. Supplementation with trans10cis12-conjugated linoleic acid induces hyperproinsulinaemia in obese men: close association with impaired insulin sensitivity. *Diabetologia* 2004; 47: 1016–1019.

25 Riserus U, Vesby B, Amer P, Zethelius B. Effects of cis-9, trans-11 conjugated linoleic acid supplementation on insulin sensitivity, lipid peroxidation and proinflammatory markers in obese men. *Am J Clin Nutr* 2004; 80: 279–283.

26 Cesano A, Visonneau S, Scimeca JA, *et al.* Opposite effects of linoleic acid and conjugated linolenic acid on human prostatic cancer in SCID mice. *Anticancer Res* 1998; 18 (3A): 1429–1434.

27 Thompson H, Zhu Z, Banni S, *et al.* Morphological and biochemical status of the mammary gland influenced by conjugated linoleic acid: implication for a reduction in mammary cancer risk. *Cancer Res* 1997; 57: 5067–5072.

28 Parodi PW. Cow's milk fat components as potential carcinogenic agents. *J Nutr* 1997; 127: 1055–1060.

29 Petrik MB, McEntee MF, Johnson BT, *et al.* Highly unsaturated (n-3) fatty acids, but not alpha linolenic, conjugated linoleic or gamma-linolenic acids, reduce tumourigenesis in Apc(Min/+) mice. *J Nutr* 2000; 130: 2434–2443.

30 Doyle C, Jewell C, Mullen A, *et al.* Effect of dietary supplementation with conjugated linoleic acid on markers of calcium and bone metabolism in healthy adult men. *Eur J Clin Nutr* 2005; 59: 432–440.

31 Tricon S, Burdge GC, Kew S, *et al.* Effects of cis-9, trans-11 and trans-10, cis-12 conjugated linoleic acid on immune cell function in healthy humans. *Am J Clin Nutr* 2004; 80: 1626–1633.

32 Nugent AP, Roche HM, Noone EJ, *et al.* The effects of conjugated linoleic acid supplementation on immune function in healthy volunteers. *Eur J Clin Nutr* 2005; 59: 742–750.

Copper

Description

Copper is an essential trace mineral.

Human requirements

See Table 1 for Dietary Reference Values for copper.

Dietary intake

In the UK, the average adult diet provides: for men, 1.82 mg daily; for women, 1.31 mg.

Action

Copper functions as an essential component of several enzymes (e.g. superoxide dismutase) and other proteins. It plays a role in bone formation and mineralisation, and in the integrity of the connective tissue of the cardiovascular system. Copper promotes iron absorption and is required for the synthesis of haemoglobin. It is involved in melanin pigment formation, cholesterol metabolism and glucose metabolism. In the central nervous system (CNS), it is required for the formation of myelin and is important for normal neurotransmission. Copper has pro-oxidant effects *in vitro* but antioxidant effects *in vivo*; there is accumulating evidence that adequate copper is required to maintain anti-oxidant effects within the body.[1]

Dietary sources

See Table 2 for dietary sources of copper.

Table 1 Dietary Reference Values for copper (mg/day)

			EU RDA = none	
Age	UK		USA	
	RNI	EVM	Safe intake	TUL
0–3 months	0.3		0.2	–
4–6 months	0.3		0.22	–
7–12 months	0.3		0.22	–
1–3 years	0.4		0.34	1.0
4–6 years	0.6		1.0–1.5	–
4–8 years	–		0.44	3.0
7–10 years	0.7		–	–
9–13 years	–		0.7	5.0
14–18 years	–		0.89	8.0
Males				
11–14 years	0.8		–	–
15–18 years	1.0		–	–
19–50+ years	1.2	5	0.9	10.0
Females				
11–14 years	0.8		–	–
15–18 years	1.0		–	–
19–50+ years	1.2	5	0.9	10.0
Pregnancy	*		1.0	10.0[2]
Lactation	+0.3		1.0[1]	10.0[2]

* No increment.

[1] ≤18 years, 1.3 mg.

[2] ≤18 years, 8.0 mg.

Note: No EAR, LRNI or FAO/WHO RNIs have been derived for copper.

EVM = Safe upper level from supplements alone.

TUL = Tolerable Upper Intake Level from diet and supplements.

Table 2   Dietary sources of copper

Food portion	Copper content (mg)
Breakfast cereals	
1 bowl All-Bran (45 g)	*0.2*
1 bowl Bran Flakes (45 g)	*0.1*
1 bowl muesli (95 g)	*0.3*
2 pieces Shredded Wheat	*0.2*
2 Weetabix	*0.2*
Cereal products	
Bread, brown, 2 slices	0.1
white, 2 slices	0.1
wholemeal, 2 slices	*0.2*
1 chapati	0.1
Pasta, brown, boiled (150 g)	*0.3*
white, boiled (150 g)	0.1
Rice, brown, boiled (165 g)	*0.5*
white, boiled (165 g)	0.2
Meat	
Meat, average, cooked (100 g)	0.2
Liver, lambs, cooked (90 g)	9.0
calf, cooked (90 g)	11.0
Kidney, lambs, cooked (75 g)	*0.4*
Vegetables	
Chick peas, lentils, or red kidney beans, cooked (105 g)	*0.2*
Potatoes, boiled (150 g)	0.1
Mushrooms, cooked (100 g)	**0.4**
Green vegetables (100 g)	0.02
Fruit	
1 banana	*0.3*
1 orange	0.1
2 handfuls raisins	0.1
8 dried apricots	*0.2*
Nuts	
20 almonds	0.2
10 Brazil nuts	*0.4*
30 hazelnuts	*0.4*
30 peanuts	*0.3*
Milk chocolate (100 g)	*0.3*
Plain chocolate (100 g)	**0.7**

Excellent sources (**bold**); good sources (*italic*).

Metabolism

Absorption

Copper is absorbed mainly in the small intestine, with a small amount absorbed in the stomach; absorption is probably by a saturable carrier-mediated mechanism at low levels of intake, and by passive diffusion at high levels of intake.

Distribution

Copper is rapidly taken up by the liver and incorporated into caeruloplasmin. It is stored primarily in the liver. Copper is transported bound to caeruloplasmin.

Elimination

Elimination is mainly via bile into the faeces; small amounts are excreted in the urine, sweat and via epidermal shedding.

Bioavailability

Absorption may be reduced by phytate (present in bran and high-fibre foods) and non-starch polysaccharides (dietary fibre), but recommended intakes of fibre-containing foods are unlikely to compromise copper status.

Deficiency

Deficiency of copper is rare, but may lead to hypochromic and microcytic anaemias, leucopenia, neutropenia, impaired immunity and bone demineralisation. Deficiency may also be caused by Menke's syndrome (an X-linked genetic disorder in which copper absorption is defective); this disease is characterised by a reduced level of copper in the blood, liver and hair, progressive mental deterioration, defective keratinisation of the hair and hypothermia.

Marginal deficiency may result in elevated cholesterol levels, impaired glucose tolerance, defects in pigmentation and structure of the hair, and demyelination and degeneration of the nervous system. In infants and children, copper deficiency can lead to skeletal fragility and increased susceptibility to infections, especially those of the respiratory tract.

Copper deficiency has been linked to many of the processes, including atherosclerosis and thrombosis, associated with ischaemic heart disease. Whether this relationship is important in humans remains unanswered. More information is required concerning possible mild copper deficiency in human populations.

Possible uses

Copper has been claimed to be protective against hypercholesterolaemia. In various animal species, it has been demonstrated that feeding a copper-deficient diet results in increased serum cholesterol levels,[1] but studies in humans have shown inconsistent results.[1-3] A recent study in 16 young women (mean age 24 years) found that copper supplementation 3 or 6 mg daily improved copper status and that the concentration of fibrinolytic factor plasminogen activator inhibitor type 1 was significantly reduced by about 30% after supplementation with copper 6 mg daily.[4]

Claims for the value of copper supplements in rheumatoid arthritis and psoriasis have not been proved.

Conclusion

There are no proven benefits in taking copper supplements unless there is a proven deficiency, which should be treated under medical supervision.

Precautions/contraindications

Copper should not be used in Wilson's disease (the disorder may be exacerbated); or hepatic and biliary disease.

Pregnancy and breast-feeding

No problems have been reported with normal intakes.

Adverse effects

With excessive doses (unlikely from supplements): epigastric pain, anorexia, nausea, vomiting and diarrhoea; hepatic toxicity and jaundice; hypotension; haematuria (blood in urine, pain on urination, lower back pain); metallic taste; convulsions and coma.

Copper toxicity may also occur in patients with Wilson's disease (an inherited disorder in which patients exhibit a deficiency of plasma caeruloplasmin and an excess of copper in the liver and bloodstream). There is a theoretical possibility of copper toxicity in women who use copper-containing intrauterine contraceptive devices (further studies required).

Interactions

Drugs

Penicillamine: reduces absorption of copper and vice versa; give 2 h apart.
Trientine: reduces absorption of copper and vice versa; give 2 h apart.

Nutrients

Iron: large doses of iron may reduce copper status and vice versa; give 2 h apart.
Vitamin C: large doses of vitamin C (> 1 g daily) may reduce copper status.
Zinc: large doses of zinc may reduce absorption of copper and vice versa; give 2 h apart.

Dose

Copper supplements are available in the form of tablets and capsules, but mostly they are found in multivitamin and mineral supplements. The copper content of various commonly used salts is: copper amino acid chelate (20 mg/g); copper gluconate (140 mg/g); copper sulphate (254 mg/g).

There is no established use or dose for copper as an isolated supplement.

Upper safety levels

The UK Expert Group on Vitamins and Minerals (EVM) has identified a safe total intake of copper for adults from supplements alone of 5 mg daily.

The US Tolerable Upper Intake Level (UL) for copper, the highest total amount from diet and supplements unlikely to pose no risk for most people, is 10 mg daily for adults, 8 mg daily for youngsters aged 14–18, 5 mg daily for youngsters aged 9–13, 3 mg daily for children aged 4–8, and 1 mg daily for children aged 1–3.

References

1 Klevay LM, Inman L, Johnson LK, *et al*. Increased cholesterol in plasma in a young man during experimental copper depletion. *Metabolism* 1984; 33: 1112–1118.

2 Medeiros D, Pellum L, Brown B. Serum lipids and glucose as associated with haemoglobin levels and copper and zinc intake in young adults. *Life Sci* 1983; 32: 1897–1904.

3 Shapcott D, Vobecky JS, Vobecky J, Demers PP. Plasma cholesterol and the plasma copper/zinc ratio in young children. *Sci Total Environ* 1985; 42: 197–200.

4 Bugel S, Harper A, Rock E, *et al*. Effect of copper supplementation on indices of copper status and certain CVD risk markers in young healthy women. *Br J Nutr* 2005; 94: 231–236.

Creatine

Description

Creatine is an amino acid synthesised from the amino acid precursors arginine, glycine and methionine. The kidneys use arginine and glycine to make guanidinoacetate, which the liver methylates to form creatine. The highest concentrations of creatine are found in skeletal muscle, but high concentrations are also found in heart and smooth muscle, as well as brain, kidney and spermatozoa.

Action

Creatine combines readily with phosphate to form creatine phosphate, which is a source of high-energy phosphate that is released during the anaerobic phase of muscle contraction. The phosphorus from creatine phosphate is transferred to adenosine diphosphate (ADP), creating adenosine triphosphate (ATP) and releasing creatine. Stored creatine phosphate can fuel the first 4–5 s of a sprint, but another fuel must provide the energy to sustain the activity.

Creatine supplements increase the storage of creatine phosphate, thus making more ATP available for the working muscles and enabling them to work harder before becoming fatigued. There appears to be an upper limit for creatine storage in muscle, and supplementation increases levels most in athletes with low stores of creatine, rather than those with high levels.

Dietary sources

Creatine is found in food, and the average omnivorous diet supplies about 1–2 g creatinine daily, although vegetarians consume less. This is because creatine is found principally in animal foods, such as fish and meat. Only trace amounts are found in plant foods. If the dietary supply is limited, creatine can be synthesised endogenously.

Possible uses

Creatine has been investigated for a possible role in sports and athletics.

Exercise performance

Supplementation increases levels of creatine in plasma and skeletal muscle, and it is used to enhance exercise performance. A study in 1992 was the first to show that creatine supplementation (5 g four to six times a day) for several consecutive days increased the creatine concentration of skeletal muscle; the authors concluded that creatine supplementation might enhance exercise performance in humans.[1]

The first published investigation into the effect of oral creatine supplementation on exercise performance in humans showed that ingestion of creatine (20 g daily for 5 days) was found to improve performance during repeated bouts of maximal isokinetic knee-extensor exercise, reducing fatigue by 6%.[2]

In a subsequent more invasive study, subjects performed two bouts of maximal isokinetic cycling exercise before and after creatine ingestion at identical dose (20 g daily for 5 days). Each exercise bout lasted 30 s, and the recovery period between bouts was 4 min. Total work performance increased during both bouts of exercise after creatine supplementation and was related to muscle creatine uptake.[3]

A randomised, placebo-controlled trial involving 16 male subjects investigated the effects of creatine supplementation (20 g daily for 5 days) on the ability to perform kayak ergo-meter performances of different durations. The results indicated that creatine could significantly increase the amount of work accomplished at durations ranging from 90 to 300 s.[4]

In a double-blind crossover study, 12 subjects were either creatine loaded (25 g daily for 5 days), or were creatine loaded and took extra creatine (5 g/hour) during an exercise test or placebo on three occasions followed by a 5-week wash-out period. Each subject underwent a 2.5-hour endurance test on their own bicycle followed by five maximal 10-s sprints separated by 2-min recovery intervals. Creatine loading for 5 days, but not creatine loading plus acute ingestion, significantly increased peak and mean sprint power for all five sprints, but endurance time to exhaustion was not affected by either creatine regimen.[5]

Ten physically active but untrained college-age males received creatine (5 g four times a day) or placebo for 5 days in a double-blind, randomised, balanced, crossover design and were assessed during maximal and three repeated submaximal bouts of isometric knee extension and handgrip exercises. Creatine significantly increased maximal isometric strength during knee extension, but not during handgrip exercise, and increased time to fatigue during all bouts of exercise. The authors concluded that improvements in maximal isometric strength following creatine supplementation were restricted to movements performed with a large muscle mass.[6]

Further studies have confirmed the ability of creatine supplements to improve performance during heavy resistance training,[7] ice hockey,[8] bicycle exercise,[9] soccer[10] and squash.[11]

However, several studies have reported no effects of creatine supplementation on exercise performance. There was no effect on power output during two bouts of 15-s maximal exercise separated by a recovery of 20 min, but this finding may reflect the design in that several bouts of exercise and a shorter recovery time may have been needed to show an effect of creatine supplementation.[12] However, in another study where subjects were assigned to recovery intervals of 30, 60, 90 or 120 s, creatine 20 g daily for 5 days still had no effect on the subjects' ability to reproduce or maintain a high percentage of peak power during the second of two bouts of high-intensity cycling.[13] This was also the case in a study that showed no effect of creatine supplementation on performance during a single 20-s bout of maximal exercise.[14]

Another study showed no effect of creatine supplementation on performance during single bouts of maximal exercise lasting 15, 30 and 60 s in elite swimmers,[15] and in a further study, no effect of creatine supplementation on performance during a single 30-s bout of maximal exercise,[16] but this may also have reflected the short supplementation period of 3 days. In a further study, no changes in performance were found after a small dose of creatine (2 g daily) taken over several weeks.[17]

Miscellaneous

There is preliminary evidence that creatine may improve strength in people with CHF,[18] chronic obstructive pulmonary disease (COPD),[19] and in neuromuscular diseases.[20] Creatine supplements may also be an effective adjunct to vitamin supplements for lowering plasma homocysteine.[21]

Preliminary evidence suggests that supplementation may be a useful therapeutic strategy for older adults to attenuate loss in muscle strength and performance in functional living tasks.[22] In addition, when combined with resistance training, creatine supplementation has been shown to increase lean tissue mass and improves leg strength, endurance, and average power in older men.[23]

Precautions/contraindications

Creatine should be used with caution in renal or hepatic disease. However, the increase in urinary excretion of creatinine observed with creatine supplementation does not indicate renal impairment. Rather, it correlates with the increase in muscle creatine storage and the increased rate of muscle creatine degradation to creatinine.

Creatine is not on the International Olympic Committee Drug List, but some consider it to be in the 'grey zone' between doping and substances allowed to enhance performance.

> **Conclusion**
> Despite a large number of clinical trials, there remains a dearth of high-quality research on creatine supplementation. Investigations of the effect of creatine on performance, strength and endurance in laboratory studies have yielded roughly equal numbers of studies showing positive effects and no effect. Field studies (i.e. of individuals participating in normal sports activities) have shown less impressive results than laboratory studies.
>
> Creatine supplementation improves performance during exercise of high to maximal intensity, and its use could potentially benefit sports involving either single bouts of high-intensity exercise (e.g. sprint running, swimming, rowing, cycling) or multiple bouts (e.g. soccer, rugby, hockey). It also has the potential to benefit an athlete involved in training that involves repetitive bouts of high-intensity exercise. However, there is no evidence that creatine can benefit prolonged, submaximal exercise (e.g. middle- or long-distance running), and it may impair endurance exercise by contributing to weight gain.

Pregnancy and breast-feeding

No problems have been reported. However, there have not been sufficient studies to guarantee the safety of creatine in pregnancy and breast-feeding. Creatine is best avoided.

Adverse effects

No serious toxic effects have been documented. In a survey of 52 college athletes supplementing with creatine, 16 reported diarrhoea, 13 reported muscle cramps and seven dehydration.[24] Another survey, which involved 28 male baseball players and 24 male football players aged 18–23, found that 16 (31%) experienced diarrhoea, 13 (25%) experienced muscle cramps,

seven (13%) reported unwanted weight gain, seven (13%) reported dehydration and 12 reported various other side-effects.[25] In the same survey, 39 (75%) exceeded the maintenance dose of 2–5 g daily.

In a placebo-controlled trial involving 175 subjects and lasting 310 days, creatine monohydrate supplementation 10 g daily did not result in significant differences in adverse effects compared with placebo. Occurrence of nausea, gastrointestinal discomfort and diarrhoea was similar in both groups. After 2 months of treatment, oedematous limbs were seen more often in subjects using creatine, probably because of water retention. Severe diarrhoea and severe nausea caused three subjects in the creatine group to stop taking it, after which these adverse events subsided.[26]

In another report a patient with nephrotic syndrome who had been supplementing with creatine experienced deterioration in renal function,[27] and a previously healthy 20-year-old man developed interstitial nephritis after taking creatine (20 g daily) for 4 weeks.[28]

Chronic administration of a large quantity of creatine can increase the production of formaldehyde. Formaldehyde is well known to crosslink proteins and DNA, and may cause potentially serious side-effects.[29]

Creatine supplementation often causes weight gain, which can be mistaken for increase in muscle mass. Increasing intracellular creatine may cause an osmotic influx of water into the cell because creatine is an osmotically active substance. It is therefore possible that the weight gained is due to water retention and not increased muscle.

The safety of prolonged use of creatine is of concern. Individuals should be advised not to take the loading dose of 20 g daily for more than 5 days and not to supplement for a total period of longer than 30 days until effects are better known.

Interactions

No known drug interactions. Caffeine may reduce or abolish the ergogenic effects of creatine.

Dose

Creatine is available mainly in the form of powder. A review of 13 US products showed that 11 of them contained the weight of creatine claimed. One of the products was found to contain less than the claimed amount and one failed to meet its claim of being free from the impurity dicyandiamide.[30]

The usual dose regimen used in studies is 5 g creatine monohydrate four times a day for the first 5 days as a loading dose, then 2–5 g daily as maintenance. These doses should not be exceeded because of the risk of adverse effects (see above).

References

1 Harris RC, Soderlund K, Hultman E. Elevation of creatine in resting and exercised muscle of normal subjects by creatine supplementation. *Clin Sci* 1992; 83: 367–374.

2 Greenhaff PL, Casey A, Short AH, *et al.* Influence of oral creatine supplementation on muscle torque during repeated bouts of maximal voluntary exercise in man. *Clin Sci* 1993; 84: 565–571.

3 Casey A, Constantin-Teodosiu D, Howell S, *et al.* Creatine ingestion favorably influences exercise performance and muscle metabolism during maximal exercise in humans. *Am J Physiol* 1996; 27: E31–E37.

4 McNaughton LR, Dalton B, Tarr J. The effects of creatine supplementation on high-intensity exercise performance in elite performers. *Eur J Appl Physiol Occup Physiol* 1998; 78: 236–240.

5 Vandebuerie F, Vanden Eynde B, Vandenberghe K, Hespel P. Effect of creatine loading on endurance capacity and sprint power in cyclists. *Int J Sports Med* 1998; 19: 490–495.

6 Urbanski RL, Vincent WJ, Yaspelkis BB III. Creatine supplementation differentially affects maximal isometric strength and time to fatigue in large and small muscle groups. *Int J Sport Nutr* 1999; 9: 136–145.

7 Volek JS, Duncan ND, Mazzetti SA, *et al.* Performance and muscle fiber adaptation to creatine supplementation and heavy resistance training. *Med Sci Sports Exerc* 1999; 31: 1147–1156.

8 Jones AM, Atter T, Georg TP. Oral creatine supplementation improves multiple sprint performance in elite ice-hockey players. *J Sports Med Phys Fitness* 1999; 39: 189–196.

9 Rici-Sanz J, Mendez Marco MT. Creatine enhances oxygen uptake and performance during alternating intensity exercise. *Med Sci Sports Exerc* 2000; 32: 379–385.

10 Mujika I, Padilla S, Ibanez J, *et al.* Creatine supplementation and sprint performance in soccer players. *Med Sci Sports Exerc* 2000; 32: 518–525.

11 Romer LM, Barrington JP, Jeukendrup AE. Effects of oral creatine supplementation on high intensity, intermittent exercise performance in competitive squash players. *Int J Sports Med* 2001; 22: 546–552.

12 Cooke WH, Grandjean PW, Barnes WS. Effect of oral creatine supplementation on power output and fatigue during bicycle egometry. *J Appl Physiol* 1995; 78: 670–673.

13 Cooke WH, Barnes WS. The influence of recovery duration on high intensity exercise performance after oral creatine supplementation. *Can J Appl Physiol* 1997; 22: 454–467.

14 Snow RJ, McKenna MJ, Selig SE, *et al.* Effect of creatine supplementation on sprint exercise performance and muscle metabolism. *J Appl Physiol* 1998; 84: 1667–1673.

15 Mukija I, Chatard JC, Lacoste L, *et al.* Creatine supplementation does not improve sprint performance in competitive swimmers. *Med Sci Sports Exerc* 1996; 28: 1435–1441.

16 Odland LM, MacDougall JD, Tarnopolsky MA, *et al.* Effect of oral creatine supplementation on muscle (PCr) and short-term maximum power output. *Med Sci Sports Exerc* 1997; 29: 216–219.

17 Thompson CH, Kemp GJ, Sanderson AL, *et al.* Effect of creatine on aerobic and anaerobic metabolism in skeletal muscle in swimmers. *Br J Sports Med* 1996; 30: 222–225.

18 Andrews R, Greenhaff P, Curtis S, *et al.* The effect of dietary creatine supplementation on skeletal muscle metabolism in congestive heart failure. *Eur Heart J* 1998; 19: 617–622.

19 Fuld JP, Kilduff LP, Neder JA, *et al.* Creatine supplementation during pulmonary rehabilitation in chronic obstructive pulmonary disease. *Thorax* 2005; 60: 531–537.

20 Tarnoplosky M, Martin J. Creatine monohydrate increases strength in patients with neuromuscular disease. *Neurology* 1999; 52: 854–857.

21 Korzun WJ. Oral creatine supplements lower plasma homocysteine concentrations in humans. *Clin Lab Sci* 2004; 17: 102–106.

22 Gotshalk LA, Volek JS, Staron RS, *et al.* Creatine supplementation improves muscular performance in older men. *Med Sci Sports Exerc* 2002; 34: 537–543.

23 Chrusch MJ, Chilibeck PD, Chad KE, *et al.* Creatine supplementation combined with resistance training in older men. *Med Sci Sports Exerc* 2001; 33: 2111–2117.

24 Juhn MS, Tarnopolsky M. Potential side effects of oral creatine supplementation: a critical review. *J Am Diet Ass* 1998; 8: 298–304.

25 Juhn MS, O'Kane JW, Vinci DM. Oral creatine supplementation in male college athletes: a survey of dosing habits and side effects. *J Am Diet Assoc* 1999; 99: 593–595.

26 Groenveld GJ, Beijer C, Veldink JH, *et al.* Few adverse effects of long-term creatine supplementation in a placebo-controlled trial. *Int J Sports Med* 2005; 26: 307–313.

27 Pritchard NR, Kalra PA, Renal dysfunction accompanying oral creatine supplements. *Lancet* 1998; 351: 1252–1253.

28 Koshy KM, Griswold E, Schneeberger EE. Interstitial nephritis in a patient taking creatine. *N Engl J Med* 1999; 340: 814–815.

29 Yu PH, Deng Y. Potential cytotoxic effect of chronic administration of creatine, a nutrition supplement to augment athletic performance. *Med Hypotheses* 2000; 54: 726–728.

30 Consumerlab. Product review. Creatine. http://www.consumerlab.com (accessed 13 November 2006).

Dehydroepiandrosterone

Description

Dehydroepiandrosterone (DHEA) is the most abundant hormone secreted by the adrenal glands. It is a steroid hormone and secreted by the zona reticularis of the adrenals. DHEA circulates in the blood as dehydroepiandrosterone-3-sulphate (DHEAS), which is converted as required to DHEA. Production of DHEA in humans normally peaks between the ages of 20 and 30 years, and then begins a steady progressive decline.[1]

Action

DHEA and DHEAS are the precursors for other hormones, including oestrogens and androgens. The degree of androgenic versus oestrogenic effect of DHEA may depend on the individual's hormonal status. For example, there is some evidence that DHEA has different effects in pre-menopausal and post-menopausal women.[2]

DHEA has also been shown to stimulate insulin growth factor-1 (IGF-1),[3] a hormone that stimulates anabolic metabolism, enhances insulin sensitivity, accelerates muscle growth and enhances energy production.

Possible uses

Supplementation with DHEA has been claimed to produce several health benefits including enhancement of immune function, increased muscle mass, improvements in memory and mood, improvement in symptoms of auto-immune disorders such as lupus erythematosus, and to have a general anti-ageing effect. However, evidence for a beneficial effect of DHEA supplements in all these conditions is inconclusive.

Immunity

The first *in vivo* evidence of an immuno-modulatory effect of DHEA came from a prospective, randomised, double-blind, crossover study involving 11 post-menopausal women with 3-week treatment arms. Results showed that DHEA supplementation reduced T helper cell populations and increased natural killer cell populations.[4]

In a single-blind, placebo-controlled study, nine healthy men (mean age 63 years) were supplemented with a placebo for 2 weeks, followed by DHEA 50 mg daily for 20 weeks.[5] DHEA stimulated immune function by significantly increasing the number of monocyte and B cells, stimulating B- and T-cell mitogenic response, interleukin-2 secretion and the number and cytotoxicity of natural killer cells. The authors acknowledged that the results of this study had limited application because post-treatment immune response was not measured.

However, in two other studies,[6,7] DHEA produced no significant effects on antibody response to influenza vaccine.

Body composition

In a double-blind, placebo-controlled study, 10 healthy men were randomised to receive either 1600 mg DHEA or placebo daily for 28 days. Compared with placebo, body fat was reduced significantly, by 31% in the supplemented group, but there was no change in body weight. There was also a 7.5% reduction in LDL cholesterol.[8] Furthermore, in another randomised, double-blind, placebo-controlled study in morbidly obese adolescents,[9] 40 mg DHEA twice a day had no effect on body weight. In two other studies,[10,11] DHEA 1600 mg daily for 4 weeks had no significant effect on body weight or lean body mass.

Memory, mood and depression

In a double-blind, placebo-controlled crossover study, 30 healthy subjects aged 40–70 years were randomised to receive in random order either 50 mg DHEA or placebo daily for 3 months each. During DHEA supplementation there was a significant increase in perceived physical and psychological well-being. There was no effect on insulin sensitivity, body fat or libido.[12]

In a double-blind, placebo-controlled crossover study, 17 healthy, elderly male subjects received 50 mg DHEA daily or a placebo for 2 weeks. There was no change in memory or mood in the supplemented group.[13]

A Cochrane systematic review[14] investigated the effect of DHEA supplementation on cognition and well-being. Five studies matched the reviewers' criteria, four of which were short-term (DHEA administered for 2 weeks or less) and one where DHEA was given for 3 months. There was no significant change in ability to perform cognitive tests, or mood or well-being (as assessed by standard scales) in the short-term studies. In the longer-term study, results of an open-ended questionnaire showed that 67% of men and 82% of women reported enhanced well-being with DHEA compared with placebo. The reviewers concluded that present data offer limited support for a beneficial effect of DHEA on well-being, but not on memory or cognitive function.

In a double-blind, placebo-controlled study,[15] 32 patients with severe depression, either medication-free or stabilised on anti-depressants, received either DHEA (maximum dose 90 mg daily) or placebo for 6 weeks. DHEA was associated with a significantly greater decrease in the Hamilton depression rating scale than placebo, and five of the 11 patients treated with DHEA compared with none of the 11 subjects in the placebo group showed a 50% or greater reduction in symptoms of depression.

In a small double-blind RCT, DHEA (50 mg twice a day) did not significantly improve cognitive performance or overall ratings of change

in severity. A transient effect on cognitive performance may have been seen at month 3, but this narrowly missed significance.[16]

A study in patients with schizophrenia found that DHEA (up to 100 mg daily) was associated with significant improvement in negative symptoms as well as in depressive and anxiety symptoms in individuals receiving DHA.[17]

Plasma levels of DHEA fall with the progression of HIV diseases and DHEA is being investigated for potential benefit. A study in 32 patients with advanced HIV disease found improved mental function scores with DHEA 50 mg daily for 4 months.[18]

Systemic lupus erythematosus

In a double-blind, placebo-controlled study,[19] 28 women with mild to moderate systemic lupus erythematosus (SLE) were randomised to receive 200 mg DHEA or placebo daily for 3 months. In the supplemented group, there were insignificant improvements in SLE Disease Activity Index scores, physicians' assessment of disease activity and a reduction in the dose of prednisone used. There was a significant improvement in patients' assessment of disease activity with DHEA compared with placebo.

In an open study, 50 women with mild to moderate SLE were treated with 50–200 mg of DHEA daily for 6–12 months. Supplementation was associated with a significant reduction in disease activity and significant improvement in patient and physician assessment compared to baseline.[20]

In a double-blind RCT, 120 adult women with active SLE received oral DHEA (200 mg daily) or placebo for 24 weeks. DHEA treatment was well tolerated, significantly reduced the number of SLE flares and improved patients' global assessment of disease activity.[21]

Miscellaneous

There is no evidence that DHEA supplements prevent ageing in humans. Reports have suggested that DHEA might reduce the risk of heart disease. Epidemiological studies have been conflicting, and although some animal and human studies have shown that DHEA may reduce LDL cholesterol and platelet aggregation, controlled trials are needed to assess the effects of DHEA supplementation on cardiovascular risk.

DHEA has also been reported to improve insulin sensitivity and reduce blood glucose levels, but again results from studies have been conflicting. One small study in 24 men found that DHEA 25 mg daily improved insulin sensitivity and vascular endothelial function and decreased the plasma activator inhibitor type 1 concentration. The authors concluded that these beneficial changes have the potential to attenuate the development of age-related disorders such as CVD.[22]

DHEA has also been investigated for an effect on bone turnover. An RCT in young women with anorexia nervosa compared the effects of DHEA with hormone replacement therapy (HRT). In initial analyses, total hip BMD increased significantly and similarly in both treatment groups. Bone formation markers increased transiently at 6–9 months in the DHEA compared with the HRT group and both treatments significantly reduced bone resorption markers. However, both groups gained weight and after correcting for weight gain, there was no treatment effect. In addition, DHEA was associated with improvement in specific psychological parameters.[23] In another study in middle-aged to elderly men, oral DHEA did not affect bone turnover when used for a 6-month period.[24]

It is often claimed that individuals can enhance their muscle capacity by boosting DHEA levels through oral supplementation. A 12-month study in 280 healthy men and women (aged 60–89 years) found that the supplement restored DHEA levels to the normal range for young adults. However, there were no beneficial effects on muscle state.[25]

Conclusion

The role of DHEA supplements in all conditions studied is inconclusive. Some studies have shown that DHEA improves the immune response while others have not. There is no good evidence that DHEA helps to reduce body weight. There is limited evidence that it may improve well-being and reduce symptoms of depression, but it seems to have no effect on memory or cognition. Preliminary evidence suggests that DHEA could improve symptoms of SLE.

Precautions/contraindications

DHEA is contraindicated in individuals who have (or have a history of) prostate cancer or oestrogen-dependent tumours (e.g. breast or uterine cancer). It should be used with caution in patients with diabetes mellitus (because it may alter blood glucose regulation). Blood glucose and doses of insulin and oral hypoglycaemics should be monitored in patients with diabetes.

Pregnancy and breast-feeding

The effects of DHEA in pregnancy and breast-feeding are unknown. It is probably best avoided.

Adverse effects

There is no known toxicity or serious side-effects. However, the safety of long-term administration is unknown. DHEA alters the levels of other hormones, and has both oestrogenic and androgenic activity. Potential side-effects in women are therefore increased facial hair and increased loss of head hair, menstrual irregularities and deepening of the voice. The risk of breast cancer may also be increased, but results from studies are conflicting, with some showing that DHEA may reduce risk while others show that it may increase risk. A review concluded that prolonged intake of DHEA may promote breast cancer in post-menopausal women.[26] Potential side-effects in men include an increased risk of prostate cancer.

A study in 22 healthy men[27] suggested that doses up to 200 mg daily for 4 weeks were safe and well tolerated. Another study[28] in 24 healthy elderly men and women (67.8 ± 4.3 years) suggested that daily doses of 25 or 50 mg DHEA are safe in elderly subjects. There were no large increases in blood levels of androgens and oestrogens in this study.

Interactions

None reported, but theoretically DHEA could interact with insulin, oral hypoglycaemic agents, oestrogens (including HRT) and androgens.

Dose

DHEA is available in the form of tablets and capsules.

The dose is not established. Dietary supplements tend to provide 5–50 mg daily.

References

1 Nafziger AN, Bowlin SJ, Jenkins PL, *et al*. Longitudinal changes in dihydroepiandrosterone sulfate and concentrations in men and women. *J Lab Clin Med* 1998; 131: 316–323.

2 Ebeling P, Koivisto VA. Physiological importance of dehydroepiandrosterone. *Lancet* 1994: 343; 1479–1481.

3 Casson PR, Santoro N, Elkind-Hirsch K, *et al*. Postmenopausal dehydroepiandrosterone administration increases free insulin-like growth factor-1 and decreases high density lipoprotein: a six-month trial. *Fertil Steril* 1998; 70: 107–110.

4 Casson PR, Andersen RN, Herrod HG, *et al*. Oral dehydroepiandrosterone in physiologic doses modulates immune function in postmenopausal women. *Am J Obstet Gynecol* 1993; 169: 1536–1539.

5 Khorram O, Vu L, Yen SS. Activation of immune function by dehydroepiandrosterone (DHEA) in age-advanced men. *J Gerontol A Biol Sci Med Sci* 1997; 52: M1–M7.

6 Degelau J, Guay D, Hallgren H. The effect of DHEAS on influenza vaccine in aging adults. *J Am Geriatr Soc* 1997; 45: 747–751.

7 Ben-Yehuda A, Daneberg HD, Zakay-Rones Z, *et al*. The influence of sequential annual vaccination and of DHEA administration on the efficacy of the immune response to influenza vaccine in the elderly. *Mech Ageing Dev* 1998: 102: 299–306.

8 Nestler JE, Barlascini CO, Clore JN, *et al*. Dehydroepiandrosterone reduces serum low density lipoprotein levels and body fat but does not alter insulin sensitivity in normal men. *J Clin Endocrinol Metab* 1988; 66: 57–61.

9 Vogiatzi MG, Boeck MA, Vlachopapadopoulou E, *et al*. Dehydroepiandrosterone in morbidly obese adolescents: effects on weight, body composition, lipids and insulin resistance. *Metabolism* 1996; 45: 1011–1015.

10 Welle S, Jozefowicz R, Statt M. Failure of dehydroepiandrosterone to influence energy and protein metabolism in humans. *J Clin Endocrinol Metab* 1990; 71: 1259–1264.

11 Usiskin KS, Butterworth S, Clore JN, *et al*. Lack of effect of dehydroepiandrosterone in obese men. *Int J Obes* 1990; 14: 457–463.

12 Morales AJ, Nolan JJ, Nelson JC, *et al*. Effects of replacement dose of DHEA in men and women of advancing age. *J Clin Endocrinol Metab* 1994; 78: 1360–1367.

13 Wolf OT, Naumann E, Helhammer DH, *et al*. Effects of dehydroepiandrosterone replacement in elderly men on event-related potentials, memory and well being. *J Gerontol A Biol Med Sci Med Sci* 1998; 53: M385–M3990.

14 Huppert FA, Van Nickerk JK, Herbert J. Dehydroepiandrosterone (DHEA) supplementation for cognition and well being. Cochrane database, issue 2, 2000. London: Macmillan.

15 Wolkowitz OM, Reus VI, Keebler A, *et al*. Double-blind treatment of major depression with dehydroepiandrosterone. *Am J Psychiatry* 1999; 156: 646–649.

16 Wolkowitz OM, Kramer JH, Reus VI, *et al*. DHEA treatment of Alzheimer's disease: a randomized, double-blind, placebo-controlled study. *Neurology* 2003; 60: 1071–1076.

17 Strous RD, Maayan R, Lapidus R, *et al*. Dehydroepiandrosterone augmentation in the management of negative, depressive, and anxiety symptoms in schizophrenia. *Arch Gen Psychiatry* 2003; 60: 133–141.

18 Piketty C, Jayle D, Leplege A, *et al*. Double-blind placebo-controlled trial of oral dehydroepiandrosterone in patients with advanced HIV disease. *Clin Endocrinol* 2001; 55: 325–330.

19 Van Vollenhoven RF, Engleman EG, McGuire GL, *et al*. Dehydroepiandrosterone in systemic lupus erythematosus. Results of a double-blind, placebo-controlled, randomised clinical trial. *Arthritis Rheum* 1995; 38: 1826–1831.

20 Van Vollenhoven RF, Morabito LM, Engleman EG, *et al*. Treatment of systemic lupus erythematosus with dehydroepiandrosterone: 50 patients treated up to 12 months. *J Rheumatol* 1998; 25: 285–289.

21 Chang DM, Lan JL, Lin HY, Luo SF. Dehydroepiandrosterone treatment of women with mild-to-moderate systemic lupus erythmatosus: a multicenter, randomized, double-blind, placebo-controlled trial. *Arthritis Rheum* 2002; 46: 2924–2927.

22 Kawano H, Yasue H, Kitagawa A, *et al*. Dehydrocpiandrosterone supplementation improves endothelial function and insulin sensitivity in men. *J Clin Endocrinol Metab* 2003; 88: 3190–3195.

23 Gordon CM, Grace E, Emans SJ, *et al*. Effects of oral dehydroepiandrosterone on bone density in young women with anorexia nervosa: a randomized trial. *J Clin Endocrinol Metab* 2002; 87: 4935–4941.

24 Kahn AJ, Halloran B, Wolkowitz O, Brizendine L. Dehydroepiandrosterone supplementation and bone turnover in middle-aged to elderly men. *J Clin Endocrinol Metab* 2002; 87: 1544–1549.

25 Percheron G, Hogrel JY, Denot-Ledunois S, *et al*. Effect of 1-year oral administration of dehydroepiandrosterone to 60 to 80-year-old individuals on muscle function and cross-sectional area: a double-blind placebo-controlled trial. *Arch Intern Med* 2003; 163: 720–727.

26 Stoll BA. Dietary supplements of dehydroepiandrosterone in relation to breast cancer risk. *Eur J Clin Nutr* 1999; 53: 771–775.

27 Davidson M, Marwah A, Sawchuk RJ, *et al*. Safety and pharmacokinetic study with escalating doses of 3-acetyl-7-oxo-dehydroepiandrosterone in healthy male volunteers. *Clin Invest Med* 2000; 23: 300–310.

28 Legrain S, Massien C, Lahlou N, *et al*. Dehydroepiandrosterone replacement administration: pharmacokinetic and pharmacodynamic studies in healthy elderly subjects. *J Clin Endocrinol Metab* 2000; 85: 328–317.

Evening primrose oil

Description

Evening primrose oil is derived from the seeds of *Oenothera biennis* and other species.

Constituents

Evening primrose oil contains gamma-linolenic acid (GLA) and linoleic acid. Starflower oil (borage oil) and blackcurrant oil are also used as sources of GLA in dietary supplements. Evening primrose oil contains 8–11% GLA. Starflower oil contains 20–25% GLA, but the biological activity of starflower oil may be no greater than that of evening primrose oil, i.e. on a weight-for-weight basis, starflower oil has not been proved to be twice as active as evening primrose oil. Blackcurrant oil contains 15–25% GLA.

Action

GLA is not an essential dietary component. It is normally synthesised in the body by the action of delta-6-desaturase on linoleic acid (obtained in the diet from vegetable and seed oils, e.g. sunflower oil).

GLA is a precursor of dihomogamma-linolenic acid (DGLA) and the series 1 prostaglandins (PG), and also of arachidonic acid (see Figure 1). Most of the DGLA formed from GLA is metabolised to PG1s; conversion of DGLA to arachidonic acid is very slow. Arachidonic acid is normally obtained from meat in the diet.

Supplementation with GLA increases the ratio of DGLA to arachidonic acid. DGLA levels are elevated to a greater extent by the administration of GLA than by the administration of linoleic acid (for reasons that are not entirely clear).

Prostaglandin PGE_1 (produced from DGLA) inhibits platelet aggregation and is also a vasodilator; it has less potent inflammatory effects than prostaglandins of the PG2 series, thromboxane A_2 and series 4 leukotrienes (produced from arachidonic acid).

The efficacy of GLA is thus thought to be due, in part, to the increased production of PG1 series prostaglandins at the expense of PG2 series prostaglandins, thromboxane A_2 and series 4 leukotrienes.

Deficiency

Patients with diabetes mellitus or eczema may be at risk of GLA deficiency. Despite some claims, there is little evidence that foods rich in saturated fat and sugar, drinking alcohol, stress, pollution, high blood cholesterol, ageing, viral infections and hormone imbalances lead to GLA deficiency.

Possible uses

Evening primrose oil is used widely as a dietary supplement for various disorders, including PMS, hypertension, asthma and angina. It is claimed to reduce blood cholesterol levels and to act as a slimming aid.

Disorders for which evening primrose oil has been tested in controlled clinical trials include atopic dermatitis, diabetic neuropathy, mastalgia and breast cysts, menopausal flushing, Reynaud's phenomenon, rheumatoid arthritis, schizophrenia, Sjogren's syndrome, ulcerative colitis and various cancers. Evening primrose oil is being investigated in a range of other disorders including multiple sclerosis and hyperactivity in children.

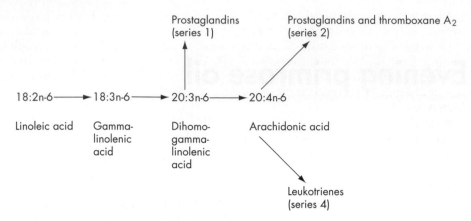

Figure 1   Metabolism of gamma-linolenic acid arachidonic acid.

Skin conditions

The efficacy of evening primrose oil in inflammatory skin conditions such as eczema is difficult to judge, because several trials have shown improvements in both the treatment and placebo groups. However, results indicate that for efficacy, high doses and long-term treatment are necessary. Evening primrose oil may work in these conditions not only by supplying precursors of prostaglandins but also by supplying the essential fatty acids to maintain cell membranes.

A double-blind crossover study involving 99 patients showed improvement in symptoms of eczema with doses of 4–6 g daily of evening primrose oil in adults and 2 g daily in children.[1] Another trial involving 25 patients showed that evening primrose oil (45 mg gamma-linolenic acid per capsule) improved symptoms of eczema. Although there was also an improvement in the placebo group, this was not as great as in the evening primrose oil group.[2] A further double-blind crossover study showed no clinical benefit in the use of evening primrose oil for atopic eczema in a mixed group of adults and children.[3] Adult doses in this study were 12 or 16 500-mg capsules each day. Another study in patients with chronic dermatitis of the hands[3] showed no difference between the effects of evening primrose oil (12 500-mg capsules each day) or placebo (sunflower oil capsules). Similarly conflicting results have been found in studies in children.[4,5]

A double-blind RCT investigated the possible preventive effect of GLA supplementation on the development of atopic dermatitis in infants at risk. One hundred and eighteen formula-fed infants with a maternal history of atopic disease received borage oil supplement (100 mg GLA) or sunflower oil supplement for the first 6 months of life. The intention-to-treat analysis showed a favourable trend for severity of atopic dermatitis associated with GLA supplementation, but no significant effects in the other atopic outcomes, including serum immunoglobulin E (IgE). The authors concluded that early supplementation with GLA in children at high familial risk does not prevent the expression of atopy, but it tends to alleviate the severity of atopic dermatitis in later infancy in these children.[6]

Premenstrual syndrome and the menopause

Evening primrose oil has been studied for its effect on the physical and psychological symptoms of PMS in some women. However, few good studies have been carried out. A review of four studies[7] concluded that evening primrose oil is effective for the treatment of PMS. However, another study in 38 women[8] showed no differences between the effect of placebo and evening primrose oil on symptoms such as fluid retention, breast pain or swelling or mood changes.

Some trials with evening primrose oil in cyclical mastalgia and breast tenderness have shown positive results.[9,10] However, the response can be slow, and it can take several months to decide whether or not treatment is successful. A recent study in 555 women with moderate to severe mastalgia found that GLA (Efamast) efficacy did not differ from that of placebo fatty acids and the presence or absence of antioxidant vitamins made no difference.[11]

Trial data on the effects of evening primrose oil during the menopause are conflicting. In one of the most recent studies,[12] involving 56 post-menopausal women suffering hot flushes, gamma-linolenic acid offered no benefit over placebo.

Rheumatoid arthritis

Results from trials with evening primrose oil in rheumatoid arthritis have been mixed. In one study of 20 patients, treatment with non-steroidal anti-inflammatory drugs (NSAIDs) was stopped and administration of evening primrose oil resulted in no significant changes in symptoms of arthritis.[13] In another study involving 49 patients,[14] treatment with evening primrose oil (equivalent to 540 mg GLA daily) or a combination of evening primrose oil and fish oil (450 mg GLA plus 240 mg eicosapentaenoic acid) allowed for a significant reduction in dose of NSAIDs. However, another study in 20 patients[15] who received either evening primrose oil or olive oil twice daily for 12 weeks, showed no significant differences in terms of prostaglandin levels, therapeutic response or laboratory parameters. However, those individuals whose pro-inflammatory prostaglandin and thromboxane levels were reduced tended to have better therapeutic responses.

Miscellaneous

Encouraging findings have been reported with trials of evening primrose oil in diabetic neuropathy,[16,17] but not in asthma,[18,19] hypercholesterolaemia,[20,21] or obesity.[22]

Recent studies have also been conducted into the potential benefit of GLA in dry eye syndrome and periodontal disease. A preliminary study in 26 patients found that GLA, or linoleic acid, or tear substitutes reduced ocular surface inflammation and improved dry eye syndrome.[23] In a small study involving 30 adults with periodontitis, GLA was found to have beneficial effects, which were more impressive than those for omega-3 fatty acids and lower doses of the two supplements in combination.[24] Further studies will be necessary to more fully assess the potential of GLA in these conditions.

> ### Conclusion
> Results of clinical studies with gamma-linolenic acid (GLA) in skin conditions, including atopic dermatitis, as well as PMS and rheumatoid arthritis, have produced conflicting results. However, some individuals with these conditions do appear to benefit. Preliminary research indicates that GLA may be beneficial in diabetic neuropathy.

Precautions/contraindications

Evening primrose oil should be avoided in patients with epilepsy and in those taking epileptogenic drugs, e.g. phenothiazines. There is some evidence that GLA may increase the risk of seizures in these patients.[25]

Pregnancy and breast-feeding

Caution should be used in pregnancy (because of possible hormonal effects). No problems have been reported in breast-feeding.

Adverse effects

Toxicity appears to be low. The only adverse effects reported are nausea, diarrhoea and headache. However, one report[26] has warned of a potential risk of inflammation, thrombosis and immunosuppression due to slow accumulation of tissue arachidonic acid after prolonged use of GLA for more than 1 year.

Interactions

Drugs
Phenothiazines: increased risk (small) of epileptic fits.

Dose

Evening primrose oil and other supplements containing GLA are generally available in the form of capsules.

Symptomatic relief of eczema: 320–480 mg (as GLA) daily; child 1–12 years, 160–320 mg daily.

Symptomatic relief of cyclical and non-cyclical mastalgia: 240–320 mg (as GLA) daily for 12 weeks (then stopped if no improvement).

Dietary supplements provide 40–300 mg (as GLA) per daily dose.

Note: doses are given in terms of GLA; evening primrose oil supplements are not identical; they provide different amounts of GLA.

References

1 Wright S, Burton JL. Oral evening primrose seed oil improves atopic eczema. *Lancet* 1982; 2: 1120–1122.
2 Schalin-Karrila M, Mattila L, Jansen CT. Evening primrose oil in the treatment of atopic eczema: effect on clinical status, plasma phospholipid fatty acids and circulating blood prostaglandins. *Br J Dermatol* 1987; 117: 11–19.
3 Bamford JT, Gibson RW, Renier CM. Atopic eczema unresponsive to evening primrose oil. *J Am Acad Dermatol* 1985; 13: 959–965.
4 Biagi PL, Bordoni A, Masi M. A long-term study on the use of evening primrose oil (Efamol) in atopic children. *Drugs Exp Clin Res* 1988; 14: 285–290.
5 Hederos CA, Berg A. Epogam evening primrose oil treatment in atopic dermatitis and asthma. *Arch Dis Child* 1996; 75: 494–497.
6 van Gool CJ, Thijs C, Henquet CJ, *et al.* Gamma-linolenic acid supplementation for prophylaxis of atopic dermatitis – a randomized controlled trial in infants at high familial risk. *Am J Clin Nutr* 2003; 77: 943–951.
7 Horrobin DF. The role of essential fatty acids and prostaglandins in the premenstrual syndrome. *J Reprod Med* 1983; 28: 465–468.
8 Khoo SK, Munro C, Battistutta D. Evening primrose oil and treatment of pre-menstrual syndrome. *Med J Austr* 1990; 153: 189–192.
9 McFayden IJ, Forrest AP, Chetty U. Cyclical breast pain – some observations and the difficulties in treatment. *Br J Gen Pract* 1992; 46: 161–164.
10 Steinbrunn BS, Zera RT, Rodriguez JL. Mastalgia – tailoring treatment to type of breast pain. *Postgrad Med* 1997; 102: 183–188.
11 Goyal A, Mansel RE, on behalf of the Efamast Study Group. A randomized multicenter study of gamolenic acid (Efamast) with and without antioxidant vitamins and minerals in the management of mastalgia. *Breast J* 2005; 11: 41–47.
12 Chenoy S, Hussain S, Tayob Y, *et al.* Effect of oral gamolenic acid from evening primrose oil on menopausal flushing. *BMJ* 1994; 308: 501–503.
13 Belch JJ, Ansell D, Madhock R, *et al.* The effects of altering dietary essential fatty acids on requirements for non-steroidal anti-inflammatory drugs in patients with rheumatoid arthritis. *Ann Rheum Dis* 1988; 47: 96–104.
14 Hansen TM, Lerche A, Kassis V, *et al.* Treatment of rheumatoid arthritis with prostaglandin E1 precursors cis-linoleic acid and gamma-linolenic acid. *Scand J Rheumatol* 1983; 12: 85–88.
15 Janntti J, Seppala E, Vapaatalo H. Evening primrose oil and olive oil in the treatment of rheumatoid arthritis. *Clin Rheumatol* 1989; 8: 238–244.
16 16. Gamma-Linolenic Acid Multicenter Trial Group. Treatment of diabetic neuropathy with gamma-linolenic acid. *Diabetes Care* 1993; 16: 8–15.
17 Jamal GA, Carmichael H. The effect of gamma-linolenic acid on human diabetic peripheral neuropathy: a double-blind placebo-controlled trial. *Diabetic Med* 1990; 7: 319–323.
18 Ebden P, Bevan C, Banks J. A study of evening primrose seed oil in atopic asthma. *Prostaglandins Leukot Essent Fatty Acids* 1989; 35: 69–72.
19 Stenius-Aarniala B, Aro A, Hakulinen A. Evening primrose and fish oil are ineffective as supplementary treatment of bronchial asthma. *Ann Allergy* 1989; 62: 534–537.
20 Viikari J, Lehtonen A. Effect of evening primrose oil on serum lipids and blood pressure in hyperlipidemic subjects. *Int J Clin Pharmacol Ther Toxicol* 1986; 24: 668–670.
21 Boberg M, Vessby B, Selenius I. Effects of dietary supplementation with n-6 and n-3 long-chain polyunsaturated fatty acids on serum lipoproteins and platelet function in hypertriglyceridaemic patients. *Acta Med Scand* 1986; 220: 153–160.
22 Haslett C, Douglas JG, Chalmers SR. A double-blind evaluation of evening primrose oil as an anti-obesity agent. *Int J Obesity* 1983; 7: 549–553.
23 Barabino S, Rolando M, Camicione P, *et al.* Systemic linoleic acid and gamma-linolenic acid therapy in dry eye syndrome with an inflammatory component. *Cornea* 2003; 22: 77–101.
24 Rosenstein ED, Kushner LJ, Kramer N, Kazandjian G. Pilot study of dietary fatty acid supplementation in the treatment of adult periodontitis. *Prostaglandins Leukot Essent Fatty Acids* 2003; 68: 213–218.
25 Miller LG. Herbal medicines. Selected clinical considerations focusing on known or potential drug-herb interactions. *Arch Intern Med* 1998; 158: 2200–2211.
26 Phinney S. Potential risk of prolonged gamma-linolenic acid use. *Ann Intern Med* 1994; 120, 692.

Fish oils

Description

There are two types of fish oil supplements:

- Fish liver oil: this is generally obtained from the liver of the cod, halibut or shark.
- Fish body oil: this is normally derived from the flesh of the herring, sardine or anchovy.

Constituents

Fish liver oil is a rich source of vitamins A and D; concentrations in cod liver oil liquids normally range between 750 and 1200 µg (2500–4000 units) vitamin A per 10 ml and 2.5–10 µg (100–400 units) vitamin D per 10 ml; halibut and shark liver oils are more concentrated sources of these vitamins. Fish body oil is low in vitamins A and D. Vitamin E is also present in both types of fish oil and extra vitamin E is normally added to supplements.

Both fish liver oil and fish body oil are sources of polyunsaturated fatty acids (PUFAs) of the omega-3 series [eicosapentaenoic acid (EPA) and docosahexaenoic acid (DHA)].

Human requirements

EPA and DHA can be synthesised in the body (in small amounts) from alpha-linolenic acid (contained in vegetable oils, e.g. soya bean, linseed and rapeseed oils). However, this conversion may be inefficient in some individuals.

Recommended intakes

Various recommendations, both in the UK and elsewhere, have been made for the intake of very-long-chain n-3 fatty acids (EPA/DHA) as follows:

UK Department of Heath:[1]	200 mg daily
British Nutrition Foundation:[2]	1250 mg daily
International Society for the Study of Fatty Acids and Lipids:[3]	650 mg daily
The Danish Ministry of Health	300 mg daily
Deutsche Gesellschaft für Ernährung (DGE)	1500 mg daily

Dietary sources

Oily fish is the best source, but some so-called 'functional foods' including eggs, bread, margarines and milk are fortified with EPA/DHA. Algae are good sources of EPA/DHA and are being investigated as sources for supplements and functional foods (Table 1). However, the technological expertise is not yet available.

Action

Fish oils have several effects. These include:

- Alteration of lipoprotein metabolism. Fish oils reduce both fasting and post-prandial plasma triacylglycerols and VLDL cholesterol. With moderate intakes of fish oils, both HDL and LDL cholesterol tend to increase. High intakes reduce HDL cholesterol and may increase LDL in some patients. A meta-analysis of published human trials (that each provided 7 g daily of fish oils for at least 2 weeks) showed that serum cholesterol is unaffected by long-chain n-3 fatty acid consumption. However, triacylglycerols fell by 25–30%, LDL increased by 5–10% and HDL fell by 1–3%.[4]
- Inhibition of atherosclerosis. Fish oils reduce the plasma concentrations of several

Table 1 Typical very-long-chain n-3 fatty acid (EPA and DHA) content of fish and fish oils

Food	Average serving(g)	Total EPA/DHA per serving[1]
Kippers	130	3.37
Mackerel	160	3.09
Pilchards (canned in tomato sauce)	110	2.86
Trout	230	2.65
Salmon (fresh)	100	2.2
Sardines (canned in tomato sauce)	100	1.67
Herring	119	1.56
Salmon (canned in brine, drained)	100	1.55
Crab (canned)	85	0.85
Plaice	130	0.39
Tuna, fresh	120	0.3–1.5
Cod	120	0.30
Mussels	40	0.24
Haddock	120	0.19
Tuna (canned in oil, drained)	45	0.17
Tuna (canned in brine, drained)	45	0.08
Prawns	60	0.06
Cod liver oil liquid[2]	10 ml	1.5–3.0
Cod liver oil capsules[2]	Varies	0.1–0.4
Fish oil capsules[2]	Varies	0.1–0.4

[1] Source (except 2): Holland B, Brown J, Buss DH. Fish and fish products; the third supplement to *McCance & Widdowson's The Composition of Food*, 5th edn. London: HMSO, 1993.

[2] Source: product labels. Doses and amounts of EPA/DHA vary between products.

atherogenic lipoproteins (see above), but other mechanisms may be important. Thus, these effects may be associated with reduced synthesis of cytokines and interleukin 1α and through stimulation of the endothelial production of nitric oxide.[5]

- Prevention of thrombosis. Thrombosis is a major complication of coronary atherosclerosis, which can lead to myocardial infarction. The n-3 fatty acids have anti-thrombotic actions through inhibiting the synthesis of thromboxane A_2 from arachidonic acids in platelets.[6] Thromboxane A_2 causes platelet aggregation and vasoconstriction and as a result fish oil increases bleeding time and reduces the 'stickiness' of the platelets. Fish oil also enhances the production of prostacyclin, which leads to vasodilatation and less 'sticky' platelets. These effects help to reduce the risk of thrombosis.

- Inhibition of inflammation. Diets rich in omega-3 fatty acids appear to reduce the inflammatory response.[7]

- Inhibition of the immune response. Immune reactivity is generally reduced by omega-3 fatty acids.[8,9]

- Reduction in heart rate. A meta-analysis of 30 RCTs found that fish oil decreased heart rate by 1.6 beats per minute compared with placebo. In trials where initial heart beat was high and/or the study period was long, reduction in heart rate averaged 2.5 beats per minute. Heart rate reduction did not significantly vary with dosage of fish oil.[10]

- Influence on arrhythmias. Fish oil may reduce the incidence of lethal myocardial infarction and sudden death. This may be due to the prevention of fatal cardiac arrhythmias. Evidence from some studies indicates an anti-arrhythmic action of fish oil,[11] while evidence from other studies does not.[12–14] In patients undergoing coronary artery bypass surgery (CABG), omega-3 fatty acids (2 g daily) substantially reduced the incidence of post-operative atrial fibrillation.[15] In a further study in patients with a recent episode of sustained ventricular arrhythmia and an implantable cardioverter defibrillator (ICD), fish oil did not reduce the risk of ventricular tachycardia and ventricular fibrillation and there was evidence of a pro-arrhythmic effect in some patients.[16]

Mechanism of action
Fish oils appear to act by:

- modulation of pro-inflammatory and pro-thrombotic eicosanoid (prostaglandin, thromboxane and leukotriene) production; and
- reduction in interleukin-1 and other cytokines.

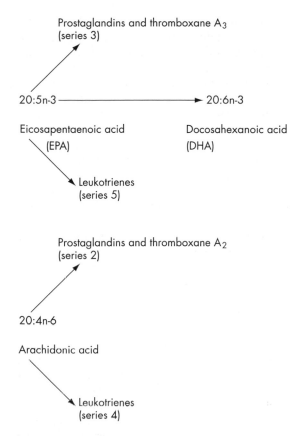

Prostaglandins and thromboxane A₃
(series 3)

20:5n-3 ──────────────→ 20:6n-3

Eicosapentaenoic acid   Docosahexanoic acid
  (EPA)   (DHA)

          Leukotrienes
          (series 5)

Prostaglandins and thromboxane A₂
(series 2)

20:4n-6

Arachidonic acid

          Leukotrienes
          (series 4)

Figure 1   Metabolism of eicosapentaenoic acid and arachidonic acid.

Eicosanoid production
The effects of omega-3 fatty acids are thought to be due to the partial replacement of arachidonic acid with EPA in cell membrane lipids. This leads to increased production of PG3 series prostaglandins, thromboxane A_3 and series 5 leukotrienes at the expense of PG2 series prostaglandins, thromboxane A_2 and series 4 leukotrienes (see Figure 1).

Thromboxane A_3 (produced from EPA) is less effective at stimulating platelet aggregation than thromboxane A_2 (produced from arachidonic acid). Prostaglandins of the PG3 series have less potent inflammatory effects than prostaglandins of the PG2 series. In addition, DHA inhibits the formation of the more inflammatory prostaglandins of the PG2 series, while EPA acts as a substrate for the synthesis of the less inflammatory prostaglandins of the PG3 series.

Series 5 leukotrienes (produced by EPA) have weaker inflammatory effects than series 4 leukotrienes (produced by arachidonic acid).

Possible uses

Fish liver oils are used as a source of vitamins A and D. Both fish liver oils and fish body oils are used as a source of EPA and DHA.

In addition, fish oils appear to have a role in the prevention and management of certain conditions such as CHD and stroke, rheumatoid arthritis, inflammatory bowel disease, psoriasis and asthma, mental disorders such as depression, schizophrenia and Alzheimer's disease, nephropathy, various cancers and diabetes mellitus.

Cardiovascular disease
The consumption of fish is associated with lower rates of CHD in many epidemiological studies. Seminal findings in Eskimos have been confirmed and extended to Western populations, and in most studies there is an inverse relationship between the intake of fish or n-3 fatty acids and total mortality or cardiovascular mortality.[17–21] However, some studies[22,23] have not shown any benefit, possibly because fish intake was higher in the studied population as a whole.

Intervention studies, in which the intake of fish or fish oil was increased, have also shown beneficial effects. One classic study[24] investigated 2000 Welsh men who had just recovered from their first heart attack. The men were randomised to a 'fish advice group', in which they were asked to eat at least two portions of oily fish a week, or failing this fish oil in capsule form, or a 'no fish advice group'. After 2 years, there was a 29% reduction in mortality in the fish/fish oil group, which was attributable to a reduction in CHD deaths. However, although there were fewer fatal heart attacks in the fish group, the total number of heart attacks did not decrease.

The GISSI Prevenzione trial[25] investigated the effects of n-3 PUFAs (1 g daily), vitamin E (300 mg daily) or both as supplements in a study involving 11 324 patients surviving recent myocardial infarction. Treatment with n-3 PUFAs, but not vitamin E, reduced total deaths and cardiovascular deaths, and the effect of the combined treatment was similar to that for n-3 PUFAs alone.

In a double-blind, placebo-controlled study in India,[26] 360 patients with suspected myocardial infarction were randomised to receive fish oil (1.09 g EPA/DHA daily), mustard oil (2.9 g alpha-linolenic acid daily) or placebo for 1 year. Total cardiac events, including cardiac arrhythmias, and also angina pectoris and left ventricular enlargement, were significantly reduced in both the fish oil and mustard oil groups compared with placebo. Fish oil, but not mustard oil, was significantly correlated with fewer cardiac deaths than placebo.

Overall, a consistent body of evidence derived from several hundred studies has indicated that a daily ingestion of at least 1 g of EPA and DHA results in a reduction in total mortality, cardiovascular mortality and morbidity.[27] The American Heart Association recommends that patients with CHD should consume 1 g EPA + DHA per day, preferably from oily fish, although if this is difficult to achieve from diet alone, a fish oil supplement may form part of the dietary and lifestyle change.

However, a more recent large trial involving 3114 men with angina found a higher risk of cardiac death in men consuming fish oil. Subjects in the trial were allocated to four groups: (i) advised to eat two portions of oily fish each week or take fish oil capsules; (ii) advised to eat more fruit, vegetables and oats; (iii) advised to eat oily fish and more fruit, vegetables and oats; and (iv) no specific dietary advice. Mortality was evaluated after 3–9 years. All-cause mortality was not reduced by any form of advice. Risk of cardiac death was higher among subjects advised to take oily fish than among those not so advised. The excess risk was largely found in those taking fish oil capsules. The authors concluded that the result is unexplained; that it may arise from risk compensation or some other effect on the behaviour of patients or doctors.[28]

Recent meta-analyses and systematic reviews have considered this issue. A meta-analysis of 11 RCTs that compared dietary or non-dietary intake of n-3 fatty acids with placebo in patients with CHD found that dietary and non-dietary intake of n-3 fatty acids reduces overall mortality, mortality due to myocardial infarction and sudden death in patients with CHD.[29]

A systematic review[30,31] investigated the role of omega-3 fatty acids for prevention and treatment of CVD using both RCT and cohort studies. RCTs were included where omega-3 intake or advice was randomised and unconfounded and study duration was at least 6 months. Cohort studies were included where a cohort was followed up for at least 6 months and omega-3 intake estimated. Forty-eight RCTs and 41 cohort studies were included. Pooled trial results did not show a reduction in the risk of total mortality or combined cardiovascular events in those taking additional omega-3 fats (with significant statistical heterogeneity). Sensitivity analysis, retaining only studies at low risk of bias, reduced heterogeneity and again suggested no significant effect of omega-3 fats. Restricting analysis to trials increasing fish-based omega-3 fats, or those increasing short-chain omega-3s, did not suggest significant effects on mortality or cardiovascular events in either group. Subgroup analysis by dietary advice or supplementation, baseline risk of CVD or omega-3 dose suggested no clear effects of these factors on primary outcomes. The reviewers concluded that: 'It is not clear that dietary or supplemental omega-3 fats alter total mortality, or combined cardiovascular events in people with, or at high risk of, CVD in the general population. There is no evidence that people should be advised to stop taking rich sources of omega-3 fats, but further high quality trials are needed to confirm suggestions of a protective effect of omega-3 fats on CV health. There is no clear evidence that omega-3 fats differ in effectiveness according to fish or plant sources, dietary or supplemental sources, dose or presence of placebo.'

These results are discussed in a further paper where the suggestion is made that fish oil could have either anti- or pro-arrhythmic effects depending on the medical status of the individual, and that this could explain conflicting results.[32] However, this systematic review has attracted criticism on the basis that it did not include several cohort trials, it analysed primary and secondary prevention trials together and included studies involving alpha-linolenic acid and fish oils.

A second review of the effects of omega-3 fatty acids on CVD[33] includes prevention studies, including 11 RCTs and one prospective cohort study that reported outcomes on CVD populations (n = 16 000 patients). Trials lasted from 1.5 to 5 years. Eleven secondary prevention studies were considered in this review. Four trials used fish oil (EPA + DHA) supplements in doses of 0.27–4.8 g daily and were of good methodological quality. The largest trial reported that fish oil supplements reduce all-cause mortality and CVD outcomes but do not affect stroke. A fifth RCT compared mustard seed oil[26] (containing alpha-linolenic acid), fish oil and non-oil placebo and found that both oils were efficacious in reducing CVD outcomes compared to placebo but found no difference between supplements. However, the methodological quality of this trial was considered by the reviewers to be poor. Six trials reported contradictory data on stroke, with three trials using omega-3 supplements reporting increased strokes and three diet/dietary advice trials reporting reduced strokes. One study, which randomised a total of 300 patients to 1.7 g daily of EPA and DHA or an equivalent amount of corn oil for 1.5 years, reported no beneficial effect of omega-3 fats on any CVD outcomes.

Primary prevention studies considered in this review included 22 prospective cohort studies, four case-control studies, one cross-sectional study and one RCT, which reported data on outcomes in the general population. These studies were conducted in many parts of the world, the methodological quality was generally good, most of the cohort studies had several thousand subjects and study duration ranged from 4 to 30 years. Most of the large cohort studies reported that fish consumption reduces all-cause mortality and CVD events, although some studies reported no significant or negative effects. Benefits in primary prevention of stroke were not clearly seen. The review also indicated that the relative effect of alpha-linolenic acid versus fish oil is not clear and that there are few data concerning the needs of different high-risk populations.

A further US systematic review[34] looked at the effect of omega-3 fatty acids on cardiovascular risk factors. The strongest and most consistent effect of omega-3 fatty acids was found on lowering triglyceride levels. The effect of omega-3 fatty acids on other lipids was weaker. In general, LDL cholesterol and HDL cholesterol were found to rise to a small extent. No consistent effect was found on levels of lipoprotein A. Total apolipoprotein B and apolipoprotein B-100 levels fell, while LDL apolipoprotein B levels increased. There was no consistent effect on markers of inflammation and thrombosis, including C-reactive protein (CRP), fibrinogen, factor VII, factor VIII, and platelet aggregation. There was an overall trend towards a net reduction of relative risk of 14% in coronary artery restenosis, while data on the effect of omega-3 fatty acids on carotid artery intima-media thickness were found to be conflicting. The review suggested that fish oil consumption may benefit exercise capacity and heart rate variability (which may reduce the incidence of ventricular arrhythmias) among people with coronary artery disease.

Rheumatoid arthritis

Fish oils appear to alleviate the symptoms of rheumatoid arthritis, and this is commensurate with the role of n-3 fatty acids in suppression of the production of inflammatory eicosanoids. Several studies have shown that very-long-chain n-3 fatty acids reduce pain and morning stiffness[35] and decrease the need for NSAIDs.[36–38] Moreover, a meta-analysis of 10 double-blind, placebo-controlled randomised trials in 395 patients showed that fish oil taken for 3 months was associated with a statistically significant reduction in joint tenderness and morning stiffness, but no significant improvements in joint swelling, grip strength or erythrocyte sedimentation rate (ESR, a marker of inflammation).[39]

However, a US review conducted for the Office of Dietary Supplements, National Institutes of Health, on the effects of omega-3 fatty acids on rheumatoid arthritis concluded that from nine studies reporting outcomes in patients with rheumatoid arthritis, omega-3 fatty acids had no effect on patient reports of pain, swollen joint count, ESR and patients' global assessment by meta-analysis.[40]

A Dutch double-blind, placebo-controlled, parallel-group study in 66 patients with rheumatoid arthritis using 1.4 g EPA, 0.211 g DHA and 0.5 g gamma-linolenic acid (GLA) with micronutrients found no significant change from baseline in tender joint count, swollen joint count, visual analogue scales for pain and disease activity, grip strength, functionality scores and morning stiffness. The conclusion was that this study adds information regarding doses of omega-3 fatty acids below which anti-inflammatory effects in rheumatoid arthritis are not seen.[41]

Inflammatory bowel disease

Fish oil has been found to have some benefits in patients with Crohn's disease or ulcerative colitis, but no real conclusions can be drawn. A review of five studies[42] investigating the effect of n-3 fatty acids in Crohn's disease was inconclusive, but a later study[43] showed that an enteric-coated preparation of very-long-chain n-3 fatty acids significantly reduced the rate of relapse in patients with Crohn's disease in remission.

In patients with ulcerative colitis, fish oil supplements have been found to reduce corticosteroid requirements,[44] improve gastrointestinal histology,[45] and reduce disease activity index.[46]

A US review[39] among 13 studies reporting outcomes in patients with inflammatory bowel disease found variable effects of omega-3 fatty acids on clinical score, sigmoidoscopic score, histologic score, induced remission and relapse. In ulcerative colitis, omega-3 fatty acids had no effect on the relative risk of relapse in a meta-analysis of three studies. There was a statistically non-significant reduction in requirement for corticosteroids for omega-3 fatty acids relative to placebo in two studies. No studies included in this review evaluated the effect of omega-3 fatty acids on requirement for other immunosuppressive agents.

A further systematic review in 13 controlled trials assessed the effects of n-3 fatty acids on clinical, sigmoidoscopic or histologic scores, rates of remission or relapse, or requirements for steroids and other immunosuppressive agents in Crohn's disease or ulcerative colitis. Most clinical trials were of good quality. Fewer than six were identified that assessed the effects of n-3 fatty acids on any single outcome of clinical, endoscopic or histologic scores or remission or relapse rates. Consistent across three studies was the finding that n-3 fatty acids reduce corticosteroid requirements, although statistical significance was shown in only one of these studies. The conclusion of the review was that the available data are insufficient to draw conclusions about the effects of n-3 fatty acids on clinical, endoscopic or histologic scores or remission or relapse rate.[47]

Psoriasis

Fish oils have been claimed to be beneficial in some individuals with psoriasis, leading to reduced itching and erythema. However, six RCTs produced inconclusive results.[48–53]

Asthma

Because asthma is an inflammatory condition, which appears to involve eicosanoids, it is biologically plausible that fish oil could be of benefit. However, results of studies have been discouraging and there is no clear evidence that fish oils are beneficial in asthma. One study has suggested that fish oil could be protective in suppressing exercise-induced bronchoconstriction in athletes,[54] and another that fish oil may be beneficial in children with bronchial asthma.[55]

A US systematic review including 31 reports (describing 26 unique studies) stated that it is impossible to conclude anything with respect to the value of using omega-3 fatty acid supplementation in the management and/or prevention of asthma for adults or children either in or beyond North America. This is due to the lack of sufficiently consistent evidence, as well as the paucity of evidence from well-designed, well-conducted and adequately powered studies. Further research is needed to establish or refute the value of omega-3 fatty acids to prevent or treat asthma in children and adults.[56]

A Cochrane review assessed the effect of omega-3 fatty acids in asthma. Nine RCTs were included. There was no consistent effect on any of the analysable outcomes: FEV_1, peak flow rate, asthma symptoms, asthma medication use or bronchial hyper-reactivity. One of the trials in children, which combined dietary manipulation with fish oil supplementation, showed improved peak flow and reduced asthma medication use. There were no adverse effects associated with fish oil supplements. The authors concluded that there is little evidence to recommend that people with asthma supplement or modify dietary intake of marine omega-3 fatty acids in order to improve their asthma control. Equally there is no evidence that they are at risk if they do so.[57]

Diabetes

Although fish oil has been linked with deterioration in glucose and insulin control in patients with diabetes mellitus, results from studies with fish oil in such patients have been inconsistent. Treatment with n-3 fatty acids led to a small increase in blood glucose levels in diabetes in one study,[58] but not in another.[59] However, a meta-analysis concluded that fish oil has no adverse effects on glucose or insulin metabolism in patients with diabetes, and lowers triacylglycerol levels effectively by 30%.[60]

A US systematic review[40] including 18 studies of type 2 diabetes or the metabolic syndrome concluded that omega-3 fatty acids had a favourable effect on triglyceride levels, but had no effect on total cholesterol, HDL cholesterol, LDL cholesterol, fasting blood sugar, or glycosylated haemoglobin, by meta-analysis. Omega-3 fatty acids had no effect on plasma insulin or insulin resistance in patients with type 2 diabetes or the metabolic syndrome.

A Cochrane review looked at 18 trials and 823 participants followed for a mean of 12 weeks taking doses of fish oils ranging from 3 to 18 g daily. Outcomes studied were glycaemic control and lipid levels. Meta-analysis of pooled data demonstrated a significant effect of fish oil on lowering triglycerides by 0.56 mmol/L (95% CI: −0.71 to −0.4) and raising LDL cholesterol by 0.21 mmol/L (95% CI: 0.02 to 0.41). No statistically significant effect was observed for fasting glucose, HbA1c, total or HDL cholesterol. The triglyceride lowering effect and the elevation in LDL cholesterol were most marked in those trials that recruited people with hypertriglyceridaemia and used higher doses of fish oil. No adverse effects were reported. The reviewers concluded that fish oil supplementation in type 2 diabetes lowers triglycerides, may raise LDL cholesterol (especially in hypertriglyceridaemic patients on high doses of fish oil) and has no significant effect on glycaemic control.[61]

Mental health

The potential role of fish oil in mental disorders is now being investigated. A number of studies have found low levels of n-3 fatty acids in cell membranes of patients with depression, schizophrenia and Alzheimer's disease, and it has been suggested that low dietary intakes of n-3 fatty acids or an imbalance in the n-6:n-3 ratio might be associated with these conditions.

A Cochrane review including five short, small trials concluded that there are no clear effects of omega-3 fatty acids in schizophrenia and that large, well-conducted trials are needed.[62] A US systematic review of the effects of omega-3 fats on mental health found that evidence was somewhat suggestive of benefit for omega-3 fatty acids as a short-term intervention for schizophrenia. However, the trials need replication with better methodology. One of the included trials demonstrated a clinical effect in depressive symptoms (rather than depressive disorders) and should not be taken to support the idea that omega-3 fatty acids are beneficial for depressive disorders. The review concluded that there is insufficient evidence to recommend omega-3 fatty acids as a supplemental treatment for any other psychiatric disorders or as a primary treatment for any of the conditions considered in the review (i.e. mainly schizophrenia and depression).[63]

A double-blind, placebo-controlled trial in 28 patients with major depressive disorder found that omega-3 PUFAs (6.6 g daily) significantly decreased the score on the 21-item Hamilton Rating Scale for Depression. The authors concluded that from the preliminary findings in this study, omega-3 PUFAs could improve the short-term course of illness and were well tolerated in patients with major depressive disorder.[64]

A further double-blind, placebo-controlled trial of fish oil involved 77 participants who were randomly allocated to receive 8 g of either fish oil or olive oil per day for 12 weeks in addition to their existing antidepressant therapy. Mood increased significantly in both groups within the first 2 weeks of the study and this improvement was sustained throughout. However, there was no evidence that fish oil improved mood when compared with placebo oil, despite an increase in circulating omega-3 polyunsaturated fatty acids.[65]

Cognitive function and neurological conditions

A US systematic review that included 12 articles concluded that fish consumption was only weakly associated with a reduced risk of cognitive impairment and had no association with cognitive decline. Fish consumption was associated with a reduced risk of Alzheimer's disease (which was significant in only one of the included studies), while omega-3 consumption and consumption of DHA (but not ALA or EPA) were associated with a significant reduction in the incidence of Alzheimer's. There were no significant associations for Parkinson's disease and effects in multiple sclerosis varied considerably from no benefit to increased disability with omega-3 fatty acids.[66]

A Cochrane review of omega-3 fatty acids for prevention of dementia found that a growing body of evidence from biological, observational and epidemiological studies suggests a protective effect of omega-3 fatty acids against dementia. However, the reviewers found no randomised trials that met their selection criteria and they concluded there is no good evidence to support the use of dietary or supplemental omega-3 fatty acids for the prevention of cognitive impairment or dementia.[67]

A more recent 12-month double-blind RCT in 31 patients with multiple sclerosis found that a low-fat diet supplemented with omega-3 PUFA can have moderate benefits in relapse-remitting multiple sclerosis patients on concurrent disease-modifying therapies.[68]

Child and maternal health

Claims are increasingly made that an increase in maternal omega-3 fatty acid intake has the potential to influence both maternal health during pregnancy and also foetal health and birth weight. Results of studies conducted in the Faroe Islands suggest that marine diets, which contain omega-3 fatty acids, increase birth weight either by prolonging pregnancy or by increasing foetal growth rate. In addition it has been hypothesised that marine oils may reduce the risks of certain pregnancy complications, including pre-term delivery, intrauterine growth retardation, pre-eclampsia and gestational diabetes.

Similarly, it has also been suggested that accumulation of omega-3 fatty acids in the child post-delivery can affect the development and health of the child. Infants fed with human milk have improved neurocognitive development compared to formula-fed infants and it has been suggested that one of the contributing factors may be the availability of long-chain derivatives of linoleic acid and alpha-linolenic acid, which are present naturally only in human milk. Infant formulae containing omega-3 long-chain PUFAs are now on the UK market.

A US systematic review has addressed these issues.[69] Various outcomes, including pregnancy outcomes, growth pattern outcomes, neurological development outcomes, visual function outcomes and cognitive development outcomes were considered. Fifteen RCTs, all poor quality, addressed pregnancy outcomes in relation to omega-3 intake in the mother. No difference was found in duration of gestation in 10 studies, while four very poor-quality studies found that omega-3 fatty acids increased the duration of gestation compared with placebo. There was no significant effect on the proportion of premature deliveries in 10 studies. Meta-analysis of the incidence of premature deliveries showed inconsistent evidence of the use of omega-3 fatty acid supplements during the second or third trimester of pregnancy to reduce the incidence of premature pregnancies in both high- and low-risk populations. No significant effects were found for omega-3 fatty acids on the incidence of gestational hypertension and pre-eclampsia. There were no significant differences in birth weight between supplemented and non-supplemented groups of mothers.

Maternal intake of omega-3 fatty acids was also investigated for an effect on growth pattern outcomes in the infant. Overall effects on infant growth patterns were found to be non-significant in infants from birth to 12 months of age. Analysis of studies in which pre-term infants were fed formula milk containing omega-3 fatty acids resulted in non-significant findings for growth parameters. In formula-fed term infants, meta-analysis demonstrated a non-significant overall effect of formulae containing DHA and arachidonic acid compared with control formula on growth patterns at 4 and 12 months.

Neurological development outcomes from studies included in the review were not significantly affected by maternal intake during pregnancy or the omega-3 content of breast milk. No significant differences in neurological outcomes were found in either pre-term infants or term infants fed supplemented formula milk compared with control formula.

According to this review, visual function in the infant was not significantly affected by either maternal intake during pregnancy or the omega-3 content of breast milk. Variable results in visual function according to formula intake in both pre-term and term infants have been found. Better or faster maturation of visual acuity has been found in some studies but not all.

Effects on cognitive development in infants according to maternal intake of omega-3 during pregnancy, the omega-3 content of maternal breast milk, and whether pre-term and term formulae were supplemented with omega-3 were also inconsistent.

In summary, this systematic review concluded that pregnancy outcomes were either unaffected by omega-3 fatty acid supplementation or the results were inconclusive. Results suggested an absence of effects with respect to the impact of supplementation on gestational hypertension, pre-eclampsia or eclampsia. Results concerning the impact of the intake of omega-3 fatty acids on the development of infants are primarily, although not uniformly, inconclusive.

More recent trials have shown: a small effect of DHA levels in breast milk on early language development in breast-fed infants;[70] a positive effect of maternal n-3 supplementation on child growth at 2.5 years;[71] a positive effect

of DHA supplementation in mothers on child neurodevelopment as measured by the Bayley Psychomotor Development Index at 30 months of age (but with no other advantages before, at or after this age);[72] and a positive effect of formula supplemented with long-chain PUFAs on visual acuity.[73]

There is also some evidence that maternal dietary n-3 PUFA intake can reduce the risk of development of allergy in the infant.[74,75]

Behavioural problems

Fatty acids have been the subject of a great deal of attention over their potential benefit in children with various behavioural disorders. There is growing evidence that a relative lack of certain polyunsaturated fatty acids may contribute to related neurodevelopmental and psychiatric disorders such as dyslexia and attention deficit hyperactivity disorder (ADHD).

An RCT in 117 children with developmental coordination disorder (DCD) found that supplementation with omega-3 and omega-6 fatty acids resulted in significant improvements in reading, spelling and behaviour over 3 months of treatment. No effect on motor skills was apparent in this study.[76]

In a study involving 40 children (aged 6–12 years) with ADHD, DHA supplementation (3.6 g/week) for 2 months did not improve ADHD-related symptoms.[77] A further study in 60 children with ADHD found that DHA supplementation (345 mg daily) did not reduce symptoms of ADHD.[78]

Fish oil (providing 3600 mg DHA + 840 mg EPA per week) for 3 months was associated in one study with reduced physical aggression, particularly in girls.[79]

Renal disease

Fish oil has been investigated for potential benefit in kidney disease. In a placebo-controlled, multicentre trial, 106 patients were randomised to receive either 12 g of fish oil daily over a period of 2 years or placebo.[80] The rate of loss of kidney function was retarded in the supplemented group and the beneficial effect was suggested to be due to the impact of n-3 fatty acids on eicosanoid production and other factors. However, other studies have shown no such benefits and more work is needed. A more recent RCT investigated the effect of low-dose omega-3 PUFAs (0.85 g EPA and 0.57 g DHA) in 14 patients with IgA nephropathy. The supplement was effective in slowing renal progression in these high-risk patients.[81]

A US systematic review, which included nine studies assessing the effect of omega-3 fatty acids in renal disease, found there were varying effects on serum creatinine and creatinine clearance and no effect on progression to end-stage renal disease. In a single study that assessed the effect on haemodialysis graft patency, graft patency was better with fish oil than with placebo. No studies in this review assessed the effects of omega-3 fatty acids on requirements for corticosteroids.[40]

Cancers

In animal studies, fish oils have been shown to reduce cell proliferation and pre-cancerous cell changes, and some epidemiological studies in humans have suggested that fish oils might be protective against cancer. A US systematic review concluded that evidence from the large body of literature does not suggest a significant association between omega-3 fatty acids and cancer incidence. From a small body of literature no significant association was found between omega-3 fatty acids and clinical outcomes after tumour surgery.[82] Another systematic review of 38 papers (published between 1966 and October 2005) did not provide any evidence to suggest a significant association between omega-3 fatty acids and cancer incidence.[83]

Miscellaneous

A US systematic review considered the role of omega-3 fatty acids in SLE. Among the three studies included in the review, variable effects on SLE were found. Omega-3 fatty acids had no effect on corticosteroid requirements in one study. No studies were identified that assessed the effects of omega-3 fatty acids on requirements for other immunosuppressive drugs for SLE. None of the studies used a measure of disease activity that incorporates both subjective and objective measures of disease activity.[40]

Omega-3 fatty acids have also been investigated for a role in prevention of osteoporosis. A review that included five reviews and 11 *in vivo* studies (eight in animals and three RCTs in humans) found that two of the human RCTs showed a positive effect of a low n-6/n-3 ratio on bone, while the third human study showed no effect. The authors concluded that these data, though preliminary, suggest that a diet with a low n-6/n-3 ratio may have beneficial effects on BMD.[84] A US systematic review[37] including five human studies concluded that the effect of omega-3 fatty acids on bone was variable.

A US systematic review has looked at the effects of omega-3 fatty acids in eye health. Sixteen studies were identified, of which only two were RCTs. The review concluded that from the studies identified, no conclusions could be reached about the effect of omega-3 fatty acids as a primary or secondary prevention in eye health, including ARMD, retinitis pigmentosa, cataract, and also vascular disease of the retina in patients with and without diabetes.[85]

There is also growing interest in the role of n-3 fatty acids in other conditions affecting respiration, including hay fever, COPD and cystic fibrosis.

Conclusion

Fish oil appears to reduce the risk of CHD. It may help to: reduce the risk of thrombosis by increasing bleeding tendency; reduce blood levels of triacylglycerols; prevent atherosclerosis and arrhythmias; and reduce blood pressure. Fish oil could have beneficial effects in inflammatory conditions such as rheumatoid arthritis, Crohn's disease and inflammatory bowel disorders, but evidence of benefit in asthma and psoriasis is poor. Fish oil may have a role in various mental disorders, such as depression, schizophrenia and Alzheimer's disease, but research in this area is in its infancy. Evidence of benefit of fish oil in maternal and child health, including child development and visual acuity, is conflicting. Evidence of value of omega-3 fatty acids in childhood behavioural disorders, such as developmental coordination disorder, is increasing.

Precautions/contraindications

Patients with blood clotting disorders or those taking anticoagulants should be monitored while taking fish oils.

Pregnancy and breast-feeding

Use in pregnancy should be supervised (because of the potential for vitamin A toxicity with excessive intakes of fish liver oil).

Adverse effects

Vitamin A and D toxicity (fish liver oil only). The unpleasant taste of fish liver oil liquids may be masked by mixing with fruit juice or milk.

Fish oil supplements are generally safe, and in one prospective study involving 295 people aged 18–76 years,[86] 10–20 ml of fish oil providing 1.8–3.6 g EPA/DHA for 7 years was not associated with any serious adverse effects. The safety of n-3 fatty acids from fish oil (derived from menhaden) was reviewed by the US Food and Drug Administration (FDA) in 1997. After reviewing more than 2600 articles, the FDA concluded that dietary intakes of up to 3 g daily of EPA/DHA from menhaden oil were generally regarded as safe (GRAS).[87] The FDA came to this conclusion after considering three main issues related to the safety of fish oils: firstly, the risk of deteriorating glycaemic control in type 2 diabetes; secondly, prolonged bleeding times; thirdly, the risk of increasing LDL levels in patients with hypertriglyceridaemia.

Many fish oil supplements (e.g. cod liver oil, halibut liver oil) contain vitamin A and vitamin D – fat-soluble vitamins that can be toxic in excessive amounts. However, the amount of these vitamins contained, for example, in an average multivitamin supplement containing no more than 100% of the RDAs together with the amounts in a recommended dose of, say, ordinary cod liver oil are unlikely to be harmful. However, care should be taken in pregnancy not to take excessive amounts of vitamin A, and product labels should be checked.

Other safety concerns expressed in relation to fish oils include the potential to increase bleeding time (a beneficial effect in relation to prevention of CHD) and the possibly of altering glycaemic control in diabetes. However, it is unlikely that any of these effects is a problem, particularly with intakes of <3 g EPA/DHA daily. Nevertheless, patients taking anticoagulant medication or those with blood clotting disorders should be monitored while taking fish oils. This does not mean that such patients have to avoid fish oils – just that their doctor should be aware of it.

There is also concern about industrial contaminants in fish oil supplements. These include dioxins and polychlorinated biphenyls (PCBs). There is no immediate danger to health, but risks come from long exposure to high levels. In 2001, the UK Committee on Toxicity (COT) set a tolerable daily intake for dioxins and dioxin-like PCBs of 2 pg TEQ/kg/bw/day. (For comparison the EU Scientific Committee on Food (SCF) set a tolerable weekly intake of 14 pg/kg/body weight). Since July 2002 it has been an offence to place on the market any fish oil supplements containing higher contaminant levels.

Interactions

Drugs

Anticoagulants: may increase the risk of bleeding; use of fish oils should be medically supervised, but fish oils need not be avoided in patients taking anticoagulants.
Aspirin: may increase the risk of bleeding; use of fish oils in patients on long-term treatment with aspirin should be medically supervised.
Dipyridamole: may increase the risk of bleeding; use of fish oils should be medically supervised.

Nutrients

Vitamin E: fish oils increase the requirement for vitamin E (absolute additional requirements not established, but 3–4 mg vitamin E per gram of total EPA/DHA appears to be adequate; sufficient amounts of vitamin E are added to most fish oil supplements; there is unlikely to be a need for any extra). Theoretically, vitamin E may be synergistic in increasing the bleeding tendency with fish oil, although there is no evidence for this.

Supplements

Gingko biloba: may increase the bleeding tendency with fish oils, although there is no evidence for this.

Ginseng: may increase the bleeding tendency with fish oils, although there is no evidence for this.

Dose

Fish oil supplements are available in the form of capsules and liquids.

The dose is not established. Dietary supplements provide 100–1500 mg combined EPA/DHA per dose; clinical trials of fish oil supplements showing beneficial effects have often used 3–4 g daily (combined EPA/DHA), but doses of 1–2 g daily may be adequate.

Note 1: Intake of cod liver oil should not be increased above the doses recommended on the product label to achieve higher intakes of EPA/DHA (risk of vitamin A and D toxicity). Several capsules of cod liver oil could be required to provide the same amount of EPA/DHA as a single dose of cod liver oil liquid. There is no risk of vitamin toxicity with one dose of cod liver oil liquid, but toxicity is likely if several capsules are ingested (vitamin concentration is usually higher in capsules).

Note 2: Fish oil supplements are not identical; they provide different amounts of EPA/DHA.

References

1 Department of Health. *Report on Health and Social Subjects, No. 46. Nutritional Aspects of Cardiovascular Disease*. Report of the Cardiovascular Review Group Committee on Medical Aspects of Food Policy. London: HMSO, 1994.

2 British Nutrition Foundation. *Unsaturated Fatty acids: Nutritional and Physiological Significance*. Task Force Report. London: HMSO, 1992.

3 International Society for the Study of Fatty Acids and Lipids. Full text of statement can be seen on www.issfal.org.uk (accessed 30 October 2006).

4 Harris WS. n-3 fatty acids and serum lipoproteins: human studies. *Am J Clin Nutr* 1997; 65 (Suppl.): S1645–S1654S.

5 Shimokawa H, Vanhoutte PM. Dietary omega-3 fatty acids and endothelium-dependent relaxations in porcine coronary arteries. *Am J Physiol* 1989; 256: H968–H973.

6 Goodnight SH Jr, Harris WS, Connor WE, Illingworth DR. Polyunsaturated fatty acids, hyperlipidaemia and thrombosis. *Arteriosclerosis* 1982; 2: 87–113.

7 Terano T, Salmon JA, Higg GA, Moncada S. Eicosapentaenoic acid as a modulator of inflammation. Effect on prostaglandin and leukotriene synthesis. *Biochem Pharmacol* 1986; 35: 779–785.

8 Endres S, Ghorbani R, Kelley VE. The effect of dietary supplementation with n-3 polyunsaturated fatty acids on the synthesis of interleukin-1 and tumour necrosis factor by mononuclear cells. *N Engl J Med* 1989; 320: 265–271.

9 Meydani SN, Lichtenstein AH, Colwell S. Immunologic effects of national cholesterol education panel step-2 diets with and without fish-derived n-3 fatty acid enrichment. *J Clin Invest* 1993; 92: 105–113.

10 Mozaffarian D, Geelen A, Brouwer IA, *et al*. Effect of fish oil on heart rate in humans: a meta-analysis of randomized controlled trials. *Circulation* 2005; 112: 1945–1952.

11 Singer P, Wirth M. Can n-3 PUFA reduce cardiac arrhythmias? Results of a clinical trial. *Prostaglandins Leukot Essent Fatty Acids* 2004; 71: 153–159.

12 Geelen A, Brouwer IA, Zock PL, *et al*. N-3 fatty acids do not affect electrocardiographic characteristics of healthy men and women. *J Nutr* 2002; 132: 3051–3054.

13 Geelen A, Brouwer IA, Schouten EG, *et al*. Effects of n-3 fatty acids from fish on premature ventricular complexes and heart rate in humans. *Am J Clin Nutr* 2005; 81: 416–420.

14 Geelen A, Zock PL, Brouwer IA, *et al*. Effect of n-3 fatty acids from fish oil on electrocardiographic characteristics in patients with frequent premature ventricular complexes. *Br J Nutr* 2005; 93: 787–790.

15 Calo L, Bianconi L, Colivicchi F, *et al*. N-3 fatty acids for the prevention of atrial fibrillation after coronary artery bypass surgery: a randomized controlled trial. *J Am Coll Cardiol* 2005; 45: 1723–1728.

16 Raitt MH, Connor WE, Morris C, *et al*. Fish oil supplementation and risk of ventricular tachycardia and ventricular fibrillation in patients with implantable defibrillators: a randomized controlled trial. *JAMA* 2005; 293: 2884–2891.

17 Dolecek TA. Epidemiological evidence of relationships between dietary polyunsaturated fatty acids and mortality in the multiple risk factor intervention trial. *Proc Soc Exp Biol Med* 1992; 200: 177–182.

18 Ascherio A, Rimm RB, Stampfer MJ, *et al*. Dietary intake of marine n-3 fatty acids, fish intake and the risk of coronary disease among men. *N Engl J Med* 1995; 332: 977–982.

19 Siscovick DS, Raghunathan TE, King I, *et al*. Dietary intake and cell membrane levels of long chain fatty

acids and the risk of primary cardiac arrest. *JAMA* 1995; 274: 1363–1367.

20 Daviglus ML, Stamler J, Orencia AJ, *et al*. Fish consumption and the 30-year risk of fatal myocardial infarction. *N Engl J Med* 1997; 336: 1046–1052.

21 Albert CM, Hennekens CH, O'Donnell CJ, *et al*. Fish consumption and risk of sudden cardiac death. *JAMA* 1998; 279: 23–28.

22 Lapidus L, Andersson H, Bengtsson C, Bosaeus I. Dietary habits in relation to incidence of cardiovascular disease and death in women: a 12-year follow-up of participants in the population study of women in Gothenburg, Sweden. *Am J Clin Nutr* 1986; 44: 444–448.

23 Morris MC, Mason JE, Rosner B, *et al*. Fish consumption and cardiovascular disease in the Physicians' Health Study: a prospective study. *Am J Epidemiol* 1995; 142: 166–175.

24 Burr ML, Fehily AM, Gilbert JF, *et al*. Effects of changes in fat, fish and fibre intakes on death and myocardial infarction: diet and reinfarction trial (DART). *Lancet* 1989; ii: 757–761.

25 Gruppo Italiano per lo Studio della Sopravvivenza nell'Infarto miocardico. Dietary supplementation with n-3 polyunsaturated fatty acids and vitamin E after myocardial infarction: results of the GISSI-Prevenzione trial. *Lancet* 1999; 354: 447–455.

26 Singh RB, Niaz MA, Sharma JP, *et al*. Randomized, double-blind, placebo controlled trial of fish oil and mustard oil in patients with suspected acute myocardial infarction: the Indian experiment of infarct survival – 4. *Cardiovasc Drugs Ther* 1997; 11: 485–491.

27 von Schacky C. The role of omega-3 fatty acids in cardiovascular disease. *Curr Atheroscler Rep 5*; 2003: 139–145.

28 Burr ML, Asffield-Watt PA, Dunstan FD, *et al*. Lack of benefit of dietary advice to men with angina: results of a controlled trial. *Eur J Clin Nutr* 2003; 57: 193–200.

29 Bucher HC, Hengstler P, Schindler C, *et al*. N-3 polyunsaturated fatty acids in coronary heart disease: a meta-analysis of randomized controlled trials. *Am J Med* 2002; 112: 298–304.

30 Hooper L, Thompson RA, Harrison CD, *et al*. Omega-3 fatty acids for prevention and treatment of cardiovascular disease. Cochrane database, issue 4, 2004. London: Macmillan.

31 Hooper L, Thompson RL, Harrison RA, *et al*. Risks and benefits of omega 3 fats for mortality, cardiovascular disease, and cancer: systematic review. *BMJ* 2006; 332: 752–760. Epub 2006 22 March.

32 Burr ML, Dunstan FDJ, George CH. Is fish oil good or bad for heart disease? Two trials with apparently conflicting results. *J Membr Biol* 2005; 206: 155–163.

33 Wang C, Chung M, Balk E, *et al*. *Effects of Omega-3 Fatty Acids on Cardiovascular Disease*. Agency for Healthcare Research and Quality Evidence Report/Technology Assessment: Number 94; 2004. Available from http://www.ahcpr.gov/clinic/epcsums/o3cardsum.htm (accessed 30 October 2006).

34 Balk E, Chung M, Lichenstein A, *et al*. *Effects of Omega-3 Fatty Acids on Cardiovascular Risk Factors and Intermediate Markers of Cardiovascular Disease*. Agency for Healthcare Research and Quality. Evidence Report/Technology Assessment: Number 93; 2004. Available from http://www.ahcpr.gov/clinic/epcsums/o3cardrisksum.htm (accessed 30 October 2006).

35 Kremer JM. Effects of modulation of inflammatory and immune parameters in patients with rheumatic and inflammatory disease receiving dietary supplements of n-3 and n-6 fatty acids. *Lipids* 1996; 31: S243–S247.

36 Lau CS, Morely KD, Belch JJ. Effects of fish oil supplementation on non-steroidal anti-inflammatory drug requirements in patients with mild rheumatoid arthritis – a double blind placebo-controlled study. *Br J Rheumatol* 1993; 32: 982–989.

37 Geusens P, Wouters C, Nijs J, *et al*. Long term effect of omega-3 fatty acid supplementation in active rheumatoid arthritis. *Arthritis Rheum* 1994; 37: 824–829.

38 Fortin PR, Lew RA, Liang MH, *et al* Validation of a meta-analysis: the effects of fish oil on rheumatoid arthritis. *J Clin Epidemiol* 1995; 48: 1379–1390.

39 Kremer JM, Lawrence DA, Petrillo GF, *et al*. Effects of high-dose fish oil on rheumatoid arthritis after stopping nonsteroidal antiinflammatory drugs. Clinical and immune correlates. *Arthritis Rheum* 1995; 38: 1107–1114.

40 MacLean CH, Mojica WA, Morton SC, *et al*. *Effects of Omega-3 Fatty Acids on Lipids and Glycemic Control in Type II Diabetes and the Metabolic Syndrome and on Inflammatory Bowel Disease, Rheumatoid Arthritis, Renal Disease, Systemic Lupus Erythematosus and Osteoporosis*. Evidence Report/Technology Assessment: Number 89; 2004. Available from http://www.ahcpr.ogv/clinic/epcsums/o3lipidsum.htm (accessed 30 October 2006).

41 Remans PH, Sont JK, Wagenaar LW, *et al*. Nutrient supplementation with polyunsaturated fatty acids and micronutrients in rheumatoid arthritis: clinical and biochemical effects. *Eur J Clin Nutr* 2004; 58: 839–845.

42 Young-In K. Can fish oil maintain Crohn's disease in remission? *Nutr Rev* 1996; 54: 248–257.

43 Belluzzi A, Brignola C, Campieri M, *et al*. Effect of enteric-coated fish oil preparation on relapses

in Crohn's disease. *N Engl J Med* 1996; 334: 1557–1560.

44 Hawthorne AB, Daneshmend TK, Hawkey CJ, *et al*. Treatment of ulcerative colitis with fish oil supplementation: a prospective 12-month randomized controlled trial. *Gut* 1992; 33: 922–928.

45 Stenson WF, Cort D, Rodgers J, *et al*. Dietary supplementation with fish oil in ulcerative colitis. *Ann Intern Med* 1992; 116: 609–614.

46 Aslan A, Triadafilopoulos G. Fish oil fatty acid supplementation in active ulcerative colitis: a double-blind, placebo-controlled, crossover study. *Am J Gastroenterol* 1992; 87: 432–437.

47 MacLean CH, Mojca WA, Newberry SJ, *et al*. Systematic review of the effects of n-3 fatty acids in inflammatory bowel disease. *Am J Clin Nutr* 2005; 82: 611–619.

48 Mayser P, Mrowietz U, Arenberger P, *et al*. Omega-3 fatty acid-based lipid infusion in patients with chronic plaque psoriasis: results of a double-blind, randomised, placebo-controlled, multicenter trial. *J Am Acad Dermatol* 1998; 38: 539–547.

49 Veale DJ, Torley HI, Richards IM, *et al*. A double-blind placebo controlled trial of Efamol Marine on skin and joint symptoms of psoriatic arthritis. *Br J Rheumatol* 1994; 33: 954–958.

50 Soyland E, Funk J, Rajka G, *et al*. Effect of dietary supplementation with very long chain fatty acids in patients with psoriasis. *N Engl J Med* 1993; 328: 1812–1816.

51 Gupta AK, Ellis CN, Goldfarb MT, *et al*. The role of fish oil in psoriasis. A randomised, double-blind, placebo-controlled study to evaluate the effect of fish oil and topical steroid therapy in psoriasis. *Int J Dermatol* 1990; 29: 591–595.

52 Gupta AK, Ellis CN, Tellner DC, *et al*. Double-blind, placebo-controlled study to evaluate the efficacy of fish oil and low dose UVB in the treatment of psoriasis. *Br J Dermatol* 1989; 120: 801–807.

53 Bjorneboe A, Smith AK, Bjorneboe GE, *et al*. Effect of dietary supplementation with n-3 fatty acids on clinical manifestations of psoriasis. *Br J Dermatol* 1988; 118: 77–83.

54 Mickleborough TD, Murray RL, Inoescu AA, Lindley MR. Fish oil supplementation reduces severity of exercise-induced bronchoconstriction in elite athletes. *Am J Respir Crit Care Med* 2003; 168: 1181–1189.

55 Nagakura T, Matsuda S, Shicchijyo K, *et al*. Dietary supplementation with fish oil rich in omega-3 polyunsaturated fatty acids in children with bronchial asthma. *Eur Respir J* 2000; 16: 861–865.

56 Schachter H, Reisman J, Tran K, *et al*. *Health Effects of Omega-3 Fatty Acids on Asthma*. Agency for Healthcare Research and Quality. Evidence Report/Technology Assessment: Number 91; 2004. Available from http://www.ahcpr. gov/clinic/epcsums/o3asthsum.htm (accessed 30 October 2006).

57 Thien FCK, Woods R, De Luca S, Abramson MJ. Dietary marine fatty acids (fish oil) for asthma in adults and children. Cochrane database, issue 2, 2002. London: Macmillan.

58 Vessby B, Karlstrom B, Boberg M, *et al*. Polyunsaturated fatty acids may impair blood glucose control in type 2 diabetic patients. *Diabet Med* 1992; 9: 126–133.

59 Toft I, Bonaa KH, Ingebretsen OC, *et al*. Effects of n-3 polyunsaturated fatty acids on glucose homeostasis and blood pressure in essential hypertension. A randomized, controlled trial. *Ann Intern Med* 1995; 123: 911–918.

60 Friedberg CE, Janssen MJ, Heine RJ, Grobbee DE. Fish oil and glycaemic control in diabetes. *Diabetes Care* 1998; 21: 494–500.

61 Farmer A, Montori V, Dinneen S, Clar C. Fish oil in people with type 2 diabetes mellitus. Cochrane database, issue 4, 2001.

62 Joy CB, Mumby-Croft R, Joy LA. Polyunsaturated fatty acid (fish or evening primrose oil) for schizophrenia. Cochrane database, issue 2, 2003. London: Macmillan.

63 Schachter HM, Kourad K, Merali Z, *et al*. *Effects of Omega-3 Fatty Acids on Mental Health*. Agency for Healthcare Research and Quality. Evidence Report/Technology Assessment: Number 116; 2005. Available from http://www.ahcpr. gov/clinic/epcsums/o3mentsum.htm (accessed 30 October 2006).

64 Su KP, Huang SY, Chiu CC, Shen WW. Omega-3 fatty acids in major depressive disorder. A preliminary double-blind, placebo-controlled trial. *Eur Neuropsychopharmacol* 2003; 13: 267–271.

65 Silvers KM, Wolley CC, Hamilton FC, *et al*. Randomised double-blind placebo-controlled trial of fish oil in the treatment of depression. *Prostaglandins Leukot Essent Fatty Acids* 2005; 72: 211–218.

66 MacLean CH, Issa AM, Mojica WA, *et al*. *Effects of Omega-3 Fatty Acids on Cognitive Function with Aging, Dementia and Neurological Diseases*. Agency for Healthcare Research and Quality. Evidence Report/Technology Assessment: Number 114; 2005. Available from http:// www.ahcpr.gov/clinic/epcsums/o3cognsum.htm (accessed 30 October 2006).

67 Lim WS, Gammack JK, Van Niekerk J, *et al*. Omega 3 fatty acid for the prevention of dementia. Cochrane database, issue 1, 2006. London: Macmillan.

68 Weinstock-Gutman B, Baier M, Park Y, *et al*. Low fat dietary intervention with omega-3 fatty acid supplementation in multiple sclerosis patients. *Prostaglandins Leukot Essent Fatty Acids* 2005; 73: 397–404.

69 Lewin G, Schachter HM, Yuen D, *et al. Effects of Omega-3 Fatty Acids on Child and Maternal Health*. Agency for Healthcare Research and Quality. Evidence Report/Rechnology Assessment: Number 118; 2005. Available from http://www.ahcpr.gov/clinic/epcsums/o3mchsum.htm (accessed 30 October 2006).

70 Lauritzen L, Jorgensen MH, Olsen SE, *et al.* Maternal fish oil supplementation in lactation: effect on developmental outcomes in breast fed infants. *Reprod Nutr Dev* 2005; 45: 535–547.

71 Lauritzen L, Hoppe C, Staarup EM, Michaelsen KF. Maternal fish oil supplementation in lactation and growth during the first 2.5 years of life. *Pediatr Res* 2005; 58: 235–242.

72 Jensen CL, Voigt RG, Prager TC, *et al.* Effects of maternal docosahexaenoic acid intake on visual function and neurodevelopment in breastfed term infants. *Am J Clin Nutr* 2005; 82: 125–132.

73 Birch EE, Castaneda YS, Wheaton DH, *et al.* Visual maturation of term infants fed long-chain polyunsaturated fatty acid supplemented or control formula for 12 months. *Am J Clin Nutr* 2005; 81: 879–879.

74 Denburg JA, Hatfield HM, Cyr MM, *et al.* Fish oil supplementation in pregnancy modifies neonatal progenitors in infants at risk of atopy. *Pediatr Res* 2005; 57: 276–281.

75 Dunstan JA, Mori TA, Barden A, *et al.* Fish oil supplementation in pregnancy modifies neonatal allergen-specific immune responses and clinical outcomes in infants at high risk of atopy: a randomized controlled trial. *J Allergy Clin Immunol* 2003; 112: 1178–1184.

76 Richardson AJ, Montgomery P. The Oxford-Durham study: a randomized, controlled trial of dietary supplementation with fatty acids in children with developmental disorder. *Pediatrics* 2005; 115: 1360–1366.

77 Hirayama S, Hamazaki T, Terasawa K. Effect of docosahexaenoic acid-containing food administration on symptoms of attention-deficit/hyperactivity disorder – a placebo-controlled double-blind study. *Eur J Clin Nutr* 2004; 58: 467–473.

78 Voigt RG, Llorente AM, Jensen CL, *et al.* A randomized, double-blind, placebo-controlled trial of docosohexaenoic acid supplementation in children with attention-deficit/hyperactivity disorder. *J Pediatr* 2001; 139: 173–174.

79 Itomura M, Hamazaki K, Sawazaki S, *et al.* The effect of fish oil on physical aggression in schoolchildren – a randomized, double-blind, placebo-controlled trial. *J Nutr Biochem* 2005; 16: 163–171.

80 Donadio JV, Bergstralh EJ, Offord KP, *et al.* A controlled trial of fish oil in IgA nephropathy. Mayo Nephrology Collaborative Group. *N Engl J Med* 1994; 331: 1194–1199.

81 Alexopoulos E, Stangou M, Pantzaki A, *et al.* Treatment of severe IgA nephropathy with omega-3 fatty acids: the effect of a "very low dose" regimen. *Ren Fail* 2004; 26: 453–459.

82 MacLean CH, Issa A, Khanna P, *et al. Effects of Omega-3 Fatty Acids on Cancer*. Agency for Healthcare Research and Quality. Evidence Report/Technology Assessment: Number 191; 2005. Available from http://www.ahcpr.gov/clinic/epcsums/o3cansum.htm (accessed 30 October 2006).

83 MacLean CH, Newberry SJ, Mojica WA, *et al.* Effects of omega-3 fatty acids on cancer risk. *JAMA* 2006; 295: 403–415.

84 Albertazzi P, Coupland K. Polyunsaturated fatty acids. Is there a role in postmenopausal osteoporosis prevention? *Maturitas* 2002; 42: 13–22.

85 Hodge W, Barnes D, Schachter HM, *et al. Effects of Omega-3 Fatty Acids on Eye Health*. Agency for Healthcare Research and Quality. Evidence Report/Technology Assessment: Number 117; 2005. Available from http://www.ahcpr.gov/clinic/epcsums/o3eyesum.htm (accessed 30 October 2005).

86 Saynor R, Gillott T. Changes in blood lipids and fibrinogen with a note on safety in a long term study on the effects of n-3 fatty acids in subjects receiving fish oil supplements and followed for seven years. *Lipids* 1992; 27: 533–538.

87 Food and Drug Administration Final Rule. Substances affirmed as generally recognized as safe: menhaden oil. *Fed Reg* 1997; 62: 30750–30757.

Flavonoids

Description

Flavonoids (or bioflavonoids) are a large group of polyphenolic compounds, ubiquitously present in foods of plant origin. Some flavonoids (e.g. quercetin, rutin) are available as dietary supplements.

Constituents

Bioflavonoids are a group of polyphenolic antioxidants, which often occur as glycosides. Flavonoids can be further subdivided into five main groups:

- flavonols (e.g. kaempferol, quercetin and myricetin)
- flavones (e.g. apigenin and luteolin)
- flavonones (e.g. hesperetin, naringenin, eriodictyol)
- flavan-3-ols (e.g. (+)-catechin, (+)-gallocatechin, (–)-epicatechin, (–)-epigallocatechin)
- anthocyanins (e.g. cyanidin, delphinidin, malvidin, pelargonidin, peonidin, petunidin)
- proanthocyanidins.

More than 4000 flavonoids have been identified, and many have been studied in the laboratory and in animal studies, but apart from quercetin, few have been studied in humans. Most flavonoids are colourless but some are responsible for the bright colours of many fruit and vegetables. Flavonoids are distinguished from the carotenoids (see Carotenoids), which are the red, yellow and orange pigments found in fruit and vegetables. Unlike carotenoids, flavonoids are water-soluble.

Action

Flavonoids appear to display several effects.[1] They:

- act as scavengers of free radicals, including superoxide anions, singlet oxygen, and lipid peroxyl radicals (they have antioxidant properties);
- sequester metal ions;
- inhibit *in vitro* oxidation of LDL cholesterol;
- inhibit cyclo-oxygenase, leading to lower platelet aggregation, decreased thrombotic tendency and reduced anti-inflammatory activity;
- inhibit histamine release;
- improve capillary function by reducing fragility of capillary walls and thus preventing abnormal leakage; and
- inhibit various stages of tumour development (animal studies only).

The activities of flavonoids are dependent on their chemical structure.

Human requirements

No proof of a dietary need exists.

Dietary intake

Estimates of dietary flavonoid intake vary from 10 to 100 mg daily, depending on the population studied, the technique used and the number and identity of flavonoids measured. If all flavonoids are included, intake may be several hundreds of milligrams a day, particularly if red wine is consumed in large amounts.

Table 1 Flavonoid content of selected foods (mg/100 g)

Food	Flavonols	Flavones	Flavanones	Flavan-3-ols	Anthocyanidins	Pro-anthocyanidins
Apples	4.42	0	–	9.09	–	80–130
Bananas	–	–	–	0	–	3.37
Beans, kidney	–	–	–	2.01	–	510
Blackberries	–	–	–	–	–	23.31
Blackcurrants	13.50	–	–	1.17		149.7
Blueberries	3.93	–	–	1.11	112.55	176.49
Broccoli, cooked	2.44	–	–	–	–	0
Cherries, raw	1.25	0	–	11.70	117.42	19.13
Chocolate bar, dark	–	–	–	53.49	–	170
Chocolate bar, milk	–	–	–	13.45	–	70
Elderberry, raw	42.00	–	–	–	749.24	–
Grapefruit juice	0.1	–	24.13	–	–	0
Grapes, black	2.8	0	–	20.9	–	–
Grapes, green	1.32	0	–	4.92	–	81.54
Kale, raw	34.45	0	–	–	–	–
Kiwi	–	–	–	0.45	–	1.83
Lemon juice, raw	–	0	18.33	–	–	–
Nectarines	–	–	–	2.74	–	29.36
Onions, cooked	19.71	–	–	–	–	0
Onions, red, raw	37.87	0	–	–	13.14	–
Orange juice	–	–	5.08	–	–	0
Orange	–	–	43.88	–	–	0
Parsley, raw	8.85	303.24	0	–	–	0
Peaches	0	0	0	2.33	–	71.75
Pears	0.3	0	–	3.53	–	42.3
Plums, black	1.2	0	–	6.19	–	220.66
Pomegranate	–	–	–	–	–	1.10
Raspberries	0.83	–	–	9.23	47.6	25.07
Strawberries	1.44	0	–	4.47		141.67
Tea, black, brewed	3.86	0	–	73.44		13.34
Tea, green, brewed	5.21	0.34	–	132.43		
Tomato, cherry	2.87	–	–	–		0
Tomato, raw	0.64	0	–	–		0
Thyme, fresh	–	56.00				
Wine, table red	1.64	0	–	11.9	9.19	61.63
Wine, table white	0.06	0	–	1.38	0.06	0.81

USDA database: http://www.nal.usda.gov/fnic/foodcomp

–, not analysed to date

Dietary sources

Flavonoids are found in the white segment or ring of fruit (especially citrus fruit) and vegetables, and also in tea and red wine. In the UK, tea, apples and onions seem to be major sources. Flavonoid content of foods varies widely (see Table 1). Cherry tomatoes contain higher concentrations than normal-sized tomatoes, and Lollo Rosso lettuce more than iceberg lettuce.[1] The flavonoid content of red wine may also vary widely, depending on the source, growing conditions and harvesting of the grapes.[2] Chocolate is also a good source of flavonoids (including flavonols, flavanols, catechins, epicatechins and proanthocyanidins).

Possible uses

Flavonoids have been investigated for a potential role in the prevention of CVD, cancer and cataracts. The totality of evidence suggests a role for flavonoids in prevention of CVD, cancer and possibly other chronic diseases.[3,4]

Cardiovascular disease

Epidemiological studies have suggested that consumption of fruit and vegetables may protect against CVD. That such a benefit could occur as a result of dietary antioxidant vitamins is well known, but the presence of flavonoids in these foods may also account for these findings.

Bioflavonoids may help to reduce the risk of heart disease (possibly by helping to dilate the coronary arteries and by preventing atherosclerosis). The Zutphen study from the Netherlands[5] demonstrated a reduced risk of CHD and a reduced incidence of myocardial infarction in men aged 65–84 years associated with increased ingestion of dietary flavonoids. The major dietary sources of flavonoids in this study were tea (61%), onions (13%) and apples (10%). Flavonoid intake was inversely associated with CHD mortality, with a 68% reduction in risk for intake >19 mg daily. There was, however, no correlation between flavonoid intake and CHD incidence among those with no history of myocardial infarction. The researchers later updated their results,[6] extending follow-up to 10 years. Similar results for CHD mortality were found, but a smaller risk reduction and a borderline significant trend ($P = 0.08$) for the incidence of CHD existed.

Another part of the Zutphen study[7] investigated a cohort of men aged 50–69 years, following them up for 15 years. Dietary flavonoids (mainly quercetin) were inversely associated with stroke incidence after adjustment for potential confounders, including antioxidant vitamins. The relative risk of stroke for the highest versus the lowest quartile of flavonoid intake was 0.27. A lower stroke risk was also observed for the highest quartile of beta-carotene intake,

but vitamins C and E were not associated with stroke risk. Black tea contributed about 70% to flavonoid intake. The relative risk for daily consumption of 4.7 cups or more of tea versus less than 2.6 cups of tea was 0.31 (95% CI, 0.12 to 0.84).

However, the Caerphilly study in Wales showed no reduced risk of heart disease with increasing flavonoid consumption.[8] This investigation involved 1900 men aged 45–59 who were studied for up to 14 years. Tea provided 82% of the flavonoid intake, and was strongly and positively associated with risk of CHD.

Baseline flavonoid intake was estimated in 16 cohorts of the Seven Countries Study,[9] and mortality from CHD, cancer and all causes was investigated after 25 years of follow-up. Average intake of flavonoids was inversely associated with mortality from CHD and explained about 25% of the variance in CHD rates in the 16 cohorts. Flavonoid intake was not independently associated with mortality from other causes, including cancer.

Two studies used data from American cohorts of men and women. One study investigated the relationship between flavonoid intake and CHD risk in 34 789 men aged 40–75 in 1986 with a follow-up of 6 years.[10] The main sources of flavonoids were tea and onions. Flavonoid intake > 40 mg daily was not associated with reduced CHD risk. The Iowa Womens' Health Study[11] investigated 34 492 postmenopausal women aged 55–69 for subsequent risk of CHD over a 10-year follow-up period. Compared to women in the lowest quintile (<5.8 mg daily) of flavonoid intake, those in the highest quintile (18.7 mg daily) had a significant 32% reduced risk of CHD death.

The association of tea intake with aortic atherosclerosis has also been investigated in a Dutch study.[12] In a prospective study of 3454 men and women aged 55 and older, who were free of CVD at baseline, tea intake was inversely correlated with severe (but not mild or moderate) aortic atherosclerosis.

A meta-analysis of seven prospective cohort studies published before 2001 included 2087 fatal CHD events. Comparison of those in the top third with those in the bottom third of dietary flavonol intake yielded a combined risk ratio of 0.8 (95% CI, 0.69 to 0.93) after adjustment for known CHD risk factors and other dietary components. The authors concluded that high dietary intakes of flavonols from a small number of fruits and vegetables, tea and red wine may be associated with reduced risk of CHD mortality in free-living populations.[13]

A prospective study in 38 445 women (free of CVD and cancer) with a mean follow-up period of 6.9 years found no significant linear trend for CVD and important vascular events across quintiles of flavonoid intake. No individual flavonol or flavone was associated with CVD. Broccoli and apple consumption were associated with non-significant reductions in CVD risk. A small proportion of women (1185) consuming four or more cups of tea a day had a reduction in the risk of important vascular events but with a non-significant linear trend. In this study flavonoid intake was not strongly associated with risk of CVD.[14]

In the SU.VI.MAX study (an 8-year trial evaluating the effect of antioxidant supplementation on the incidence of major chronic disease), flavonoid-rich food in women was inversely associated with systolic blood pressure. No such relationship was seen in men. Women in the highest tertile of flavonoid-rich food consumption were at lower risk for CVD (OR 0.31; 95% CI, 0.14 to 0.68), while a positive tendency was observed in men. In this study, a high consumption of flavonoid-rich food appeared to reduce cardiovascular risk in women.[15]

Chocolate has attracted attention for its possible role in preventing CVD. A systematic review of 136 publications, mainly short-term feeding trials, suggested that cocoa and chocolate may exert benefit on cardiovascular risk via lowering blood pressure, anti-inflammatory effects, anti-platelet function, raising HDL and decreasing LDL oxidation. An associated meta-analysis of flavonoid intake suggests that these compounds may lower cardiovascular mortality.[16]

Intervention trials have shown that flavonoids can reverse endothelial dysfunction. Endothelial dysfunction appears to be important in the pathogenesis of CVD so any improvement could reduce the risk of coronary events. However, there is considerable variation in the response in endothelial function to flavonoids and this may be related to inter-individual differences in flavonoid metabolism.[17]

Cancer

Activity of flavonoids against malignant cells has been demonstrated *in vitro*,[18–20] and there is much current interest in the potential use of bioflavonoids in the prevention and treatment of cancer.

In a Finnish study involving 9959 men and women (initially cancer-free) aged from 15 to 99, high dietary flavonoid intake was shown to reduce the risk of cancer.[21] Researchers involved in the Iowa Women's Health Study showed that in 35 000 post-menopausal women, those who drank more than two cups of tea a day were 32% less likely to have cancers of the mouth, oesophagus, stomach, colon and rectum. Risk of urinary tract cancer was reduced by 60%. In those who drank more than four cups of tea a day, the risk of cancer was lowered by 63%.[22] Onions are high in flavonoids, which might explain the reduced risk of stomach cancer among those with a high intake of onions in a group of 120 852 men and women aged 55 to 69 years.[23]

A review of data from four cohort studies and six case-control studies examining associations between flavonoid intake and cancer risk found consistent evidence that flavonoids, especially quercetin, may reduce the risk of lung cancer.[24]

In the Nurses Health Study II, validated food frequency questionnaires from 90 630 women showed no associations between flavonols and breast cancer risk and there were no associations between individual flavonols such as kaempferol, quercetin and myricetin and breast cancer risk. However there was a significant inverse association between breast cancer and beans and lentils.[25]

Cataract

There may be a role for flavonoids in preventing diabetes-related cataract formation. In diabetes mellitus, excess sorbitol or dulcitol is produced by the conversion of glucose by aldose reductase. The dulcitol cannot be further metabolised and therefore forms a hard crystalline layer in the lens, which forms the cataract. Flavonoids are potent inhibitors of the enzyme,[26] but further studies are required before flavonoids could be recommended for cataract prevention.

Miscellaneous

Experimental studies have demonstrated that some flavonoids prevent ulcer formation,[27] and that they may be useful in treating ulcers.

Flavonoids have been investigated for potential anti-viral activity. *In vitro* tests have shown some activity against rhinovirus (responsible for 50% of common colds), but little activity against herpes simplex and influenza virus.[28]

Many claims have been made for the usefulness of bioflavonoids in a range of disorders, including haemorrhoids, allergy, asthma, menopausal symptoms and the prevention of habitual abortion, but scientific studies are required to investigate these claims. The suggestion has been made that flavonoids may reduce the occurrence of type 2 diabetes. However, a prospective study in 38 018 women aged over 45 and free of CVD, cancer and diabetes with an average 8.8-year follow-up found that total flavonols, flavones or individual compounds were associated with risk of type 2 diabetes, although apple and tea consumption was inversely associated with diabetes risk.[29]

Quercetin

As a dietary supplement, quercetin is promoted for prevention and treatment of atherosclerosis and hyperlipidaemia, diabetes, cataracts, hay fever, peptic ulcer, inflammation, prevention of cancer and for treating prostatitis. A preliminary, double-blind, placebo-controlled trial in chronic non-bacterial prostatitis showed that quercetin reduced pain and improved quality of life, but had no effect on voiding dysfunction.[30] However, there is insufficient reliable information about the effectiveness of quercetin for other indications.

Rutin

As a dietary supplement, rutin is used to reduce capillary permeability and treat symptoms of varicose veins. In combination with bromelain and trypsin, rutin is used to treat osteoarthritis. In one double-blind trial, 73 patients with osteoarthritis of the knee were randomly assigned to a combination enzyme product (containing rutin, bromelain and trypsin) or diclofenac. The enzyme product had a similar effect on reducing pain and mobility of the knee to diclofenac.[31] However, there is insufficient reliable information about the effectiveness of rutin for other indications.

> ### Conclusion
> High dietary intakes of flavonoids have been linked with a reduced risk of CHD, cancer and cataracts. However, although a number of supplements (e.g. quercetin, rutin) are now available, there is currently only limited evidence that supplements are beneficial in any condition.

Pregnancy and breast-feeding

No problems have been reported.

Adverse effects

None reported. However, there are no long-term studies assessing the safety of flavonoid supplements.

Interactions

None reported.

Dose

Flavonoids (e.g. quercetin, rutin) are available in the form of tablets and capsules.

The dose is not established; dietary supplements of quercetin and rutin provide around 500 mg in a single dose.

References

1 Crozier A, McDonald MS, Lean MEJ, Black C. Quantitative analysis of the flavonoid content of tomatoes, onions, lettuce and celery. *J Agric Food Chem* 1997; 45: 590–595.
2 McDonald MS, Hughes M, Burns J, *et al*. A survey of the free and conjugated flavonol content of sixty five red wines of different geographical origin. *J Agric Food Chem* 1998; 46: 368–375.

3 Knekt P, Kumpulainen J, Jarvinen R, *et al*. Flavonoid intake and risk of chronic diseases. *Am J Clin Nutr* 2002; 76: 560–568.

4 Graf BA, Milbury PE, Blumberg JB. Flavonols, flavones, flavonones and human health. *J Med Food* 2005; 8: 281–290.

5 Hertog MGL, Feskens EJM, Hollman PCH, *et al*. Dietary antioxidant flavonoids and risk of coronary heart disease: the Zutphen elderly study. *Lancet* 1993; 342: 1007–1011.

6 Hertog MG, Feskens EJ, Hollman PC, *et al*. Antioxidant flavonols and coronary heart disease risk (letter). *Lancet* 1997; 349: 699.

7 Keli SO, Hertog MG, Feskens EJ. Dietary flavonoids, antioxidant vitamins and the incidence of stroke; the Zutphen study. *Arch Intern Med* 1996; 156: 637–642.

8 Hertog MG, Sweetman PM, Fehily AM, *et al*. Antioxidant flavonols and ischaemic heart disease in a Welsh population of men: the Caerphilly Study. *Am J Clin Nutr* 1997; 65: 1489–1494.

9 Hertog MG, Kromhout D, Aravanis C, *et al*. Flavonoid intake and long-term risk of coronary heart disease and cancer in the seven countries study. *Arch Intern Med* 1995; 155: 381–386.

10 Rimm EB, Katam MB, Ascherio A, *et al*. Relation between intakes of flavonoids and risk for coronary heart disease in male health professionals. *Ann Intern Med* 1996; 125: 384–389.

11 Yochum L, Kushi LH, Meyer K, Folsom AR. Dietary flavonoid intake and risk of cardiovascular disease in postmenopausal women. *Am J Epidemiol* 1999; 149: 943–949.

12 Geleijinse JM, Launer LJ, Hofman A, *et al*. Tea flavonoids may protect against atherosclerosis. *Arch Intern Med* 1999; 159: 2170–2174.

13 Huxley RR, Neil HA. The relation between dietary flavonol intake and coronary heart disease mortality: a meta-analysis of prospective cohort studies. *Eur J Clin Nutr* 2003; 57: 904–908.

14 Sesso HD, Gaziano JM, Liu S, Buring JE. Flavonoid intake and the risk of cardiovascular disease in women. *Am J Clin Nutr* 2003; 77: 1440–1448.

15 Mennen LI, Saphino D, de Bree A, *et al*. Consumption of foods rich in flavonoids is related to a decreased cardiovascular risk in apparently healthy women. *J Nutr* 2004; 134: 923–926.

16 Ding EL, Hutfless SM, Ding X, Girotra S. Chocolate and prevention of cardiovascular disease: a systematic review. *Nutr Metab* 2006; 3: 2.

17 Hodgson J, Puddey IB, Burke V, Croft KD. Is reversal of endothelial dysfunction by tea related to flavonoid metabolism? *Br J Nutr* 2006; 95: 14–17.

18 Havsteen B. Flavonoids. A class of natural products of high pharmacological potency. *Biochem Pharmacol* 1983; 32: 1141.

19 Tripathi VD, Rastogi RP. Flavonoids in biology and medicine. *J Sci Ind Res* 1981; 40: 116.

20 Kandaswami C, Perkins E, Soloniuk DS, *et al*. Antiproliferative effects of citrus flavonoids on a human squamous cell carcinoma *in vitro*. *Cancer Lett* 1991; 56: 147–152.

21 Knekt P, Jarvinen R, Seppanen R, *et al*. Dietary flavonoids and the risk of lung cancer and other malignant neoplasms. *Am J Epidemiol* 1997; 146: 223–230.

22 Zheng W, Doyle TJ, Kushi LH. Tea consumption and cancer incidence in a prospective cohort study of postmenopausal women. *Am J Epidemiol* 1996; 144: 175–182.

23 Dorant E, van den Brandt PA, Goldbohm RA. Consumption of onions and a reduced risk of stomach carcinoma. *Gastroenterology* 1996; 110: 12–20.

24 Neuhouser ML. Dietary flavonoids and cancer risk: evidence from human population studies. *Nutr Cancer* 2004; 50: 1–7.

25 Adebamowo CA, Cho E, Sampson L, *et al*. Dietary flavonol-rich foods intake and the risk of breast cancer. *Int J Cancer* 2005; 114: 628–633.

26 Wagner H. Phenolic compounds of pharmaceutical interest. In: *Recent Advances in Phytochemistry, Vol 12, Biochemistry of Plant Phenolics*, 1977: 589.

27 Farkas L, Gabor M, Kallay F, Wagner H. Flavonoids and bioflavonoids. Proceedings, International Bioflavonoid Symposium, Munich. Amsterdam: Elsevier, 1977.

28 Tshuiya Y, Shimuzu M, Hiyama Y, *et al*. Antiviral activity of naturally occurring flavonoids *in vitro*. *Chem Pharm Bull* 1985; 33: 3881.

29 Song Y, Manson JE, Buring JE, *et al*. Associations of dietary flavonoids with risk of type 2 diabetes and markers of insulin resistance and systemic inflammation in women: a prospective study and cross-sectional analysis. *J Am Coll Nutr* 2005; 24: 376–384.

30 Shoskes DA, Zeitlin SI, Shahed A, Rajfer A. Quercetin in men with category III chronic prostatitis: a preliminary prospective, double-blind, placebo-controlled trial. *Urology* 1999; 54: 960–963.

31 Klein G, Kullich W. Short-term treatment of painful osteoarthritis of the knee with oral enzymes. *Clin Drug Invest* 2000; 19: 15–23.

Flaxseed oil

Description

Flaxseed is the soluble fibre mucilage obtained from the fully developed seed of *Linus usitatissimum*.

Constituents

Flaxseed is a rich source of alpha-linolenic acid and lignans. Alpha-linolenic acid is an essential fatty acid of the n-3 (omega-3) series, which must be supplied by the diet. It can be converted into longer-chain fatty acids of the n-3 series, such as eicosapentaenoic acid (EPA) and docosahexaenoic acid (DHA), the fatty acids found in fish oils (see Fish oils).

Action

Fatty acids of the n-3 series (like those of the n-6 series) are precursors to a range of prostaglandins, thromboxanes and leukotrienes, and those formed from the n-3 series are generally less pro-inflammatory and atherogenic than those formed from the n-6 series. In addition, there is competition between the fatty acids of both series for the enzyme systems that effect chain elongation, suggesting that a balance between the two types of fatty acids is important; it is estimated that an optimal ratio between n-3 and n-6 fatty acid is 1:4. However, changes in food production and advice to consume polyunsaturated fats has led to an increase in the n-6 fatty acids at the expense of the n-3 fats, and the ratio of n-3 to n-6 fats is between 1:10 and 1:30. Flaxseed oil, which contains approximately three times more n-3 than n-6 fatty acids, may help to reverse the imbalance between n-3 and n-6 fats.

Lignans are a type of phytoestrogen. They are digested in the colon to produce enterodiol and enterolactone, lignans that are thought to be protective against cancer.

Possible uses

Traditionally, flaxseed has been used for constipation and other bowel disorders such as diverticulitis and irritable bowel syndrome (IBS). In theory, it may also be useful as a source of n-3 fatty acids for the same conditions (e.g. CVD and other inflammatory disorders) where fish oil has benefit. It is also a useful oil for vegetarians, to help improve the balance between omega-3 and omega-6 fatty acids, because vegetarians tend to consume significant quantities of omega-6 fatty acids.

Cardiovascular disease

In a small trial, 11 healthy male subjects were randomly assigned to receive 40 g flaxseed oil or sunflower seed oil for 23 days.[1] A statistically significant reduction in platelet aggregation response to collagen was found in subjects supplemented with flaxseed but not with sunflower seed. The authors noted that the higher percentage of energy from fat in the sunflower oil might have skewed the results. In spite of this limitation, the conclusion was that oils rich in alpha-linolenic acid may offer increased protection in CVD (via reduction in platelet aggregation) compared with oils rich in linoleic acid.

In a randomised, double-blind study, 32 healthy subjects received either 35 mg flaxseed oil or 35 mg fish oil for 3 months.[2] In contrast to fish oil, flaxseed had no effect on serum triglyceride or cholesterol levels, but the authors concluded that the dose may have been insufficient or that conversion of alpha-linolenic acid to EPA was inadequate.

In a double-blind crossover study, 29 subjects with hyperlipidaemia were given (in random order) muffins containing either 50 g partially defatted flaxseed or wheat bran (control) each day for 3 weeks. Flaxseed significantly reduced total serum cholesterol by 4.6% and LDL cholesterol by 7.6%, but there were no effects on HDL cholesterol.[3]

In a double-blind, placebo-controlled study, 11 patients with well-controlled type 2 diabetes were given flaxseed oil or fish oil capsules for 3 months each, in random order. Fish oil, but not flaxseed oil, reduced serum triglycerides, but there were no significant differences between the two oils in relation to total, LDL and HDL cholesterol levels.[4]

In a study involving post-menopausal women who were not on HRT, flaxseed supplementation (40 g with 1 g of calcium and 400 units of vitamin D daily) lowered both serum total cholesterol and non-HDL cholesterol by 6% whereas the comparative control regime had no such effect. Flaxseed reduced serum levels of both LDL and HDL cholesterol by 4.7% and triglyceride by 12.8% (although these did not reach statistical significance). Serum apolipoprotein B concentrations were significantly reduced by 6.0% and 7.5% respectively by the flaxseed regimen. Markers of bone formation and resorption were not affected.[5]

A trial in 25 menopausal women with total cholesterol > 6.2 mmol/L, a cholesterol:HDL cholesterol ratio > 4.5 and triglycerides < 3.5 mmol/L compared 40 g crushed flaxseed daily with 0.625 mg of conjugated equine oestrogens alone or combined with progesterone. Both HRT and flaxseed produced similar decreases in menopausal symptoms and glucose and insulin levels. However, only HRT significantly improved cholesterol profile and favourably modified markers related to cardiovascular health.[6]

A meta-analysis of five cohort studies and three clinical trials on alpha-linolenic acid and heart disease, together with nine cohort and case-control studies on alpha-linolenic acid (ALA) and prostate cancer found that high ALA intake was associated with reduced risk of fatal heart disease in prospective cohort studies. Three open-label trials also indicated that ALA may protect against heart disease. However, epidemiological studies in this meta-analysis also showed an increased risk of prostate cancer in men with a high intake or blood level of ALA.[7]

More recently, an RCT in 199 menopausal women found that flaxseed (40 g daily) reduced serum total cholesterol and HDL cholesterol compared with placebo. There was no significant change in BMD or menopausal symptoms.[8] A further RCT in 57 men with an atherogenic lipoprotein phenotype found that fish oil produced predictable changes in plasma lipids and small dense LDL that were not reproduced by a diet enriched with ALA.[9]

A systematic review of 14 studies found that ALA supplementation may cause small decreases in fibrinogen concentrations and plasma glucose, but most cardiovascular risk markers do not appear to be affected. The reviewers concluded that supplementation with ALA to reduce CVD cannot be recommended.[10]

Cancer

There is some evidence from animal studies that flaxseed inhibits tumour growth, particularly mammary tumours,[11,12] but clinical trials are needed to assess whether flaxseed has anti-cancer properties in humans.

Autoimmune disorders

In a double-blind, placebo-controlled study involving 22 patients with rheumatoid arthritis, 30 g flaxseed powder daily for 3 months had no effect on clinical subjective parameters of the disorder compared with sunflower oil.[13]

A small study in eight patients with SLE, present as lupus nephritis, found that flaxseed in a dose of 30 g daily improved renal function and inflammatory mediators and was well tolerated.[14]

> **Conclusion**
>
> Theoretically, flaxseed as a source of n-3 fatty acids could benefit the same conditions as those indicated for fish oil. However, research data are currently insufficient to make recommendations for supplements for reduction in risk of heart disease and cancer or management of rheumatoid arthritis and other inflammatory conditions.

Precautions/contraindications

No problems have been reported.

Pregnancy and breast-feeding

No problems have been reported, but there have not been sufficient studies to guarantee the safety of flaxseed in pregnancy and breast-feeding.

Adverse effects

There are no known toxicity or serious side-effects, but no long-term studies have assessed the safety of flaxseed. Flaxseed contains cyanogenic glycosides, which are naturally-occurring toxicants. The long-term effects of these compounds are unknown, but high doses could increase plasma thiocyanate levels.

Interactions

None reported.

Dose

Flaxseed oil is available in the form of a liquid and in capsules.

The dose is not established. Manufacturers suggest one tablespoon of flaxseed oil daily.

References

1   Allman MA, Pena NM, Pang D. Supplementation with flaxseed oil versus sunflower oil in healthy young men consuming a low fat diet: effects on platelet composition and function. *Eur J Clin Nutr* 1995; 49: 169–178.

2   Layne KS, Goh YK, Jumpsen JA, *et al.* Normal subjects consuming physiological levels of 18:3(n-3) and 20:5(n-3) from flaxseed or fish oils have characteristic differences in plasma lipid and lipoprotein fatty acid levels. *J Nutr* 1996; 126: 2130–2140.

3   Jenkins DJA, Kendall CWC, Vidgen E, *et al.* Health aspects of partially defatted flaxseed, including effects on serum lipids, oxidative measures, and ex vivo androgen and progestin activity: a controlled crossover trial. *Am J Clin Nutr* 1999; 69: 395–402.

4   McManus RM, Jumpson J, Finegood DT. A comparison of the effects of n-3 fatty acids from linseed oil and fish oil in well-controlled type II diabetes. *Diabetes Care* 1996; 19: 463–467.

5   Lucas AE, Wild RD, Hammond LJ, *et al.* Flaxseed improves lipid profile without altering biomarkers of bone metabolism in postmenopausal women. *J Clin Endocrinol Metab* 2002; 87: 1527–1532.

6   Lemay A, Dodin S, Kadri N, *et al.* Flaxseed dietary supplement versus hormone replacement therapy in hypercholesterolemic menopausal women. *Obstet Gynecol* 2002; 100: 495–504.

7   Brouwer IA, Katan MB, Zock PL. Dietary alpha-linolenic acid is associated with reduced risk of fatal coronary heart disease, but increased prostate cancer: a meta-analysis. *J Nutr* 2004; 134: 919–922.

8   Dodin S, Lemay A, Jaques H, *et al.* The effects of flaxseed dietary supplement on lipid profile, bone mineral density, and symptoms in menopausal women: a randomized, double-blind, wheat germ placebo-controlled clinical trial. *J Clin Endocrinol Metab* 2005; 90: 1390–1397.

9   Wilkinson P, Leach C, Ah-Sing EE, *et al.* Influence of alpha-linolenic acid and fish-oil on markers of cardiovascular risk in subjects with an atherogenic lipoprotein profile. *Atherosclerosis* 2005; 181: 115–124.

10 Wendland E, Farmer A, Glasziou P, Neil A. Effect of alpha linolenic acid on cardiovascular risk markers: a systematic review. *Heart* 2006; 92: 166–169.

11 Serraino M, Thompson LU. The effect of flaxseed supplementation on the initiation and promotional stages of mammary tumorigenesis. *Nutr Cancer* 1992; 17: 153–159.

12 Thompson LU, Rickard SE, Orcheson LJ, *et al.* Flaxseed and its lignan and oil components reduce mammary tumour growth at a late stage of carcinogenesis. *Carcinogenesis* 1996; 17: 1373–1376.

13 Nordstrom DC, Honkanen VE, Nasu Y, *et al.* Alpha-linolenic acid in the treatment of rheumatoid arthritis. A double-blind placebo controlled and randomized study; flaxseed versus safflower seed. *Rheumatol Int* 1995; 14: 231–234.

14 Clark WF, Parbtani A, Huff MW, *et al.* Flaxseed: a potential treatment for lupus nephritis. *Kidney Int* 1995; 48: 475–480.

Fluoride

Description

Fluoride is a trace element.

Human requirements

There does not appear to be a physiological requirement for fluoride and, in the UK, no Reference Nutrient Intake has been set, but a safe and adequate intake, for infants only, is 0.05 mg/kg daily.

Action

Fluoride has a marked affinity for hard tissues, and forms calcium fluorapatite in teeth and bone. It protects against dental caries and may have a role in bone mineralisation. It helps remineralisation of bone in pathological conditions of demineralisation.

Dietary sources

Foods high in fluoride include seafoods and tea. Cereals and milk are poorer sources. An important source of fluoride is fluoridated drinking water. In the UK, tea provides 70% of the total intake; if the water is fluoridated, consumption of large volumes of tea can result in fluoride intakes of 4–12 mg daily.

Metabolism

Absorption

Oral fluoride is rapidly absorbed by passive transport from the gastrointestinal tract; some is absorbed from the stomach, and some from the small intestine.

Distribution

Fluoride is found principally in bones and teeth.

Elimination

Elimination is mainly via the urine, with small amounts lost in sweat (especially in warm climates) and bile.

Deficiency

No essential function has been clearly established; low levels of fluoride in drinking water are associated with dental caries.

Possible uses

Dental caries

Fluoride is recommended for the prophylaxis of dental caries in infants and children (see Dose, below).

Osteoporosis

Evidence for a role of fluoride in osteoporosis and prevention of fracture is conflicting. In one study,[1] there was a higher incidence of fractures in an area of Italy with a lower concentration of fluoride in the water than in another area. In another study,[2] women with continuous exposure to fluoridated water for 20 years were compared with those with no exposure. In those with exposure, BMD was 2.6% higher at the femoral neck, 2.5% higher at the lumbar spine and 1.9% lower at the distal radius. In addition, the risk of hip fracture was slightly reduced, as was the risk of vertebral fracture. However, there was no difference in the risk of humerus fracture and a non-significant trend towards an increased risk of wrist fracture.

Table 1   Daily doses[1] of fluoride (expressed as fluoride ion) in infants and children

Fluoride content of water	Under 6 months	6 months–3 years	3–6 years	Over 6 years
<300 μg	none	250 μg	500 μg	1 mg
300–700 μg	none	none	250 μg	500 μg
>700 μg	none	none	none	none

[1] Recommended by the British Dental Association, the British Society of Paediatric Dentistry and the British Association for the Study of Community Dentistry (*Br Dent J* 1997 ; 182: 6–7).

In an intervention study,[3] sodium fluoride (75 mg daily) was no more effective than placebo in retarding progression of spinal osteoporosis. Another study in 202 post-menopausal women[4] with vertebral fractures showed that sodium fluoride 75 mg daily was not an effective treatment. Yet another intervention study[5] showed that fluoride (as sodium fluoride 50 mg daily or monofluorophosphate 200 mg or 150 mg daily) was no more effective than calcium and vitamin D in preventing new vertebral fractures in women with post-menopausal osteoporosis. A trial comparing etidronate with fluoride[6] in the treatment of post-menopausal osteoporosis showed that although fluoride was more effective at increasing lumbar bone mass, there were no differences in fracture incidence.

Precautions/contraindications

The British Association for Community Dentistry advises that fluoride is unnecessary for infants under 6 months and that fluoride should not be given in areas where the drinking water contains fluoride levels that exceed 700 μg/L.

Adverse effects

Chalky white patches on the surface of the teeth (may occur with recommended doses); yellow-brown staining of teeth, stiffness and aching of bones (with chronic excessive intake). Symptoms of acute overdose include diarrhoea, nausea, gastrointestinal cramp, bloody vomit, black stools, drowsiness, weakness, faintness, shallow breathing, tremors and increased watering of mouth and eyes.

Interactions

None reported.

Dose

Systemic fluoride supplements should not be prescribed without reference to the fluoride content of the local water supply (information available from the local Water Board). See Table 1 for daily fluoride doses in infants and children.

References

1   Fabiani L, Leoni V, Vitali M. Bone-fracture incidence rate in two Italian regions with different fluoride concentration levels in drinking water. *J Trace Elem Med Biol* 1999; 13: 232–237.
2   Phipps KR, Orwoll ES, Mason JD, Cauley JA. Community water fluoridation, bone mineral density, and fractures: prospective study of effects in older women. *BMJ* 2000; 321: 860–864.
3   Kleerekoper M, Peterson EL, Nelson DA, *et al*. A randomized trial of sodium fluoride as a treatment for osteoporosis. *Osteoporosis Int* 1991; 1: 155–161.
4   Riggs BL, Hodgson SF, O'Fallon M, *et al*. Effect of fluoride treatment on the fracture rate in postmenopausal women with osteoporosis. *N Engl J Med* 1990; 322: 802–809.
5   Meunier PJ, Sebert JL, Reginster JY, *et al*. Fluoride salts are no better at preventing new vertebral fractures than calcium-vitamin D in postmenopausal osteoporosis; the FAVO study. *Osteoporosis Int* 1998; 8: 4–12.
6   Guanabens N, Farrerons J, Perez-Edo L, *et al*. Cyclical etidronate versus sodium fluoride in established postmenopausal osteoporosis: a randomized 3 year trial. *Bone* 2000; 27: 123–128.

Folic acid

Description

Folic acid is a water-soluble vitamin of the vitamin B complex.

Nomenclature

Folic acid (pteroylglutamic acid) is the parent compound for a large number of derivatives collectively known as folates. Folate is the generic term used to describe the compounds that exhibit the biological activity of folic acid; it is the preferred term for the vitamin present in foods that represents a mixture of related compounds (folates).

Human requirements

See Table 1 for Dietary Reference Values for folic acid.

Dietary intake

In the UK, the average adult diet provides: for men, 322 µg daily; for women, 224 µg daily.

Action

Folates are involved in a number of single carbon transfer reactions, especially in the synthesis of purines and pyrimidines (and hence the synthesis of DNA), glycine and methionine. They are also involved in some amino acid conversions and the formation and utilisation of formate. Deficiency leads to impaired cell division (effects most noticeable in rapidly regenerating tissues).

Dietary sources

See Table 2 for dietary sources of folic acid.

Metabolism

Absorption

Absorption of folate takes place mainly in the jejunum.

Distribution

Folate is stored mainly in the liver. Entero-hepatic recycling is important for maintaining serum levels.

Elimination

Excretion of folate is largely renal, but folates may also be eliminated in the faeces (mainly as a result of folate synthesis by the gut microflora). Folates are also found in breast milk.

Bioavailability

Folates leach into cooking water and are destroyed by cooking or food processing at high temperatures.

Deficiency

Folate deficiency results in reduction of DNA synthesis and hence in reduction of cell division. While DNA synthesis occurs in all dividing cells, deficiency is most easily seen in tissues with high rates of cell turnover such as erythrocytes (red blood cells). The main clinical observation associated with folate deficiency is, therefore, megaloblastic anaemia.

The main causes of folate deficiency are as follows:

- Decreased dietary intake. This occurs in people eating inadequate diets, such as some

Table 1   Dietary Reference Values for folic acid (µg/day)

							EU RDA = 200 µg
Age	UK				USA		FAO/WHO
	LRNI	EAR	RNI	EVM	RDA	TUL	RNI
0–3 months	30	40	50		65	–	80
4–6 months	30	40	50		65	–	80
7–12 months	30	40	50		80	–	80
1–3 years	35	50	70		150	300	150
4–6 years	50	75	100		–	–	200
4–8 years	–	–	–		200	400	–
7–10 years	75	110	150		–	–	300[a]
9–13 years	–	–	–		300	600	400
14–18 years	–	–	–		400	800	400
Males							
11–14 years	100	150	200		–	–	–
15–50+ years	100	150	200	1000	400	1000	400
Females							
11–14 years	100	150	200		–	–	–
15–50+ years	100	150	200	1000	400	1000	400
Pregnancy			+100[1]		600	1000[2]	600
Lactation			+60		500	1000[2]	600

[a] 7–9 years.

[1] The Department of Health recommends that all women who are pregnant or planning a pregnancy should take a folic acid supplement (see dose).

[2] ≤ 18 years = 800 µg daily.

EVM = Likely safe daily intake from supplements alone.

TUL = Tolerable Upper Intake Level (not determined for thiamine).

elderly people, those on low incomes, and alcoholics who substitute alcoholic drinks for good sources of nutrition.

- Decreased intestinal absorption. Patients with disorders of malabsorption (e.g. coeliac disease) may suffer folate deficiency.
- Increased requirements. Increased requirement for folate, and hence an increased risk of deficiency, can occur in pregnancy, during breast-feeding, in haemolytic anaemia and leukaemia.
- Alcoholism. Chronic alcoholism is a common cause of folate deficiency. This may occur as a result of poor dietary intake, reduced absorption or increased excretion by the kidney. The presence of alcoholic liver disease increases the likelihood of folate deficiency.

- Drugs. Long-term use of certain drugs (e.g. phenytoin, sulfasalazine) is associated with folate deficiency.

Signs and symptoms include megaloblastic, macrocytic anaemia, weakness, tiredness, irritability, forgetfulness, dyspnoea, anorexia, diarrhoea, weight loss, headache, syncope, palpitations and glossitis. In babies and young children, growth may be affected.

Possible uses

Pregnancy and pre-pregnancy

The risk of neural tube defects (NTDs) can be reduced by increased folic acid intake during the periconceptual period.[1–5] These findings gave rise to recommendations in several countries

Table 2	Dietary sources of folic acid

Food portion	Folate content (µg)
Breakfast cereals	
1 bowl All-Bran (45 g)	80
1 bowl Bran Flakes (45 g)	**110**
1 bowl Corn Flakes (30 g)	70
1 bowl muesli (95 g)	**130**
1 bowl Start (40 g)	**140**
Cereal products	
Bread, brown, 2 slices	30
white, 2 slices	25
wholemeal 2 slices	30
fortified, 2 slices	**70**
1 chapati	10
Milk and dairy products	
½ pint (280 ml) milk, whole, semi-skimmed, or skimmed	15
½ pint (280 ml) soya milk	50
1 pot yoghurt (150 g)	25
Cheese, average (50 g)	15
Camembert (50 g)	50
Meat	
Liver, lambs, cooked (90 g)	**220**
Kidney, lambs, cooked (75 g)	60
Vegetables	
Broccoli, boiled (100 g)	65
Brussels sprouts, boiled (100 g)	**110**
Cabbage, boiled (100 g)	30
Cauliflower, boiled (100 g)	50
Kale, boiled (100 g)	90
Lettuce (30 g)	20
Peas, boiled (100 g)	50
Potatoes, boiled (150 g)	**145**
Spinach, boiled (100 g)	**100**
1 small can baked beans (200 g)	45
Chickpeas, cooked (105 g)	**110**
Red kidney beans (105 g)	90
Fruit	
1 orange	45
1 large glass orange juice	40
Half a grapefruit	20
Yeast	
Brewer's yeast (10 g)	**400**
Marmite, spread on 1 slice bread	50

Excellent source (**bold**); good source (*italics*).

that women intending to become pregnant should consume additional folic acid. The reason for the beneficial effect of folic acid is unclear. Although it may be a result of deficiency, a genetic defect in the methylene tetrahydrofolate reductase (MTHFR) gene, estimated to occur in about 5–15% of white populations, appears to result in an increased requirement for folates and an increased risk of recurrent early pregnancy loss and NTDs.[6,7] In addition, elevated levels of plasma homocysteine have been observed in mothers producing offspring with NTDs,[8] and the possibility that this factor could have toxic effects on the foetus at the time of neural tube closure is currently under further investigation.

Whether folic acid taken throughout pregnancy has any benefit on birth outcome is unclear. Re-analysis of data from a large randomised trial, combined with trials from an updated Cochrane review, found no association between folic acid supplementation and birth weight, placental weight or gestational age. Folic acid at high dose (5 mg daily) was associated with reduced risk of low birth weight (pooled relative risk 0.73 (95% CI, 0.53 to 0.99). Overall there was no conclusive evidence of benefit for folic acid supplementation in pregnant women given from time of booking onwards.[9]

Results from some trials have suggested that folic acid is associated with an increase in twin pregnancies. A Hungarian study involving 38 151 women found that both pre- and post-conceptual supplementation of a high dose of folic acid and multivitamins are associated with a slight increase in the incidence of twin pregnancies.[10] A British prospective cohort study involving 602 women undergoing fertility treatment found that the likelihood of a twin birth after in vitro fertilisation rose with increased concentrations of plasma folate and red-cell folate. There was no association between folate and vitamin B_{12} levels and the likelihood of a successful pregnancy, but the MTHFR genotype was associated with the women's potential to produce healthy embryos.[11]

Cardiovascular disease

Marginal folate status is also associated with elevated plasma homocysteine levels, a known risk factor for CVD mortality.[12-14] Mechanisms by which plasma homocysteine may be associated with increased risk of CVD have not been clearly established, but possibilities include:[15]

- oxidative damage to the vascular endothelium;
- inhibition of endothelial anticoagulant factors, resulting in increased clot formation;
- increased platelet aggregation; and
- proliferation of smooth muscle cells, resulting in increased vulnerability of the arteries to obstruction.

Homocysteine is derived from dietary methionine, and it is removed by conversion to cystathionine, cysteine and pyruvate, or by remethylation to methionine. Rare inborn errors of metabolism can cause severe elevations in plasma homocysteine levels. One example is homocystinuria, which occurs as a result of a genetic defect in the enzyme, cystathione beta-synthase. Genetic changes in the enzymes involved in the remethylation pathway, including MTHFR and methionine synthase, are also associated with increase in plasma homocysteine concentrations. All such cases are associated with premature vascular disease, thrombosis and early death.

However, such genetic disorders are rare and cannot account for the raised homocysteine levels observed in many patients with CVD. However, attention is now being given to the possibility that deficiency of the various vitamins that act as cofactors for the enzymes involved in homocysteine metabolism could result in increased homocysteine concentrations. In particular, folate is required for the normal function of MTHFR, vitamin B_{12} for methionine synthase and vitamin B_6 for cystathione beta-synthase.

In theory, lack of any one of these three vitamins could cause hyperhomocysteinaemia, and could therefore increase the risk of CVD. In the Framingham Heart Study,[16] a cohort study on vascular disease, it was shown that folic acid, vitamin B_6 and vitamin B_{12} are determinants of plasma homocysteine levels, with folic acid showing the strongest association.

The question of whether increased vitamin intake can reduce cardiovascular risk was examined in the Nurse's Health Study,[17] which showed that those with the highest intake of folate had a 31% lower incidence of heart disease than those with the lowest intake. For vitamin B_6, those with the highest intake had a 33% lower risk of heart disease, while in those with the highest intake of both folate and vitamin B_6, the risk of heart disease was reduced by 45%. The risk of heart disease was reduced by 24% in those who regularly used multivitamins. In a large Australian study involving 1419 men and 1531 women aged 20–90, the risk of fatal CVD was not associated with serum folate and serum B_{12} concentrations.[18]

Another question is whether homocysteine levels can be lowered with folate and other B vitamins. Folic acid (250 µg daily), in addition to usual dietary intakes of folate, significantly decreased plasma homocysteine concentrations in healthy young women,[19] and breakfast cereal fortified with folic acid reduced plasma homocysteine in men and women with coronary artery disease.[20] Another study has demonstrated that the addition of vitamin B_{12} to folic acid supplements or enriched foods (400 µg folic acid daily) maximises the reduction of homocysteine.[21] Furthermore, two meta-analyses[22,23] suggest that administration of folic acid reduces plasma homocysteine concentrations and that vitamin B_{12} but not vitamin B_6 may have an additional effect.[23] Vitamin B_6 alone also seems to be less effective than a combination of folic acid and B_{12} in lowering plasma homocysteine concentrations in patients with coronary artery disease.[24,25]

A meta-analysis of 25 RCTs involving 2595 subjects found that the proportional reductions in plasma homocysteine concentrations produced by folic acid were greater at higher homocysteine and lower folate pretreatment concentrations. They were also greater in women than men. Vitamin B_{12} produced further reduction in homocysteine, but vitamin B_6 had no significant effect. The conclusion of this meta-analysis was that daily doses ≥ 0.8 mg folic acid are required to achieve maximal reduction in homocysteine concentrations produced by folic acid. Doses of 0.2 mg and 0.4 mg were associated with 60% and 90% respectively, of this maximal effect.[26] A more recent RCT also found that the homocysteine lowering effect of B vitamins (folate, B_6 and B_{12}) was maximal in those with high homocysteine and low B_{12} levels.[27]

Although high homocysteine levels are associated with CVD, the question as to whether lowering homocysteine reduces cardiovascular risk has not been clearly answered. A meta-analysis in 2002 found strong evidence that the association between homocysteine and CVD is causal, and calculated that lowering homocysteine concentrations by 3 μmol/L (achievable by increasing folic acid intake) would reduce the risk of ischaemic heart disease by 16%, deep vein thrombosis by 25% and stroke by 24%.[28]

However, a more recent meta-analysis that investigated the association between the MTHFR gene and CHD found no strong evidence to support this association, concluding that the possible benefit of folic acid in preventing CVD, through lowering homocysteine, is in some doubt.[29]

In addition, a recent RCT in Singaporean stroke patients found that the MTHFR gene polymorphism (MTHFR C677T) did not significantly influence the effect of vitamin therapy on homocysteine levels. In this study, the magnitude of the reduction in homocysteine levels at 12 months was similar, irrespective of MTHFR genotype.[30]

In another trial, moderate reduction of total homocysteine after non-disabling cerebral infarction had no effect on vascular outcomes during 2 years of follow-up.[31] Further trials of homocysteine lowering with folic acid either alone or in combination with other B vitamins have shown no significant effects on biomarkers of inflammation, endothelial dysfunction and hypercoagulablity,[32–34] or inflammatory and thrombogenic markers in smokers.[35] One trial found that folate (5 mg daily) and B_{12} (500 μg daily) improved insulin resistance and endothelial dysfunction in patients with metabolic syndrome.[36] Another study showed no improvement in markers of endothelial dysfunction and low-grade inflammation in patients with type 2 diabetes,[37] while another found that short-term folic acid supplementation (5 mg daily) significantly enhances endothelial function in type 2 diabetes.[38]

Two large RCTs (the Heart Outcomes Prevention Evaluation[39] and the NORVIT Trial[40]) found that B_{12}, folic acid and B_6 in combination reduced plasma homocysteine, but did not reduce the risk of major cardiovascular events in patients with CVD,[39] and did not reduce the risk of recurrent CVD after acute myocardial infarction.[40]

Cancer

Marginal folate status also appears to be associated with certain cancers,[41] notably colon cancer, although it is at present unclear as to whether it is folate or some other nutritional factors that could be involved. Data, including those from two prospective studies[42,43] and four case-control studies,[44–47] indicate that inadequate intake of folate may increase risk of colon cancer. However, a recent prospective study has indicated that low plasma folate concentrations may protect against colorectal cancer. A bell-shaped curve was observed between plasma folate and colorectal cancer risk. The MTHFR C677T polymorphism was associated with a reduced risk of colorectal cancer that was independent of folate status.[48]

There is some evidence – albeit limited – that use of supplements containing folic acid could reduce the risk of colon cancer.[49,50] More recent studies have also found a lower incidence of colorectal adenomas in people with higher intakes of and plasma concentrations of folate and lower homocysteine.[51]

A meta-analysis of seven cohort and nine case-control studies also added support for the hypothesis that folate has a small protective effect against colorectal cancer.[52]

There is also evidence that high folate intake may have a particular effect in reducing colorectal cancer risk in people with high alcohol intake,[53,54] or in smokers.[55] In women with high alcohol intake, there is also a strong inverse relationship between dietary folate intake and ovarian cancer risk.[56] Higher folate intake has also been shown to reduce breast cancer risk in women with loss of oestrogen receptor (ER) gene expression, but not in those with oestrogen receptor (ER+) gene expression.[57] A study investigating the effect of folate taken in pregnancy on breast cancer found that women taking high doses of folate throughout pregnancy may be more likely to die of breast cancer in later life than women taking no folate.

The authors suggested that this could be a chance finding, so further studies should be conducted.[58]

Mental disorders

There is an apparent increase in mental disorders associated with reduced folate status.[59] Recent studies have found that Alzheimer's disease is associated with low blood levels of folate and vitamin B_{12} and elevated homocysteine levels.[60–68] However, a meta-analysis of four randomised controlled intervention trials provide no evidence that folic acid, with or without vitamin B_{12}, has a beneficial effect on cognitive function or mood in cognitively impaired older people.[69]

Evidence exists of a link between depression and low folate levels and some RCTs have found folate supplements helpful when added to conventional antidepressants. A recent US study amongst 110 patients with major depressive disorder compared levels of folate, B_{12} and homocysteine with the time taken to respond to the antidepressant fluoxetine. The 15% of patients who initially had low folate levels took longer to onset of clinical improvement than those with normal folate. Initial levels of B_{12} and homocysteine had no relationship to response onset.[70]

A systematic review of three RCTs of folate supplementation suggests that folate may have a potential role as a supplement to other treatments for depression. Low folate patients given extra folate had reduced Hamilton Depression Rating Scale scores and increased odds of a 50% score improvement compared to placebo. Folate given to patients with initially normal folate had no significant impact.[71] Two other recent RCTs in which average folate status was normal or not measured also found no evidence that folate supplements helped depression.[72,73]

A UK study has investigated a genetic factor in the link between folate and depression. A cross-sectional observational study of 3478 women (from a heart health study) compared the presence of the MTHFR C677T genotype with the presence of depressive symptoms. Eight other similar studies were meta-analysed together with the new results. Depression was found to be associated with the C677T genotype.[74]

In summary, it is clear that a proportion of depressed patients have low folate status and that this can be associated with a worse response to antidepressants. Whether low folate is the cause or effect of depression in these patients is less clear. Evidence to date from RCTs of folate supplementation in depression is minimal but positive. Patients with depression should be tested for red cell folate and supplemented when folate is low, particularly if they are elderly or have co-existing nutritional risk.

Hip fracture

Preliminary evidence from one RCT in 628 patients in Japan aged 65 or older with stroke found that daily oral treatment with folic acid 5 mg and mecobalamin 1500 µg reduced plasma homocysteine and the risk of hip fracture.[75]

Conclusion

There is good evidence that folic acid reduces the risk of neural tube defects, and supplementation is recommended pre-conceptually and during the first 12 weeks of pregnancy. There is increasing evidence that folic acid reduces elevated plasma homocysteine levels, a risk factor for CVD. However, it is still not clear whether folic acid, with or without other B vitamins, reduces the risk of CVD. This may be confused by the MTHFR gene, defects in which may influence the effect of folic acid. Epidemiological studies have shown an inverse relationship between serum folate levels and colon cancer. Poor folate status has also been demonstrated in some people with depression and a few RCTs have found supplementation helpful when added to conventional antidepressants. Depressed patients should be tested for folate and supplemented when folate is low. However, controlled trials are required to determine whether supplements reduce the risk of cancer.

Precautions/contraindications

In pernicious anaemia, folic acid will correct the haematological abnormalities, but neuropathy may be precipitated. Doses of folic acid > 400 μg daily are not recommended until pernicious anaemia has been ruled out.

Pregnancy and breast-feeding

No problems have been reported. Supplements are required during pregnancy and when planning a pregnancy (see Dose).

Adverse effects

Folic acid is generally considered to be safe even in high doses, but it may lead to convulsions in patients taking anticonvulsants and may precipitate neuropathy in pernicious anaemia. Some gastrointestinal disturbance and altered sleep pattern has been reported at doses of 15 mg daily. Allergic reactions (shortness of breath, wheezing, fever, erythema, skin rash, itching) have been reported rarely.

Interactions

Drugs

Anticonvulsants: requirements for folic acid may be increased, but concurrent use of folic acid may antagonise the effects of anticonvulsants; an increase in anticonvulsant dose may be necessary in patients who receive supplementary folic acid (monitoring required).

Antibiotics: may interfere with the microbiological assay for serum and erythrocyte folic acid (falsely low results).

Colestyramine: may reduce the absorption of folic acid; patients on prolonged colestyramine therapy should take a folic acid supplement 1 h before colestyramine administration.

Methotrexate: acts as a folic acid antagonist; risk significant with high dose and/or prolonged use.

Oestrogens (including oral contraceptives): may reduce blood levels of folic acid.

Pyrimethamine: acts as a folic acid antagonist; risk significant with high dose and/or prolonged use; folic acid supplements should be given in pregnancy.

Sulfasalazine: may reduce the absorption of folic acid; requirements for folic acid may be increased.

Trimethoprim: acts as a folic acid antagonist; risk significant with high dose and/or prolonged use.

Nutrients

Adequate amounts of all B vitamins are required for optimal functioning; deficiency or excess of one B vitamin may lead to abnormalities in the metabolism of another.

Zinc: folic acid may reduce the absorption of zinc.

Dose

Folic acid is available in the form of tablets.

For prevention of first occurrence of NTDs in women who are planning a pregnancy, oral, 400 μg daily before conception until 12th week of pregnancy.

For prevention of recurrence of NTDs, oral, 5 mg daily before conception until 12th week of pregnancy.

For prophylaxis during pregnancy (after 12th week), oral, 200–500 μg daily. A Cochrane review concluded that folate supplementation in pregnancy appears to improve haemoglobin status and folate status.[76]

In women with diabetes mellitus, oral, 5 mg daily before conception until the 12th week. This is because women with diabetes are at significantly increased risk of having a baby with NTDs. This dose has been recommended by Diabetes UK (2005), the British Medical Association (2004) and the Society of Obstetricians and Gynaecologists (2003).[77]

As a dietary supplement, oral, 100–500 μg daily.

When co-prescribed with methotrexate, in patients who suffer mucosal or gastrointestinal side-effects with this drug, folic acid 5 mg each week may help to reduce the frequency of such side-effects. This dose has been recommended by ATTRACT, the British National Formulary and PRODIGY.[78]

Upper safety levels

The UK Expert Group on Vitamins and Minerals (EVM) has identified a likely safe total intake of folic acid for adults from supplements alone of 1000 µg daily.

References

1 Laurence KM, James N, Miller MH, *et al*. Double-blind randomised controlled trial of folate treatment before conception to prevent recurrence of neural tube defects. *BMJ* 1981; 282: 1509–1511.

2 Smithells RW, Seller MJ, Harris R, *et al*. Further experience of vitamin supplementation for prevention of neural tube defect recurrences. *Lancet* 1983; i: 1027–1031.

3 Medical Research Council Vitamin Study Research Group. Prevention of neural tube defects: results of the Medical Research Council Vitamin Study. *Lancet* 1991; 338: 131–137.

4 Czeizel AE, Dudas I. Prevention of the first occurrence of neural tube defects by periconceptual vitamin supplementation. *N Engl J Med* 1992; 327: 1832–1835.

5 Weller MM, Shapiro S, Mitchel AA, *et al*. Periconceptual folic acid exposure and risk of occurrent neural tube defects. *JAMA* 1993; 269: 1257–1261.

6 Molloy AM, Daly S, Mills JL, *et al*. Thermolabile variant of 5,10-methylenetetrahydrofolate reductase associated with low red cell folates: implications for folate intake recommendations. *Lancet* 1997; 349: 1591–1593.

7 Nelen WLDM, Van der Molen EF, Blom HJ, *et al*. Recurrent early pregnancy loss and genetic related disturbances in folate and homocysteine metabolism. *Br J Hosp Med* 1997; 58: 511–513.

8 Mills JL, McPartlin P, Kirke PM, *et al*. Homocysteine metabolism in pregnancies complicated by neural tube defects. *Lancet* 1995; 345: 149–151.

9 Charles DH, Ness AR, Campbell D, *et al*. Folic acid supplements in pregnancy and birth outcome: re-analysis of a large randomised controlled trial and update of Cochrane review. *Paediatr Perinat Epidemiol* 2005; 19: 112–124.

10 Czeizel AE, Vargha P. Preconceptual folic acid/multivitamin supplementation and twin pregnancy. *Am J Obstet Gynecol* 2004; 191: 790–794.

11 Haggarty P, McCallum H, McBain H, *et al*. Effect of B vitamins and genetics on success of in-vitro fertilisation: prospective cohort study. *Lancet* 2006; 367: 1513–1519.

12 Alfthan G, Aro A, Gey KF. Plasma homocysteine and cardiovascular disease mortality. *Lancet* 1997; 349: 397.

13 Nygard O, Nordrehaug JE, Refsum H, *et al*. Plasma homocysteine levels and mortality in patients with coronary artery disease. *N Engl J Med* 1997; 337: 230–236.

14 Wald NJ, Watt HC, Law MR, *et al*. Homocysteine and ischaemic heart disease: results of a prospective study with implications on prevention. *Arch Intern Med* 1998; 158: 862–867.

15 Weir DG, Scott JM. Homocysteine as a risk factor for cardiovascular and related disease: nutritional implications. *Nutr Res Rev* 1998; 11: 311–338.

16 Selhub J, Jacques PF, Wilson PWF, *et al*. Vitamin status and intake as primary determinants of homocysteinaemia in an elderly population. *JAMA* 1993; 270: 2693–2698.

17 Rimm EB, Willett WC, Hu FB, *et al*. Folate and vitamin B_6 from diet and supplements in relation to risk of coronary heart disease among women. *JAMA* 1998; 279: 359–364.

18 Hung J, Beilby JP, Knuiman MW, Divitini M. Folate and vitamin B-12 and risk of fatal cardiovascular disease: cohort study from Busselton, Western Australia. *BMJ* 2003; 326: 131–135.

19 Brouwer IA, van Dusseldorp M, Thomas CMG, *et al*. Low-dose folic acid supplementation decreases plasma homocysteine concentrations: a randomized trial. *Am J Clin Nutr* 1999; 69: 99–104.

20 Malinow MR, Duell PB, Hess DL, *et al*. Reduction of plasma homocysteine levels by breakfast cereal fortified with folic acid in patients with coronary heart disease. *N Engl J Med* 1998; 338: 1009–1015.

21 Bronstrup A, Hages M, Prinz-Langenohl R, Pietrzik K. Effects of folic acid and combinations of folic acid and vitamin B-12 on plasma homocysteine concentrations in healthy young women. *Am J Clin Nutr* 1998; 68: 1104–1110.

22 Boushey CJ, Beresford SAA, Omenn GS, Motulsky AG. A quantitative assessmemt of plasma homocysteine as a risk factor for vascular disease: probable benefits of increasing folic acid intake. *JAMA* 1995; 274: 1049–1057.

23 Homocysteine Lowering Trialists' Collaboration. Lowering blood homocysteine with folic acid based supplements: meta-analysis of randomised trials. *BMJ* 1998; 316: 894–898.

24 Lee BJ, Huang MC, Chung LJ, *et al*. Folic acid and vitamin B12 are more effective than vitamin B6 in lowering fasting plasma homocysteine concentration in patients with coronary artery disease. *Eur J Clin Nutr* 2004; 58: 481–487.

25 Stott DJ, MacIntosh G, Lowe GD, *et al*. Randomized controlled trial of homocysteine-lowering vitamin treatment in elderly patients with vascular disease. *Am J Clin Nutr* 2005; 82: 1320–1326.

26 Homocysteine Lowering Trialists' Collaboration. Dose-dependent effects of folic acid on blood

concentrations of homocysteine: a meta-analysis of the randomized trials. *Am J Clin Nutr* 2005; 82: 806–812.

27 Flicker L, Vasikaran SD, Thomas J, *et al*. Efficacy of B vitamins in lowering homocysteine in older men. *Stroke* 2006; 37: 547.

28 Wald DS, Law M, Morris JK. Homocysteine and cardiovascular disease: evidence on causality from a meta-analysis. *BMJ* 2002; 325: 1202–1204.

29 Lewis SJ, Ebrahim S, Davey Smith G. Meta-analysis of MTHFR 677CT polymorphism and coronary heart disease: does totality of evidence support a causal role for homocysteine and preventive potential of folate? *BMJ* 2005; 331: 1053–1058.

30 Ho GYH, Eikelboom JW, Hankey GJ, *et al*. Methylenetetrahydrofolate reductase polymorphisms and homocysteine-lowering effect of vitamin therapy in Singaporean stroke patients. *Stroke* 2006; 37: 456.

31 Toole JF, Malinow MR, Chambless LE, *et al*. Lowering homocysteine in patients with ischemic stroke to prevent recurrent stroke, myocardial infarction, and death: the Vitamin Intervention for Stroke Prevention (VISP) randomized controlled trial. *JAMA* 2004; 291: 565–575.

32 Peeters AC, van der Molen EF, Blom HJ, den Heijer M. The effect of homcysteine reduction by B-vitamin supplementation on markers of endothelial dysfunction. *Thromb Haemost* 2004; 92: 1086–1091.

33 Dusitanond P, Eikelboom JW, Hankey JG, *et al*. Homocysteine-lowering treatment with folic acid, cobalamin, and pyridoxine does not reduce blood markers of inflammation, endothelial dysfunction, or hypercoagulability in patients with previous transient ischaemic attack or stroke: a randomized substudy of the VITATOPS trial. *Stroke* 2005; 36: 144–146.

34 Durga J, van Tits LJ, Schouten EG, *et al*. Effect of lowering of homocysteine levels on inflammatory markers: a randomized controlled trial. *Arch Intern Med* 2005; 165: 1388–1394.

35 Mangoni AA, Arya R, Ford E, *et al*. Effects of folic acid supplementation on inflammatory and thrombogenic markers in chronic smokers. A randomised controlled trial. *Thromb Res* 2003; 110: 13–17.

36 Setola A, Mont LD, Galluccio E, *et al*. Insulin resistance and endothelial function are improved after folate and vitamin B12 therapy in patients with metabolic syndrome: relationship between homocysteine levels and hyperinsulinaemia. *Eur J Endocrinol* 2004; 151: 483–489.

37 Spoelstra-de MA, Brouwer CB, Terheggen F, *et al*. No effect of folic acid on markers of endothelial dysfunction or inflammation in patients with type 2 diabetes mellitus and mild hyperhomocysteinaemia. *Neth J Med* 2004; 62: 246–253.

38 Mangoni AA, Sherwood RA, Asonganyi B, *et al*. Short-term oral folic acid supplementation enhances endothelial function in patients with type 2 diabetes. *Am J Hypertens* 2005; 18 (2 Pt 1): 220–226.

39 Lonn E, Yusuf S, Arnold MJ, on behalf of the Heart Outcomes Prevention Evaluation (HOPE) 2 Investigators. Homocysteine lowering with folic acid and B vitamins in vascular disease. *N Engl J Med* 2006; 354: 1567–1577. Epub 2006 March 12.

40 Bonaa KH, Njolstad I, Ueland PM, on behalf of the NORVIT Trial Investigators. Homocysteine lowering and cardiovascular events after acute myocardial infarction. *N Engl J Med* 2006; 354: 1578–1588. Epub 2006 March 12.

41 Mason JB. Folate status: Effects on carcinogenesis. In: Bailey LB, ed. *Folates in Health and Disease*. New York: Marcel Dekker, 1995: 361–378.

42 Giovannucci E, Rimm EB, Ascherio A, *et al*. Alcohol, low methionine, low folate diets and risk of colon cancer in men. *J Natl Cancer Inst* 1995; 87: 265–273.

43 Glynn SA, Albanes D, Pietinen P, *et al*. Colorectal cancer and folate status: a nested case-control study among male smokers. *Cancer Epidemiol Biomarkers Prev* 1996; 5: 487–494.

44 Benito E, Stigglebout A, Bosch FX, *et al*. Nutritional factors in colorectal cancer risk: a case-control study in Majorca. *Int J Cancer* 1991; 49: 161–167.

45 Meyer F, White E. Alcohol and nutrients in relation to colon cancer in middle-aged adults. *Am J Epidemiol* 1993; 138: 225–236.

46 Ferraroni M, La Vecchia C, D'Avanzo B, *et al*. Selected micronutrient intake and the role of colon cancer. *Br J Cancer* 1994; 70: 1150–1155.

47 Freudenheim JL, Graham S, Marshall JR, *et al*. Folate intake and carcinogenesis of the colon and rectum. *Int J Epidemiol* 1991; 20: 368–374.

48 Van Guelpen B, Hultdin J, Johansson I, *et al*. Low folate levels may protect against colorectal cancer. *Gut* 2006; 55: 1387–1389.

49 White E, Shannon JS, Patterson RE. Relationship between vitamin and calcium supplement use and colon cancer. *Cancer Epidemiol Biomarkers Prev* 1997; 6: 769–774.

50 Giovannucci E, Stampfer MJ, Colditz GA, *et al*. Multivitamin use, folate and colon cancer in women in the nurses' health study. *Ann Intern Med* 1998; 129: 517–524.

51 Martinez ME, Henning SM, Alberts DS. Folate and colorectal neoplasia: relation between plasma and dietary markers of folate and adenoma recurrence. *Am J Clin Nutr* 2004; 79: 691–697.

52 Sanjoaquin MA, Allen N, Couto E, *et al*. Folate intake and colorectal cancer risk: a meta-analytical approach. *Int J Cancer* 2005; 113: 825–828.

53 Boyapati SM, Bostick RM, McGlynn KA, *et al*. Folate intake, MTHFR C677T polymorphism,

alcohol consumption, and risk for sporadic colo-rectal adenoma (United States). *Cancer Causes Control* 2004; 15: 493–501.

54 Le Marchand L, Wilkens LR, Kolonel LN, Henderson BE. The MTHFR C677T polymorphism and colorectal cancer: the multiethnic cohort study. *Cancer Epidemiol Biomarkers Prev* 2005; 14: 1198–1203.

55 Larrson SC, Giovannucci E, Wolk A. A prospective study of dietary folate intake and risk of colorectal cancer: modification by caffeine intake and cigarette smoking. *Cancer Epidemiol Biomarkers Prev* 2005; 14: 740–743.

56 Larrson SC, Giovannucci E, Wolk A. Dietary folate intake and incidence of ovarian cancer: the Swedish Mammography Cohort. *J Natl Cancer Inst* 2004; 96: 396–402.

57 Zhang SM, Hankinson SE, Hunter DJ, *et al*. Folate intake and risk of breast cancer characterized by hormone receptor status. *Cancer Epidemiol Biomarkers Prev* 2005; 14: 2004–2008.

58 Charles D, Ness AR, Campbell D, *et al*. Taking folate in pregnancy and risk of maternal breast cancer. *BMJ* 2004; 329: 1375–1376.

59 Bottiglieri ET, Crellin RF, Reynolds EH. Folates and neuropsychiatry. In: Bailey L, ed. *Folate in Health and Disease*. New York: Marcel Dekker, 1995: 435–462.

60 Joosten E, Lesaffre E, Riezler R, *et al*. Is metabolic evidence for vitamin B_{12} and folate deficiency more frequent in elderly patients with Alzheimer's disease? *J Gerontol A Biol Sci Med* 1997; 52: M76–M79.

61 Clarke R, Smith AD, Jobst KA, *et al*. Folate, vitamin B_{12} and serum homocysteine levels in confirmed Alzheimer's disease. *Arch Neurol* 1998; 11: 1449–1455.

62 Wang HX, Wahlin A, Basun H, *et al*. Vitamin B(12) and folate in relation to the development of Alzheimer's disease. *Neurology* 2001; 56: 1188–1194.

63 Luchsinger JA, Tang MX, Shea S, *et al*. Plasma homocysteine levels and risk of Alzheimer disease. *Neurology* 2004; 62: 1972–1976.

64 Quadri P, Fragiacomo C, Pezzati R, *et al*. Homocysteine, folate and vitamn B-12 in mild cognitive impairment, Alzheimer disease, and vascular dementia. *Am J Clin Nutr* 2004; 80: 114–122.

65 Ellinson M, Thomas J, Patterson A. A critical evaluation of the relationship between serum vitamin B, folate and total homocysteine with cognitive impairment in the elderly. *J Hum Nutr Diet* 2004; 17: 371–383.

66 Kado DM, Karlamangla AS, Huang MH, *et al*. Homcysteine versus the vitamins folate, B6, and B12 as predictors of cognitive function and decline in older high-functioning adults: MacArthur Studies of Successful Aging. *Am J Med* 2005; 118: 161–167.

67 Ravaglia G, Forti P, Maioli F, *et al*. Homocysteine and folate as risk factors for dementia and Alzheimer disease. *Am J Clin Nutr* 2005; 82: 636–643.

68 Tucker KL, Qiao N, Scott T, *et al*. High homocysteine and low B vitamins predict cognitive decline in aging men: the Veterans Affairs Normative Aging Study. *Am J Clin Nutr* 2005; 82: 627–635.

69 Malouf R, Grimley Evans J, Areosa Sastre A. Folic acid with or without vitamin B12 for cognition and dementia. Cochrane database, issue 4, 2003. London: Macmillan.

70 Papakostas GI, Petersen T, Lebowitz BD, *et al*. The relationship between serum folate, vitamin B12, and homocysteine levels in major depressive disorder and the timing of improvement with fluoxetine. *Int J Neuropsychopharmacol* 2005; 8: 523–528.

71 Taylor MJ, Carney SM, Goodwin GM, Geddes JR. Folate for depressive disorders: systematic review and meta-analysis of randomized controlled trials. *J Psychopharmacol* 2004 18: 251–256.

72 Williams E, Stewart-Knox B, Bradbury I, *et al*. Effect of folic acid supplementation on mood and serotonin response in healthy males. *Br J Nutr* 2005; 94: 602–608.

73 Bryan J, Calvaresi E. Association between dietary intake of folate and vitamins B-12 and B-6 and self-reported psychological well-being in Australian men and women in midlife. *J Nutr Health Aging* 2004; 8: 226–232.

74 Lewis SJ, Lawlor DA, Davey Smith G, *et al*. The thermolabile variant of MTHFR is associated with depression in the British Women's Heart and Health Study and a meta-analysis. *Mol Psychiatry* 2006; 11: 352–360 (Epub 2006 10 Jan).

75 Sato Y, Honda Y, Iwamoto J, *et al*. Effect of folate and mecobalamin on hip fractures in patients with stroke: a randomized controlled trial. *JAMA* 2005; 293: 1082–1088.

76 Mahomed K. Folate supplementation in pregnancy. Cochrane database, issue 3, 1997. London: Macmillan.

77 National Health Service. National Library for Health. http://www.clinicalanswers nhs.uk/index.cfm?question=1473 (accessed 31 October 2006).

78 National Health Service. National Library for Health. http://www.clinicalanswers.nhs.uk/index.cfm?question=248 (accessed 31 October 2006).

Gamma-oryzanol

Description

Gamma-oryzanol is one of several lipid fractions obtained from rice bran oil.

Constituents

Gamma-oryzanol is a mixture of phytosterols (plant sterols), including campesterol, cyclo-artanol, cycloartenol, beta-sitosterol, stigmasterol, and also ferulic acid.

Action

Phytosterols appear to reduce lipid levels and ferulic acid has antioxidant properties. Gamma-oryzanol has also been suggested to have anabolic properties, but evidence is conflicting.

Possible uses

Gamma-oryzanol has been investigated for a role in lipid lowering and improving exercise performance.

Lipid lowering

Several animal studies[1-3] have shown a lipid-lowering effect with gamma-oryzanol supplementation, but one study did not.[4]

In two uncontrolled studies in humans with hyperlipidaemia, gamma-oryzanol was shown to reduce serum cholesterol levels. One study involved 80 patients with hyperlipidaemia who were given gamma-oryzanol for 6 months. In those with type IIa and IIb hypercholesterolaemia, serum cholesterol fell by 12% and 13% respectively, but the reduction was significant only after 3 months. Plasma triglycerides reduced significantly after 3 months and there was a non-significant increase in HDL cholesterol.[5]

In the other study, 20 patients with chronic schizophrenia with dyslipidaemia were given 300 mg gamma-oryzanol daily for 16 weeks. Both total and LDL cholesterol fell significantly, but there was no significant change in HDL levels.[6]

Exercise

In a double-blind, placebo-controlled study, 22 weight-trained men were given 500 mg gamma-oryzanol daily or placebo for 9 weeks. There were no differences between the groups for measures of circulating concentrations of testosterone, cortisol, oestradiol, growth hormone, insulin or beta-endorphin, blood lipids, calcium, magnesium and albumin. Resting cardiovascular variables decreased in both groups and vertical jump power and one-repetition maximum muscle strength (bench press and squat) increased in both groups. The authors concluded that gamma-oryzanol 500 mg for 9 weeks did not influence either performance or physiological parameters in moderately weight-trained men.[7]

> **Conclusion**
> Preliminary evidence from animal studies and uncontrolled studies indicates that gamma-oryzanol may reduce serum cholesterol levels. There is no good evidence that it improves exercise performance. Further research is required.

Precautions/contraindications

None have been reported.

Pregnancy and breast-feeding

No problems have been reported, but there have not been sufficient studies to guarantee the safety of gamma-oryzanol in pregnancy and breast-feeding.

Adverse effects

There are no long-term studies assessing the safety of gamma-oryzanol in humans. There is some evidence from a Japanese study that doses up to 600 mg daily cause dry mouth, somnolence, hot flushes, irritability and headaches.[8]

Interactions

None reported.

Dose

Gamma-oryzanol is available in the form of tablets and capsules.

The dose is not established. Dietary supplements provide 100–500 mg daily.

References

1   Seetharamaiah GS, Chandrasekhara N. Studies on hypercholesterolemic activity of rice bran oil. *Atherosclerosis* 1989; 78: 219–223.
2   Rukmini C, Raghuram TC. Nutritional and biochemical aspects of the hypolipidemic action of rice bran oil: a review. *J Am Coll Nutr* 1991; 10: 593–601.
3   Rong N, Ausman LM, Nicolosi RJ. Oryzanol decreases cholesterol absorption and fatty streaks in hamsters. *Lipids* 1997; 32: 303–309.
4   Sugano M, Tsuji E. Rice bran oil and cholesterol metabolism. *J Nutr* 1997; 127: S521S–S524.
5   Yoshino G, Kazumi T, Amano M, *et al*. Effects of gamma-oryzanol and probucol on hyperlipidemia, *Curr Ther Res* 1989; 45: 975–982.
6   Sasaki J, Takada Y, Handa K, *et al*. Effects of gamma-oryzanol on serum lipids and apolipoproteins in dyslipidemic schizophrenics receiving major tranquillisers. *Clin Ther* 1990; 12: 263–268.
7   Fry AC, Bonner E, Lewis DL, *et al*. The effects of gamma-oryzanol supplementation during resistance exercise training. *Int J Sport Nutr* 1997; 7: 318–329.
8   Takemoto T. Clinical trial of Hi-Z fine granules (gamma-oryzanol) on gastrointestinal symptoms at 375 hospitals. *Shinyaku To Rinsho* 1977; 26 (in Japanese).

Garlic

Description

Garlic is the fresh bulb of *Allium sativum*, which is related to the lily family (Liliaceae).

Constituents

The major constituents of garlic include alliin, allicin, diallyl disulphide and ajoene, but these compounds form only a small proportion of the compounds that have been isolated from crushed, cooked and dried garlic.

Alliin, present in fresh garlic, is converted by the enzyme allinase into allicin when the garlic bulb is crushed. Allicin can be converted (by heat) into diallyldisulphide, which in turn is converted into various sulphide-containing substances that cause the typical smell of garlic. Allicin and diallyldisulphide combine to form ajoene.

Possible uses

Garlic has been cultivated for thousands of years for medicinal purposes, such as bites, tumours, wounds, headache, cancer and heart disease, and but has also been used as a pungent flavouring agent for cooking.

Evidence for the beneficial effects of garlic is accumulating but is still incomplete. Interpretation of trials is made difficult by the fact that different forms of garlic are used and that active ingredients may be lost in processing.[1] The use of standardised dried garlic preparations or fresh garlic appears to provide the most beneficial effects. Extracts or oils prepared by steam distillation or organic solvents, or 'odourless' garlic preparations, may have little activity.[2] Any preparation that produces no odour whatsoever may be clinically ineffective, because release of the biologically active allicin has not occurred. However, allicin is rapidly destroyed even by crushing the fresh bulb, and some suggest that although allicin may be important for cholesterol lowering, it may not be important for protecting against cancer.

Cardiovascular disease

Hyperlipidaemia

Many studies have looked at the potential effects of garlic on serum lipid levels. In a placebo-controlled, double-blind study of 40 patients with hypercholesterolaemia,[3] total cholesterol, triglycerides and blood pressure decreased significantly in the group receiving garlic. Daily doses of 900 mg of a garlic powder preparation (equivalent to 2700 mg fresh garlic) were administered over 16 weeks, and differences were significant after 4 weeks of treatment.

In a randomised, double-blind, placebo-controlled study of 42 healthy adults, 300 mg of a standardised garlic preparation three times daily showed a significantly greater reduction in total and LDL cholesterol than placebo.[4] In a study of eight healthy males, ingestion of a garlic clove (approximately 3 g a day for 16 weeks) resulted in an approximately 20% reduction in serum cholesterol.[5]

In another study, serum levels of total cholesterol, LDL and triglycerides decreased significantly after administration of 400 mg garlic three times a day for a month.[5] In a study involving 56 men, administration of an aged garlic extract (7.2 g daily) resulted in a 7% reduction in total cholesterol compared with baseline and a 6% reduction compared with placebo.[6] In a multicentre, placebo-controlled,

141

double-blind study carried out in Germany[7] using standardised dried garlic tablets, total cholesterol fell by 11%.

In 35 renal transplant patients, garlic 680 mg twice daily (equivalent to 4080 μg allicin) or placebo was administered over 12 weeks.[8] After 6 weeks, total and LDL cholesterol had fallen, changes that were maintained at 12 weeks. Garlic had no effect on triglyceride or HDL levels. Yet other studies using garlic 700 mg daily for 8 weeks,[9] 200 mg three times a day for 12 weeks,[10] or 1000 mg a day for 24 weeks[11] have resulted in 12–14% reductions in serum cholesterol. Other studies[12–15] demonstrated no effect of garlic on hyperlipidaemia, however.

A meta-analysis of studies[16] evaluating the effect of garlic on serum cholesterol included five of the above studies.[3,7,9–11] The garlic dose was 600–1000 mg daily for 8–24 weeks. The pooled results of the meta-analysis indicated that patients treated with garlic achieved mean total serum cholesterol concentrations of 230–290 mg/L lower than patients in placebo groups. Since the investigators used a range of dose regimens, the optimum dose for garlic could not be identified.

More recently another meta-analysis,[17] which included 13 trials, found that garlic reduced total cholesterol level from baseline significantly more than placebo. The weighted mean difference was 0.41 mmol/L (157 mg/L). However, when the trials with the highest scores for methodological quality were analysed alone, the differences in cholesterol levels between garlic and placebo were non-significant. The authors concluded that garlic is superior to placebo in reducing cholesterol levels, but the robustness of the data is questionable and any effect likely to be small. The use of garlic for hypercholesterolaemia was therefore debatable.

Garlic has been evaluated for an effect in various psychopathological parameters in patients with hypercholesterolaemia. In a 16-week prospective, double-blind, placebo-controlled trial, 33 patients with hypercholesterolaemia and no evidence of CVD were randomly assigned to receive garlic or placebo. Garlic in the form of alliin 22.4 mg daily was given to 13 patients and placebo to 20. Both groups received dietary counselling. No significant changes were observed in levels of total cholesterol, LDL, HDL and triglycerides, or in the psychopathologic parameters evaluated.[18]

An RCT in 15 men with angiographically proven coronary artery disease (CAD) investigated the role of aged garlic in endothelial function. Aged garlic was used because it contains antioxidant compounds that increase nitric oxide production and decrease the output of inflammatory cytokines from cultured cells. Oxidative stress and increased systemic inflammation may contribute to endothelial dysfunction. During supplementation, flow-mediated endothelium-dependent dilatation (FMD) increased significantly from the baseline and mainly in those men with lower baseline FMD. Markers of oxidant stress (plasma-oxidised LDL and peroxides), systemic inflammation (plasma C-reactive protein and interleukin-6) and endothelial activation did not change significantly during the study. The authors concluded that short-term treatment with aged garlic extract may improve endothelial function in men with CAD treated with aspirin and a statin.[19]

A systematic review of garlic's effects on cardiovascular risk concluded that there are insufficient data to draw conclusions regarding garlic's effects on clinical cardiovascular outcomes such as claudication and myocardial infarction. Garlic preparations may have a small positive short-term effect on lipids. Whether effects are sustainable beyond 3 months is unclear.[20]

Hypertension

Several studies have evaluated the efficacy of garlic in hypertension. In a multicentre, randomised, placebo-controlled, double-blind study of 47 patients with mild hypertension, garlic powder tablets, 200 mg three times a day for 12 weeks, produced significant reductions in blood pressure as well as total cholesterol and triglycerides.[10] In an acute pilot study of nine patients with severe hypertension, single doses of 2400 mg of a garlic powder preparation (standardised to release 0.6% allicin) produced a significant reduction in diastolic blood pressure 5–14 h after administration.[21]

A meta-analysis of studies[22] evaluated the efficacy of garlic on blood pressure. Only prospective, randomised studies with two or more treatment group comparisons and a duration of at least 4 weeks were included, and eight studies met the defined criteria. Six of the studies were placebo-controlled, one compared garlic with a diuretic and reserpine, and another compared garlic with bezafibrate. All but one of the studies were supposedly double-blind, but with the odour of garlic being difficult to mask, it is not clear whether the studies really were blinded. All eight studies used the same dried garlic powder in doses of 600–900 mg daily (equivalent to 1.8–2.7 g of fresh garlic daily) for 1–12 months. The pooled mean reduction in systolic blood pressure was 7.7 mmHg and the pooled mean diastolic pressure 5.0 mmHg more with garlic. However, there have not been enough trials with different garlic doses for the optimum dose to be defined.

In a systematic review,[20] consistent reductions in blood pressure with garlic were not found and no effects on glucose or insulin sensitivity were found.

Peripheral artery disease

A Cochrane review assessed the effects of garlic for the treatment of peripheral arterial occlusive disease. One eligible trial (small, of short duration) found no statistically significant effect of garlic on walking distance.[23]

Cancer

Preliminary data from *in vitro* animal and epidemiological studies suggest that garlic may have a protective effect in cancer development and progression. Results of epidemiological case-control studies in China[24] and Italy[25] suggest that garlic may reduce the risk of gastric cancer. Epidemiological studies cannot by themselves establish causal relationships and prospective data on this possible effect of garlic on cancer risk are required.

Garlic consumption has been associated with a reduced risk of colon cancer in some studies,[26,27] but not others.[28] However, in another study, garlic consumption was not associated with reduced risk of stomach cancer,[29] breast cancer[30] or prostate cancer.[31] A meta-analysis of the relation between cooked garlic, raw garlic or both raw and cooked garlic on the risk of colorectal and stomach cancers showed that garlic may be associated with a protective effect against both types of cancer.[32]

A systematic review[20] found that garlic supplementation for less than 3–5 years was not associated with decreased risk of breast, lung, gastric, colon or rectal cancer. Some case-control studies suggest that high dietary garlic consumption may be associated with decreased risks of laryngeal, gastric, colorectal and endometrial cancers and adenomatous colorectal polyps.

Antimicrobial activity

Garlic is being investigated for antibacterial, antifungal and antiviral activity, but current evidence is too limited to recommend garlic for the prevention of infections.

Conclusion

There is evidence from meta-analyses that garlic supplements reduce blood cholesterol and blood pressure. However, authors of meta-analyses have criticised studies for poor methodology, small numbers of subjects and short duration. There is preliminary evidence that garlic reduces platelet aggregation and may reduce the risk of cancer, but controlled clinical trials are needed to confirm this. Garlic has been used for centuries for antibacterial and antiviral effects. Although such effects have been demonstrated *in vitro*, controlled clinical studies are needed to confirm these findings.

Precautions/contraindications

Hypersensitivity to garlic.

Pregnancy and breast-feeding

No problems have been reported. However, there have not been sufficient studies to guarantee the safety of garlic supplements in pregnancy and breast-feeding.

Adverse effects

Unpleasant breath odour; indigestion; hypersensitivity reactions including contact dermatitis and asthma have been reported occasionally. A spinal haematoma (isolated report) has been attributed to the antiplatelet effects of garlic.

Interactions

None reported. Theoretically, garlic could increase bleeding with anticoagulants, aspirin and antiplatelet drugs.

Dose

Garlic supplements are available in the form of tablets and capsules.

The dose is not established, but 400–1000 mg (equivalent to 2–5 g fresh garlic or one to two cloves) daily of a standardised garlic product has been used in several studies. Dietary supplements provide 400–1000 mg dried garlic daily. Standardised products may be standardised for allicin potential. However, allicin is now known not to be the only improtant active ingredient in garlic. One clove of fresh garlic is equivalent to 4000 µg allicin potential.

References

1 Kleijnen J, Knipschild P, Ter Riet G. Garlic, onions and cardiovascular risk factors. A review of the evidence from human experiments with emphasis on commercially available preparations. *Br J Clin Pharmacol* 1989; 28: 533–544.

2 Mansell P, Reckless JP. Garlic. *BMJ* 1991; 303: 379–380.

3 Vorberg G, Schneider B. Therapy with garlic: results of a placebo-controlled, double-blind study. *Br J Clin Pract* 1990; 44 (Suppl. 69): 7–11.

4 Jain AK, Vargas R Gotzkowsky S, McMahon FG. Can garlic reduce levels of serum lipids? A controlled clinical study. *Am J Med* 1993; 94: 632–635.

5 Ali M, Thompson M. Consumption of a garlic clove a day could be beneficial in preventing thrombosis. *Prostaglandins Leukot Essent Fatty Acids* 1995; 53: 211–212.

6 Steiner M, Khan AH, Holberd D, *et al*. A double-blind crossover study in moderately hypercholesterolemic men that compared the effect of aged garlic extract and placebo administration on blood lipids. *Am J Clin Nutr* 1996; 64: 866–870.

7 Mader FH. Treatment of hyperlipidaemia with garlic-powder tablets. *Arzneimittelforschung* 1990; 40: 3–8.

8 Silagy S, Neil A. Garlic as a lipid lowering agent – a meta-analysis. *J R Coll Physicians London* 1994; 28: 39–45.

9 Plengvidhya C, Chinayon S, Sitprija S, *et al*. Effects of spray dried garlic preparation on primary hyperlipoproteinaemia. *J Med Ass Thai* 1988; 71: 248–252.

10 Auer W, Eiber A, Hertkorn E, *et al*. Hypertension and hyperlipidaemia: garlic helps in mild cases. *Br J Clin Pract* 1990; 44 (Suppl. 69): 3–6.

11 Lau BH, Lam F, Wang-Chen R. Effect of an odor modified garlic preparation on blood lipids. *Nutr Res* 1987; 7: 139–149.

12 Luley C, Lehmann-Leo W, Moeller B, *et al*. Lack of efficacy of dried garlic in patients with hyperlipoproteinaemia. *Arzneimittelforschung* 1986; 36: 766–768.

13 Berthold HK, Sudhop T, von Bergmann K. Effect of a garlic oil preparation on serum lipoproteins and cholesterol metabolism: a randomized controlled trial. *JAMA* 1998; 279: 1900–1902.

14 Isaacsohn JL, Moser M, Stein EA, *et al*. Garlic powder and plasma lipids and lipoproteins: a multi-center, randomized, placebo-controlled trial. *Arch Intern Med* 1998; 158: 1189–1194.

15 Simons LA, Balasubramaniam S, von Konigsmark M, *et al*. On the effect of garlic on plasma lipids and lipoproteins in mild hypercholesterolaemia. *Atherosclerosis* 1995; 113: 219–225.

16 Warshafsky S, Kamer RS, Sivak SL. Effect of garlic on total serum cholesterol: a meta-analysis. *Ann Intern Med* 1993; 119: 599–605.

17 Stevinson C, Pittler M, Ernst E. Garlic for treating hypercholesterolaemia. *Ann Intern Med* 2000; 133: 420–429.

18 Peleg A, Hershcovici T, Lipa R, *et al*. Effect of garlic on lipid profile and psychpathologic parameters in people with mild to moderate hypercholesterolaemia. *Isr Med Ass J* 2003; 5: 637–640.

19 Williams MJ, Sutherland WH, McCormick MP, *et al*. Aged extract improves endothelial function in men with coronary artery disease. *Phytother Res* 2005; 19: 314–319.

20 Mulrow C, Lawrence V, Ackermann A, *et al. Garlic: Effects on Cardiovascular Risks and Disease, Protective Effects Against Cancer, and Clinical Adverse Effects*. Evidence Report/Technology Assessment: Number 20; 2000. Available from http://www.ahcpr.gov/clinic/epcsums/garlicsum.htm (accessed 30 October 2006).

21 McMahon GF, Vargas R. Can garlic lower blood pressure? A pilot study. *Pharmacotherapy* 1993; 13: 406–407.

22 Silagy CA, Neil HAW. A meta-analysis of the effect of garlic on blood pressure. *J Hypertens* 1994; 12: 463–468.

23 Jepson RG, Kleijnen J, Leng GC. Garlic for peripheral arterial occlusive disease. Cochrane database, issue 2, 2005. London: Macmillan.

24 You WC, Blot WJ, Chang YS. Allium vegetables and reduced risk of stomach cancer. *J Natl Cancer Inst* 1989; 81: 162–164.

25 Buiatti E, Palli D, Declari A. A case control study of gastric cancer and diet in Italy. *Int J Cancer* 1989; 44: 611–616.

26 Steinmetz KA, Kushi LH, Bostick RM, *et al*. Vegetables, fruit, and colon cancer in the Iowa Woman's Health Study. *Am J Epidemiol* 1994; 139: 1–15.

27 Witte JS, Longnecker MP, Bird CL, *et al*. Relation of vegetable, fruit, and grain consumption to colorectal adenomatous polyps. *Am J Epidemiol* 1996; 144: 1015–1025.

28 Le Marchand L, Hankin JH, Wilkens LR, *et al*. Dietary fiber and colorectal cancer risk. *Epidemiology* 1997; 8: 658–665,

29 Dorant E, van den Brandt PA, Goldbohm RA. Allium vegetable consumption, garlic supplement intake, and female breast carcinoma incidence. *Breast Cancer Res Treat* 1995; 33: 163–170.

30 Dorant E, van den Brandt PA, Goldbohm RA, *et al*. Consumption of onions and a reduced risk of stomach carcinoma. *Gastroeneterology* 1996; 110: 12–20.

31 Key TJA, Silcocks PB, Davey GK, *et al*. A case-control study of diet and prostate cancer. *Br J Cancer* 1997; 76: 678–687.

32 Fleischauer AT, Poole C, Arab L. Garlic consumption and cancer prevention: meta-analyses of colorectal and stomach cancers. *Am J Clin Nutr* 2000; 72: 1047–1052.

Ginkgo biloba

Description

Ginkgo biloba is an extract from the dried leaves of *Ginkgo biloba* (maidenhair tree). In Germany, it is one of the most frequently prescribed supplements for cognitive disorders.

Constituents

The leaf contains amino acids, flavonoids and terpenoids (including bilobalide and ginkgolides A, B, C, J and M).

Action

The pharmacological properties of ginkgo biloba have been reviewed.[1,2] Ginkgo biloba extract has the following properties. It:

- antagonises platelet activating factor (PAF), reducing platelet aggregation and decreasing the production of oxygen free radicals;[3,4]
- increases blood flow, produces arterial vasodilatation and reduces blood viscosity;[5]
- has free radical scavenging properties;[6,7] and
- may influence neurotransmitter metabolism.[8]

These effects are probably due to stimulation of prostaglandin biosynthesis or by direct vasoregulatory effects on catecholamines.[6,9] In addition, ginkgo biloba acts as an antioxidant.[10]

Possible uses

Ginkgo biloba has been studied for the treatment of cerebrovascular disease and peripheral vascular insufficiency.

Memory and cognitive function

The main interest in ginkgo has focused on its use in patients with poor memory and poor cognitive function due to cerebral insufficiency, and it is licensed for this indication in Germany. A review of over 40 European clinical trials evaluated ginkgo's efficacy in the treatment of cerebral and peripheral insufficiency.[2,11] All 40 trials showed positive effects, and the authors concluded that there may have been publication bias. Of the 40 trials, eight were judged to be of good quality. The majority of studies evaluated 12 symptoms: difficulty in concentration; difficulty in memory; absent-mindedness; confusion; lack of energy; tiredness; decreased physical performance; depression; anxiety; dizziness; tinnitus and headaches. Seven of the eight trials showed statistically and clinically significant positive effects of ginkgo compared with placebo. No serious adverse effects were reported.

A meta-analysis of 11 placebo-controlled, randomised, double-blind studies (which included six of the studies) showed that ginkgo was significantly better than placebo for all symptoms associated with cerebrovascular insufficiency of old age. Of the 11 studies, one study was inconclusive, but all the rest showed positive effects.[12]

In a double-blind, placebo-controlled study, 31 patients over the age of 50 years were randomised to receive gingko biloba 40 mg or placebo three times a day. Using a range of psychometric tests, ginkgo was shown to produce a significant improvement in cognitive function at both 12 and 24 weeks.[13] More recent double-blind, placebo-controlled trials have confirmed the benefits of ginkgo on memory[14] and cognitive function.[15]

However, in a 6-week RCT, involving 98 men and 112 women over the age of 60 with no cognitive impairment, gingko biloba 40 mg three times a day did not facilitate performance on standard neuropsychological tests of learning, memory, attention and concentration, or naming and verbal fluency. The ginkgo group also did not differ from the control group in terms of self-reported memory function or global rating by spouses, friends and relatives. The authors concluded that ginkgo provides no measurable benefit in memory or related cognitive function to adults with healthy cognitive function.[16]

Effects of gingko biloba in young adults have been less well characterised. A double-blind, placebo-controlled trial in 19 men and 23 women (mean age 23.6 years) investigated the effect of ginkgo biloba (mean dose 184.5 mg daily) on various alertness, performance, affective state and chemosensory tests after meals over a 13-week period. Ginkgo biloba was found to be ineffective at alleviating the symptoms of post-lunch dip or at enhancing smell and taste function.[17]

A double-blind RCT in 52 students found that an acute dose of ginkgo significantly improved performance in tests of attention and memory. However, there were no effects on working memory, planning, mental flexibility or mood. Moreover, after 6 weeks of treatment, there were no significant effects of ginkgo on mood or any of the cognitive tests, suggesting that tolerance developed to the effects, at least in this young healthy population.[18]

Ginkgo biloba has also been investigated for effects on cognition and mood in post-menopausal women. In one small controlled trial, ginkgo 120 mg daily for 7 days was associated with significantly better non-verbal memory, sustained attention and frontal lobe function than placebo. However, the two groups did not differ in tests of planning, immediate or delayed paragraph recall, delayed recall of pictures, menopausal symptoms, sleepiness, physiological symptoms or aggressive behaviour.[19] In a further trial, post-menopausal women (aged 51–67 years) were randomly allocated to receive ginkgo 120 mg daily for 6 weeks. The only significant effects of ginkgo were limited to the test of mental flexibility, and also to those with poorer performance, who were mainly in the late stages of menopause (mean age 61 years).[20]

Peripheral vascular disease

In the review of 40 trials mentioned above,[11] 15 controlled trials evaluated the role of ginkgo in intermittent claudication, and of these, two were judged to be of reasonable quality. One showed significant increase in walking distance tolerated before pain with ginkgo,[21] and the other showed a greater reduction in pain at rest.[22]

In a multicentre, randomised, double-blind, placebo-controlled study involving 74 patients with peripheral arterial occlusive disease, pain-free walking distance improved in patients given either 120 or 240 mg ginkgo biloba daily, with a greater improvement in the group given the higher dose.[23]

In another multicentre, double-blind, placebo-controlled trial, 111 patients with peripheral occlusive arterial disease were randomised to receive 120 mg ginkgo biloba extract or placebo for 24 weeks. Pain-free walking and maximum walking distance were significantly greater in the ginkgo group and subjective assessment by the patients showed an amelioration of complaints in both groups.[24]

A meta-analysis of eight RCTs with 415 participants concluded that ginkgo biloba extract is superior to placebo in the symptomatic treatment of intermittent claudication. However, the size of the overall treatment effect is modest and of uncertain clinical relevance.[25] A more recent double-blind trial in patients with Reynaud's disease found that ginkgo biloba reduced the number of attacks of digital ischaemia by 56% whereas placebo reduced the number by 27%.[26]

Dementia

In a double-blind, placebo-controlled trial, 216 patients with Alzheimer's disease were randomised to receive either 240 mg ginkgo biloba EGb 761 extract or placebo for 24 weeks. In the 156 patients who completed the study, the frequency of responders in the two groups differed significantly in favour of EGb 761. Analysis of the results on an intention-to-treat basis showed similar results and the authors concluded that EGb 761 was beneficial in dementia of the Alzheimer type and in multi-infarct dementia.[27]

A 52-week, randomised, double-blind, placebo-controlled, parallel-design, multicentre study in 309 patients found that EGb 761 120 mg daily improved measures of cognitive function, daily living, and social performance and psychopathology. The authors concluded that ginkgo was safe and capable of maintaining, or in some cases improving, cognitive and social function in patients with dementia.[28] Of the 309 patients, 244 completed the study up to 26 weeks, but analysis on an intention-to-treat basis still showed significant benefits with ginkgo biloba.[29]

A review of 50 articles, of which four randomised, placebo-controlled, double-blind trials met the inclusion criteria, concluded that there is a small but significant effect of 3–6 months of treatment with 120–240 mg of ginkgo biloba extract on objective measures of cognitive function in Alzheimer's disease.[30]

However, in another study of 214 elderly patients with dementia or memory impairment, who were split into three groups and given one of two different doses of ginkgo biloba extract EGb 761 or a placebo, no differences were detected in memory function after 24 weeks.[31] The authors suggested that these results came about because of the effort made to find a good placebo (ginkgo has a pronounced taste and smell). However, others have questioned the validity of the study, suggesting that a positive effect would have been unlikely in such a heterogeneous population where all types of memory loss were included.[32]

Ginkgo biloba has not been directly compared to conventional medicines for dementia, but improvement seems to be similar to that found with prescription drugs (e.g. donepezil, tacrine and possibly other cholinesterase inhibitors).[33,34]

More recent trials have shown inconsistent results. A 24-week RCT in 214 patients with dementia or age-associated memory impairment did not find a significant effect of ginkgo (special extract EGb 761) treatment. There was no dose–effect relationship and no effect of prolonged ginkgo treatment.[35] However, intention-to-treat analysis of another study concluded that ginkgo (EGb 761) improves cognitive function in a clinically relevant manner in patients suffering from dementia.[36] A review comparing different doses of ginkgo biloba with cholinesterase inhibitors in the treatment of dementia found significant benefits on cognition with cholinesterase inhibitors, but only with ginkgo when all doses were pooled.[37] An RCT in 513 patients with dementia of the Alzheimer's type did not show efficacy of ginkgo. However, there was little cognitive and functional decline in the placebo-treated patients, which may have compromised the sensitivity of the trial to detect a treatment effect. This study was therefore inconclusive with respect to the efficacy of ginkgo biloba.[38] A Cochrane review concluded that overall there is promising evidence of improvement in cognition and function associated with ginkgo. However early trials, which showed beneficial results, used unsatisfactory methodology and more modern trials, with better methodology, show inconsistent results. There is need for a large trial using modern methodology with intention-to-treat analysis to provide robust estimates of the size and mechanism of any treatment effects.[39]

Tinnitus

There are many reports in the literature that ginkgo biloba may be effective in tinnitus. However, recent trials suggest there is little evidence of benefit. An RCT in 66 adults together with six further RCTs were meta-analysed, and ginkgo was found not to benefit patients with tinnitus.[40] A Cochrane review of 12 trials excluded 10 trials on methodological grounds. No trials of tinnitus in cerebral insufficiency reached a satisfactory standard for inclusion in the review and there was no evidence that ginkgo was effective for the primary complaint of tinnitus.[41]

Miscellaneous

Ginkgo biloba has been claimed to be of value in a number of other conditions, including asthma, sexual dysfunction, PMS and mountain sickness. However, there is only very limited evidence that ginkgo biloba has any benefit in these conditions. A review (which included one study) of the role of ginkgo in ARMD concluded that, although a beneficial effect was observed, only 20 people were enrolled in the trial and assessment was not masked, thus making the results equivocal.[42] A Cochrane review of ginkgo biloba for acute ischaemic stroke concluded that the methodological quality of the trials to date had been too poor to support the routine use of ginkgo biloba to promote recovery after stroke.[43] Further research is needed in all these areas.

Conclusion

Several studies have shown that gingko biloba may slow the progression of dementia, particularly in Alzheimer's disease. There is also some evidence that gingko improves memory and concentration in the elderly and increases pain-free walking and maximum walking distance in those with peripheral vascular disease. However, ginkgo should not be taken in any of these conditions without medical advice. There is no sound evidence that ginkgo is effective in other conditions.

Precautions/contraindications

Ginkgo biloba should not be used for the treatment of disease without medical supervision. It is contraindicated in hypertension. Ginkgo has been associated with increased bleeding tendency. However, a recent trial showed no evidence that EGb 761 inhibits blood coagulation, platelet aggregation and haemorrhagic complications.[44] There is anecdotal evidence that ginkgo might be associated with seizure, so until more is known, ginkgo should be avoided in epilepsy or in patients at risk of seizure. There is also preliminary evidence that ginkgo increases insulin clearance,[45] and this should be borne in mind in monitoring blood glucose in diabetes.

Pregnancy and breast-feeding

Contraindicated in pregnancy, breast-feeding and in children.

Adverse effects

There are few reports of serious toxicity. Headache, nausea, vomiting, heartburn and diarrhoea have been reported occasionally. There have been rare reports of severe allergic reactions, including skin reactions (e.g. itching, erythema and blisters) and convulsions.

Interactions

Drugs

Anticoagulants, aspirin, anti-platelet drugs: use ginkgo biloba with caution. However, a recent study showed no effect of ginkgo on the pharmacodynamics and pharmacokinetics of warfarin in healthy patients.[46]

There is preliminary evidence that ginkgo can influence cytochrome P450 and other drug-metabolising enzymes.[47] There are no reports of interactions, but ginkgo should be used with caution in any patients taking other medication.

Dose

Ginkgo biloba is available in the form of tablets, capsules and tincture. A review of 30 US ginkgo biloba products found that nearly one-quarter did have the expected chemical marker compounds for ginkgo biloba extract (e.g. flavone glycosides, terpene lactones).[48]

Most clinical trials have used a 50:1 concentrated leaf extract (EGb 761) standardised to 24% flavone glycosides and 6% terpene glycones. (A standardised 40 mg tablet should therefore contain 9.6 mg flavone glycosides and 2.4 mg terpene glycones.) Studies have used 120–240 mg daily. Dietary supplements provide 40–80 mg in a dose.

References

1 Braquet P. The ginkgolides: potent platelet activating factor antagonists isolated from *Ginkgo biloba* L.: chemistry, pharmacology and clinical applications. *Drugs of the Future* 1987; 12: 643–699.
2 Kleijnen J, Knipschild P Ginkgo biloba for cerebral insufficiency. *Br J Clin Pharmacol* 1992; 34: 352–358.

3 Chung KF, Dent G, McCusker M, *et al*. Effect of a ginkgolide mixture (BN 52063) in antagonising skin and platelet responses to platelet activating factor in man. *Lancet* 1987; 1: 248–251.

4 Braquet P, Hosford D. Ethnopharmacology and the development of natural PAF antagonists as therapeutic agents. *J Ethnopharmacol* 1991; 32: 135–139.

5 Jung F, Morowietz C, Kiesewetter H, Wenzel E. Effect of ginkgo biloba on fluidity of blood and peripheral microcirculation in volunteers. *Arzneimittelforschung* 1990; 40: 589–593.

6 Pincemail J, Dupuis M, Nasr C. Superoxide anion scavenging effect and superoxide dismutase activity of Ginkgo biloba extract. *Experientia* 1989; 45: 708–712.

7 Robak J, Gryglewski RJ. Flavonoids are scavengers of superoxide anions. *Biochem Pharmacol* 1988; 37: 837–841.

8 Defeudis FG. Ginkgo biloba *Extract (EGb 761): Pharmacological Activities and Clinical Applications*. Paris: Editions Scientifiques, Elsevier, 1991: 78–84.

9 Nemecz G, Combest WL. Ginkgo biloba. *US Pharmacist* 1997; 22: 144–151.

10 Kobuchi H. Ginkgo biloba extract. (EGB 761): inhibitory effect of nitric oxide production in the macrophage cell line RAW 264.7. *Biochem Pharmacol* 1997; 53: 897–903.

11 Kleijnen J, Knipschild P. Ginkgo biloba. *Lancet* 1992; 340: 1136–1139.

12 Hopfenmuller W. Evidence for a therapeutic effect of Ginkgo biloba special extract. Meta-analysis of 11 clinical studies in patients with cerebrovascular insufficiency in old age. *Arzneimittelforschung* 1994; 44: 1005–1013.

13 Rai GS, Shovlin C, Wesnes KA. A double-blind, placebo-controlled study of Ginkgo biloba extract ('tanakan') in elderly outpatients with mild to moderate memory impairment. *Curr Med Res Opin* 1991; 12: 350–355.

14 Rigney U, Kimber S, Hindmarch I. The effects of acute doses of standardized Ginkgo biloba extract on memory and psychomotor performance in volunteers. *Phytother Res* 1999; 13: 408–415.

15 Mix JA, Crews WD Jr. An examination of the efficacy of Ginkgo biloba extract Egb761 on the neuropsychologic functioning of cognitively intact older adults. *J Altern Complement Med* 2000; 6: 219–229.

16 Solomon PR, Adams F, Silver A, *et al*. Ginkgo for memory enhancement: a randomized controlled trial. *JAMA* 2002; 288: 835–840.

17 Mattes RD, Pawlick MK. Effects of ginkgo biloba on alertness and chemosensory function in healthy adults. *Hum Psychopharmacol* 2004; 19: 81–90.

18 Elsabagh S, Hartley DE, Ali O, *et al*. Differential cognitive effects of gingko biloba after acute and chronic treatment in healthy young volunteers. *Psychopharmacology* 2005; 179: 437–446.

19 Hartley DE, Heinze L, Elsabagh S, File SE. Effects on cognition and mood in postmenopausal women of 1-week treatment with ginkgo biloba. *Pharmacol Biochem Behav* 2003; 75: 711–720.

20 Elsabagh S, Hartley DE, File SE. Limited cognitive benefits in Stage 2 postmenopausal women after 6 weeks of treatment with ginkgo biloba. *J Psychopharmacol* 2005; 19: 173–181.

21 Bauer U. 6-month double-blind randomised clinical trial of Ginkgo biloba extract versus placebo in two parallel groups in patients suffering from peripheral arterial insufficiency. *Arzneimitteforschung* 1984; 34: 716–720.

22 Saudreau F, Serise JM, Pillet J, *et al*. Efficacité de l'extrait de Ginkgo biloba dans le traitement des artériopathies oblitérantes chroniques des membres inférieurs as stade III de la classification de fontaine. *J Mal Vasc* 1989; 14: 177–182.

23 Peters H, Kieser M, Holscher U. Demonstration of the efficacy of ginkgo biloba special extract EGb 761 on intermittent claudication – a placebo-controlled double-blind multicenter trial. *Vasa* 1998; 27: 106–110.

24 Schweizer J, Hautmann C. Comparison of two dosages of ginkgo biloba extract EGb 761 in patients with peripheral arterial occlusive disease Fontaine's stage Iib: a randomised, double-blind, multicentric clinical trial. *Arzneimittelforschung* 1999; 49: 900–904.

25 Pittler MH, Ernst E. Ginkgo biloba extract for the treatment of intermittent claudication: a meta-analysis of randomized trials. *Am J Med* 2000; 108: 276–281.

26 Muir AH, Robb R, McLaren M, *et al*. The use of ginkgo biloba in Raynaud's disease: a double-blind placebo controlled trial. *Vasc Med* 2002; 7: 265–267.

27 Kanowski S. Proof of efficacy of the ginkgo biloba special extract EGB 761 in outpatients suffering mild to moderate primary degenerative dementia of the Alzheimer type of multi-infarct dementia. *Pharmacopsychiatry* 1996; 29: 47–56.

28 Le Bars PL. A placebo-controlled, double-blind, randomized trial of an extract of Ginkgo biloba for dementia. *JAMA* 1997; 278: 1327–1332.

29 Le Bars PL, Kieser M, Itil KZ. A 26-week analysis of a double-blind placebo-controlled trial of the ginkgo biloba extract Egb 761® in dementia. *Dement Geriatr Cogn Disord* 2000; 11: 230–237.

30 Oken BS, Storzbach DM, Kaye JA. The efficacy of Ginkgo biloba on cognitive function in Alzheimer disease. *Arch Neurol* 1998; 55: 1409–1415.

31 van Dongen MC, van Rossum E, Kessels AG, *et al.* The efficacy of ginkgo for elderly people with dementia and age-associated memory impairment: new results of a randomized clinical trial. *J Am Geriatr Soc* 2000; 48: 1183–1194.

32 Weber W. Ginkgo not effective for memory loss in elderly. *Lancet* 2000; 356: 1389.

33 Itil TM, Eralp E, Ahmed I, *et al.* The pharmacological effects of ginkgo biloba, a plant extract, on the brain of dementia patients in comparison with tacrine. *Psychopharmacol Bull* 1998; 34: 391–397.

34 Wettstein A. Cholinesterase inhibitors and Ginkgo extracts – are they comparable in the treatment of dementia? Comparison of published placebo-controlled efficacy studies of at least six months' duration. *Phytomedicine* 2000; 6: 393–401.

35 van Dongen M, van Rossum E, Kessels A, *et al.* Ginkgo for elderly people with dementia and age-associated memory impairment: a randomized clinical trial. *J Clin Epidemiol* 2003; 56: 367–376.

36 Kanowski S, Hoerr R. Ginkgo biloba extract EGb 761 in dementia: intent-to-treat analyses of a 24-week, multi-center, double-blind, placebo-controlled, randomized trial. *Pharmacopsychiatry* 2003; 36: 297–303.

37 Kurz A, Van Baelen B. Ginkgo biloba compared with cholinesterase inhibitors in the treatment of dementia: a review based on meta-analyses by the Cochrane collaboration. *Dement Geriatr Cogn Disord* 2004; 18: 217–226.

38 Schneider LS, DeKosky ST, Farlow MR, *et al.* A randomized, double-blind, placebo-controlled trial of two doses of ginkgo biloba extract in dementia of the Alzheimer's type. *Curr Alzheimer Res* 2005; 2: 541–551.

39 Birks J, Grimley Evans J. Ginkgo biloba for cognitive impairment and dementia. Cochrane database, issue 4, 2002. London: Macmillan.

40 Rejali D, Sivakumar A, Balaji N. Ginkgo biloba does not benefit patients with tinnitus: a randomized placebo-controlled double-blind trial and meta-analysis of randomized trials. *Clin Otolaryngol Allied Sci* 2004; 29: 226–231.

41 Hilton M, Stuart E. Ginkgo biloba for tinnitus. Cochrane database, issue 2, 2004. London: Macmillan.

42 Evans JR. Ginkgo biloba extract for age-related macular degeneration. Cochrane database, issue 3, 1999.

43 Zeng X, Liu M, Yang Y, *et al.* Ginkgo biloba for acute ischaemic stroke. Cochrane database, issue 4, 2005.

44 Kohler S, Funk P, Kieser M. Influence of a 7-day treatment with ginkgo biloba special extract EGb 761 on bleeding time and coagulation: a randomized, placebo-controlled, double-blind study in healthy volunteers. *Blood Coagul Fibrinolysis* 2004; 15: 303–309.

45 Kudolo GB. The effect of 3-month ingestion of Ginkgo biloba extract on pancreatic beta-cell function in response to glucose loading in normal glucose tolerant individuals. *J Clin Pharmacol* 2000; 40: 647–654.

46 Jiang X, Williams KM, Liauw WS, *et al.* Effect of ginkgo and ginger on the pharmacokinetics and pharmacodynamics of warfarin in healthy subjects. *Br J Clin Pharmacol* 2005; 59: 425–432.

47 Budzinski JW, Foster BC, Vandenhoek S, *et al.* An *in vitro* evaluation of human cytochrome P450 3A4 inhibition by selected commercial herbal extracts and tinctures. *Phytomedicine* 2000; 7: 273–282.

48 Consumerlab. Product review. Ginkgo biloba. http://www.consumerlab.com (accessed 25 November 2006).

Ginseng

Description

Ginseng is the collective term used to describe several species of plants belonging to the genus *Panax*. These include the Asian ginsengs (*Panax ginseng* and *Panax japonicus*), which have been used medicinally for more than 2000 years in China, Japan and Korea. American ginseng (*Panax quinquefolius* L) grows in North America and much of it is exported to the Far East. Siberian/Russian ginseng (*Eleuthrococcus senticosus*) is not considered to be true ginseng because it is not a species of the genus *Panax*. However, as a supplement, it is often promoted alongside Asian and American ginseng products.

Constituents

Panax ginseng contains complex mixtures of saponins known as ginsenosides, which are found in the roots. At least 20 saponins have been isolated from ginseng roots. However, species vary in composition and concentration, and varying concentrations of different saponins appear to exert opposite pharmacological effects.[1,2] This may explain the conflicting results reported in clinical studies, although issues such as type of ginseng, time of harvest, storage and lack of standardisation of active ingredients may also be important. Eleutherosides are believed to be the active ingredients in Siberian ginseng, but these have different chemical structures than the ginsenosides.

Action

Ginseng has a wide range of pharmacological effects, but its clinical significance in humans has not been fully investigated. Differences in composition of the different species lead to differences in activity.

Analgesic activity, anti-pyretic activity, anti-inflammatory activity, CNS-stimulating and CNS-depressant activity, hypotensive and hypertensive activity, histamine-like activity and antihistamine activity, hypoglycaemic activity and erythropoietic activity have all been reported.[2] Opposing activities such as hypertension and hypotension are thought to be a result of different ginsenosides in one preparation.

The most consistent biochemical explanation for the effects of the ginsenosides is a facilitating influence on the hypothalamic-pituitary-adrenal axis.[3,4] Interactions with central cholinergic[5] and dopaminergic mechanisms[6] have also been demonstrated.

Possible uses

Ginseng is an ancient remedy that has been used for thousands of years in the East. A number of extravagant claims have been made for it, including aphrodisiac and anti-ageing properties. It is not claimed to cure any specific disease, but to restore general vitality. Ginseng is claimed to be useful for:

- improving stamina;
- alleviating symptoms of tiredness and exhaustion;
- headaches;
- amnesia and mental function;
- improving libido and sexual vigour and preventing impotence;
- regulating blood pressure;
- preventing diabetes mellitus;

- preventing signs of old age and extending youth;
- improving immunity; and
- reducing the risk of cancer.

Available evidence for some of these claims has come mainly from animal studies, including: increased adaptability to stress;[7] increasing stamina;[8] decreasing learning time;[9] reduction in blood pressure;[10] anti-inflammatory activity;[11] and improved sleep.[12]

Cardiovascular function

Ginseng has been suggested to influence cardiovascular function. One double-blind RCT in healthy adults investigated the potential influence of *Panax* ginseng on electrocardiographic parameters: PR, QRS, QT, QT_c and RR intervals, and QT and QT_c interval dispersion. Effects on blood pressure and heart rate were also evaluated. Thirty subjects were randomly allocated to receive 28 days of therapy with *Panax* ginseng 200 mg or placebo. *Panax* ginseng was found to significantly increase the QTc interval and decrease diastolic blood pressure 2 h after ingestion on the first day of therapy.[13]

North American ginseng has been evaluated for its effect on blood pressure. Sixteen individuals with hypertension were randomised to receive placebo treatment on two mornings or powdered North American ginseng on six mornings. After treatment, blood pressure was measured every 10 min for 160 min, and the mean obtained for the overall 160-min period. None of the North American ginsengs or their means differed from placebo in their overall effect on mean blood pressure change. None affected blood pressure versus placebo at 10-min intervals, but their mean versus placebo increased systolic and diastolic blood pressure at 100 min. The authors concluded that these findings together suggested that North American ginseng exerts a neutral acute effect on blood pressure in hypertensive individuals.[14]

A further study in 24 children undergoing heart surgery found that a ginsenosides compound injected intravenously may attenuate gastrointestinal mucosal injury and inhibit the systemic inflammatory response that occurs after cardiopulmonary bypass in patients with congenital heart disease.[15]

A systematic review of 34 studies investigating the influence of ginseng on blood pressure, lipids and/or blood glucose found mixed results, with current evidence not supporting the use of ginseng to treat cardiovascular risk factors. Some studies suggest a small reduction in blood pressure and some that ginseng improves blood lipid profiles and lowers blood glucose. However, the authors concluded that the overall picture is inconsistent and well-designed RCTs are lacking.[16] A recent 12-week RCT found that American ginseng had no effect on 24-h blood pressure.[17]

Cognitive function

In an uncontrolled study in humans, ginseng has been shown to increase stamina in athletes and concentration in radio operators.[18] In a double-blind, placebo-controlled trial, 60 elderly patients received a supplement containing *Panax* ginseng and vitamins and minerals or placebo daily for 8 weeks. There was no difference in the ability of the supplement or placebo to influence the rehabilitation of these patients, and the effects of the ginseng could not be separated from the other ingredients in the product.[19]

A more recent trial, in 30 healthy young adults given ginseng G115 200 mg, ginseng G115 400 mg or placebo, found notable behavioural effects during sustained mental activity, particularly with 200 mg ginseng. These included significantly improved subtraction task performance and significantly reduced mental fatigue. Both the ginseng treatments led to significant reductions in blood glucose levels and the authors suggested that the effects on mental performance may be related to the acute gluco-regulatory properties of the extract.[20]

Studies have also investigated the cognitive effects of *Panax* ginseng and ginkgo biloba in combination. In a trial involving 20 healthy young adults, receiving 320, 640 and 960 mg of the combination, the most striking result was a dose-dependent improvement in performance on the 'quality of memory' factor at the highest dose of the combination (960 mg).

Further analysis revealed that this effect was differentially targeted at the secondary memory rather than the working memory component. There was also a dose-dependent decrement in performance of the 'speed of attention' factor for both the 320 and 640 mg doses.[21]

A further trial by this same group investigated the influence of ginkgo 360 mg, ginseng 400 mg, 960 mg of a ginseng/ginkgo combination and a matching placebo on both mood and cognition. All three treatments were associated with improved secondary memory performance, with the ginseng treatment showing some improvement in the speed of performing memory tasks and in the accuracy of attentional tasks. Following the combination, there was improvement in some mental arithmetic tasks. No modulation of the speed of performing attention tasks was evident. Improvements in self-rated mood were also found following ginkgo and to a lesser extent the combination product.[22]

Diabetes

A small preliminary study[23] showed that American ginseng reduced blood sugar levels both in people who had diabetes mellitus and in healthy subjects. However, because the study looked only at a single time point, it is unclear what the results mean for real meals or prevention and treatment of diabetes. But the research suggests that ginseng may be useful in preventing sharp increases in blood sugar. A further study in 10 patients with type 2 diabetes showed that American ginseng reduced post-prandial glycaemia, and that no more than 3 g was required to achieve reductions.[24]

A double-blind, placebo-controlled study in 36 patients with type 2 diabetes showed that ginseng therapy (100 and 200 mg) significantly reduced fasting blood glucose and elevated mood, and the 200-mg dose resulted in a statistically significant improvement in glycated haemoglobin.[25]

Further trials have shown variable effects on blood glucose, possibly because of the variety and concentration of ginsenosides in the preparations tested. One trial showed that American ginseng reduced post-prandial glycaemia in subjects without diabetes. This reduction was time-dependent, but not dose-dependent. An effect was seen only when the ginseng was administered 40 min before the challenge. Doses within the range 1–3 g were equally effective.[26] Another trial found that American ginseng 6 g daily did not reduce post-prandial glycaemia. The authors suggested that a possible explanation for this was the reduced total ginsenosides in the product, indicating that the ginsenoside profile of American ginseng might play a role in its hypoglycaemic effects.[27]

A further study with Asian ginseng found both null and opposing effects on indices of acute post-prandial plasma glucose and insulin, with the authors concluding that this could be explained by the marked ginsenoside differences in the product.[28] The same research group went on to look at the effects of eight popular types of ginseng on acute post-prandial glycaemic indices in healthy humans to find again that there was some variability. They concluded that the ginsenoside content might be involved but that other components might also have an effect.[29]

Cancer

Case-control[30] and cohort[31] studies in Korean subjects have shown that incidence of cancer is lower in those who consume ginseng than in those who do not.

Sexual function

A placebo-controlled (not blinded study) included 90 patients with erectile dysfunction.[32] They were randomly assigned to receive *Panax* ginseng (300 mg daily), trazodone or placebo. Patient satisfaction, libido and penile rigidity and girth were greater in the ginseng group than in the other two groups, but changes in the frequency of intercourse, premature ejaculation and morning erections were not found in any group. None of the treatments resulted in complete remission of erectile dysfunction.

Korean ginseng has been investigated for a role in erectile dysfunction. A total of 45 patients with diagnosed erectile dysfunction were enrolled in a double-blind, placebo-controlled, crossover study in which the effects of Korean red ginseng (900 mg three times a day) were compared with placebo. Mean

International Index of Erectile Function scores and scores on penetration and maintenance were significantly higher in patients treated with Korean red ginseng. Penile tip rigidity also showed significant improvement for ginseng versus placebo. The authors concluded that Korean red ginseng can be an effective alternative for treating male erectile dysfunction.[33]

Exercise performance

Several human studies have shown an ergogenic effect in exercise, but a review concluded that such trials have been poorly controlled and not blinded, and that there is no compelling evidence that ginseng improves exercise performance in humans.[34] Double-blind, placebo-controlled trials do not support an ergogenic effect of ginseng on exercise performance,[35–38] or on the response of anabolic hormones (growth hormone, testosterone, cortisol, insulin-like growth factor 1) following resistance status.[39]

A double-blind RCT in 38 active healthy adults investigated the effect of 400 mg daily of G115 (equivalent to 2 g of *Panax* ginseng) on secretory IgA, performance and recovery after interval exercise. There was no significant change in secretory IgA (an indicator of mucosal immunity). Supplementation with ginseng failed to improve physical performance and heart rate recovery of individuals undergoing repeated bouts of exhausting exercise.[40]

A trial with *Panax* notoginseng found that a dose of 1350 mg daily for 30 days improved endurance time to exhaustion by 7 min and lowered mean blood pressure (from 113 ± 12 to 109 ± 14 mmHg) and VO2 at the 24th minute (from 32.5 ± 8 to 27.6 ± 8) during endurance cycle exercise.[41] A trial in 13 physically active male students found that supplementation with American ginseng for 4 weeks prior to exhaustive aerobic treadmill running did not enhance aerobic work capacity but significantly reduced plasma creatine kinase during the exercise. The authors concluded that the reduction in plasma creatine kinase may be due to the fact that American ginseng is effective in decreasing skeletal muscle cell membrane damage, induced by exercise during the high-intensity treadmill run.[42]

Upper respiratory tract infections

Two recent trials have investigated the potential benefit of ginseng in preventing upper respiratory tract infection. In one trial, American ginseng over 8 or 12 weeks was found to be safe, well tolerated and potentially effective in preventing acute respiratory illness caused by influenza and respiratory syncytial virus (RSC).[43] A further trial with American ginseng in 323 subjects aged 18–65 years found that supplementation for 4 months reduced the mean number of colds per person, the proportion of subjects who experienced two or more colds, the severity of symptoms and the number of days on which cold symptoms were reported.[44]

Quality of life

Both *Panax* ginseng and Siberian ginseng have been found to improve aspects of mental health and social functioning after 4 weeks of therapy, although these benefits attenuate with continued use.[45,46] In another study, *Panax* ginseng had no influence on mood or affect.[47] Siberian ginseng has been shown to have potential efficacy for patients with moderate fatigue.[48]

Conclusion

Ginseng has been used for thousands of years, but there are few controlled trials in humans. Many studies have produced conflicting results, perhaps due to lack of standardised products, variation in dosage, differences in harvest conditions of the plants and types of ginseng used. A 1999 systematic review[49] concluded that evidence for the efficacy of ginseng for any indication is weak. The review investigated the effect of ginseng on athletic performance, psychomotor and cognitive performance, immunomodulation, diabetes mellitus and herpes. Ginseng is taken for a range of other indications but there is little evidence that ginseng slows the ageing process, helps mental or physical functioning in the elderly, increases exercise performance or improves sexual function.

Precautions/contraindications

Ginseng should be avoided by children and used with caution by patients with CVD (including hypertension), diabetes mellitus, asthma, schizophrenia and other disorders of the nervous system. Because of a possible effect on blood glucose, the effect of ginseng on glucose measurement in diabetes should be borne in mind.

Pregnancy and breast-feeding

Ginseng should be avoided.

Adverse effects

Ginseng is relatively non-toxic, but in high doses (>3 g ginseng root daily) can give rise to the following symptoms: insomnia, nervous excitation, euphoria; nausea and diarrhoea (especially in the morning); skin eruptions; oedema; oestrogenic effects (e.g. breast tenderness; temporary return of menstruation in post-menopausal women).[50,51]

A systematic review of the adverse effects and drug interactions of *Panax* ginseng concluded that the incidence of adverse effects with ginseng monopreparations is similar to that with placebo. The most commonly experienced adverse events are headache, sleep and gastro-intestinal disorders. The possibility of more serious adverse events is indicated in isolated case reports and data from reporting schemes. However, causality is often difficult to determine from the evidence provided. Combination products containing ginseng as one of several constituents have been associated with serious adverse events and even fatalities. Possible interactions include ginseng and warfarin and ginseng and phenelzine.[52]

Interactions

Drugs

Tranquillisers: ginseng may reverse the effects of sedatives and tranquillisers.
Digoxin: ginseng may increase blood levels of digoxin.[53]
Warfarin: ginseng may influence the effect of warfarin.[54–57]

Dose

Ginseng is available in the form of tablets, capsules, teas, powders and tinctures. Red ginseng is derived from steam-treated ginseng roots and white ginseng from air-dried roots. Surveys have found that the ginsenoside concentrations in different products vary enormously.[1,58] A review of 21 US products found that seven had less than the required concentration of ginsenosides, two products contained lead above acceptable levels and eight contained unacceptable levels of quintozene and hexachlorobenzene.[59]

The dose is not established. Manufacturers tend to recommend 0.5–3 g daily of the dried root or its equivalent.

References

1   Cui J, Garle M, Eneroth P, Bjorkhem L. What do commercial ginseng preparations contain? *Lancet* 1994; 344: 134.

2   Hikino H. Traditional remedies and modern assessment: the case for ginseng. In: Wijesekera ROB, ed. *The Medicinal Plant Industry*. Boca Raton, FL: CRC Press, 1991: 149–166

3   Filaretov AA, Bogdanova TS, Podvigina TT, Bogdanov AL. Role of pituitary-adrenocortical system in body adaption possibilities. *Exp Clin Endocrinol* 1988; 92: 129–136.

4   Fulder S. Ginseng and the hypothalamic control of stress. *Am J Chinese Med* 1981; 9: 112–118.

5   Benishin CG, Lee R, Wang LCH, Liu HJ. Effects of ginsenoside Rb-1 on central cholinergic metabolism. *Pharmacology* 1991; 42: 223–229.

6   Watanebe H, Ohta-Himamura L, Asakura W, *et al.* Effect of *Panax* ginseng on age-related changes in the spontaneous motor activity and dopaminergic system in rat. *Jpn J Pharmacol* 1991; 55: 51–56.

7   Bittles AH, Fulder SJ, Grant EC, Nicholls W. The effect of ginseng on lifespan and stress response in mice. *Gerontology* 1979; 25: 125–131.

8   Brekhman II, Dardymov IV. New substances of plant origin which increase non-specific stress. *Ann Rev Pharmacol* 1969; 9: 419–430.

9   Saito H, Tschuiya M, Naka S, Takugi K. Effects of *Panax* ginseng root on conditioned avoidance response in rats. *Jpn J Pharmacol* 1977; 27: 509–516.

10 Lee DC, Lee MO, Kim CY, Clifford DH. Effect of ether, ethanol, and aqueous extracts of ginseng on cardiovascular function in dogs. *Can J Comp Med* 1981; 45: 182–185.

11 Yuan WX, Gui LH, Zhou JY, *et al*. Some pharmaco-logical effects of ginseng saponins. *Zhongguo Yaoli Zuebo* 1983; 4: 124–128.

12 Lee SP, Honda K, Ho-Rhee Y, Inoue S. Chronic intake of *Panax* ginseng extract stabilises sleep and wakefulness in sleep-deprived rats. *Neurosci Lett* 1990; 111: 217–221.

13 Caron MF, Hotsko AL, Robertson S, *et al*. Electro-cardiographic and hemodynamic effects of *Panax* ginseng. *Ann Pharmacother* 2002; 36: 758–763.

14 Stavro PM, Woo M, Heim TF, *et al*. North American ginseng exerts a neutral effect on blood pressure in individuals with hypertension. *Hypertension* 2005; 46: 406–411.

15 Xia ZY, Liu XY, Zhan LY, *et al*. Ginsenosides com-pound (shen-fu) attenuates gastrointestinal injury and inflammatory response after cardiopulmonary bypass in patients with congenital heart disease. *J Thorac Cardiovasc Surg* 2005; 130: 258–264.

16 Buettner C, Yeh GY, Phillips RS, *et al*. Systematic review of the effects of ginseng on cardiovascular risk factors. *Ann Pharmacother* 2006; 40: 83–95.

17 Stavro PM, Woo M, Leiter L, *et al*. Long-term intake of North American ginseng has no effect on 24-hour blood pressure and renal function. *Hypertension* 2006; 47; 791.

18 Medvedev MA. The effect of ginseng on the working performance of radio operators. In: *Papers on the study of ginseng and other medicinal plants of the Far East, Vol 5*. Vladivostok: Primorskoe Knizhnoe Izdatelsvo, 1963.

19 Thommessen B, Laake K. No identifiable effect of ginseng (Gericomplex) as an adjuvant in the treatment of geriatric patients. *Aging (Milano)* 1996; 8: 417–420.

20 Reay JL, Kennedy DO, Scholey AB. Single doses of *Panax* ginseng (G115) reduce blood glucose levels and improve cognitive performance during sus-tained mental activity. *J Psychopharmacol* 2005; 19: 357–365.

21 Kennedy DO, Scholey AB, Wesnes KA. Differen-tial, dose dependent changes in cognitive perfor-mance following acute administration of a ginkgo biloba/panax ginseng combination to healthy young volunteers. *Nutr Neurosci* 2001; 4: 399–412.

22 Kennedy DO, Scholey AB, Wesnes KA. Modulation of cognition and mood following administration of single doses of ginkgo biloba, ginseng, and a ginkgo/ginseng combination to healthy young adults. *Physiol Behav* 2002; 75: 739–751.

23 Vuksan V, Sievenpiper JL, Koo VVY, *et al*. American ginseng (*Panax quinquefolius* L) reduces postpran-dial glycemia in nondiabetic subjects and subjects with type 2 diabetes mellitus. *Arch Intern Med* 2000; 160: 1009–1013.

24 Vuksan V, Stavro MP, Sievenpiper JL, *et al*. Similar postprandial glycemic reductions with escalation

of dose and administration time of American gin-seng in type 2 diabetes. *Diabetes Care* 2000; 23: 1221–1226.

25 Sotaniemi EA, Haapakoski E, Rautio A. Ginseng therapy in non-insulin-dependent diabetic patients. *Diabetes Care* 1995; 18: 1373–1375.

26 Vuksan V, Sievenpiper JL, Wong J, *et al*. Amer-ican ginseng (*Panax quinquefolius* L) attenuates postprandial glycemia in a time-dependent but not dose-dependent manner in healthy individuals. *Am J Clin Nutr* 2001; 73: 753–758.

27 Sievenpiper JL, Arnason JT, Leiter LA, Vuksan V. Variable effects of American ginseng: a batch of American ginseng (*Panax quinquefolius* L.) with a depressed ginsenoside profile does not affect postprandial glycemia. *Eur J Clin Nutr* 2003; 57: 243–248.

28 Sievenpiper JL, Arnason JT, Leiter LA, Vuksan V. Null and opposing effects of Asian ginseng (*Panax ginseng* C.A. Meyer) on acute glycaemia: results of two acute dose escalation studies. *J Am Coll Nutr* 2003; 22: 524–532.

29 Sievenpiper JL, Arnason JT, Leiter LA, Vuksan V. Decreasing, null and increasing effects of eight popular types of ginseng on acute postprandial glycemic indices in healthy humans: the role of ginsenosides. *J Am Coll Nutr* 2004; 23: 248–258.

30 Yun TK, Choi SY. Preventive effect of ginseng intake against various human cancers: a case-control study on 1,987 matched pairs. *Cancer Epidemiol Biomarkers Prev* 1995; 4: 401–408.

31 Yun TK. Experimental and epidemiological evidence of the cancer preventive effects of *Panax* ginseng CA Meyer. *Nutr Rev* 1996; 54 (11 pt 2): S71–S81.

32 Choi HK, Seong DH, Rha KH. Clinical efficacy of Korean red ginseng for erectile dysfunction. *Int J Impot Res* 1995; 7: 181–186.

33 Hong B, Ji YH, Hong JH, *et al*. A double-blind crossover study evaluating the efficacy of Korean red ginseng in patients with erectile dys-function: a preliminary report. *J Urol* 2002; 168: 2070–2073.

34 Bahrke MS, Morgan WP. Evaluation of ergogenic properties of ginseng. *Sports Med* 1994; 18: 229–248.

35 Allen JD, McLung J, Nelson AG, *et al*. Ginseng supplementation does not enhance healthy adults' peak aerobic exercise performance. *J Am Coll Nutr* 1998; 17: 462–466.

36 Engels HJ, Wirth JC. No ergogenic effects of ginseng (*Panax ginseng* CA Meyer) during graded maximal aerobic exercise. *J Am Dietet Assoc* 1997; 97: 1110–1115.

37 Morris AC, Jacobs I, McLellan TM, *et al*. No ergogenic effect of ginseng ingestion. *Int J Sport Nutr* 1996; 6: 263–271.

38 Engels HJ, Kolokouri I, Cieslak TJ 2nd, Wirth JC. Effects of ginseng supplementation on supramaximal exercise performance and short-term recovery. *J Strength Cond Res* 2001; 15: 290–295.

39 Youl Kang H, Hwan Kim S, Jun Lee W, Byrne HK. Effects of ginseng ingestion on growth hormone, testosterone, cortisol, and insulin-like growth factor 1 responses to acute resistance exercise. *J Strength Cond Res* 2002; 16: 179–183.

40 Engels HJ, Fahlman MM, Wirth JC. Effects of ginseng on secretory IgA, performance and recovery from interval exercise. *Med Sci Sports Exerc* 2003; 35: 690–696.

41 Liang MT, Podolka TD, Chuang WJ. *Panax* notoginseng supplementation enhances physical performance during endurance exercise. *J Strength Cond Res* 2005; 19: 108–114.

42 Hsu CC, Ho MC, Lin LC, *et al.* American ginseng supplementation attenuates creatine kinase level induced by submaximal exercise in human beings. *World J Gastroenterol* 2005; 14: 5327–5331.

43 McElhaney JE, Gravenstein S, Cole SK, *et al.* A placebo-controlled trial of a proprietary extract of North American ginseng (CVT-E002) to prevent acute respiratory illness in institutionalized older adults. *J Am Geriatr Soc* 2004; 52: 13–19.

44 Predy GN, Goel V, Lovlin R, *et al.* Efficacy of an extract of North American ginseng containing poly-furanosyl-pyranolsyl-saccharides for preventing upper respiratory tract infections: a randomized controlled trial. *CMAJ* 2005; 173: 1043–1048.

45 Ellis JM, Reddy P. Effects of *Panax* ginseng on quality of life. *Ann Pharmacother* 2002; 36: 375–379.

46 Cicero AF, Derosa G, Brilliante R, *et al.* Effects of Siberian ginseng (*Eleutherococcus senticosus maxim.*) on elderly quality of life: a randomized clinical trial. *Arch Geriatr Suppl* 2004: 9: 69–73.

47 Cardinal BJ, Engels HJ. Ginseng does not enhance psychological well-being in healthy, young adults: results of a double-blind, placebo-controlled, randomized clinical trial. *J Am Diet Assoc* 2001; 101: 655–660.

48 Hartz AJ, Bentler S, Noyes R, *et al.* Randomized controlled trial of Siberian ginseng for chronic fatigue. *Psychol Med* 2004; 34: 51–61.

49 Volger BK, Pittler MH, Ernst E. The efficacy of ginseng. A systematic review of randomised clinical trials. *Eur J Clin Pharmacol* 1999; 55: 567–575.

50 Siegel RK. Ginseng abuse syndrome: problems with the panacea. *JAMA* 1979; 241: 1614–1615.

51 Greenspan EM. Ginseng and vaginal bleeding. *JAMA* 1983; 249: 2018.

52 Coon JT, Ernst E. Panax ginseng: a systematic review of adverse effects and drug interactions. *Drug Saf* 2002; 25: 323–344.

53 McRae S. Elevated serum digoxin levels in a patient taking digoxin and Siberian ginseng. *CMAJ* 1996; 155: 293–295.

54 Janetzky K. Probable interaction between warfarin and ginseng. *Am J Health Syst Pharm* 1997; 54: 692–693.

55 Cheng TO. Ginseng–warfarin interaction. *ACC Curr J Rev* 2000; 9: 84.

56 Palop-Larrea V, Gonzalvez-Perales JL, Catalan-Oliver C, *et al.* Metrorrhagia and ginseng. *Ann Pharmacother* 2000; 34: 1347–1348.

57 Yuan CS, Wei G, Dey L, *et al.* Brief communication: American ginseng reduces warfarin's effect in healthy patients: a randomized controlled trial. *Ann Intern Med* 2004; 141: 23–27.

58 American Botanical Council. Ginseng Evaluation Program. http://www.herbalgram.org/default.asp?c=ginseng_eval (accessed 26 January 2006).

59 Consumerlab. Product review. Asian and American ginseng. http://www.consumerlab.com (accessed 26 November 2006).

Glucosamine

Description

Glucosamine is a natural substance found in mucopolysaccharides, mucoproteins and chitin. It is found in relatively high concentrations in the joints. Some foods, such as crabs, oysters and the shells of prawns, are relatively rich in glucosamine, but supplements are the best source of additional glucosamine. It is available as a synthetically manufactured dietary supplement in the form of glucosamine sulphate and glucosamine hydrochloride.

Constituents

Glucosamine is a hexosamine sugar and a basic building block for the biosynthesis of glycoprotein, glycolipids, hyaluronic acid, glycosaminoglycans and proteoglycans, which are important constituents of articular cartilage. Chondroitin sulphate (sometimes found together with glucosamine in supplements), which is synthesised by the chondrocytes, is one example of a glycosaminoglycan.

Action

Glucosamine is important for maintaining the elasticity, strength and resilience of cartilage in joints. This helps to reduce damage to the joints. In addition to supporting cartilage and other connective tissue, glucosamine enhances both the production of hyaluronic acid and its anti-inflammatory action.

The mechanism of action is not fully understood, but administration of glucosamine is believed to stimulate production of cartilage components and allow rebuilding of damaged cartilage. *In vitro* studies have found that glucosamine can increase mucopolysaccharide and collagen synthesis in fibroblast tissue.[1] Glucosamine also appears to activate core protein synthesis in human chondrocytes.[2]

Possible uses

Glucosamine is used to promote the maintenance of joint function and to treat pain, increase mobility, and help repair damaged joints in individuals with osteoarthritis and other joint disorders. It is sometimes provided in supplements with chondroitin, with which it may act synergistically. Both substances have anti-inflammatory activities,[3,4] and both affect cartilage metabolism *in vitro*.[5,6] Animal studies have also demonstrated that glucosamine has anti-arthritic effects.[7,8]

Since 1990, more than 50 studies have examined the effects of glucosamine on osteoarthritis. However, many of these studies have been short, and many have major design flaws and critical problems with data analysis and interpretation of results. Some of the largest RCTs are discussed below.

In a double-blind trial involving 80 inpatients with established arthritis randomly split into two groups, the first group received two 250-mg capsules of glucosamine sulphate and the second group an indistinguishable placebo.[9] Each dose was given three times daily for 30 days. Articular pain, joint tenderness and restriction of movement were scored on a scale of 1 to 4 at 1-week intervals. Any adverse reactions were similarly scored. Safety was monitored by haematology; results of urine analysis and occult faecal blood were recorded before and after treatment. Samples of articular cartilage from two patients of each group and from one healthy subject were submitted for scanning electron microscopy after the end of treatment. Patients treated with glucosamine sulphate experienced a reduction in overall symptoms that was almost twice as great and twice as fast as those who had placebo. The results were supported by the electron microscopy findings.

Another double-blind trial used 252 outpatients who had suffered arthritis in the knee to a measurable amount for at least 6 months.[10] The trial randomly allocated the patients to two groups, one receiving 250-mg tablets of glucosamine sulphate and the other placebo, three times daily. The trial was for 4 weeks, with assessment at enrolment and weekly thereafter. A statistically significant difference between glucosamine and placebo was observed, but only after the fourth week of treatment, and the clinical significance of the difference is open to debate.

A total of 155 outpatients with osteoarthritis of the knee were involved in another double-blind trial.[11] Inclusion criteria included a requirement to have been suffering from symptoms for at least 6 months. The two groups, consisting of 79 and 76 patients, received 400 mg glucosamine sulphate and placebo respectively, administered as intramuscular injection twice weekly for 6 weeks. Assessment was carried out at enrolment, at 2-weekly intervals during the trial and once after the trial had been concluded. At the end of the trial the patients were assessed by the investigator and classified as good, moderate, unchanged, or worse. Safety was monitored by a number of biochemical tests. A significant improvement in symptoms was noted compared with placebo, but this occurred only during weeks 5 and 6 of the treatment. This may have been related to the twice-weekly dosing, or to the slow onset of action. However, methodological problems of lack of randomisation and missing data, such as symptom severity at baseline, make the clinical significance of the improvement questionable, and the observed differences may be meaningless.

In a further double-blind trial in patients with osteoarthritis of the knee, 80 subjects were randomised to receive either glucosamine sulphate 1500 mg daily for 6 months or placebo. Patients'

global assessment of pain in the affected knee did not differ between placebo and glucosamine. There was a statistically significant difference between the two groups in knee flexion, but the difference was small and could have been due to measurement error. Overall, as a symptom modifier in osteoarthritis patients with a wide range of severities, glucosamine sulphate was no more effective than placebo.[12]

A Czech trial involving 202 patients investigated the effect of glucosamine sulphate 1500 mg daily or placebo on progression of osteoarthritis of the knee. With placebo there was progressive narrowing of the joint space after 3 years, but no average change with glucosamine sulphate use, with a significant difference between groups. Symptoms improved modestly with placebo use but as much as 20–25% with glucosamine sulphate use. Safety was good, with no difference between groups. In this study, long-term treatment with glucosamine sulphate slowed the progression of knee osteoarthritis, possibly by influencing disease modification.[13]

A further study involving 212 patients over a period of 3 years investigated the effect of glucosamine sulphate on future progression of osteoarthritis. Patients with less severe radiographic knee osteoarthritis were found to experience, over 3 years, the most dramatic disease progression in terms of joint space narrowing. In these patients with mild osteoarthritis, glucosamine sulphate was associated with a trend ($P = 0.01$) towards a significant reduction in joint space narrowing, while in those with severe disease, joint space narrowing did not differ between glucosamine and placebo.[14]

In a trial involving 319 post-menopausal women, those taking glucosamine sulphate showed no joint space narrowing while participants in the placebo group experienced a narrowing of 0.33 mm, with a statistically significant difference between the two groups after 3 years.[15]

A more recent trial investigated the effect of continued use of glucosamine or placebo in 137 users of glucosamine with knee osteoarthritis who had experienced at least moderate improvement in knee pain after starting glucosamine. After 6 months, no differences were found between glucosamine and placebo patients in severity and time to disease flare, use of paracetamol and use of NSAIDs.[16]

Another trial recruited 205 patients with symptomatic knee arthritis from the Internet. Participants were randomly assigned to glucosamine 1500 mg daily or placebo. After 12 weeks, there was no difference between treatment and control groups in terms of change in pain score, stiffness, physical function or analgesic use.[17]

A trial in 142 patients suffering from knee osteoarthritis compared the efficacy and safety of glucosamine sulphate (1500 mg daily) with that of glucosamine hydrochloride (1440 mg daily). Symptoms improved in both groups, but there were no significant differences in efficacy and safety between the two groups. Glucosamine hydrochloride was as effective and safe as glucosamine sulphate in the treatment of knee osteoarthritis.[18]

Other trials have compared the efficacy of glucosamine with ibuprofen[19,20] and piroxicam.[21] Oral glucosamine sulphate 500 mg three times a day was reported to be at least as effective as oral ibuprofen 400 mg three times a day in a study involving 40 patients with osteoarthritis of the knee.[19] Pain scores decreased significantly in both groups, but the onset of action was more rapid with ibuprofen, with maximum effectiveness reached after 2 weeks, whereas glucosamine was associated with a gradual, progressive improvement throughout the trial.

In a randomised, double-blind, parallel-group study,[20] glucosamine 500 mg three times daily was as effective as ibuprofen 400 mg three times daily for 4 weeks in the treatment of 200 inpatients with osteoarthritis of the knee. Again, therapeutic effect was generally obtained sooner with ibuprofen, but glucosamine was significantly better tolerated than ibuprofen. A total of six patients reported adverse effects (versus 35 with ibuprofen) and one discontinued treatment (versus seven with ibuprofen). However, the definition of treatment response, as well as short duration of the study, leave the results open to debate as to their clinical significance.

Glucosamine sulphate was as effective as piroxicam alone or a combination of glucosamine and piroxicam in a randomised multicentre, double-blind, placebo-controlled trial involving 329 patients.[21] Glucosamine sulphate 1500 mg daily, piroxicam 20 mg daily, a combination of glucosamine and piroxicam, or placebo was given for 60 days, followed by a 60-day observation period without treatment. Glucosamine appeared to have a persistent treatment effect after withdrawal compared to piroxicam, and significantly fewer adverse effects were recorded for glucosamine.

Several meta-analyses and systematic reviews have investigated the benefits of glucosamine in the treatment of osteoarthritis. One evaluated the benefit of both glucosamine and chondroitin for osteoarthritis symptoms.[22] It used a meta-analysis combined with systematic quality assessment of clinical trials of these preparations in knee and/or hip osteoarthritis. Reviewers performed data extraction and scored each trial using a quality assessment instrument. Of the 37 trials identified, only 15 met their criteria of being double-blind (published or unpublished), randomised, placebo-controlled or of 4 or more weeks' duration that tested glucosamine or chondroitin for knee or hip osteoarthritis and reported extractable data on the effect of treatment on symptoms. Of the 15 trials analysed, only six concerned glucosamine; the remaining nine, almost all of which were manufacturer-sponsored, were judged to be of inadequate quality by the authors. Nevertheless, they concluded that trials of glucosamine and chondroitin preparations for osteoarthritis symptoms did show moderate to large beneficial effects, but acknowledged that quality issues and likely publication bias might have exaggerated these benefits.

A further meta-analysis[23] included 10 trials (three of which were also included in the above meta-analysis[22]). The trials included looked at glucosamine alone – not chondroitin. The method employed was a scoring system,[24] and only five of the 10 trials achieved the arbitrary pass mark. The major problems in most of the trials in this meta-analysis were a lack of participants, a lack of detail about the randomisation process, and no monitoring of patients after the trial period had finished. Of the 10 clinical trials, six compared glucosamine sulphate to placebo.

Of the remaining four trials, two compared glucosamine to ibuprofen and the other two used glucosamine sulphate alone. The results of this meta-analysis were in broad agreement with those of the above study[22] and were positive. However, the authors concluded that the variations in study methodology made it difficult to reach a firm decision as to the overall effectiveness of glucosamine for the treatment of osteoarthritis.

A mini-review compared the effectiveness of oral glucosamine with ibuprofen for relief of joint pain in arthritis. From the two RCTs included in the review, there were no significant differences between the two treatments with respect to pain reduction. Both were efficacious treatments and glucosamine appeared to be at least as effective as ibuprofen.[25]

A further meta-analysis assessed the structural and symptomatic efficacy of glucosamine sulphate and chondroitin sulphate in knee osteoarthritis through their effects on joint space narrowing, Lequesne Index, Western Ontario McMaster University Osteoarthritis Index (WOMAC), visual analogue scale for pain, mobility, safety and response to treatment. Suitable clinical trials performed between January 1980 and March 2002 were included. There was a highly significant effect of glucosamine on all outcomes, including joint space narrowing and WOMAC. Chondroitin was found to be effective on Lequesne Index, visual analogue scale pain, mobility and responding status. Joint mobility also improved markedly, with one person responding for every five patients treated (number needed to treat = 4.9). Safety was good for both compounds.[26]

Another meta-analysis investigated the structural and symptomatic efficacy and safety of glucosamine in knee osteoarthritis. Suitable trials up to August 2004 were included. Studies were included if they were double-blind RCTs, lasting at least 1 year, that evaluated oral glucosamine and reported symptom severity and disease progression as assessed by joint space narrowing. Glucosamine sulphate was more effective than placebo in delaying structural progression in knee osteoarthritis, reducing pain and improving physical function. Glucosamine sulphate caused no more adverse events than placebo. The authors concluded that due to the sparse data on structural efficacy and safety, more studies are warranted.[27]

A Cochrane review of 20 RCTs evaluating the effectiveness and toxicity of glucosamine in osteoarthritis found glucosamine more favourable than placebo, with a 28% improvement in pain and 21% improvement in function, using the Lequesne Index. However, the trials did not show uniformly positive results. In the 10 RCTs in which the Rotta (name of manufacturer) preparation of glucosamine was compared to placebo, glucosamine was found to be superior for pain and function. In those trials where a non-Rotta preparation of glucosamine was compared to placebo, statistical significance was not reached. In the four RCTs where the Rotta preparation of glucosamine was compared to a NSAID, glucosamine was superior in two and equivalent in two. Two RCTs using the Rotta preparation showed that glucosamine was able to slow radiological progression of osteoarthritis of the knee over a 3-year period. Glucosamine and placebo were of equivalent safety in terms of the number of subjects reporting adverse reactions.[28]

The multicentre, double-blind, placebo- and celecoxib-controlled Glucosamine/chondroitin Arthritis Intervention Trial (GAIT) evaluated the efficacy and safety of glucosamine and chondroitin as a treatment for knee pain from osteoarthritis. A total of 1583 patients with symptomatic knee osteoarthritis were randomised to receive 1500 mg glucosamine daily, 1200 mg chondroitin sulphate daily, both glucosamine and chondroitin sulphate, 200 mg of celecoxib daily or placebo for 24 weeks. Overall, glucosamine and chondroitin sulphate were not significantly better than placebo in reducing knee pain by 20%. The rate of response to glucosamine was 3.9% higher than placebo, the rate of response to chondroitin was 5.3% higher, the rate of response to combined treatment was 6.5% higher and the rate of response to celecoxib was 10% higher. However, for the subgroup of patients with moderate to severe knee pain at baseline, the rate of response was significantly higher with combined therapy than with placebo (79.2% vs 54.3%, $P = 0.002$).

This suggests that glucosamine and chondroitin in combination may be effective in the group of patients with moderate to severe knee pain, but not in patients overall with osteoarthritis of the knee.[29]

A blinded RCT compared a topical cream containing glucosamine, chondroitin sulphate and camphor with placebo. The study included 63 patients with osteoarthritis of the knee. Intention-to-treat analysis showed that after 4–8 weeks, reduction in pain was greater in the treatment group than the placebo group.[30]

Conclusion

Glucosamine and also chondroitin are likely to be effective therapies for the symptoms of osteoarthritis, but the degree of benefit apparent in the literature is probably overestimated because of methodological flaws in the studies. Further long-term, adequately designed, rigorous controlled studies are required before the role of glucosamine in the treatment of bone and joint disorders can be fully determined. In addition, further trials are needed to determine whether glucosamine can significantly modify the radiological progression of osteoarthritis.

Precautions/contraindications

Glucosamine may alter glucose regulation/insulin sensitivity.[31,32] However, more recent research reports no significant effects on haemoglobin A1c levels in patients with type 2 diabetes after 90 days' therapy,[33] nor on serum insulin, plasma glucose and glycated haemoglobin after 12 weeks.[34] However, until further studies are conducted, it would appear prudent for patients with diabetes taking glucosamine to be aware of its potential influence on glucose metabolism.

Pregnancy and breast-feeding

No problems have been reported, but there have not been sufficient studies to guarantee the safety of glucosamine in pregnancy and breast-feeding. Glucosamine is probably best avoided.

Adverse effects

Glucosamine is relatively non-toxic, and does not appear to be associated with serious side-effects. Side-effects reported include constipation, diarrhoea, heartburn, nausea, drowsiness, headache and rash.

Interactions

Drugs

None are known, but in theory insulin or oral hypoglycaemics may be less effective.

Dose

Glucosamine is available in the form of tablets, capsules and powders as glucosamine sulphate, glucosamine hydrochloride and N-acetyl-D-glucosamine (NAG). It is also available in the form of cream. A review of 10 products containing glucosamine found that all products contained the labelled amounts of glucosamine, but six out of 13 products containing glucosamine and chondroitin did not pass, all due to low chondroitin levels.[35]

The dose is not definitely established. However, a dose of glucosamine sulphate 500 mg three times a day (1500 mg daily) has been used in most studies and this is the dose recommended by many manufacturers. Full therapeutic benefit may take more than 4 weeks.

References

1 McCarty MF. The neglect of glucosamine as treatment for osteoathritis. *Med Hypotheses* 1994; 42: 323–327.

2 Bassleer C, Henroitin Y, Franchimont P. *In vitro* evaluation of drugs proposed as chondroprotective agents. *Int J Tissue React* 1992; 14: 231–241.

3 Sentnikar I, Cereda R, Pacini MA, Revel L. Antireactive properties of glucosamine sulphate. *Arznemittelforschung* 1991; 41: 157–161.

4 Ronca F, Palmieri L, Panicucci P, Ronca G. Anti-inflammatory activity of chondroitin sulphate. *Osteoarthritis Cartilage* 1998; 6 (Suppl. A): 14–21.

5 Bassleer CT, Combal JP, Bougaret S, Malaise M. Effects of chondroitin sulphate and interleukin-1 beta on human articular chondrocytes cultivated

in clusters. *Osteoarthritis Cartilage* 1998; 6: 196–204.

6 Bassleer CT, Rovati L, Franchimont P. Stimulation of proteoglycan production by glucosamine sulphate in chondrocytes isolated from human osteoarthritic articular cartilage *in vitro*. *Osteoarthritis Cartilage* 1998; 6: 196–204.

7 Setnikar I, Pacini MA, Revel L. Antiarthritic effects of glucosamine sulfate studied in animal models. *Arzneimittelforschung* 1991; 41: 542–545.

8 Uebelhart D, Thonar EJ, Zhang J, Williams JM. Protective effect of exogenous chondroitin 4,6-sulfate in the acute degradation of articular cartilage in the rabbit. *Osteoarthritis Cartilage* 1998; 6 (Suppl. A) 6–13.

9 Drovanti A, Bignamini AA, Rovati AL. Therapeutic activity of oral glucosamine sulphate in osteoarthritis: a placebo controlled double blind investigation. *Clin Ther* 1980; 3: 260–272.

10 Noack W, Fischer M, Forster K, *et al*. Glucosamine in osteoarthritis of the knee. *Osteoarthritis Cartilage* 1994; 2: 51–59.

11 Reichelt A, Forster KK, Fischer M, *et al*. Efficacy and safety of intramuscular glucosamine sulphate in osteoarthritis of the knee. *Arzneimittelforschung* 1994; 44: 75–80.

12 Hughes R, Carr A. A randomized, double-blind, placebo-controlled trial of glucosamine sulphate as an analgesic in osteoarthritis of the knee. *Rheumatology (Oxford)* 2002; 41: 279–284.

13 Pavelka K, Gatterova J, Olejarova M, *et al*. Glucosamine sulfate use and delay of progression of knee osteoarthritis: a 3-year, randomized, placebo-controlled, double-blind study. *Arch Intern Med* 2002; 162: 2113–2123.

14 Bruyere O, Honore A, Ethgen O, *et al*. Correlation between radiographic severity of knee osteoarthritis and future disease progression. Results from a 3-year prospective, placebo-controlled study evaluating the effect of glucosamine sulfate. *Osteoarthritis Cartilage* 2003; 11: 1–5.

15 Bruyere O, Pavelka K, Rovati LC, *et al*. Glucosamine sulfate reduces osteoarthritis progression in postmenopausal women with knee osteoarthritis: evidence from two 3-year studies. *Menopause* 2004; 11: 134–135.

16 Cibere J, Kopec JA, Thorne RA, *et al*. Randomized, double-blind, placebo-controlled glucosamine discontinuation trial in knee osteoarthritis. *Arthritis Rheum* 2004; 51: 738–745.

17 McAlindon T, Formica M, LaValley M, *et al*. Effectiveness of glucosamine for symptoms of knee osteoarthritis: results from an internet-based randomized double-blind controlled trial. *Am J Med* 2004; 117: 643–649.

18 Qui GX, Weng XS, Zhang K, *et al*. A multi-central, randomized, controlled clinical trial of glucosamine hydrochloride/sulfate in the treatment of knee osteoarthritis. *Zhingua Yi Xue Za Zhi* 2005; 85: 3067–3070 (in Chinese)

19 Vaz AL. Double-blind clinical evaluation of the relative efficacy of ibuprofen and glucosamine sulphate in the management of osteoarthritis of the knee in outpatients. *Curr Med Res Opin* 1983; 3: 145–149.

20 Muller-Fassbender H, Bach G, Haase W, *et al*. Glucosamine sulphate compared with ibuprofen in osteoarthritis of the knee. *Osteoarthritis Cartilage* 1994; 2: 61–69.

21 Rovati LC, Giacovelli G, Annefeld M, *et al*. A large, randomized, placebo-controlled, double-blind study of glucosamine sulfate vs piroxicam and vs their association on the kinetics of the symptomatic effect in knee osteoarthritis (abstract). *Osteoarthritis Cartilage* 1994; 2 (Suppl. 1): 56.

22 McAlindon TE, LeValley MP, Gulin JP, Felson DT. Glucosamine and chondroitin for treatment of osteoarthritis. A systematic quality assessment and meta-analysis. *JAMA* 2000; 283: 169–175.

23 Kayne SB, Wadeson K, MacAdam A. Glucosamine – an effective treatment for osteoarthritis? A meta-analysis. *Pharm J* 2000; 265: 759–763.

24 Kleijnen J, Knipschild P, ter Riet G. Clinical trials of homoeopathy. *BMJ* 1991; 302: 316–323.

25 Ruane R, Griffiths P. Glucosamine therapy compared to ibuprofen for joint pain. *Br J Community Nurs* 2002; 7: 148–152.

26 Richy F, Bruyere O, Ethgen O, *et al*. Structural and symptomatic efficacy of glucosamine and chondroitin in knee osteoarthritis: a comprehensive meta-analysis. *Arch Intern Med* 2003; 163: 1514–1522.

27 Poolsup N, Suthisisang C, Channark, P Kittikulsuth W. Glucosamine long-term treatment and the progression of knee osteoarthritis: systematic review of randomized controlled trials. *Ann Pharmacother* 2005; 39: 1080–1087.

28 Towheed TE, Maxwell L, Anastassiades TP, *et al*. Glucosamine therapy for treating osteoarthritis. Cochrane database, issue 2, 2005. London: Macmillan.

29 Clegg DO, Reda DJ, Harris CL, *et al*. Glucosamine, chondroitin sulfate and the two in combination for painful knee osteoarthrtitis. *N Engl J Med* 2006; 354: 795–808.

30 Cohen M, Wolfe R, Mai T, *et al*. A randomized, double blind, placebo controlled trial of a topical cream containing glucosamine sulfate, chondroitin sulfate, and camphor for osteoarthritis of the knee. *J Rheumatol* 2003; 30: 523–528.

31 Balkan B, Dunning BE. Glucosamine inhibits glucokinase *in vitro* and produces a glucose-specific

impairment of *in vivo* insulin secretion in rats. *Diabetes* 1994; 43: 1173–1179.

32 Shankar RR, Zhu JS, Baron AD. Glucosamine infusion in mice mimics the beta-cell dysfunction of non-insulin dependent diabetes mellitus. *Metabolism* 1998; 47: 573–577.

33 Scroggie DA, Albright A, Harris MD. The effect of glucosamine-chondroitin supplementation on glycosylated hemoglobin levels in patients with type 2 diabetes mellitus: a placebo-controlled, double-blinded, randomized controlled trial. *Arch Intern Med* 2003; 163: 1587–1590.

34 Tannis AJ, Barban J, Conquer JA. Effect of glucosamine supplementation on fasting and non-fasting plasma glucose and serum insulin concentrations in healthy individuals. *Osteoarthritis Cartilage* 2004; 12: 506–511.

35 Consumerlab. Product review. Glucosamine and chondroitin. http://www.consumerlab.com (accessed 6 November 2006).

Grape seed extract

Description

Grape seed extract is an extract from the tiny seeds of red grapes.

Constituents

Grape seed extract is a source of oligomeric proanthocyanidin complexes (OPCs), sometimes known as proanthocyanidins, which are one of the categories of flavonoids (see Flavonoids). Proanthocyanidins are polyphenol oligomers derived from flavan-3-ols and flavan-3,4-diols. Grape seed extract contains OPCs made up of dimers or trimers of catechin and epicatechin. Additional active ingredients in grape seed extract include essential fatty acids and tocopherols.

Action

Grape seed is a potent antioxidant. Proanthocyanidins are thought to:[1]

- neutralise free radicals, including hydroxyl groups and lipid peroxides, blocking lipid peroxidation and stabilising cell membranes;
- inhibit the destruction of collagen by stabilising the activity of 1-antitrypsin, which inhibits the activity of destructive enzymes such as elastin and hyaluronic acid (this is thought to prevent fluid exudation by allowing red blood cells to cross the capillaries);
- inhibit the release of inflammatory mediators, such as histamine and prostaglandins; and
- inhibit platelet aggregation.

In addition, they are thought to have antibacterial, antiviral and anticarcinogenic actions.

Possible uses

Grape seed extract is promoted as an antioxidant to prevent CHD and stroke, and to strengthen fragile capillaries and improve circulation to the extremities. It is promoted for the treatment of conditions associated with poor vascular function such as diabetes mellitus, varicose veins, impotence and tingling in the arms and legs. Anecdotally it has been reported to be useful for treating inflammatory conditions, varicose veins and cancer. It has also been suggested to be useful for helping to prevent macular degeneration and cataracts.

Cardiovascular disease

Oral administration of proanthocyanidins from grape seed extract reduced serum cholesterol in a high-cholesterol animal feed model.[2] Specifically, it prevented the increase of total and LDL cholesterol.

In a double-blind study, 71 patients with peripheral venous insufficiency received 300 mg daily OPCs from grape seed. A reduction in functional symptoms was observed in 75% of the treated patients compared to 41% of the patients given a placebo.[3]

In a double-blind clinical trial, a group of elderly patients with either spontaneous or drug-induced poor capillary resistance were treated with 100–150 mg OPCs from grape extract daily, or placebo. There was a significant improvement in capillary resistance in the treated group after approximately 2 weeks.[4]

A further trial evaluated the effect of a standardised formulation of a polyphenolic extract of grapes on LDL susceptibility to oxidation in a group of heavy smokers. This was a randomised, double-blind, crossover study involving 24 healthy male heavy smokers aged 50 years or over. Subjects were given two capsules (containing 75 mg of a grape procyanidin extract) twice daily for 4 weeks. This was followed by a washout period of 3 weeks and placebo for 4 weeks. Subjects did not show significant modification of total cholesterol, triglycerides, HDL or LDL cholesterol during grape seed extract treatment. However, among oxidative indices, the concentration of thiobarbituric acid reactive substances was significantly reduced in subjects taking grape seed extract compared with placebo and basal values. The authors concluded that the antioxidant potential of grape seed extract polyphenols may prove effective as a model of oxidative stress (smoking). However, more investigational data are needed before use in wider clinical settings can be recommended.[5]

Miscellaneous

Grape seed extract is increasingly being investigated for other conditions. A double-blind RCT investigated the effect of grape seed extract in the treatment of seasonal allergic rhinitis. Patients with seasonal allergic rhinitis and skin prick test sensitivity to ragweed were randomised to 8 weeks' treatment with grape seed extract 100 mg twice daily or placebo, which was begun before the ragweed pollen season. Over the period of the study, no significant differences were observed between active and placebo groups in rhinitis quality of life assessments, symptom diary scores or requirements for rescue antihistamine. No significant laboratory abnormalities were detected. Overall, this study showed no trends towards supporting the efficacy of grape seed extract in the treatment of seasonal allergic rhinitis.[6]

Grape seed extract has been shown to stimulate lipolysis *in vitro* and reduce food intake in rats. Leading on from these findings, a study has assessed the efficacy of grape seed extract with respect to energy intake and satiety. In a randomised, placebo-controlled, double-blind crossover study, 51 subjects (aged 18–65 years, body mass index 22–30) were given a grape seed supplement for 3 days, 30–60 min prior to *ad libitum* lunch and dinner in a university restaurant. In the total study population, no difference in 24-hour energy intake was found between grape seed extract and placebo. However, in a subgroup of subjects ($n = 23$) with an energy requirement ≥ 7.5 MJ/day, energy intake was reduced by 4% after grape seed compared to placebo. There were no significant differences in macronutrient composition, attitude towards eating, satiety, mood or tolerance. The authors concluded that these findings suggest that grape seed could be effective in reducing 24-hour energy intake in normal to overweight dietary unrestrained subjects and could therefore play a role in body weight management.[7]

Conclusion
Preliminary evidence suggests that grape seed extract might lower lipid levels, improve symptoms of venous insufficiency and capillary resistance, reduce oxidative stress and play a role in body weight management. However, there are no well-controlled studies, and evidence for efficacy is promising but not yet robust.

Precautions/contraindications

No known contraindications, but based on the potential pharmacological activity of OPCs, i.e. that they may inhibit platelet aggregation, grape seed extract should be used with caution in patients with a history of bleeding or haemostatic disorders. It is probably wise to discontinue use 14 days before any surgery, including dental surgery.

Pregnancy and breast-feeding

No problems have been reported, but there have not been sufficient studies to guarantee the safety of grape seed extract in pregnancy and breast-feeding.

Adverse effects

None reported. However, there are no long-term studies assessing the safety of grape seed extract.

Interactions

Drugs
None reported, but in theory bleeding tendency may be increased with anticoagulants, aspirin and anti-platelet drugs.

Dose

Grape seed extract is available in the form of tablets and capsules. Supplements should be standardised (and labelled) to contain 92–95% proanthocyanidins or OPCs.

The dose is not established, but doses of 100–300 mg daily have been used in studies.

References

1   Murray M, Pizzorono J. Procyanidolic oligomers. In: Murray M, Pizzorono J, eds. *The Textbook of Natural Medicine*, 2nd edn. London: Churchill Livingstone, 1999: 899–902.

2   Tebib K, Bessanicon P, Roaunet J. Dietary grape seed tannins affect lipoproteins, lipoprotein lipases and tissue lipids in rats fed hypercholesterolemic diets. *J Nutr* 1994; 124: 2451–2457.

3   Thebaut JF, Thebaut P, Vin F. Study of Endotolon in functional manifestations of peripheral venous insufficiency. *Gaz Med France* 1985; 92: 96–100.

4   Dartenuc JY, Marache P, Choussat H. Capillary resistance in geriatry. A study of a microangioprotector – Endotolon. *Bord Med* 1980; 13: 903–907.

5   Vigna GB, Costantini F, Aldini G, *et al.* Effect of standardized grape seed extract on low-density lipoprotein susceptibility to oxidation in heavy smokers. *Metabolism* 2003; 52: 1250–1257.

6   Bernstein DI, Bernstein CK, Deng C, *et al.* Evaluation of the clinical efficacy and safety of grapeseed extract in the treatment of fall seasonal allergic rhinitis: a pilot study. *Ann Allergy Asthma Immunol* 2002; 88: 272–278.

7   Vogels N, Nijs IM, Westerterp-Plantenga MS. The effect of grape-seed extract on 24 h energy intake in humans. *Eur J Clin Nutr* 2004; 58: 667–673.

Green-lipped mussel

Description

Green-lipped mussel extract comes from *Perna canaliculata*, a salt-water shellfish indigenous to New Zealand.

Constituents

Green-lipped mussel extract contains a weak prostaglandin inhibitor that exerts an anti-inflammatory effect, as well as amino acids, fats, carbohydrates and minerals. Omega-3 fatty acids may be the key to its anti-inflammatory activity.

Possible uses

Rheumatoid arthritis

Green-lipped mussel extract is claimed to be effective in the treatment of rheumatoid arthritis. The small number of human studies published have generally shown that green-lipped mussel is not effective in arthritis,[1–3] but two studies have shown positive effects.[4,5] A more recent study has indicated that green-lipped mussel, added to a complete dry diet, can help alleviate symptoms of arthritis in dogs.[6]

A systematic review of studies using freeze-dried green-lipped mussel found mixed outcomes and was not conclusive. Of five RCTs, only two attested benefits for rheumatoid and osteoarthritic patients. Similarly, animal studies have yielded mixed findings. In both cases, according to the authors, this could be due to lack of stabilisation of the omega-3 fatty acids in the product. Overall there is little consistent and compelling evidence to date to show the therapeutic value of green-lipped mussel supplements, such as Seatone™, in arthritis. The authors conclude that there is a need for further investigations.[7]

Asthma

Experimental studies have shown that lipid extract of green-lipped mussel is effective at inhibiting 5′-lipoxygenase and cyclo-oxygenase pathways responsible for production of eicosanoids, including leukotrienes and prostaglandins, and it has been suggested that this compound could help patients with asthma. An RCT assessed the effect of green-lipped mussel on asthma symptoms, peak expiratory flow and hydrogen peroxide as a marker of airway inflammation in patients in expired breath condensate as a marker of airway inflammation. Forty-six patients with atopic asthma received two capsules of a lipid extract of green-lipped mussel or placebo three times a day for 8 weeks. Each capsule of extract contained 50 mg omega-3 polyunsaturated fatty acids and 100 mg olive oil, while the placebo contained only 100 mg olive oil. There was a significant decrease in daytime wheeze, the concentration of exhaled hydrogen peroxide and an increase in morning peak expiratory flow rate. The authors concluded that lipid extract of New Zealand green-lipped mussel may have some beneficial effect in patients with atopic asthma.[8]

Adverse effects

Green-lipped mussel is relatively non-toxic, but allergic reactions (e.g. gastrointestinal discomfort, nausea and flatulence) have been reported occasionally.

Interactions

None reported.

Dose

Green-lipped mussel extract is available in the form of capsules.

The dose is not established; dietary supplements provide approximately 1 g per daily dose.

References

1 Caughey DE, Grigor RR, Caughey EB. *Perna canaliculus* in the treatment of rheumatoid arthritis. *Eur J Rheumatol Inflamm* 1983; 6: 197–200.
2 Huskisson EC, Scott J, Bryans R. Seatone is ineffective in arthritis. *BMJ* 1981; 282: 1358–1359.
3 Larkin JG, Capell HA, Sturrock RD. Seatone in rheumatoid arthritis: a six-month placebo-controlled study. *Ann Rheum Dis* 1985; 44: 199–201.
4 Gibson RG, Gibson SL. Seatone in arthritis. *BMJ* 1981; 282: 1795.
5 Gibson RG, Gibson SL, Conway V, Chapell D. *Perna canaliculus* in the treatment of arthritis. *Practitioner* 1980; 224: 955–960.
6 Bui LM, Bierer TL. Influence of green lipped mussels (*Perna canaliculus*) in alleviating signs of arthritis in dogs. *Vet Ther* 2003; 4: 397–407.
7 Cobb CS, Ernst E. Systematic review of a marine nutraceutical supplement in clinical trials for arthritis: the effectiveness of the New Zealand green-lipped mussel *Perna canaliculus*. *Clin Rheumatol* 2005; 12: 1–10.
8 Emelyanov A, Fedoseev G, Krasnoschekova O, *et al.* Treatment of asthma with lipid extract of New Zealand green-lipped mussel: a randomised clinical trial. *Eur Respir J* 2002; 20: 596–600.

Green tea extract

Description

Green tea is prepared from the steamed and dried leaves of *Camellia sinensis*. It is different from black tea in that black tea is produced from leaves that have been withered, rolled, fermented and dried. The lack of fermentation gives green tea its unique flavour and also preserves the naturally present flavonoids, which are antioxidants.

Constituents

Green tea contains flavonoids, a large group of polyphenolic compounds with antioxidant properties. Of the flavonoids found in green tea, catechins make up 30–50% of the dry tea leaf weight. These include epigallocatechin gallate, epicatechin and epicatechin gallate. Green tea also contains flavonols, tannins, minerals, free amino acids, and methylxanthines (caffeine, theophylline and theobromine).

Action

Green tea appears to have the following effects:

- An antioxidant effect. Green tea may protect against oxidative damage to cells and tissues.
- A chemoprotective effect. This is attributed to the catechins, compounds that are thought to inhibit cell proliferation. *In vitro* studies have shown that green tea polyphenols induce programmed cell death (apoptosis) in human cancer cells[1,2] and block tumour growth by inhibition of tumour necrosis factor-α as well as a variety of other potential anti-cancer effects.[3-7] Animal studies have also shown the inhibitory effect of green tea against carcinogens.[8-10]
- Antibacterial and antiviral activity. *In vitro* studies have demonstrated that green tea polyphenols block the growth of micro-organisms that cause diarrhoea[11] and influenza.[12]
- Reduction of serum cholesterol.
- Reduction in LDL cholesterol oxidation. Two *in vitro* studies[13,14] showed that green tea can inhibit oxidation of LDL.
- Inhibition of platelet aggregation.

Possible uses

Green tea has been investigated mainly for supposed protective effects in cancer and CVD.

Cancer

A review of 31 epidemiological studies of green tea consumption and cancer risk found no overall consistent effect.[6] Of the total studies reviewed, 17 showed reduced cancer risk, seven increased risk, three no association and five an increased risk. Of the 10 studies on stomach cancer, six suggested a reduced risk and three an increased risk. Of the nine studies investigating colorectal cancer, four suggested a reduced risk and three an increased risk. Both studies on bladder cancer showed a reduced risk, and two out of the three studies on pancreatic cancer showed reduced risk. Studies examining oesophageal cancer showed mixed results, but very hot or scalding tea was associated with increased risk.

In a study of 472 Japanese patients with stage I, II and III breast cancer,[15] the level of green tea consumption before clinical diagnosis of cancer was evaluated. Increased consumption of green tea was significantly associated with decreased numbers of axillary lymph node metastases

171

among pre-menopausal patients with stage I and II breast cancer and increased expression of progesterone receptor and oestrogen receptor in post-menopausal patients. In a follow-up study, increased consumption of green tea was correlated with reduced recurrence of stage I and II breast cancer; the recurrence rate was 16.7% among those consuming five or more cups daily or 24.3% in those consuming four or more cups daily. However, no improvement was seen in those with stage III breast cancer.

Green tea may block the frequency of sister chromatid exchange (SCE), a biomarker of mutagenesis. A study in 52 Korean smokers[16] showed that SCE rates were significantly higher in smokers than non-smokers. However, the frequency of SCE in smokers who consumed green tea was comparable to that of non-smokers.

A systematic review and meta-analysis of observational studies linking green tea with breast cancer found that the pooled relative risk of developing breast cancer for the highest levels of green tea consumption in cohort studies was 0.89 (95% CI, 0.71 to 1.1; $P = 0.28$), and in case-control studies, the odds ratio was 0.44 (95% CI, 0.14 to 1.31; $P = 0.14$). The pooled relative risk of cohort studies for breast cancer recurrence in all stages was 0.75 (95% CI, 0.47 to 1.19; $P = 0.22$). The authors' conclusion was that, to date, the epidemiological data indicate that consumption of five or more cups of green tea a day shows a non-statistically significant trend towards the prevention of breast cancer. There is some evidence that green tea consumption may help to prevent breast cancer recurrence in early stage (I and II) cancers.[17]

Genetic factors may play a role in the influence of green tea on breast cancer. A case-control study involving 297 incident breast cancer cases and 665 control subjects in Singapore found no association of green tea consumption and breast cancer among all women or those with low activity of angiotensin-converting enzyme (ACE) genotype. However, among women with high activity of ACE genotype, frequency of intake for green tea was associated with a significantly decreased risk of breast cancer.[18]

Cardiovascular disease

A cross-sectional study of the effects of drinking green tea on cardiovascular and liver disease[19] in 1371 Japanese men aged over 40 showed that increased consumption of green tea was associated with reduced serum concentrations of total cholesterol and triglyceride and an increased proportion of HDL cholesterol, with a decreased proportion of low and very LDL cholesterol. In addition, increased consumption of green tea was associated with reduced concentrations of hepatic markers in serum (aspartate aminotransferase, alanine transferase and ferritin).

However, another cross-sectional study in 371 individuals from five districts of Japan[20] showed that green tea was not associated with serum concentrations of total cholesterol, triglycerides or HDL cholesterol.

Another study examined the relation between green tea consumption and arteriographically determined coronary atherosclerosis.[21] The subjects were 512 patients (302 men and 210 women) aged 30 years or older, who had undergone coronary arteriography for the first time between September 1996 and August 1997. Green tea consumption tended to be inversely associated with coronary atherosclerosis in men but not in women.

A further study investigated the impact of theaflavin-enriched green tea extract on the lipids and lipoproteins of subjects with mild to moderate hypercholesterolaemia. A total of 240 men and women aged 18 or over on a low-fat diet with mild to moderate hypercholesterolaemia were randomly assigned to receive a daily capsule containing theaflavin-enriched green tea extract (375 mg) or placebo for 12 weeks. In the green tea group, mean total cholesterol fell by 11.3% and mean LDL cholesterol by 16.4%, both statistically significant changes compared with baseline. There were no significant changes in the placebo group. The authors concluded that the green tea extract studied is an effective adjunct to a low-saturated fat diet to reduce LDL cholesterol in hypercholesterolaemic adults and is well tolerated.[22] Green tea has also been shown to improve overall antioxidant status and to protect against oxidative damage in human beings,[23] and to attenuate the increase in plasma triacylglycerol (triglyceride) levels following a fat load.[24]

Body weight

Green tea is being increasingly investigated for its potential influence on body weight. One study found that weight maintenance after 7.5% body weight loss was not affected by green tea treatment.[25] In another study, a green tea/caffeine mixture improved weight maintenance, partly through thermogenesis and fat oxidation, but only in habitual low caffeine consumers.[26] Further evidence for a thermogenic effect of green tea was found in another study where there was an increase in 24-h energy expenditure with mixtures of caffeine and epigallocatechin-3-gallate (EGCG), a catechin in green tea.[27] However, green tea had no significant effect on body weight in Chinese obese women with polycystic ovary syndrome.[28]

Miscellaneous

Green tea has been studied for its effect on insulin resistance, blood glucose level, HbA1c level and markers of inflammation, but without any clear effects.[29] Green tea polyphenols have been postulated to protect human skin from photoageing, but clinically significant changes were not detected in one study.[30]

A further study found that green tea extracts can be a potential therapy for patients with human papilloma virus (HPV) infected cervical lesions.[31] This study evaluated the influence of green tea extracts delivered in the form of an ointment or capsules in 51 patients with HPV-infected cervical lesions. Overall, a 69% response rate was noted for treatment with green tea extracts compared with a 10% response rate from untreated controls.

A recent Japanese cross-sectional study has evaluated the effect of green tea on cognitive function. The frequency of green tea consumption was examined in 1003 Japanese subjects aged 70 or over. Higher consumption of green tea was associated with lower levels of cognitive impairment.[32]

Conclusion

Green tea has been investigated for protective effects in CVD and cancer, in which it shows some promise. There is also some evidence that it helps to maintain body weight after weight loss. However, there is still a dearth of good-quality controlled trials and firm conclusions must await results from such trials.

Precautions/contraindications

No known contraindications, but based on the potential pharmacological activity of polyphenols (i.e. that they may inhibit platelet aggregation), green tea extract should be used with caution in patients with a history of bleeding or haemostatic disorders. It is probably wise to discontinue use 14 days before any surgery, including dental surgery.

Pregnancy and breast-feeding

No problems have been reported, but there have been insufficient studies to guarantee the safety of green tea supplements in pregnancy and breast-feeding.

Adverse effects

There is a lack of tolerance and safety data on supplements of this substance. However, green tea has been consumed safely in China for more than 4000 years. Recently there have been case reports of green tea extracts (not the beverage) being associated with liver toxicity. As with any plant-containing substance, this may be due to the presence of contaminants.

Interactions

Drugs

None are known, but in theory bleeding tendency may be increased with anticoagulants, aspirin and anti-platelet drugs.

Dose

Green tea is available in the form of capsules as well as tea for drinking.

The dose is not established, but doses of 250–300 mg daily have been used. Supplements should be standardised (and labelled) to contain 50–97% polyphenols, containing per dose at least 50% (–)epigallocatechin-3-gallate. Four to six cups of freshly brewed green tea should provide similar levels of polyphenols.

References

1 Ahmad N, Feyes DK, Niemenen Al, *et al*. Green tea constituent epigallocatechin-3-gallate and induction of apoptosis and cell cycle arrest in human carcinoma cells. *J Natl Cancer Inst* 1997; 89: 1881–1886.

2 Hibasami H, Komiya T, Achiwa Y, *et al*. Induction of apoptosis in human stomach cancer cells by green tea catechins. *Oncol Rep* 1998; 5: 527–529.

3 Kuroda Y, Hara Y. Antimutagenic and anticarcinogenic activity of tea polyphenols. *Mutat Res* 1999; 436: 69–97.

4 Leanderson P, Faresjo AO, Tagesson C. Green tea polyphenols inhibit oxidant-induced DNA strand breakage in cultured lung cells. *Free Rad Biol Med* 1997; 310: 235–242.

5 Fujiki H, Suganuma M, Okabe S, *et al*. Mechanistic findings of green tea as cancer preventive for humans. *Proc Soc Exp Biol Med* 1999; 220: 225–228.

6 Bushman JL. Green tea and cancer in humans: a review of the literature. *Nutr Cancer* 1998; 31: 151–159.

7 Nihal A, Hasan M. Green tea polyphenols and cancer: biological mechanisms and practical implications. *Nutr Rev* 1999; 57: 78–83.

8 Yang CS, Yang GY, Landau JM, *et al*. Tea and tea polyphenols inhibit cell proliferation, lung tumorigenesis and tumour progression. *Exp Lung Res* 1998; 24: 629–639.

9 Wang ZY, Huang MT, Ferraro T, *et al*. Inhibitory effect of green tea in the drinking water on tumorigenesis by ultraviolet light and 12-o-tetradecanoylphorbol-13-acetate in the skin of SKH-1 mice. *Cancer Res* 1992; 52: 1162–1170.

10 Paschka GA, Butler R, Young CY. Induction of apoptosis in prostate cancer lines by the green tea component (–)epigallocatechin-3-gallate. *Cancer Lett* 1998; 130: 1–7.

11 Shetty M, Subbannaya K, Shivananda PG. Antibacterial activity of tea (*Camellia sinensis*) and coffee (*Coffee arabica*) with special reference to *Salmonella typhimurium*. *J Commun Dis* 1994; 26: 147–150.

12 Nakayama M, Suzuki K, Toda M, *et al*. Inhibition of the infectivity of influenza virus by tea polyphenols. *Antiviral Res* 1993; 21: 289–299.

13 van het Kof KH, de Boer HS, Wiseman SA, *et al*. Consumption of green or black tea does not increase resistance of low-density lipoprotein to oxidation in humans. *Am J Clin Nutr* 1997; 66: 1125–1132.

14 Yokozawa T, Dong E. Influence of green tea and its three major components upon low density lipoprotein oxidation. *Exp Toxicol Pathol* 1997; 49: 329–335.

15 Nakachi K, Suemasu K, Suga K, *et al*. Influence of drinking green tea on breast cancer malignancy among Japanese patients. *Jpn J Cancer Res* 1998; 89: 254–261.

16 Lee IP, Kim JH, Kang MH, *et al*. Chemoprotective effect of green tea (*Camellia sinensis*) against cigarette smoke-induced mutations (SCE) in humans. *J Cell Biochem Suppl* 1997; 27: 68–75.

17 Seely D, Mills EJ, Wu P, *et al*. The effects of green tea consumption on incidence of breast cancer and recurrence of breast cancer: a systematic review and meta-analysis. *Integr Cancer Ther* 2005; 4: 144–155.

18 Yuan J-M, Koh W-P, Sun C-L, *et al*. Green tea intake, ACE gene polymorphism and breast cancer risk among Chinese women in Singapore. *Carcinogenesis* 2005; 26: 1389–1394.

19 Imai K, Nakachi K. Cross sectional study of effects of drinking green tea on cardiovascular and liver disease. *BMJ* 1995; 310: 693–696.

20 Tsubono Y, Tsugane S. Green tea intake in relation to serum lipid levels in middle-aged Japanese men and women. *Ann Epidemiol* 1997; 7: 280–284.

21 Sasazuki S, Kodama H, Yoshimasu K, *et al*. Relation between green tea consumption and the severity of coronary atherosclerosis among Japanese men and women. *Ann Epidemiol* 2000; 10: 401–408.

22 Maron DJ, Lu GP, Cai NS, *et al*. Cholesterol-lowering effect of a theaflavin-enriched green tea extract: a randomized controlled trial. *Arch Intern Med* 2003; 163: 1448–1453.

23 Erba D, Riso P, Bordoni A, *et al*. Effectiveness of moderate green tea consumption on antioxidative status and plasma lipid profile in humans. *J Nutr Biochem* 2005; 16: 144–149.

24 Unno T, Tago M, Suzuki Y, *et al*. Effect of tea catechins on postprandial plasma lipid responses in human subjects. *Br J Nutr* 2005; 93: 543–547.

25 Kovacs EM, Lejeune MP, Nijs I, Westerterp-Plantenga MS. Effects of green tea on weight maintenance after body-weight loss. *Br J Nutr* 2004; 91: 431–437.

26 Westerterp-Plantenga MS, Lejeune MP, Kovacs EM. Body weight loss and weight maintenance in relation to habitual caffeine intake and green tea supplementation. *Obes Res* 2005; 13: 1195–1204.

27 Berube-Parent S, Pelletier C, Dore J, Tremblay A. Effects of encapsulated green tea and guarana extracts containing a mixture of epigallocatechin-3-gallate and caffeine on 24 h expenditure and fat oxidation in men. *Br J Nutr* 2005; 94: 432–436.

28 Chan CC, Koo MW, Ng EH, *et al.* Effects of Chinese green tea on weight, and hormonal and biochemical profiles in obese patients with polycystic ovary syndrome – a randomized placebo-controlled trial. *J Soc Gynecol Investig* 2006; 13: 63–68.

29 Fukino Y, Shimbo M, Aoki N, *et al.* Randomized controlled trial for an effect of green tea consumption on insulin resistance and inflammation markers. *J Nutr Sci Vitaminol (Tokyo)* 2005; 51: 335–342.

30 Chiu AE, Chan JL, Kern DG, *et al.* Double-blind, placebo-controlled trial of green tea extracts in the clinical and histology appearance of photo-aging skin. *Dermatol Surg* 2005; 31(7 Pt 2): 855–860.

31 Ahn WS, Yoo J, Huh SW, *et al.* Protective effects of green tea extracts (polyphenon E and EGCG) on human cervical lesions. *Eur J Cancer Prev* 2003; 12: 383–390.

32 Kuriyama S, Hozawa A, Ohmori K, *et al.* Green tea consumption and cognitive function: a cross sectional study from the Tsurugaya Project. *Am J Clin Nutr* 2006; 83: 355–361.

Guarana

Description

Guarana is produced from the dried and powdered seeds of a South American shrub, *Paullinia cupana*.

Constituents

Guarana contains a substance called guaranine (a synonym for caffeine). It also contains theobromine, theophylline and tannins.

Action

Guarana acts as a CNS stimulant, increases heart rate and contractility, increases blood pressure, inhibits platelet aggregation, stimulates gastric acid secretion, causes diuresis, relaxes bronchial smooth muscle and stimulates the release of catecholamines.

Possible uses

Guarana is claimed to:

- improve mental alertness, endurance, vitality, immunity, stamina in athletes and sexual drive;
- retard ageing;
- alleviate migraine, diarrhoea, constipation and tension; and
- act as an appetite suppressant to aid slimming.

Because of it caffeine content, guarana is likely to be effective when taken as a CNS stimulant, but it has not been subjected to controlled trials. There is no good evidence that guarana improves stamina and performance in athletes. There is insufficient reliable information about the effectiveness of guarana for other indications.

Precautions/contraindications

Guarana should be avoided by people with heart conditions, peptic ulcer, anxiety disorders, and renal impairment. It should also not be taken within 2 h of bedtime.

Pregnancy and breast-feeding

Guarana should be avoided during pregnancy and breast-feeding.

Adverse effects

High doses of guarana may cause insomnia, nervousness, irritability, palpitations, gastric irritation, flushing and elevated blood pressure.

Interactions

None have been reported.

Dose

Guarana is available in the form of tablets and capsules, either in isolation or with vitamins and minerals in other dietary supplements.

The dose is not established. Guarana should not be recommended. Dietary supplements provide 50–200 mg.

Iodine

Description

Iodine is an essential trace element.

Human requirements

See Table 1 for Dietary Reference Values for iodine.

Dietary intake

In the UK, the average adult diet provides: for men, 220 µg daily; for women, 159 µg.

Action

Iodine is an essential part of the thyroid hormones thyroxine (T_4) and triiodothyronine (T_3).

Dietary sources

See Table 2 for dietary sources of iodine.

Metabolism

Absorption
Inorganic iodine is rapidly and efficiently absorbed. Organically bound iodine is less well absorbed.

Distribution
Iodine is transported to the thyroid gland (for the synthesis of thyroid hormones), and to a lesser extent to the salivary and gastric glands.

Elimination
Excretion of inorganic iodine is mainly via the urine. Some organic iodine is eliminated in the faeces. Iodine is excreted in the breast milk.

Deficiency

Iodine deficiency leads to goitre and hypothyroidism.

Possible uses

Supplements containing iodine may be required by vegans (strict vegetarians who consume no dairy products). In a study in Greater London that included 38 vegans,[1] intakes of iodine in the vegan individuals were below the DRVs. The authors of the study concluded that the impact of these low iodine intakes should be studied further and that vegans should use appropriate dietary supplements. Further studies have confirmed a markedly reduced iodine intake with a lactovegetarian diet compared with an ordinary diet,[2] and a higher prevalence of iodine deficiency in vegans and vegetarians.[3]

Precautions/contraindications

None reported.

Pregnancy and breast-feeding

Doses exceeding the RDA should not be used (they may result in abnormal thyroid function in the infant).

Table 1 Dietary Reference Values for iodine (µg/day)

						EU RDA = 150 µg
Age	UK			USA		WHO/FAO
	LNRI	RNI	EVM	RDA	TUL	RNI
0–3 months	40	50		110[1]	–	90
4–6 months	40	60		110[1]	–	90
7–12 months	40	60		130	–	90
1–3 years	40	70		90	200	90
4–6 years	50	100		–	–	–
4–8 years	–	–		90	300	
7–10 years	55	110		–	–	120[3]
9–13 years	–	–		120	600	–
14–18 years	–	–		150	900	150[4]
Males and females						
11–14 years	65	130		–	–	–
15–18 years	70	140		–	–	–
19–50+	70	140	500[1]	150	1100	150
Pregnancy	*	*		220	1100[2]	200
Lactation	*	*		290	1100[2]	200

[1] Adequate Intakes (AIs). [2] < 18 years, 90 µg. [3] 6–12 years. [4] 13–18 years.
EVM = Likely upper safe daily intake from supplements alone.
TUL = Tolerable Upper Intake Level.

Adverse effects

High iodine intake may induce hyperthyroidism (particularly in those over the age of 40 years) and toxic modular goitre or hypothyroidism in autoimmune thyroid disease. There is a risk of hyperkalaemia with prolonged use of high doses. Toxicity is rare with intakes below 5000 µg daily and extremely rare at intakes below 1000 µg daily.

Hypersensitivity reactions including headache, rashes, symptoms of head cold, swelling of lips, throat and tongue, and arthralgia (joint pain) have been reported.

Interactions

Drugs

Antithyroid drugs: iodine may interfere with thyroid control.

Table 2 Dietary sources of iodine

Food portion	Iodine content (µg)
Milk and dairy products	
½ pint milk, whole, semi-skimmed or skimmed	*45*
1 pot yoghurt (150 g)	90
Cheese (50 g)	*25*
Fish	
Cod, cooked (150 g)	**150**
Haddock, cooked (150 g)	**300**
Mackerel, cooked (150 g)	**200**
Plaice, cooked (150 g)	*50*

Excellent sources (**bold**); good sources (*italics*).
Note: Iodised salt contains 150µg/5 g.

Dose

Iodine is available mostly as an ingredient in multivitamin and mineral products.

Dietary supplements usually provide 50–100% of the RDA.

Upper safety levels

The UK Expert Group on Vitamins and Minerals (EVM) has identified a likely safe total intake of iodine for adults from supplements alone of 500 µg daily.

References

1 Draper A, Lewis J, Malhotra N, Wheeler E. The energy and nutrient intakes of different types of vegetarian: a case for supplements? *Br J Nutr* 1993; 69: 3–19.
2 Remer T, Neubert A, Manz F. Increased risk of iodine deficiency with vegetarian nutrition. *Br J Nutr* 1999; 81: 45–49.
3 Krajovicova-Kuldlackova M, Buckova K, Klimes I, Sebokova E. Iodine deficiency in vegetarians and vegans. *Ann Nutr Metab* 2003; 47: 183–185.

Iron

Description

Iron is an essential trace mineral.

Human requirements

See Table 1 for Dietary Reference Values of iron.

Dietary intake

In the UK, the average adult diet provides: for men 13.2 mg daily; for women, 10.0 mg. Dietary iron consists of haem and non-haem iron; in animal foods, about 40% of the iron is haem iron and 60% is non-haem iron; all the iron in vegetable products is non-haem iron.

Action

Iron is a component of haemoglobin, myoglobin and many enzymes that are involved in a variety of metabolic functions, including transport and storage of oxygen, the electron transport chain, DNA synthesis and catecholamine metabolism.

Dietary sources

See Table 2 for dietary sources of iron.

Metabolism

Absorption

Absorption of iron occurs principally in the duodenum and proximal jejunum. Absorption of food iron varies between 5% and 15%. Haem iron is more efficiently absorbed than non-haem iron. Body iron content is regulated mainly through changes in absorption.

Distribution

Iron is transported in the blood bound to the protein transferrin, and is stored in the liver, spleen and bone marrow as ferritin and haemosiderin.

Elimination

The body has a limited capacity to eliminate iron, and it can accumulate in the body to toxic amounts. Small amounts are excreted in the faeces, urine, skin, sweat, hair, nails and menstrual blood.

Bioavailability

The absorption of non-haem iron is enhanced by concurrent ingestion of meat, poultry and fish, and by various organic acids, especially ascorbic acid; it is inhibited by phytates (found in bran and high-fibre cereals), tannins (found in tea and coffee), egg yolk and by some drugs and nutrients (see Interactions). Ferrous salts are more efficiently absorbed than ferric salts.

Deficiency

Iron deficiency leads to microcytic, hypochromic anaemia. Symptoms include fatigue, weakness, pallor, dyspnoea on exertion and palpitations. Non-haematological effects include impairment in work capacity, intellectual performance, neurological function and immune function and, in children, behavioural disturbances. Gastrointestinal symptoms are also fairly common and the fingernails may become lustreless, brittle, flattened and spoon-shaped.

Table 1   Dietary Reference Values for iron (mg/day)

EU RDA = 14 mg

Age	UK			EVM	USA		FAO/WHO RNI[4]
	LNRI	EAR	RNI		RDA	TUL	
0–3 months	0.9	1.3	1.7		0.27[2]	40	–
4–6 months	2.3	3.3	4.3		0.27[2]	40	–
7–12 months	4.2	6.0	7.8		11	40	6.2–18.6
1–3 years	3.7	5.3	6.9		7	40	3.9–11.6
4–6 years	3.3	4.7	6.1		–	–	4.2–12.6
4–8 years	–	–	–		10	40	–
7–10 years	4.7	6.7	8.7		10	–	5.9–17.8[a]
9–13 years	–	–	–		8	40	–
Males							
11–14 years	6.1	8.7	11.3		–	–	9.7–29.2[b]
15–18 years	6.1	8.7	11.3		–	–	12.5–37.6
14–18 years	–	–	–		11	45	–
19–50+ years	4.7	6.7	8.7	17	8	45	9.2–27.4
Females							
11–14 years	8.0	11.4	14.8[1]		–	–	9.3–28.0[5b]/21.8–65.4[6b]
14–18 years	–	–	–		15	45	–
15–50+ years	8.0	11.4	14.8[1]	17	–	–	–
19–50 years	–	–	–		18	45	19.6–58.8
50+ years	4.7	6.7	8.7		8	45	9.1–27.4
Pregnancy	*	*	*		27	45	NS
Lactation	*	*	*		9[3]	45	10.0–30.0
Post-menopause						8	
Pre-menopause					18		

* No increment.
[a] 7–9 years.   [b] 10–14 years.
[1] Insufficient level for women who have high menstrual losses who may need iron supplements.   [2] Adequate Intakes (AIs).
[3] aged < 18 years, 10 mg daily.   [4] Requirement depends on iron bioavailability of the diet.   [5] Pre-menarche.   [6] Post-menarche.
EVM = Likely safe daily intake from supplements alone.
TUL = Tolerable Upper Intake Level from diet and supplements.

Possible uses

Requirements may be increased and/or supplements needed in:

- infants and children from the age of 6 months to 4 years;
- early adolescence;
- the female reproductive period;
- pregnancy; and
- vegetarians.

Precautions/contraindications

Iron supplements should be avoided in conditions associated with iron overload (e.g. haemochromatosis, haemosiderosis, thalassaemia); gastrointestinal disease, particularly

Table 2   Dietary sources of iron

Food portion	Iron content (mg)	Food portion	Iron content (mg)
Breakfast cereals		**Liver, lambs, cooked (90 g)**	**9**
1 bowl All-Bran (45 g)	**5**	**Kidney, lambs, cooked (75 g)**	**9**
1 bowl Bran Flakes (45 g)	**9**	*Fish*	
1 bowl Corn Flakes (30 g)	*2*	**Cockles (80 g)**	**21**
1 bowl muesli (95 g)	**5**	**Mussels (80 g)**	**6**
2 pieces Shredded Wheat	*2*	*Pilchards, canned (105 g)*	*2.8*
1 bowl Special K (35 g)	*4*	*Sardines, canned (70 g)*	*3*
1 bowl Start (30 g)	**5**	*Vegetables*	
1 bowl Sultana Bran (35 g)	**5**	*Green vegetables, average, boiled (100 g)*	*1.5*
2 Weetabix	*3*	*Potatoes, boiled (150 g)*	*0.5*
Cereal products		*1 small can baked beans (200 g)*	*3*
Bread, brown, 2 slices	*1.5*	*Lentils, kidney beans or other pulses (105 g)*	*2*
white[1], 2 slices	*1*	**Dahl, chickpea (155 g)**	**5**
wholemeal, 2 slices	*2*	*lentil (155 g)*	*2.5*
1 chapati	*1.5*	*Soya beans, cooked (100 g)*	*3*
1 naan bread	*3.5*	*Fruit*	
Pasta, brown, boiled (150 g)	*2.0*	*8 dried apricots*	*2*
white, boiled (150 g)	*1.0*	*4 figs*	*2.5*
Rice, brown, boiled (165 g)	*0.7*	*½ an avocado pear*	*1.5*
white, boiled (165 g)	*0.3*	*Blackberries (100 g)*	*1*
Dairy products		*Blackcurrants (100 g)*	*1*
1 egg, size 2 (60 g)	*1*	*Nuts*	
Meat		*20 almonds*	*1*
Red meat, roast (85 g)	*2.5*	*10 Brazil nuts*	*1*
1 beef steak (155 g)	**5.4**	*1 small bag peanuts (25 g)*	*0.5*
Minced beef, lean, stewed (100 g)	**3**	*Milk chocolate (100 g)*	*1.6*
1 chicken leg (190 g)	*1*	*Plain chocolate (100 g)*	*2.4*

White bread is supplemented with additional iron in the UK.
Excellent sources (**bold**); good sources (*italics*).

inflammatory bowel disease, intestinal stricture, diverticulitis and peptic ulcer.

Pregnancy and breast-feeding

The Reference Nutrient Intake for iron during pregnancy is no greater than for other adult women. Requirements during pregnancy are partly offset by lack of menstruation and partly by increased efficiency of absorption. Routine iron supplementation is not required in pregnancy, but iron status should be monitored.

Adverse effects

Iron supplements may cause gastrointestinal irritation, nausea and constipation, which may lead to faecal impaction, particularly in the elderly. Patients with inflammatory bowel disease may suffer exacerbation of diarrhoea. Any reduced incidence of side-effects associated with modified-release preparations may be due to the fact that only small amounts of iron are released in the intestine. Liquid iron preparations may stain the teeth.

Table 3   Iron content of commonly used iron supplements

Iron salt	Iron(mg/g)	Iron(%)
Ferrous fumarate	330	33
Ferrous gluconate	120	12
Ferrous glycine sulphate	180	18
Ferrous orotate	150	15
Ferrous succinate	350	35
Ferrous sulphate	200	20
Ferrous sulphate, dried	300	30
Iron amino acid chelate	100	10

Interactions

Drugs

Antacids: reduced absorption of iron; give 2 h apart.

Bisphosphonates: reduced absorption of bisphosphonates; give 2 h apart.

Co-careldopa: reduced plasma levels of carbidopa and levodopa.

Levodopa: absorption of levodopa may be reduced.

Methyldopa: reduced absorption of methyldopa.

Penicillamine: reduced absorption of penicillamine.

4-Quinolones: absorption of ciprofloxacin, norfloxacin and ofloxacin reduced by oral iron; give 2 h apart.

Tetracyclines: reduced absorption of iron and vice versa; give 2 h apart.

Trientine: reduced absorption of iron; give 2 h apart.

Nutrients

Calcium: calcium carbonate or calcium phosphate may reduce absorption of iron; give 2 h apart (absorption of iron in multiple formulations containing iron and calcium is not significantly altered).

Copper: large doses of iron may reduce copper status and vice versa.

Manganese: reduced absorption of manganese.

Vitamin E: large doses of iron may increase requirement for vitamin E; vitamin E may impair haematological response to iron in patients with iron-deficiency anaemia.

Zinc: reduced absorption of iron and vice versa.

Dose

Iron is best taken on an empty stomach, but food reduces the possibility of stomach upsets; oral liquid preparations should be well diluted with water or fruit juice and drunk through a straw.

As a dietary supplement, 10–17 mg daily.

Upper safety levels

The UK Expert Group on Vitamins and Minerals (EVM) has identified a likely safe total intake of iron for adults from supplements alone of 17 mg daily.

Note: doses are given in terms of elemental iron; patients should be advised that iron supplements are not identical and provide different amounts of elemental iron; iron content of various iron salts commonly used in supplements is shown in Table 3.

Isoflavones

Description

Isoflavones belong to the class of compounds known as flavonoids, and they are found principally in soya beans and products made from them, including soya flour, soya milk, tempeh and tofu. They are present in varying amounts depending on the type of soya product and how it is processed. Isoflavones are also found in dietary supplements.

Constituents

The principal isoflavones in the soya bean are genistein, daidzein and glycetin, which are present mainly as glycosides. After ingestion, the glycosides are hydrolysed in the large intestine by the action of bacteria to release genistein, daidzein and glycetin. Daidzein can be metabolised by the bacteria in the large intestine to form either equol, which is oestrogenic, or O-desmethylangolensin, which is non-oestrogenic, while genistein is metabolised to the non-oestrogenic P-ethyl phenol. Variation in the ability to metabolise daidzein could therefore have an influence on the health effects of isoflavones.

Action

Isoflavones are naturally-occurring weak oestrogens, also known as phyto-oestrogens, which are capable of binding to oestrogen receptors where, depending on the hormonal status of the individual, they may seem to exert either oestrogenic or anti-oestrogenic effects. Pre-menopausally, isoflavones may therefore be anti-oestrogenic, while post-menopausally they could act oestrogenically, although further research is required to confirm this concept.

There are two types of oestrogen receptors – alpha and beta – and different tissues appear to have different ratios of each type. Thus, alpha-receptors appear to predominate in breast, uterus and ovary, while beta-receptors appear to predominate in prostate, bone and vascular tissue. Phyto-oestrogens, although less potent than endogenous or synthetic oestrogens, have been shown to bind to beta-oestrogen receptors, raising the possibility that phyto-oestrogens could produce beneficial effects on, for example, bone and vascular tissue, without causing adverse effects on the breast and ovary.

In addition to these hormonal effects, animal and *in vitro* evidence indicates that isoflavones arrest growth of cancer cells through inhibition of DNA replication, interference of signal transduction pathways and reduction in the activity of various enzymes. Isoflavones also exhibit antioxidant effects, suppress angiogenesis and inhibit the actions of various growth factors and cytokines.[1]

Possible uses

Isoflavones have been investigated for a potential role in CVD, cancer, osteoporosis and menopausal symptoms.

Cardiovascular disease

Soya protein
Products containing soya protein have been shown to reduce both total and LDL cholesterol in some – but not all – studies in animals and humans with raised cholesterol levels. The mechanisms by which soya foods could reduce

cholesterol are being investigated, but may include enhancement of bile acid secretion and reduced cholesterol metabolism. Other mechanisms, independent of cholesterol lowering, by which soya could be cardioprotective, include reduction of platelet aggregation and clot formation, and inhibition of atherosclerosis by an antioxidant effect and by inhibiting cell adhesion and proliferation in the arteries.[2] However, further studies are required to confirm these possibilities.

In addition, the question of which constituents of soya are actually responsible for lipid lowering is under discussion, and it is not certain that isoflavones are the components responsible for any beneficial effect. Animal studies specifically comparing the effects of isoflavone-rich soya with isoflavone-free soya on a range of blood lipids have produced conflicting results.

A meta-analysis of 38 controlled clinical trials looking at the effects of soya protein on serum lipid levels in humans showed that there was a statistically significant association between soya protein intake and improvement in serum lipid levels.[3] Of the 38 trials, 34 reported a reduction in serum cholesterol, and overall there was a 9.3% decrease in total cholesterol, a 12.9% decrease in LDL cholesterol and a 10.5% decrease in triacylglycerols. HDL cholesterol increased, but this change was not significant.

A double-blind, randomised 6-month trial involving 66 post-menopausal women with hypercholesterolaemia found that compared to control, soya protein providing either 56 or 90 mg isoflavones significantly reduced non-HDL cholesterol and raised HDL cholesterol, with no change in total cholesterol.[4]

The effects of consuming a soya protein beverage powder compared with a casein supplement were evaluated in 20 male subjects randomly allocated to the two groups.[5] There were no significant differences in plasma total and HDL cholesterol or in platelet aggregation between the groups, possibly because the men were normocholesterolaemic at entry into the study.

In a further study, soya protein was found to enhance the effect of a low-fat, low-cholesterol diet by reducing serum LDL cholesterol and increasing the ratio of LDL cholesterol to HDL

cholesterol in men with both normal and high serum lipid levels.[6]

In a double-blind, placebo-controlled trial involving 156 healthy men and women, soya protein providing 62 mg isoflavones was associated with a significant reduction in total and LDL cholesterol compared with isoflavone-free soya protein (the placebo).[7] Moreover, soya protein providing 37 mg isoflavones was also associated with a decrease in total and LDL cholesterol, but the reduction was significant only in those subjects with a baseline LDL exceeding 4.24 mmol/L. There was no effect on HDL levels or triacylglycerols. Soya protein providing a lower dose of isoflavones (27 mg daily) had no effect on any of the measured indices. In subjects with baseline LDL levels between 3.62 and 4.24 mmol/L there was no significant effect of any dose of isoflavones.

A further study, involving 81 men with moderate hypercholesterolaemia (total serum cholesterol 5.7–7.7 mmol/L) found that soya protein (20 g daily, providing 37.5 mg isoflavones) reduced non-HDL cholesterol by 2.6% and total cholesterol by 1.8% after 6 weeks.[8] Another trial involving healthy young men compared the effects of milk protein isolate, low isoflavone soya protein isolate (1.64 ± 0.19 mg aglycone isoflavones daily) and high isoflavone soya protein isolate (61.7 ± 7.4 mg aglycone isoflavones daily) on lipid levels. The differences produced by the three treatments were not significant, but the ratios of total to HDL cholesterol, LDL to HDL cholesterol and apo B to apo A-1 were significantly lower with both the soya protein treatments than with the milk protein isolate.[9]

A study in 13 pre-menopausal women with normal serum cholesterol levels found that total cholesterol, HDL cholesterol and LDL cholesterol levels changed significantly across menstrual cycle phases. During specific phases of the cycle, soya protein providing 128.7 mg isoflavones significantly lowered LDL cholesterol by 7.6–10.0%, the ratio of total to HDL cholesterol by 10.2% and the ratio of LDL to HDL cholesterol by 13.8%. Despite the high intake of isoflavones, the changes in lipid concentrations were small, but the authors concluded that over a lifetime the small effects observed could slow the development of atherosclerosis and reduce the risk of CHD in women with normal cholesterol levels.[10]

A preliminary study in six subjects investigated the effect of soya (providing genistein 12 mg and daidzein 7 mg) daily for 2 weeks on resistance of LDL to oxidation, because it appears that LDL has to be oxidised before it can damage the arteries. The results from this small study indicated that isoflavones could offer protection against LDL oxidation.[11]

A randomised crossover study in 24 subjects compared a soya-enriched diet that was providing 1.9 or 66 mg of isoflavones daily. The aim was to investigate the effects of the diets on biomarkers of lipid peroxidation and resistance of LDL to oxidation, because oxidative damage to lipids may be involved in the aetiology of atherosclerosis and CVD. The diet high in isoflavones reduced lipid peroxidation and increased the resistance of LDL to oxidation.[12]

Isoflavone supplements

Studies giving isoflavones in tablet form have yielded less positive results than those using soya protein. Forty-six men and 13 post-menopausal women not taking HRT, all with average serum cholesterol levels, participated in an 8-week randomised, double-blind, placebo-controlled trial of two-way parallel design. One tablet containing 55 mg isoflavones (predominantly in the form of genistein) or placebo was taken daily. Post-intervention, there were no significant differences in total, LDL and HDL cholesterol and lipoprotein(a).[13]

Another trial, this time in 14 pre-menopausal women, found that a supplement providing 86 mg daily for 2 months produced no change compared with placebo in plasma concentrations of total cholesterol and triacylglycerol, nor in the oxidisability of LDL.[14] A further study in 20 healthy post-menopausal women (50–70 years old) with evidence of endothelial dysfunction, found that a soya bean tablet providing 80 mg of isoflavones daily for 8 weeks produced no significant effects on plasma lipids compared to placebo.[15]

The effects of dietary isoflavone supplementation using a purified red clover supplement (containing approximately biochanin A 26 mg, formononetin 16 mg, daidzein 0.5 mg and genistein 1 mg per tablet) at doses of one to two tablets daily were compared to placebo in a three-period, randomised, double-blind, ascending-dose study in 66 post-menopausal women with moderately elevated plasma cholesterol levels (5.0–9.0 mmol/L).[16] Each of the three treatment periods lasted for 4 weeks. The dietary supplement did not significantly alter plasma total cholesterol, LDL or HDL cholesterol, or plasma triglycerides. Further trials with red clover have also shown that this preparation has no effect on blood lipids.[17,18] However, at least one trial has shown that red clover may favourably influence blood pressure and endothelial function in post-menopausal women with type 2 diabetes.[19]

Recent trials have looked at other cardiovascular risk factors besides lipids that soya isoflavones might influence. Results to date have not been promising. Isoflavones were found to have no significant effect on reducing oxidative damage.[20,21] Studies looking at effects of isoflavones on vascular function have been conflicting, some showing improved function,[22,23] while others showed no effect.[24] One trial in healthy post-menopausal women suggested a positive influence of soya isoflavones on endothelial function, as evidenced by improvement in endothelium-dependent vasodilatation and a reduction in plasma adhesion molecule levels.[25] Another trial in post-menopausal women suggested that isoflavones could have beneficial effects on C-reactive protein concentrations, but not on other inflammatory markers of cardiovascular risk in post-menopausal women. This study also assessed whether there were any differences in response according to equol production, but there were not.[26]

A study looking at the effect of a specific isoflavone – genistein – suggested that genistein may have a favourable effect on some cardiovascular markers, including fasting glucose, fasting insulin, insulin resistance and fibrinogen.[27] However, a further trial involving genistein found that after 6 months' treatment, genistein did not modify circulating homocysteine levels or C-reactive protein.[28]

Isoflavones have been studied in healthy young men and found to reduce plasma homocysteine and to have antioxidant activity.[29] Daily intake of soya isoflavones (80 mg) in high-risk, middle-aged men has been found to reduce blood pressure, total cholesterol and non-HDL cholesterol, while raising HDL cholesterol.[30]

Meta-analyses and systematic reviews

Several systematic reviews and meta-analyses evaluating the effect of soya/isoflavones on lipids and cardiovascular risk factors have now been conducted. A 2003 meta-analysis of 10 studies, which included 21 treatments in total, found that soya-associated isoflavones were not related to changes in LDL or HDL cholesterol.[31]

A 2004 meta-analysis of eight RCTs found that under conditions of identical soya protein intake, high isoflavone intake led to significantly greater decreases in serum LDL cholesterol than low isoflavone intake, demonstrating that isoflavones have LDL cholesterol-lowering effects independent of soya protein.[32]

A 2005 meta-analysis of 23 RCTs published from 1995 to 2002 found that soya protein with isoflavones intact was associated with significant decreases in serum total cholesterol, LDL cholesterol and triacylglycerols and significant increases in serum HDL cholesterol. The reductions in total and LDL cholesterol were larger in men than in women. Initial total cholesterol concentrations had a powerful effect on changes in total and HDL cholesterol, especially in subjects with hypercholesterolaemia. The strongest lowering effects on total cholesterol, LDL cholesterol and triacylglycerol occurred within the short initial period of intervention, while increases in HDL cholesterol were only observed in studies lasting longer than 12 weeks. However, tablets containing extracted soya isoflavones did not have a significant effect on total cholesterol reduction.[33]

The American Heart Association Science Advisory assessed the more recent work on soya protein and isoflavones. In the majority of 22 randomised trials, isolated soya protein with isoflavones (as compared with other proteins) decreased LDL cholesterol concentrations, but the reduction of approximately 3% was very small relative to the large amount of soya protein consumed (averaging 50 g, about half the usual total daily protein intake). No significant effects on HDL cholesterol, triglycerides or blood pressure were evident. Among 19 studies of soya isoflavones, the average effect on LDL cholesterol and other lipid risk factors was nil.[34]

A further critical analysis of investigations into the effect of soya protein and isoflavones on plasma lipoproteins concluded that the data are not quantitatively impressive and raise substantial questions about the clinical importance of the hypocholesterolaemic effects observed.[35]

Cancer

Epidemiological studies have shown that populations with high intakes of soya foods – such as in China, Japan and other Asian countries – usually have a lower risk of cancers of the breast, uterus, prostate and colon.[36,37] Epidemiological evidence from the USA suggests that dietary phyto-oestrogens (of which isoflavones are one type) are associated with a decreased risk of lung cancer.[38] Experimental evidence from in vitro and animal studies on the effects of isoflavones on cancerous cells[39–41] has led to the suggestion that isoflavones could reduce the risk of cancer in humans.

Substantial reduction in risk of breast cancer has been reported among women with high intakes of phyto-oestrogens (as evidenced from urinary excretion).[42] Lower urinary daidzein and genistein concentrations were found in post-menopausal women with recently diagnosed breast cancer compared with controls.[43] Isoflavones appear to protect against cancer by influences on growth factor, malignant cell proliferation and cell differentiation. A more recent study found no evidence that isoflavone treatment reduces colorectal epithelial cell proliferation or the average height of proliferating cells in the caecum, sigmoid colon or rectum, and that it increases cell-proliferating measures in the sigmoid colon.[44] Another study found no evidence that isoflavones alter the concentration of serum prostate-specific antigen (PSA).[45] The American Heart Association Science Advisory has concluded that the efficacy and safety of soya isoflavones for preventing or treating cancer of the breast, endometrium and prostate are not established.[34]

Osteoporosis

There is some evidence from animal studies that soya isoflavones preserve BMD.[46,47] A preliminary study in 66 hypercholesterolaemic, post-menopausal women supplemented with soya protein (providing either 1.39 or 2.2 mg isoflavones/g protein) or placebo for 6 months showed that the higher dose of isoflavones was associated with a significant increase in BMD at the lumbar spine site.[48] The lower dose was not associated with any change in BMD. HDL cholesterol (the beneficial type) increased significantly with both soya treatments.

A later study examined the effects of 24-week consumption of soya protein isolate with isoflavones (80.4 mg daily) on bone loss in peri-menopausal women.[49] The randomised double-blind study showed that soya isoflavones attenuated the reduction in lumbar spine BMD and bone mineral content, both of which occurred in the control group.

More recent studies evaluating the effect of isoflavones on bone have continued to show mixed results. One 3-month trial in 22 post-menopausal women found that isoflavones (61.8 mg daily) could slow down bone turnover as judged by decreased urinary pyridinoline excretion.[50] A further trial in 58 menopausal Japanese women found that isoflavones (40 mg daily) for 8 weeks produced a significant decrease in urinary deoxypyridoline and may therefore have a beneficial effect on bone resorption.[51] A trial in 203 Chinese women (aged 48–62 years) found that isoflavones have a mild, but significant, effect on maintenance of hip bone mineral content. This effect was more marked in women in later menopause or those with lower body weight or lower calcium intake.[52,53] A 1-year supplementation study in post-menopausal Taiwanese women found that isoflavones 100 mg daily were associated with a protective effect on oestrogen-related bone loss and the BMD of lumbar vertebrae 1–3 was increased.[54] Other trials have shown no significant effect of isoflavones on bone turnover markers[55] or calcium retention,[56] while another trial showed that isoflavones do not appear to have oestrogenic effects on markers of bone resorption.[57]

Studies conducted with ipriflavone, a synthetic isoflavone available as a dietary supplement, have found that ipriflavone reduced bone loss in post-menopausal women.[58–61] However, a large multicentre RCT in 472 post-menopausal women (aged 45–75 years) found

that ipriflavone does not prevent bone loss or affect biochemical markers of bone metabolism. In addition, in this study, ipriflavone was found to induce lymphocytopenia in a significant number of women.[62]

Menopausal symptoms

Reduction of oestrogen production in middle-aged women is associated with symptoms of the menopause, such as hot flushes, vaginal dryness and atrophic vaginitis, and is also thought to contribute to the increased risk of CHD and osteoporosis. The main symptoms of the menopause were thought to occur universally, but women in some countries, such as Japan, appear to experience symptoms such as hot flushes less frequently than women in Western countries,[63] yet far fewer Japanese women use HRT post-menopausally.[64]

Several preliminary studies on the effects of administration of soya isoflavones on menopausal symptoms indicated possible benefit. One study involved 58 post-menopausal women with at least 14 hot flushes a week.[65] They received either 45 g soya flour or wheat flour each day as a supplement to their regular diet over 12 weeks in a randomised double-blind design. Hot flushes decreased in both groups (45% in the soya group and 25% in the controls), with a rapid response in the soya group at 6 weeks. Menopausal symptoms also decreased significantly in both groups. The authors concluded that the lack of difference between the two groups could be due either to a strong placebo effect or a decline in symptoms with time.

Another study provides more persuasive evidence. One hundred and forty-five post-menopausal women were randomised to receive either three servings of soya foods daily or control for 12 weeks.[66] Menopausal symptom scores, hot flushes and vaginal dryness decreased by 50, 54 and 60%, respectively, in women on the soya diet. These three parameters also fell in the control group, but only the reduction in menopausal symptom score was significant.

More recently, a double-blind placebo-controlled study involved 104 post-menopausal women who were randomised to receive 60 g soya protein isolate containing 76 mg isoflavones, or a control.[67] In comparison with placebo, subjects on the soya supplement reported a statistically lower mean number of flushes per 24 h after 4, 8 and 12 weeks. By week three, the treated group experienced a 26% reduction in the mean number of hot flushes, a 33% reduction by week 4, and by week 12 a 45% reduction, compared with 30% in the control group.

A study in 241 women reporting vasomotor symptoms suggested that soya protein containing 42 or 58 mg of isoflavones is no more effective than isoflavone-extracted soya protein for improving the number and severity of vasomotor symptoms in peri- and post-menopausal women.[68] In another study, which evaluated the effects of a supplement containing both soya isoflavones and black cohosh, there was no statistically significant effect on climacteric effects compared with placebo in peri-menopausal women experiencing at least five vasomotor symptoms per day.[69] A 6-month study in 79 post-menopausal women comparing a soya extract providing 120 mg isoflavones with 0.625 mg conjugated equine oestrogens and placebo found that there was a decrease in symptoms in both treatment groups and that the effects of soya with isoflavones was similar to that of oestrogen. However, soya isoflavone had no effect on endometrium and vaginal mucosa during the treatment.[70]

Red clover (another source of isoflavones) has also been investigated for an effect on menopausal symptoms. An RCT in 252 women aged 45–60 years compared two red clover supplements (Promensil and Rimostil, providing 82 and 57 mg isoflavones, respectively) with placebo. The reductions in mean hot flush count at 12 weeks were similar for Promensil (5.1), Rimostil (5.4) and placebo (5.0). In comparison with the placebo group, participants in the Promensil group, but not in the Rimostil group, reduced hot flushes more rapidly. Quality of life improvements and adverse events were comparable in the three groups. The authors concluded that neither supplement had a clinically important effect on hot flushes or other symptoms of menopause.[71] Another trial in 60 post-menopausal women found that a red clover supplement (80 mg isoflavones) significantly decreased menopausal symptoms and

had a positive effect on vaginal cytology and triglyceride levels.[72]

Studies evaluating the effect of genistein have found that this compound can have a beneficial effect on menopausal hot flushes.[73,74]

Systematic reviews have considered the effects of soya and red clover isoflavones on menopausal symptoms. A UK systematic review including 10 RCTs that investigated the value of soya preparations for peri-menopausal symptoms found that the results were not conclusive. Four of the trials were positive, but six were negative, with one of these six showing a positive trend. The conclusions were that there is some evidence of benefit for soya preparations in peri-menopausal symptoms, but the heterogeneity of the studies performed to date means it is difficult to make a definitive statement.[75] A US systematic review identified 25 trials involving 2348 participants; the researchers concluded that the available evidence suggests that phyto-oestrogens available as soya foods, soya extracts and red clover extracts do not improve hot flushes or other menopausal symptoms.[76] Evidence from a further systematic review and meta-analysis suggests that frequency of hot flushes is not reduced by red clover isoflavone extracts and results were mixed for soya isoflavone extracts.[77]

Cognitive function

Isoflavones have been evaluated for effects on cognitive function. Results to date have been inconsistent. In a 6-month, double-blind RCT involving 53 women (aged 55–74 years), women taking the isoflavone supplement (110 mg) did consistently better compared with their own baseline scores and placebo responses at 6 months. Isoflavone supplementation had a favourable effect on cognitive function, particularly veral memory, in these post-menopausal women.[78] In a further 6-month trial in 30 women aged over 60, a red clover isoflavone supplement did not appear to have major cognitive effects.[79] A Dutch trial in 202 healthy post-menopausal women aged 60–65 years found that cognitive function and also BMD and plasma lipids did not differ significantly between the isoflavone and placebo groups after a year.[80]

Miscellaneous

Other symptoms and conditions have been a recent focus of trials involving isoflavones. Isoflavones have been found to have no effect on quality of life (health status, life satisfaction, depression) in elderly post-menopausal women.[81] Another study suggested that isoflavones do not have beneficial effects on body composition and physical performance in post-menopausal women.[82] A further trial found that soya isoflavones (100 mg) and 0.625 mg conjugated oestrogen equally lower fasting glucose and insulin levels in post-menopausal women.[83] Another study showed that soya isoflavones may have the potential to reduce specific premenstrual symptoms (e.g. headache, breast tenderness, cramps, swelling).[84]

Conclusion

The effects of isoflavones have been studied in many clinical trials. The scientific literature is conflicting because of inconsistencies in populations studied, lack of appropriate control groups, selection of end points and types of study. There are some data to suggest that isoflavones have beneficial physiological effects, but the clinical implications of these effects are unclear. The consumption of whole soya bean foods and soya bean protein isolates has beneficial effects on lipid markers of cardiovascular risk. The consumption of isolated isoflavones does not appear to have a significant effect on blood lipids or blood pressure, although it may improve endothelial function. For menopausal symptoms there is some evidence that soya bean protein isolates, soya foods or red clover extracts are effective, but soya bean isoflavone extracts may be effective in reducing hot flushes. There is a suggestion, but no conclusive evidence, that isoflavones may have a beneficial effect on bone health. There are too few RCTs to reach conclusions on the effects of isoflavones on breast cancer, colon cancer, diabetes or cognitive function.[85]

Precautions/contraindications

Use with caution in individuals at risk of hormone-dependent cancers.

Pregnancy and breast-feeding

No problems have been reported, but there have not been sufficient studies to guarantee the safety of isoflavones in pregnancy and breast-feeding. Because of their hormonal effects, isoflavones are probably best avoided.

Adverse effects

Soya foods have been consumed in Asian cultures for centuries. However, studies are needed to assess the long-term safety of supplemental soya protein isolates or isoflavone supplements. In addition, isoflavones are oestrogenic – albeit weakly so – and there is some evidence that they may stimulate cancer cell proliferation in women with breast cancer.[86] In a study in healthy women, soya isoflavones did not increase mammographic breast density.[87] Until more is known about these compounds, women with breast cancer should consult their doctors before taking isoflavones.

Interactions

None reported.

Dose

Supplements

Isoflavones are available in the form of tablets and capsules.

The dose is not established. Dietary supplements containing mixed isoflavones provide 50–100 mg in a dose.

Health claims

In 2002, the UK Joint Health Claims Initiative (JHCI: www.jhci.org.uk) proposed a generic health claim for soya protein that may be included on the labels of appropriate foods as follows: "The inclusion of at least 25 g soya protein per day as part of a diet low in saturated fat can help reduce blood cholesterol."

In 1999, the US Food and Drug Administration (FDA: www.fda.gov) approved a similar claim: "Diets low in saturated fat and cholesterol that include 25 g of soy protein a day may reduce the risk of heart disease. One serving of [name of food] provides _____ grams of soy protein."

References

1   Potter JD, Steinmetz K. Vegetables, fruit and phytoestrogens as preventive agents. In: Stewart BW, McGregor D, Kleihues P, eds. *Principles of Chemoprevention.* Lyon, France: International Agency for Research on Cancer, 1996: 61–90.

2   Setchell KDR. Phytoestrogens: the biochemistry, physiology, and implications for human health of soy isoflavones. *Am J Clin Nutr* 1998; 68: S1333–S1346.

3   Anderson JW, Johnstone BW, Cook-Newell ME. Meta-analysis of the effects of soy protein intake on serum lipids. *N Engl J Med* 1995; 333: 276–282.

4   Baum JA, Teng H, Erdman Jr, JW, et al. Long-term intake of soy protein improves blood lipid profiles and increases mononuclear cell low-density-lipoprotein receptor messenger RNA in hypercholesterolemic, postmenopausal women. *Am J Clin Nutr* 1998; 68: 545–551.

5   Gooderham MH, Adlercreutz H, Ojala ST, et al. A soy protein isolate rich in genistein and daidzein and its effects on plasma isoflavone concentration, platelet aggregation, blood lipids and fatty acid composition of plasma phospholipid in normal men. *J Nutr* 1996; 126: 2000–2006.

6   Wong W, O'Brian Smith E, Stuff JE, et al. Cholesterol-lowering effect of soy protein in normocholesterolemic and hypercholesterolemic men. *Am J Clin Nutr* 1998; 68: S1385–1389.

7   Crouse JR III, Morgan T, Terry JG, et al. Soy protein containing isoflavones reduces plasma concentrations of lipids. *Arch Intern Med* 1999; 27; 159: 2070–2076.

8   Teixera SR, Potter SM, Weigel R, et al. Effects of feeding 4 levels of soy protein for 3 and 6 weeks on blood lipids and apolipoproteins in moderately hypercholesterolemic men. *Am J Clin Nutr* 2000; 71: 1077–1084.

9   McVeigh BL, Dillingham BL, Lampe JW, Duncan AM. Effect of soy protein varying in isoflavone content on serum lipids in healthy young men. *Am J Clin Nutr* 2006; 83: 244–251.

10 Merz-Demlow BE, Duncan AM, Wangen KE, et al. Soy isoflavones improve plasma lipids in normocholesterolemic, premenopausal women. *Am J Clin Nutr* 2000; 71: 1462–1469.

11 Tikkanen MJ, Wahala K, Ojala S, et al. Effect of soybean phytoestrogen intake on low density lipoprotein oxidation resistance. *Proc Natl Acad Sci USA* 1998; 17: 95: 3106–3110.

12 Wiseman H, O'Reilly JD, Adlercreutz H, et al. Isoflavone phytoestrogens consumed in soy decrease F_2-isoprostane concentrations and increase resistance of low-density lipoprotein to oxidation in humans. *Am J Clin Nutr* 2000; 72: 395–400.

13 Hodgson JM, Puddey IB, Beilin LJ, et al. Supplementation with isoflavonoid phytoestrogens does not alter serum lipid concentrations: a randomized controlled trial in humans. *J Nutr* 1998; 128: 728–732.

14 Samman S, Lyons Wall PM, Chan GS, et al. The effect of supplementation with isoflavones on plasma lipids and oxidisability of low density lipoprotein in premenopausal women. *Atherosclerosis* 1999; 147: 277–283.

15 Simons LA, von Koningsmark M, Simons J, Celermajer DS. Phytoestrogens do not influence lipoprotein levels or endothelial function in healthy, postmenopausal women. *Am J Cardiol* 2000; 85: 1297–1301.

16 Howes JB, Sullivan D, Lai N, et al. The effects of dietary supplementation with isoflavones from red clover on the lipoprotein profiles of postmenopausal women with mild to moderate hypercholesterolaemia. *Atherosclerosis* 2000; 152: 143–147.

17 Blakesmith SJ, Lyons-Wall PM, George C, et al. Effects of supplementation with purified red clover (*Trifolium pratense*) isoflavones on plasma lipids and insulin resistance in healthy premenopausal women. *Br J Nutr* 2003; 89: 467–474.

18 Atkinson C, Oosthuizen W, Scollen S, et al. Modest protective effects of isoflavones from a red clover-derived dietary supplement on cardiovascular risk factors in perimenopausal woman, and evidence of an interaction with ApoE genotype in 49–65 year old women. *J Nutr* 2004; 134: 1759–1764.

19 Howes JB, Tran D, Brilliante D, Howed LG. Effects of dietary supplementation with isoflavones from red clover on ambulatory blood pressure and endothelial function in postmenopausal type 2 diabetes. *Diabetes Obes Metab* 2003; 5: 325–332.

20 Engelman HM, Alekel DL, Hanson LN, et al. Blood lipid and oxidative stress responses to soy protein with isoflavones and phytic acid in postmenopausal women. *Am J Clin Nutr* 2005; 81: 590–596.

21 Hutchins AM, McIver JE, Johnston CS. Soy isoflavones and ascorbic acid supplementation alone or in combination minimally affect plasma lipid peroxides in healthy postmenopausal women. *J Am Diet Assoc* 2005; 105: 1134–1137.

22 Kreijkamp-Kaspers S, Kok L, Bots ML, *et al*. Randomized controlled trial of the effects of soy protein containing isoflavones on vascular function in postmenopausal women. *Am J Clin Nutr* 2005; 81: 189–195.

23 Lissin LW, Okra R, Lakshmi S, Cooke JP. Isoflavones improve vascular reactivity in postmenopausal women with hypercholesesterolaemia. *Vasc Med* 2004; 9: 26–30.

24 Hermansen K, Hansen B, Jacobsen R, *et al*. Effects of soy supplementation on blood lipids and arterial function in hypercholesterolaemic subjects. *Eur J Clin Nutr* 2005; 59: 843–850.

25 Colacurci N, Chiantera A, Fornaro F, *et al*. Effects of soy isoflavones on endothelial function in healthy postmenopausal women. *Menopause* 2005; 12: 299–307.

26 Hall WL, Vafeiadou K, Hallund J, *et al*. Soy-isoflavone-enriched foods and inflammatory biomarkers of cardiovascular disease risk in postmenopausal women: interactions with genotype and equol production. *Am J Clin Nutr* 2005; 82: 1260–1268.

27 Crisafulli A, Altavilla D, Marini H, *et al*. Effects of the phytoestrogen genistein on cardiovascular risk factors in postmenopausal women. *Menopause* 2005; 12: 186–192.

28 D'Anna R, Baviera G, Corrado F, *et al*. The effect of the phytoestrogen genistein and hormone replacement therapy on homocysteine and C-reactive protein level in postmenopausal women. *Acta Obstet Gynecol Scand* 2005; 84: 474–477.

29 Chen CY, Bakhiet RM, Hart V, Holtzman G. Isoflavones improve plasma homocysteine status and antioxidant defense system in healthy young men at rest but do not ameliorate oxidative stress induced by 80% VO2pk exercise. *Ann Nutr Metab* 2005; 49: 33–41.

30 Sagara M, Kanda T, Njelekera M, *et al*. Effects of dietary intake of soy protein and isoflavones on cardiovascular risk factors in high-risk, middle-aged men in Scotland. *J Am Coll Nutr* 2004; 23: 85–91.

31 Weggermans RM, Trautwein EA. Relation between soya-associated isoflavones and LDL and HDL cholesterol concentrations in humans: a meta-analysis. *Eur J Clin Nutr* 2003; 57: 940–946.

32 Zhuo XG, Melby MK, Watanabe S. Soy isoflavone intake lowers serum LDL cholesterol: a meta-analysis of 8 randomized controlled trials in humans. *J Nutr* 2004; 134: 2395–2400.

33 Zhan S, Ho SC. Meta-analysis of the effects of soy protein containing isoflavones on the lipid profile. *Am J Clin Nutr* 2005; 81: 397–408.

34 Sacks FM, Lichtenstein A, Van Horn L, *et al*. Soy protein, isoflavones and cardiovascular health. An American Heart Association Science Advisory for Professionals from the Nutrition Committee.

35 Dewell A, Hollenbeck PL, Hollenbeck CB. Clinical review: a critical evaluation of the role of soy protein and isoflavone supplementation in the control of plasma cholesterol concentrations. *J Clin Endocrinol Metab* 2006; 91: 772–780 (Epub ahead of print 29 Dec 2005).

36 Messina MJ, Persky V, Setchell KD, *et al*. Soy intake and cancer risk: a review of the *in vitro* and *in vivo* data. *Nutr Cancer* 1994; 21: 113–131.

37 Goodman MT, Wilkens LR, Hankin JH, *et al*. Association of soy and fiber consumption with the risk of endometrial cancer. *Am J Epidemiol* 1997; 146: 294–306.

38 Schabath MB, Hernandez LM, Wu X, *et al*. Dietary phytoestrogens and lung cancer risk. *JAMA* 2005; 294: 1493–1504.

39 Barnes S. Effect of genistein on *in vitro* and *in vivo* models of cancer. *J Nutr* 1995; 125: S777–S783.

40 Hawrylewicz EJ, Zapata JJ, Blair WH. Soy and experimental cancer. *J Nutr* 1995; 125: S698–S708.

41 Kennedy AR. The evidence for soybean products as cancer preventive agents. *J Nutr* 1995; 125: S733–S743.

42 Ingram D, Sanders K, Kolybaba M, Lopez D. Case-control study of phyto-estrogens and breast cancer. *Lancet* 1997; 350: 990–994.

43 Murkies A, Dalais FS, Briganti EM, *et al*. Phytoestrogens and breast cancer in postmenopausal women: a case control study. *Menopause* 2000; 7: 289–296.

44 Adams KF, Lampe PD, Newton KM, *et al*. Soy protein containing isoflavones does not decrease colorectal epithelial cell proliferation in a randomized controlled trial. *Am J Clin Nutr* 2005; 82: 620–626.

45 Adams KF, Chen C, Newton KM, *et al*. Soy isoflavones do not modulate prostate-specific antigen concentrations in older men in a randomized controlled trial. *Cancer Epidemiol Biomarkers Prev* 2004; 13: 644–648.

46 Arjmandi BH, Alekel L, Hollis BW, *et al*. Dietary soybean protein prevents bone loss in an ovariectomized rat model of osteoporosis. *J Nutr* 1996; 126: 161–167.

47 Anderson JJ, Ambrose WW, Garner SC. Biphasic effects of genistein on bone tissue in the ovariectomized, lactating rat model. *Proc Soc Exp Biol Med* 1998; 217: 345–350.

48 Potter SM, Baum JA, Teng H, *et al*. Soy protein and isoflavones: their effects on blood lipids and bone mineral density in postmenopausal women. *Am J Clin Nutr* 1998; 68: S1375–S1379.

49 Alekel DL, St Germain A, Peterson CT, *et al*. Isoflavone-rich soy protein isolate attenuates bone

Circulation 2006; 113: 1034 (Epub ahead of print 17 Jan 2006).

loss in the lumbar spine of perimenopausal women. *Am J Clin Nutr* 2000; 72: 844–852.

50 Uesugi T, Toda T, Okuhira T, Chen JT. Evidence of estrogenic effect by the three-month intervention of isoflavone on vaginal maturation and bone metabolism in early postmenopausal women. *Endocr J* 2003; 50: 613–619.

51 Useugi S, Watanabe S, Ishiwata N, *et al*. Effects of isoflavone supplements on bone metabolic markers and climacteric symptoms in Japanese women. *Biofactors* 2004; 22: 221–228.

52 Chen YM, Ho SC, Lam SS, *et al*. Beneficial effect of soy isoflavones on bone mineral content was modified by years since menopause, body weight and calcium intake: a double-blind, randomized, controlled trial. *Menopause* 2004; 11: 246–254.

53 Chen YM, Ho SC, Lam SS, *et al*. Soy isoflavones have a favourable effect on bone mass in Chinese postmenopausal women with lower bone mass: a double-blind, randomized, controlled trial. *J Clin Endocrinol Metab* 2003; 88: 4740–4747.

54 Hui-Ying H, Hsiao-Ping Y, Hui-Ting Y, *et al*. One-year isoflavone supplementation prevents early postmenopausal bone loss but without a dose-dependent effect. *J Nutr Biochem* 2006; 17: 509–517.

55 Schult TM, Ensrud KE, Blackwell T, *et al*. Effects of isoflavones on lipids and bone turnover markers in menopausal women. *Maturitas* 2004; 48: 209–218.

56 Spence LA, Lipscomb ER, Cadogan J, *et al*. The effect of soy protein and soy isoflavones on calcium metabolism in postmenopausal women: a randomized crossover study. *Am J Clin Nutr* 2005; 81: 916–922.

57 Dalais FS, Ebeling PR, Kotsopoulos D, *et al*. The effects of soy protein containing isoflavones on lipids and indices of bone resorption in postmenopausal women. *Clin Endocrinol* 2003; 58: 704–709.

58 Agnusdei D, Crepaldi G, Isaia G, *et al*. A double-blind, placebo-controlled diet of ipriflavone for prevention of postmenopausal spinal bone loss. *Calcif Tissue Int* 1997; 61: 142–147.

59 Gambacciani M, Ciaponi M, Cappagli B, *et al*. Effects of combined low dose of the isoflavone derivative ipriflavone and estrogen replacement on bone mineral density and metabolism in postmenopausal women. *Maturitas* 1997; 28: 75–81.

60 Ohta H, Komukai S, Makita K, *et al*. Effects of 1-year ipriflavone treatment on bone mineral density and bone metabolic markers in postmenopausal women with low bone mass. *Horm Res* 1999; 51: 178–183.

61 Katase K, Kato T, Hirai Y, *et al*. Effects of ipriflavone on bone loss following a bilateral ovariectomy and menopause: a randomized placebo-controlled study. *Calcif Tissue Int* 2001; 69: 73–77.

62 Alexandersen P, Toussaint A, Chistiansen C, *et al*. Ipriflavone in the treatment of postmenopausal osteoporosis: a randomized controlled trial. *JAMA* 2001; 285: 1482–148.

63 Lock M. Contested meanings of the menopause. *Lancet* 1991; 337: 1270–1272.

64 Kurzer MS, Xu X. Dietary phytoestrogens. *Ann Rev Nutr* 1997; 17: 353–381.

65 Murkies AL, Lombard C, Strauss BJG, *et al*. Dietary flour supplementation decreases post-menopausal hot flushes: effect of soy and wheat. *Maturitas* 1995; 21: 189–195.

66 Brzezinski A, Aldercreutz H, Shaoul R, *et al*. Short-term effects of phytoestrogen-rich diet on postmenopausal women. *J North Am Menopause Soc* 1997; 4: 89–94.

67 Albertazzi P, Pansini F, Bonaccorsi G, *et al*. The effect of dietary soy supplementation on hot flushes. *Obstet Gynecol* 1998; 91: 6–11.

68 Burke GL, Legault C, Anthony M, *et al*. Soy protein and isoflavone effects on vasomotor symptoms in peri- and postmenopausal women: the Soy Estrogen Alternative Study. *Menopause* 2003; 10: 147–153.

69 Verhoeven MO, van der Mooren MJ, van de Weijer PH, *et al*. Effect of a combination of isoflavones and Actaea racemosa Linnaeus on climacteric symptoms in healthy symptomatic perimenopausal women: a 12-week randomized, placebo controlled, double-blind study. *Menopause* 2005; 12: 412–20.

70 Kaari C, Haidar MA, Junior JM, *et al*. Randomized clinical trial comparing conjugated equine estrogens and isoflavones in postmenopausal women: a pilot study. *Maturitas* 2006; 53: 49–58.

71 Tice JA, Ettinger B, Ensrud K, *et al*. Phytoestrogen supplements for the treatment of hot flashes: the Isoflavone Clover Extract (ICE) Study: a randomized controlled trial. *JAMA* 2003; 290: 207–214.

72 Hidalgo LA, Chedraui PA, Morocho N, *et al*. The effect of red clover isoflavones on menopausal symptoms, lipids and vaginal cytology in menopausal women: a randomized, double-blind, placebo-controlled study. *Gynecol Endocrinol* 2005; 21: 257–264.

73 Crisafulli A, Marini II, Bitto A, *et al*. Effects of genistein on hot flushes in early postmenopausal women: a randomized, double-blind EPT- and placebo-controlled study. *Menopause* 2004; 11: 400–404.

74 Albertazzi P, Steel SA, Bottazzi M. Effect of genistein on bone markers and hot flushes. *Climacteric* 2005; 8: 371–379.

75 Huntley AL, Ernst E. Soy for the treatment of perimenopausal symptoms – a systematic review. *Maturitas* 2004; 47: 1–9.

76 Krebs EE, Ensrud KE, MacDonald R, Wilt TJ. Phytoestrogens for treatment of menopausal symptoms:

a systematic review. *Obstet Gynecol* 2004; 104: 824–836.

77 Nelson HD, Vesco KK, Haney E, *et al*. Non-hormonal therapies for menopausal hot flashes. *JAMA* 2006; 295: 2057–2071.

78 Kritz-Silverstein D, Von Muhlen D, Barrett-Connor E, Bressel MA. Isoflavones and cognitive function in older women: the SOy and Postmenopausal Health in Ageing (SOPHIA) Study. *Menopause* 2003; 10: 196–202.

79 Howes JB, Bray K, Lorenz L, *et al*. The effects of dietary supplementation with isoflavones from red clover on cognitive function in postmenopausal women. *Climacteric* 2004; 7: 70–77.

80 Kreijkamp-Jaspers S, Kok L, Grobbee DL, *et al*. Effect of soy protein containing isoflavones on cognitive function, bone mineral density, and plasma lipids in postmenopausal women: a randomized controlled trial. *JAMA* 2004; 292: 65–74.

81 Kok L, Kreijkamp-Kaspers S, Grobbee DE, *et al*. A randomized placebo-controlled trial on the effects of soy protein containing isoflavones on quality of life in postmenopausal women. *Menopause* 2005; 12: 56–62.

82 Kok L, Kreijkamp-Kaspers S, Grobbee DE, *et al*. Soy isoflavones, body composition, and physical performance. *Maturitas* 2005; 52: 102–110.

83 Cheng SY, Shaw NS, Tsai KS, Chen CY. The hypoglycemic effects of soy isoflavones on post-menopausal women. *J Women's Health (Larchmt)* 2004; 13: 1080–1086.

84 Bryant M, Cassidy A, Hill C, *et al*. Effect of consumption of soy isoflavones on behavioural, somatic and affective symptoms in women with premenstrual symptoms. *Br J Nutr* 2005; 93: 731–739.

85 Cassidy A, Albertazzi A, Lise Nielsen I, *et al*. Critical review of health effects of soybean phyto-oestrogens in post-menopausal women. *Proc Nutr Soc* 2006; 65: 76–92.

86 McMichael-Phillips DF, Harding C, Morton M, *et al*. Effects of soy-protein supplementation on epithelial proliferation in the histologically normal human breast. *Am J Clin Nutr* 1998; 68: S1431–S1436.

87 Atkinson C, Warren RM, Sala E, *et al*. Red-clover derived isoflavones and mammographic breast density: a double-blind, randomized, placebo-controlled trial (ISRCTN42940165). *Breast Cancer Res* 2004; 6: R170–R179.

Kelp

Description

Kelp is a long-stemmed seaweed, derived from various species (e.g. *Fucus*, *Laminaria*) of brown algae, known as a preparation of dried seaweed of various species.

Constituents

Kelp is a source of several minerals and trace elements, especially iodine.

Possible uses

Kelp is claimed to be a slimming aid (some herbal products containing kelp are licensed in the UK for this purpose). Its main use is as a source of iodine.

Precautions/contraindications

Kelp should be avoided in patients with thyroid disease, unless recommended by a doctor. It may be contaminated with toxic trace elements (e.g. antimony, arsenic, lead, strontium).

Pregnancy and breast-feeding

Avoid (because of contaminants – see Precautions).

Adverse effects

A few case reports have linked hyperthyroidism to kelp ingestion.[1-5] Hypothyroidism may also be more prevalent in people who consume excess amounts of iodine in the form of kelp.[6] A US guideline on detection of thyroid dysfunction notes that patients who ingest iodine compounds (e.g. kelp) are at increased risk of developing thyroid dysfunction.[7] Nausea and diarrhoea have been reported occasionally.

Interactions

See Iodine monograph.

Dose

Kelp is available in the form of capsules, tablets, powder and liquid.

The dose is not established. Dietary supplements contain 200–500 mg kelp. The iodine content is variable and not always quoted on the label.

References

1   Shilo S, Hirsch HJ. Iodine-induced hyperthyroidism in a patient with a normal thyroid gland. *Postgrad Med J* 1986; 62: 661–662.
2   Ishizuki Y, Yamauchi K, Miura Y. Transient thyrotoxicosis induced by Japanese kombu. *Nippon Naibunpi Gakkai Zasshi* 1989; 65: 91–98.
3   de Smet PA, Stricker BH, Wilderink F, Wiersinga WM. Hyperthyroidism during treatment with kelp tablets. *Ned Tijdschr Geneeskd* 1990; 134: 1058–1059.
4   Hartmann AA. Hyperthyroidism during administration of kelp tablets. *Ned Tijdschr Geneeskd* 1990; 134: 1373.
5   Eliason BC. Transient hyperthyroidism in a patient taking dietary supplements containing kelp. *J Am Board Fam Pract* 1998; 11: 478–480.
6   Konno N, Iizuka N, Kawasaki K, *et al*. Screening for thyroid dysfunction in adults residing in Hokkaido, Japan: in relation to urinary iodide concentration and thyroid autoantibodies. *Hokkaido Igaku Zasshi* 1994; 69: 614–626.
7   Landenson PW, Singer PA, Ain KB, *et al*. American Thyroid Association Guidelines for Detection of Thyroid Dysfunction. *Arch Intern Med* 2000; 160: 1573–1575.

Lecithin

Description

Lecithin is a phospholipid and is known as phosphatidylcholine.

Constituents

Lecithin is composed of phosphatidyl esters, mainly phosphatidylcholine, phosphatidylethanolamine, phosphatidylserine and phosphatidylinositol. It also contains varying amounts of other substances such as fatty acids, triglycerides and carbohydrates. One teaspoon (3.5 g) lecithin granules provides on average: energy 117 kJ (28 kcal), phosphatidyl choline 750 mg, phosphatidyl inositol 500 mg, choline 100 mg, inositol 100 mg, phosphorus 110 mg.

Human requirements

Lecithin is not an essential component of the diet. It is synthesised from choline.

Action

Lecithin is a source of choline (see Choline) and inositol. It is an essential component of cell membranes and a precursor to acetylcholine.

Dietary sources

Soya beans, peanuts, liver, meat, eggs.

Metabolism

About 50% of ingested lecithin enters the thoracic duct intact. The rest is degraded to glycerophosphorylcholine in the intestine, and then to choline in the liver. Plasma choline levels reflect lecithin intake.

Deficiency

Not established.

Possible uses

Lecithin is claimed to be beneficial in the treatment of disease related to impaired cholinergic function (see Choline). It has also been claimed to be of benefit in lowering serum cholesterol levels and improving memory. It is sometimes taken for dementia and Alzheimer's disease.

Cholesterol

An open clinical trial in the 1970s showed that oral lecithin in large doses (20–30 g daily) led to a significant reduction in cholesterol concentration in one out of the three healthy subjects studied and three out of the seven people with hypercholesterolaemia.[1]

However, in a double-blind study, 20 hyperlipidaemic men were randomised to receive frozen yoghurt, frozen yoghurt with 20 g soya bean lecithin or frozen yoghurt with 17 g sunflower oil. Sunflower oil was used to control for the increased intake in energy and linoleic acid from the lecithin. Lecithin treatment had no independent effect on serum lipoprotein or plasma fibrinogen levels in this group of men.[2]

A review of 24 papers examining the effect of consuming lecithin on serum cholesterol raised concern about the small size and lack of control groups in many of the studies. The authors concluded that there was no evidence for a specific effect of lecithin on serum cholesterol independent of its linoleic acid content or secondary changes in food intake. The observed lecithin-induced hypocholesterolaemic effects in the studies were artefacts caused by the manner and design of the data analysis, were mediated by dietary changes or were due to the linoleic acid present in lecithin.[3]

Alzheimer's disease

A double-blind, placebo-controlled crossover study in 11 outpatients with Alzheimer's disease found that lecithin 10 g three times a day for 3 months was associated with an improvement in tests of learning ability, but there was no improvement in any of the psychological tests used.[4]

Two further double-blind studies (one in patients with Alzheimer's disease,[5] one in normal adults[6]) showed no effect of lecithin on memory.

Another double-blind RCT in 53 subjects with probable Alzheimer's disease involved the use of lecithin and tacrine or lecithin and placebo for 36 weeks. No clinically relevant improvement was found in any of the groups over 36 weeks.[7]

A Cochrane review investigating the efficacy of lecithin in the treatment of dementia or cognitive impairment found 12 RCTs involving patients with Alzheimer's disease (265 patients), Parkinsonian dementia (21 patients) and subjective memory problems (90 patients). No trials reported any clear benefit of Alzheimer's disease or Parkinsonian dementia. A dramatic result in favour of lecithin was obtained in a trial of subjects with subjective memory problems. The authors concluded that evidence from randomised trials does not support the use of lecithin in the treatment of dementia. A moderate effect could not be ruled out, but they concluded that results from the small trials to date do not indicate priority for a large randomised trial.[8]

Conclusion

Controlled clinical trials have provided no evidence that lecithin lowers cholesterol or helps to improve memory in patients with Alzheimer's disease. Claims for the value of lecithin in lowering blood pressure and also in hepatitis, gallstones, psoriasis and eczema are unsubstantiated. Further trials are needed to assess the role of lecithin.

Precautions/contraindications

None known.

Pregnancy and breast-feeding

No problems have been reported, but there have not been sufficient studies to guarantee the safety of lecithin (in amounts greater than those found in foods) in pregnancy and breast-feeding.

Adverse effects

None reported.

Interactions

None reported.

Dose

Lecithin is available in the form of tablets, capsules and powder. Lecithin supplements provide between 20 and 90% phosphatidylcholine (depending on the product).

The dose is not established. On current evidence, lecithin is unlikely to be useful. Product manufacturers recommend 1200–2400 mg daily.

References

1 Simons LA, Hickie JB, Ruys J. Treatment of hypercholesterolaemia with oral lecithin. *Aust NZ J Med* 1977; 7: 262–266.
2 Oosthuizen W, Vorster HH, Vermaak WJ, *et al*. Lecithin has no effect on serum lipoprotein, plasma fibrinogen and macromolecular protein complex levels in hyperlipidaemic men in a double-blind controlled study. *Eur J Clin Nutr* 1998; 52: 419–424.
3 Knuiman JT, Beynen AC, Katan MB. Lecithin intake and serum cholesterol. *Am J Clin Nutr* 1989; 49: 266–268.
4 Etienne P, Dastoor D, Gauthier S, *et al*. Alzheimer disease: lack of effect of lecithin treatment for 3 months. *Neurology* 1981; 31: 1552–1554.
5 Brinkman SD, Smith RC, Meyer JS, *et al*. Lecithin and memory training in suspected Alzheimer's disease. *J Gerontol* 1982; 37: 4–9.

6   Harris CM, Dysken MW, Fovall P, Davis JM. Effect of lecithin on memory in normal adults. *Am J Psychiatry* 1983; 140: 1010–1012.

7   Maltby N, Broe GA, Creasey H, *et al*. Efficacy of tacrine and lecithin in mild to moderate Alzheimer's disease: double-blind trial. *BMJ* 1994; 308: 879–883.

8   Higgins JPT, Flicker L. Lecithin for dementia and cognitive impairment. Cochrane database, issue 4, 2000. London: Macmillan.

Magnesium

Description

Magnesium is an essential mineral. It is the second most abundant intracellular cation in the body.

Human requirements

See Table 1 for Dietary Reference Values for magnesium.

Dietary intake

In the UK, the average diet provides: for males, 336 mg daily; for females, 250 mg daily.

Action

Magnesium is an essential cofactor for enzymes requiring ATP (these are involved in glycolysis, fatty acid oxidation and amino acid metabolism). It is also required for the synthesis of RNA and replication of DNA; neuromuscular transmission; and calcium metabolism.

Dietary sources

See Table 2 for dietary sources of magnesium.

Metabolism

Absorption

Absorption of magnesium occurs principally in the jejunum and ileum by active carrier-mediated processes (partly dependent on vitamin D and parathyroid hormone) and by diffusion.

Distribution

Magnesium is widely distributed in the soft tissues and skeleton.

Elimination

Excretion is largely via the urine (magnesium homeostasis is controlled mainly by the kidneys), with unabsorbed and endogenously secreted magnesium in the faeces. Small amounts are excreted in saliva and breast milk.

Bioavailability

Bioavailability appears to be enhanced by vitamin D, but is decreased by phytates and non-starch polysaccharides (dietary fibre).

Deficiency

Signs and symptoms include hypocalcaemia and hypokalaemia; muscle spasm, tremor and tetany; personality changes, lethargy and apathy; convulsions, delirium and coma; anorexia, nausea, vomiting, abdominal pain and paralytic ileus; cardiac arrhythmias, tachycardia and sudden cardiac death.

Possible uses

Magnesium has been investigated for a role in CVD (including hypertension), diabetes mellitus, migraine, osteoporosis and PMS.

Cardiovascular disease

Magnesium deficiency has been associated with CVD, and some epidemiological data have suggested a reduced mortality from coronary artery disease in populations living in hard water areas compared with those living in soft water areas.

Table 1 Dietary Reference Values for magnesium (mg/day)

EU RDA = 14 mg

Age	UK				USA		WHO RNI
	LNRI	EAR	RNI	EVM	RDA	TUL	
0–3 months	30	40	55		30	–	26–36
4–6 months	40	50	60		30	–	26–36
7–9 months	45	60	75		75	–	54
10–12 months	45	60	80		75	–	54
1–3 years	50	65	85		80	65	60
4–6 years	70	90	120		–	–	76
4–8 years	–	–	–		130	110	–
7–10 years	115	150	200		170	–	100[a]
9–13 years	–	–	–	–	240	350	–
Males							
11–14 years	180	230	280		–	–	230[b]
14–18 years	–	–	–		410	350	230
15–18 years	190	250	280		–	–	–
19–50+ years	190	250	300	300	–	–	260[1]
19–30 years	–	–	–		400	350	–
31–70+ years	–	–	–		420	350	–
Females							
11–14 years	180	230	280		–	–	220[b]
14–18 years	–	–	–		360	350	220
15–18 years	190	250	300		310	–	–
19–50 years	190	250	300	300	280	–	260[2]
50+ years	150	200	270	300	280	–	–
19–30 years	–	–	–		310	350	–
31–70+ years	–	–	–		320	350	–
Pregnancy	*	*	*		360–400	350	220
Lactation			+50		320–360	350	270

* No increment.
[a] 7–9 years. [b] 10–14 years.
[1] > 65 years = 224 mg. [2] > 65 years = 190 mg.
EVM = Likely safe daily intake from supplements alone.
TUL = Tolerable Upper Intake Level.

Other data, however, have indicated no such association, and a large cohort study[1] in which 2512 older men were followed for 10 years also provided no evidence of a protective role for magnesium in CHD.

Marginal magnesium status has been implicated in myocardial infarction, but reduced serum magnesium levels found in some myocardial infarct patients may be a result of the infarction rather than the cause of it. However, one double-blind placebo-controlled study in patients with acute myocardial infarction showed reduced serum triglyceride concentrations and tendencies towards increased HDL cholesterol concentrations after oral magnesium supplementation.[2]

Some controlled studies have suggested that intravenous magnesium given early after

Table 2   Dietary sources of magnesium

Food portion	Magnesium content (mg)
Breakfast cereals	
1 bowl All-Bran (45 g)	*90*
1 bowl Bran Flakes (45 g)	*50*
1 bowl Corn Flakes (30 g)	5
1 bowl muesli (95 g)	*90*
2 pieces Shredded Wheat	*50*
2 Weetabix	*50*
Cereal products	
Bread, brown, 2 slices	40
white, 2 slices	15
wholemeal, 2 slices	*60*
1 chapati	30
Pasta, brown, boiled (150 g)	*60*
white, boiled (150 g)	25
Rice, brown, boiled (165 g)	*60*
white, boiled (165 g)	15
Milk and dairy products	
½ pint milk, whole, semi-skimmed or skimmed	35
1 pot yoghurt (150 g)	30
Cheese (50 g)	12
1 egg, size 2 (60 g)	10
Meat and fish	
Meat, cooked (100 g)	25
Liver, lambs, cooked (90 g)	20
Kidney, lambs, cooked (75 g)	20
White fish, cooked (150 g)	30
Pilchards, canned (105 g)	40
Sardines, canned (70 g)	35
Shrimps (80 g)	*49*
Tuna, canned (95 g)	30
Vegetables	
Green vegetables, average, boiled (100 g)	20
Potatoes, boiled (150 g)	20
1 small can baked beans (200 g)	*60*
Lentils, kidney beans or other pulses (105 g)	50
Fruit	
1 banana	35
1 orange	20
Nuts	
20 almonds	*50*
10 Brazil nuts	*80*
30 hazelnuts	*50*
30 peanuts	*70*

Note: Hard drinking water may contribute significantly to intake.
Excellent sources (**bold**); good sources (*italics*).

suspected myocardial infarction could reduce the frequency of serious arrhythmias and mortality. However, magnesium has been given as a prescription medicine in these cases and not as a dietary supplement.

A more recent trial in 187 people found that magnesium 365 mg daily for 6 months increased exercise duration time compared with placebo, and decreased exercise-induced chest pain. Quality of life parameters significantly improved in the magnesium group. The authors concluded that these findings suggest that oral magnesium supplementation for 6 months in patients with coronary artery disease results in a significant improvement in exercise tolerance, exercise-induced chest pain and quality of life, suggesting a mechanism whereby magnesium could beneficially alter outcomes in patients with coronary artery disease.[3]

Blood pressure

There is some evidence that magnesium reduces blood pressure.[4] A 20 mmol increase in daily magnesium intake resulted in a diastolic blood pressure fall of 3.4 mmHg in a trial in Dutch women.[5] A reduction in blood pressure occurred with a low-sodium, high-potassium, high-magnesium salt in older patients with mild to moderate hypertension and suggested that the increased magnesium intake could have contributed to the fall in blood pressure.[6]

However, another study[7] showed that magnesium supplementation did not have an additive hypotensive effect in mild hypertensive subjects on a reduced sodium intake. Another group,[8] using a double-blind randomised crossover design, detected no fall in blood pressure with magnesium supplementation, despite a significant increase in plasma magnesium concentration.

More recent double-blind placebo-controlled trials[9,10] have shown no effect of magnesium supplementation (300–360 mg) on blood pressure in healthy subjects and those with mild to moderate hypertension.[11]

A meta-analysis of 20 randomised trials involving 1220 subjects found that magnesium supplementation produced a modest dose-dependent blood pressure lowering effect.[12] For each 250 mg daily increase in magnesium intake, systolic blood pressure fell by a further

4.3 mmHg and diastolic blood pressure by 2.3 mmHg.

Diabetes mellitus

Magnesium modulates glucose transport across cell membranes, and is a cofactor in various pathways involving enzymatic oxidation. Individuals with diabetes, especially those with glycosuria and ketoacidosis, may have excessive urinary losses of magnesium.[13,14] Hypomagnesaemia is common in these patients and can potentially cause insulin resistance.[15] One study has shown that insulin secretory capacity improved with dietary magnesium supplementation for 4 weeks.[16] The effect of diabetes on tissue content of magnesium is variable and cannot always be predicted from serum magnesium measurements. Epidemiologically, magnesium deficiency has been associated with diabetic neuropathy,[17] and although there is no evidence to indicate that magnesium supplementation can alter this complication, the magnesium status of patients at risk of magnesium depletion (e.g. those on thiazides) should be assessed. However, monitoring is difficult and a dose for patients with diabetes mellitus has not been established.

In an open trial, 11 patients with type 1 diabetes and persistently low erythrocyte magnesium levels were given 450 mg magnesium following an intravenous loading dose of magnesium. During intravenous loading, plasma magnesium decreased and erythrocyte magnesium increased. Supplementation did not normalise magnesium status, and there were no significant changes in glycated haemoglobin or serum lipid levels. The authors concluded that chronic magnesium depletion may occur in type 1 diabetes and that it is difficult to replete and maintain body stores.[18]

In a double-blind, placebo-controlled trial, 128 Brazilian patients with type 2 diabetes were randomised to receive 497 mg magnesium, 994 mg magnesium or placebo. At the start of the study, 47.7% of the patients had low plasma magnesium and 31.1% had low intramononuclear magnesium levels. Intracellular magnesium was significantly lower than in the normal population and was lower in those with peripheral neuropathy than those without. However, there was no correlation between plasma and intracellular magnesium and glycaemic control. In the groups on placebo and lower-dose magnesium, neither a change in plasma nor intracellular magnesium occurred and there was no change in glycaemic control. The higher dose of magnesium was associated with an increase in plasma and intracellular magnesium and a significant fall in fructosamine.[19]

In a placebo-controlled (not blinded) study, involving 50 patients with type 2 diabetes, supplementation with 360 mg magnesium daily over 3 months increased plasma magnesium and urinary magnesium excretion, but had no effect on glycaemic control or lipid concentration.[20]

More recent trials have shown that oral magnesium supplementation improves insulin sensitivity and metabolic control in type 2 diabetic patients with decreased serum magnesium levels,[21] and also improves insulin sensitivity in non-diabetic subjects with decreased magnesium levels.[22]

Premenstrual syndrome

Reduced magnesium levels have been reported in women affected by PMS. An Italian double-blind randomised study[23] in 32 women showed that a supplement of 360 mg magnesium daily improved premenstrual symptoms related to mood changes. More recently, a randomised, double-blind, placebo-controlled study[24] in 38 women showed no effect of magnesium supplementation (200 mg daily) in the first month, but symptoms including weight gain, swelling of extremities, breast tenderness and abdominal bloating, improved during the second month. A further study[25] in 44 women lasting 1 month showed that magnesium 200 mg daily plus vitamin B_6 50 mg daily produced a modest effect on anxiety-related premenstrual symptoms.

Migraine

There is some evidence that magnesium supplementation is effective in migraine, but results from studies are equivocal. Thus, oral magnesium was effective in reducing the frequency of migraine in a 12-week, placebo-controlled, double-blind study.[26] There was also a reduction in the average duration of pain and need for acute medication, although these changes were not significant. However, in another similar study, magnesium had no effect.[27] A further trial compared a placebo containing riboflavin 25 mg with a treatment containing riboflavin 400 mg, magnesium 300 mg and feverfew 100 mg. The placebo response in this trial was high and there was no difference between placebo and treatment.[28]

Osteoporosis

Magnesium is a constituent of bone, and supplementation has been shown to increase bone density in individuals with osteoporosis. Increased magnesium intake is associated with a lower decline in BMD after the menopause.[29] Supplements have been shown to decrease markers of bone turnover in young men,[30] but not young women.[31] Bone density increased in patients with gluten-sensitive enteropathy and associated osteoporosis,[32] and also in menopausal women[33] who were given oral magnesium.

Athletes

Magnesium supplementation has been suggested to improve athletic performance. In one double-blind, placebo-controlled study,[34] magnesium (507 mg versus 246 mg daily) improved muscular strength, and in another similar study,[35] swimming, running and cycling performance was improved. However, in a 2-week study,[36] athletes taking magnesium 500 mg daily did not demonstrate improved performance or reduced muscle tiredness.

Cancer

Epidemiological studies have shown an association between magnesium and colon cancer in women. A prospective cohort study among 61 433 Swedish women aged 40–75 years found an inverse association of magnesium intake with colorectal cancer.[37] Another prospective cohort study among 35 196 Iowa women aged 55–69 years found an inverse association between magnesium intake and colon cancer, but this association was largely lacking for rectal cancer.[38]

Pregnancy

Many women, particularly those from disadvantaged backgrounds, have intakes of magnesium below recommended levels. Magnesium supplementation has been investigated for possible benefit in reducing foetal growth retardation and pre-eclampsia, and increasing birth weight. A Cochrane review found seven trials involving 2689 women. Six of these trials randomly allocated women to either oral magnesium or control, while the largest trial with 985 women had a cluster design where randomisation was according to a study centre. The analysis was conducted with and without this trial. When all seven trials were included, oral magnesium from the 25th week of pregnancy was associated with lower frequency of pre-term birth, a lower frequency of low birth weight, fewer small for gestational age infants and fewer cases of antepartum haemorrhage compared with placebo. In the analysis excluding the cluster trial the effects were no different between treatment and placebo. Only one of the trials was judged to be of high quality, with the others likely to have resulted in a bias favouring magnesium supplementation. The review concluded that there is not enough high-quality evidence to show that dietary magnesium supplementation during pregnancy is beneficial.[39] A further review concluded that magnesium, used after threatened pre-term labour, does not reduce pre-term birth or improve the outcome for the infant.[40]

Conclusion

Epidemiological studies show an association between marginal magnesium status and CVD and hypertension. However, the effect of supplementation is equivocal and any effect appears to be small. Patients with diabetes often have poor magnesium status, but supplementation does not appear to have an effect on glucose control, possibly because it is difficult to replete and maintain adequate magnesium levels. Preliminary evidence suggests that magnesium could reduce the frequency and pain of migraine and may help the symptoms of PMS. There is no good evidence that magnesium improves performance in athletes.

Precautions/contraindications

Doses exceeding the RDA are best avoided in renal impairment.

Pregnancy and breast-feeding

No problems reported with normal intakes.

Adverse effects

Toxicity from oral ingestion is unlikely in individuals with normal renal function. Doses of 3–5 g have a cathartic effect.

Interactions

Drugs

Alcohol: excessive alcohol intake increases renal excretion of magnesium.

Loop diuretics: increased excretion of magnesium.

4-quinolones: may reduce absorption of 4-quinolones; give 2 h apart.

Tetracyclines: may reduce absorption of tetracyclines; give 2 h apart.

Thiazide diuretics: increased excretion of magnesium.

Dose

Magnesium is available in the form of tablets and capsules. It is available in isolation, in combination with calcium (and sometimes with vitamin D) and in multivitamin and mineral preparations.

The dose is not established. Dietary supplements provide 100–500 mg per dose.

References

1   The Caerphilly and Speedwell Collaborative Group. Caerphilly and Speedwell collaborative heart disease studies. *J Epidemiol Community Health* 1994; 38: 235–238.
2   Rasmussen HS, Aurup P, Goldstein K, *et al*. Influence of magnesium substitution therapy on blood lipid composition in patients with ischaemic heart disease. A double-blind, placebo controlled study. *Arch Intern Med* 1989; 149: 1050–1053.
3   Shechter M, Bairey Merz CN, Stuchlinger HG, *et al*. Effects of oral magnesium therapy on exercise tolerance, exercise-induced chest pain, and quality of life in patients with coronary artery disease. *Am J Cardiol* 2003; 91: 517–521.
4   Widman L, Webster PO, Stegmayr BK, Wirell M. The dose-dependent reduction in blood pressure through administration of magnesium. *Am J Hypertension* 1993; 6: 41–45.
5   Witteman JCM, Grobbee DE, Derkx FHM, *et al*. Reduction of blood pressure with oral magnesium supplementation in women with mild to moderate hypertension. *Am J Clin Nutr* 1994; 60: 129–135.
6   Geleijnse JM, Witteman JCM, Bak AAA, *et al*. Reduction in blood pressure with a low sodium, high potassium, high magnesium salt in older subjects with mild to moderate hypertension. *BMJ* 1994; 309: 436–440.
7   Nowson CA, Morgan TO. Magnesium supplementation in mild hypertensive patients on a moderately low sodium diet. *Clin Exp Pharmacol Physiol* 1989; 16: 299–302.
8   Cappuccio FP, Markandu ND, Beynon GW, *et al*. Lack of effect of oral magnesium on high blood pressure: a double-blind study. *BMJ* 1985; 291: 235–238.
9   Sacks FM, Willet WC, Smith A, *et al*. Effect on blood pressure of potassium, calcium and magnesium in women with low habitual intake. *Hypertension* 1998; 31: 131–138.
10 Yamamoto ME, Applegate WB, Klag MJ, *et al*. Lack of blood pressure effect with calcium and magnesium supplementation in adults with high-normal blood pressure. Reports from phase I of the Trials of Hypertension Prevention (TOHP). Trials of Hypertension Prevention (TOHP) Collaborative Research Group. *Ann Epidemiol* 1995; 5: 96–107.
11 Ferrara LA, Iannuzzi R, Castaldo A, *et al*. Long-term magnesium supplementation in essential hypertension. *Cardiology* 1992; 81: 25–33.
12 Jee SH, Miller ER III, Gullar E, *et al*. The effect of magnesium supplementation on blood pressure: a meta-analysis of randomized controlled trials. *Am J Hypertens* 2002; 15: 691–696.
13 Fujii S, Takemura T, Wada M, *et al*. Magnesium levels in plasma, erythrocyte and urine in patients with diabetes mellitus. *Horm Metab Res* 1982; 14: 161–162.
14 McNair P, Christensen MS, Christiansen C, *et al*. Renal hypomagnesaemia in human diabetes mellitus: its relation to glucose homeostasis. *Eur J Clin Invest* 1982; 12: 81–85.
15 Jain AP, Gupta NN, Kumar A. Some metabolic effects of magnesium in diabetes mellitus. *J Assoc Physicians India* 1976; 24: 827–831.

16 Paolisso G, Passariello N, Pizza G, *et al*. Dietary magnesium supplements improve β-cell response to glucose and arginine in elderly non-insulin dependent diabetic subjects. *Acta Endocrinol* 1989; 121: 16–20.

17 McNair P, Christiansen C, Madsbad S, *et al*. Hypomagnesaemia, a risk factor in diabetic nephropathy. *Diabetes* 1978; 27: 1075–1077.

18 De Leeuw I, Engelen W, Vertommen J, *et al*. Effect of intensive IV + oral magnesium supplementation on circulating ion levels, lipid parameters, and metabolic control in Mg-depleted insulin-dependent diabetic patients (IDDM). *Magnes Res* 1997; 10: 135–141.

19 Lima M de L, Cruz T, Pousada JC, *et al*. The effect of magnesium supplementation in increasing doses on the control of type 2 diabetes. *Diabetes Care* 1998; 21: 682–686.

20 de Valk HW, Verkaaik R, van Rijn HJ, *et al*. Oral magnesium supplementation in insulin-requiring Type 2 diabetic patients. *Diabet Med* 1998; 15: 503–507.

21 Rodriguez-Moran M, Guerrero-Romero F. Oral magnesium supplementation improves insulin sensitivity and metabolic control in type 2 diabetic subjects: a randomized double-blind controlled trial. *Diabetes Care* 2003; 26: 1147–1152.

22 Guerrero-Romero F, Tamez-Perez HE, Gonzalez-Gonzalez G, *et al*. Oral magnesium supplementation improves insulin sensitivity in non-diabetic subjects with insulin resistance. A double-blind placebo-controlled randomized trial. *Diabetes Metab* 2004; 30: 253–258.

23 Facchinetti F, Borella P, Sances G, *et al*. Oral magnesium successfully relieves premenstrual mood changes. *Obstet Gynecol* 1991; 78: 177–181.

24 Walker AF, De Souza MC, Vickers MF, *et al*. Magnesium supplementation alleviates premenstrual symptoms of fluid retention. *J Womens Health* 1998; 7: 1157–1165.

25 De Souza MC, Walker AF, Robinson PA, Bolland K. A synergistic effect of a daily supplement for 1 month of 200 mg magnesium plus 50 mg vitamin B6 for the relief of anxiety related premenstrual symptoms: a randomized, double-blind, crossover study. *J Women's Health Gend Based Med* 2000; 9: 131–139.

26 Peikert A, Wilimzig C, Kohne-Volland R. Prophylaxis of migraine with oral magnesium: results from a progressive multi-center, placebo-controlled and double blind randomized study. *Cephalagia* 1996; 16: 257–263.

27 Pfaffenrath V, Wessely P, Meyer C. Magnesium in the prophylaxis of migraine – a double blind, placebo-controlled study. *Cephalagia* 1996; 16: 436–440.

28 Maizels M, Blumenfeld A, Burchette R. A combination of riboflavin, magnesium, and feverfew for migraine prophylaxis: a randomized trial. *Headache* 2004; 44: 885–890.

29 Tucker AK, Hannan MT, Chen H. Potassium, magnesium, and fruit and vegetable intakes are associated with greater bone mineral density in elderly men and women. *Am J Clin Nutr* 1999; 69: 727–736.

30 Dimai HP, Porta S, Wirnsberger G. Daily oral magnesium supplementation suppresses bone turnover in young adult males. *J Clin Endocrinol Metab* 1998; 83: 2742–2748.

31 Doyle L, Flynn A, Cashman K. The effect of magnesium supplementation on biochemical markers of bone metabolism or blood pressure in healthy young adult females. *Eur J Clin Nutr* 1999; 53: 255–261.

32 Rude RK, Olerich M. Magnesium deficiency: possible role in osteoporosis associated with gluten-sensitive enteropathy. *Osteoporosis Int* 1996; 6: 453–461.

33 Stendig-Limberg G, Tepper R, Leichter R. Trabecular bone density in a two year controlled trial of peroral magnesium in osteoporosis. *Magnes Res* 1993; 6: 155–163.

34 Brilla LR, Haley TF. Effect of magnesium supplementation on strength training in humans. *J Am Coll Nutr* 1992; 11: 326–329.

35 Golf SW, Bender S, Gruttner J. On the significance of magnesium in extreme physical stress. *Cardiovasc Drugs Ther* 1998; 12 (Suppl. 2): 197–202.

36 Weller E, Backert P, Meinck HM. Lack of effect of oral Mg-supplementation on magnesium in serum, blood cells, and calf muscle. *Med Sci Sport Exerc* 1998; 30: 1584–1591.

37 Larsson SC, Bergkvist L, Wolk A. Magnesium intake in relation to risk of colorectal cancer in women. *JAMA* 2005; 293: 87–89.

38 Folsom AR, Hong Ching-Ping. Magnesium intake and reduced risk of colon cancer in a prospective study of women. *Am J Epidemiol* 2006; 163: 232–235.

39 Makrides M, Crowther CA. Magnesium supplementation in pregnancy. Cochrane database, issue 4, 2001. London: Macmillan.

40 Crowther CA, Moore V. Magnesium maintenance therapy for preventing preterm birth after threatened preterm labour. Cochrane database, issue 1, 1998. London: Macmillan.

Manganese

Description

Manganese is an essential trace mineral.

Human requirements

No Reference Nutrient Intake or Estimated Average Requirement has been set for manganese in the UK, but a safe and adequate intake is: for adults, 1.4 mg daily; infants, 10 μg daily. The UK safe upper intake from supplements alone is 5 mg daily for adults.

In the USA, the daily adequate intakes (AIs) are: for infants 0–6 months, 0.003 mg, 7–12 months, 0.6 mg; children, 1–3 years, 1.2 mg, 4–8 years, 1.5 mg; males, 9–13 years, 1.9 mg, 14–18 years, 2.2 mg, 19–70+ years, 2.3 mg; females 9–18 years, 1.6 mg, 19–70+ years, 1.8 mg, pregnancy 2.0 mg, breast-feeding 2.6 mg.

The daily Tolerable Upper Intake Level from food, water and supplements is: for children 1–3 years, 2 mg, 4–8 years, 3 mg; 9–13 years, 6 mg, 14–18 years, 9 mg, 19–70+ years, 11 mg, pregnancy, 9 mg, breast-feeding 11 mg.

Dietary intake

In the UK, the average adult diet provides 4.6–5.4 mg daily.

Action

Manganese activates several enzymes, including hydroxylases, kinases, decarboxylases and transferases. It is also a constituent of several metalloenzymes, such as arginase, pyruvate carboxylase, and also superoxide dismutase, which protects cells from free radical attack. It may have a role in the regulation of glucose homeostasis and in calcium mobilisation.

Table 1 Dietary sources of manganese

Food portion	Manganese content (mg)
Cereal products	
Bread, brown, 2 slices	**1**
white, 2 slices	0.3
wholemeal, 2 slices	**1.5**
Milk and dairy products	
Milk and cheese	Traces
Meat and fish	
Meat and fish	Traces
Liver, lambs, cooked (90 g)	0.4
Vegetables	
1 small can baked beans (200 g)	0.6
Lentils, kidney beans or other pulses (105 g)	**1–1.5**
Green vegetables, average, boiled (100 g)	0.2
Fruit	
1 banana	0.5
Blackberries, stewed (100 g)	**1.5**
Pineapple, canned (150 g)	**1.5**
Nuts	
20 almonds	0.3
10 Brazil nuts	0.4
30 hazelnuts	**1.0**
30 peanuts	0.7
Tea, 1 cup	0.3

Note: Some other foods (e.g. breakfast cereals) contain significant quantities, but there is no reliable information on the amount.
Excellent sources (>1 mg/portion) (**bold**).

Dietary sources

See Table 1 for dietary sources of manganese.

Metabolism

Absorption

Absorption of manganese occurs throughout the length of the small intestine, probably via a saturable carrier mechanism, but absorptive efficiency is believed to be poor.

Distribution

Manganese is transported in the blood bound to plasma proteins. Organs with the highest concentrations include the liver, kidney and pancreas, but 25% of the body pool is found within the skeleton. Homeostasis is maintained by hepatobiliary and intestinal secretion.

Elimination

Manganese is eliminated primarily in the faeces.

Bioavailability

Bioavailability of manganese appears to be enhanced by vitamin C and meat-containing diets, but is decreased by iron and non-starch polysaccharides (dietary fibre). Although tea contains large amounts of manganese, it is essentially unavailable to humans.

Deficiency

Manganese deficiency in individuals consuming mixed diets is very rare. Symptoms thought to be associated with deficiency (which have occurred only on semi-purified diets) include weight loss, dermatitis, hypocholesterolaemia, depressed growth of hair and nails and reddening of black hair.

Possible uses

Diabetes

Manganese has been claimed to be useful in diabetes mellitus. A relationship between dietary manganese and carbohydrate metabolism in humans has been suggested.[1] This paper described the case of a diabetic patient resistant to insulin therapy who responded to oral manganese with a consistent drop in blood glucose levels. However, there is insufficient evidence to warrant recommendation of manganese supplements to patients with diabetes.

Miscellaneous

Manganese supplements have also been used to treat inflammatory conditions such as rheumatoid arthritis, on the basis that manganese supplementation has been shown to raise levels of superoxide dismutase, which may protect against oxidative damage.[2]

Precautions/contraindications

No problems reported.

Pregnancy and breast-feeding

No problems reported at normal doses.

Adverse effects

Manganese is essentially non-toxic when administered orally. Toxic reactions in humans occur only as the result of the chronic inhalation of large amounts of manganese found in mines and some industrial plants. Signs include severe psychiatric abnormalities and neurological disorders similar to Parkinson's disease.

Interactions

None reported.

Dose

Manganese is available in the form of tablets and capsules.

The dose is not established. Dietary supplements provide 5–50 mg per dose.

Upper safety levels

The UK Expert Group on Vitamins and Minerals (EVM) has identified a likely safe total intake of manganese for adults from supplements alone of 4 mg daily.

References

1 Rubenstein AH, Levin NW, Elliot GA. Manganese-induced hypoglycaemia. *Lancet* 1962; 2: 1348–1351.
2 Pasquier C. Manganese containing superoxide dismutase deficiency in polymorphonuclear lymphocytes in rheumatoid arthritis. *Inflammation* 1984; 8: 27–32.

Melatonin

Description

Melatonin is a hormone synthesised by the pineal gland. It is synthesised from tryptophan, which is converted to serotonin and this in turn is converted to melatonin. Melatonin is secreted in a 24-h circadian rhythm, regulating the normal sleep–wake periods. Secretion starts as soon as darkness falls, normally peaking between 02:00 and 04:00, and synthesis is inhibited by exposure to light. Daily output is greatest in young adults and production declines after the age of 20 years.

Action

Melatonin has a role in the regulation of sleep, and as a supplement it can reset the sleep–wake cycle and help to promote sleep. In addition, it regulates the secretion of growth hormone and gonadotrophic hormones, and it has anti-oxidant activity. It may also have anti-cancer properties.

Possible uses

Melatonin has been investigated for jet lag, sleeping difficulties and cancer prevention.

Jet lag

A small double-blind, placebo-controlled trial evaluated 17 volunteers who flew from London to San Francisco, where they stayed for 2 weeks before returning. For 3 days before returning to London, subjects were given 5 mg melatonin or placebo at 18:00 local time. Following their return to Britain, the dose was continued for 4 more days between 14:00 and 16:00. On day 7, the volunteers were asked to rate their jet lag, and those taking melatonin reported significantly less severe jet lag than those taking placebo.[1]

In a similar study, 20 subjects flew east from Auckland, New Zealand, to London and returned after 3 weeks. Subjects took either melatonin 5 mg or placebo for the first journey and vice versa for the return journey. Less jet lag was experienced in the volunteers taking melatonin.[2]

In a further double-blind placebo-controlled trial, 52 flight crew were randomly assigned to three groups: early melatonin (5 mg melatonin for 3 days before arrival, continuing for 5 days after returning home); late melatonin (placebo for 3 days, followed by melatonin 5 mg for 5 days); and placebo. The flight was from Los Angeles to New Zealand and all subjects began taking capsules at 07:00 to 08:00 Los Angeles time (corresponding to 02:00 to 03:00 New Zealand time) 2 days before departure and continued for 5 days after arrival in New Zealand. Subjects in the late melatonin group reported less jet lag and sleep disturbance than the placebo group, while those in the early melatonin group reported a worse recovery than the placebo group. The authors concluded that the timing of melatonin appeared to influence the subjective symptoms of jet lag.[3]

In another double-blind placebo-controlled study, 257 subjects on a flight from New York to Oslo were randomised to receive either 5 mg melatonin or placebo at bedtime, 0.5 mg melatonin at bedtime or 0.5 mg melatonin taken on a shifting schedule. In this study, melatonin showed no difference from placebo. However, the authors acknowledged that the study had various limitations, including the fact that the subjects stayed only 4 days at their destination before flying back and may not have had enough time to adapt to the new time. In addition, time of sleep onset at night, awakening in the morning and daytime sleepiness were assessed rather than night-time sleep disturbance, and it is night-time disturbance that is most associated with jet lag. Moreover, subjects knew that they had three out of four chances of receiving melatonin, and the placebo effect may have been quite large, diluting the influence of melatonin.[4]

In a study in baboons (which have similar sleep patterns to humans), various doses of melatonin were given at various times of day to see if melatonin shifted circadian rhythms. Activity patterns of the baboons were constantly monitored in a darkened room. Melatonin did not shift circadian rhythms, but it did induce sleep when given at night. However, the same dose given during the day did not cause sleep.[5] The authors concluded that melatonin does not shift circadian phase in baboons using doses similar to those prescribed for treating human circadian system disorders, suggesting that melatonin may not help to overcome the effects of jet lag.

Melatonin has been compared with zolpidem and also used in combination with zolpidem for jet lag in relation to eastwards travel. In a study involving 137 people, zolpidem was rated as producing the best sleep quality during the night flight and as the most effective jet lag medication. However, all active treatments led to a decrease in jet lag. Zolpidem and the combination of zolpidem and melatonin were less well tolerated than melatonin alone. Adverse reports included nausea, vomiting, amnesia and somnambulia to the point of incapacitation. Confusion, morning sleepiness and nausea were highest in the combination group.[6]

Another trial measured the effects of slow-release caffeine and melatonin on sleep and daytime sleepiness after a seven time zone eastbound flight. Three groups of nine subjects were given either caffeine (300 mg) at 08:00 on recovery days 1 to 5, or melatonin 5 mg on the pre-flight day (at 17:00), the flight day (at 16:00) and from days 1 to 3 after the flight (at 23:00) or placebo at the same times. Compared with baseline there was a significant rebound of slow-wave sleep on nights 1 to 2 with placebo and melatonin and a significant decrease in rapid eye movement sleep on night 1 with placebo and on nights 1 to 3 with melatonin. Caffeine reduced sleepiness but also tended to affect sleep quality until the last drug day. The authors concluded that both caffeine and melatonin have positive effects on some jet lag symptoms after an eastbound flight, caffeine on daytime sleepiness and melatonin on sleep.[7]

A Cochrane review involving 10 trials found that in eight of these trials melatonin, when taken close to the target bedtime at the destination (22:00 to midnight) decreased jet lag from flights crossing five or more time zones. Daily doses of 0.5–5 mg were effective except that people fell asleep faster and slept better after 5 mg than 0.5 mg. Doses above 5 mg appear to be more effective. The relative ineffectiveness of 2 mg slow-release melatonin suggests that a short-lived higher peak concentration of melatonin works better. The reviewers said that timing of the melatonin dose is crucial. If taken early in the day, it can cause sleepiness and delay adaptation to local time. The authors concluded that melatonin is effective in preventing or reducing jet lag, and occasional short-term use appears to be safe. They also recommended it should be offered to travellers crossing five or more time zones, particularly in an easterly direction, and especially if they have experienced jet lag on previous journeys.[8]

Sleep disorders

In a study of six healthy young men, doses of 0.3 mg and 1 mg melatonin given at night produced acute hypnotic effects. There were no residual hypnotic effects the next morning, as shown from the results on mood and performance tests carried out by the volunteers.[9]

In a double-blind, placebo-controlled, crossover study, 12 elderly patients were randomised to receive 2 mg controlled-release melatonin daily for 3 weeks. There were no differences in sleep time, but there was a reduction in time to onset of sleep, and an increase in sleep quality, as measured by wrist actigraphy.[10]

In a further double-blind, placebo-controlled, crossover study, 14 patients with insomnia (55–80 years) received 0.5 mg melatonin either as an immediate-release dose 30 min before bedtime, a controlled-release dose 30 min before bedtime, an immediate-release dose 4 h after bedtime, or placebo. Each trial lasted for 2 weeks with 2-week washout periods. All melatonin doses resulted in significant reductions in time to sleep onset, but no improvement in sleep quality and no increase in sleep time.[11]

A 2001 systematic review of melatonin in older people with insomnia included six crossover RCTs. Five of the RCTs reported some positive effects, with decreased sleep latency in four studies, an increase in sleep efficiency in three studies and a decrease in wake time during sleep in two studies. Subjective sleep quality was not improved in the two studies that assessed this. There were no adverse effects with melatonin. The authors concluded that further research is required before widespread use of melatonin in geriatric populations can be advocated. They also consider it worth while investigating whether melatonin could be used to reduce the amount of benzodiazepines used by older people.[12]

A later RCT involving older people with age-related sleep maintenance problems found that 5 mg melatonin taken at bedtime did not improve sleep quality.[13] In 10 patients (aged 30–75 years) with primary insomnia, there were no differences in sleep electroencephalographic (EEG) records, the amount or subjective quality of sleep or side-effects between a placebo, 0.3 mg melatonin or 1 mg melatonin.[14] In a further study in patients (mean age 50 years) with reduced rapid eye movement (REM) sleep duration, melatonin 3 mg administered between 22:00 and 23:00 for 4 weeks significantly increased percentage of REM sleep compared with placebo.[15] Melatonin has also been found to restore sleep efficiency in individuals with mental retardation and insomnia.[16]

A 2004 systematic review of melatonin in sleep disorders concluded that melatonin is not effective in treating most primary sleep disorders with short-term use, although there is some evidence to suggest that melatonin is effective in treating delayed sleep phase syndrome with short-term use. The review also stated that evidence suggests that melatonin is not effective in treating most secondary sleep disorders with short-term use and no evidence suggests that melatonin is effective in alleviating the sleep disturbance aspect of jet lag and shift work disorder. Evidence also suggests that melatonin is safe with short-term use.[17]

A meta-analysis published in 2005 by the same group as the 2004 systematic review also suggested that melatonin is not effective in treating most primary sleep disorders with short-term use (4 weeks or less), but there is some evidence that melatonin is effective in treating delayed sleep phase syndrome with short-term use.[18] A further 2005 meta-analysis of 15 studies found that melatonin significantly reduced sleep latency by 4 min, increased sleep efficiency by 3.1% and increased sleep duration by 13.7 min.[19]

A meta-analysis published in 2006 (by the same group as the 2004 systematic review[17] and the 2005 meta-analysis[18]) included six RCTs, which showed no evidence that melatonin had an effect on sleep latency in people with secondary disorders. Analysis of nine RCTs found no evidence that melatonin had an effect on sleep latency in people with sleep disorders accompanying sleep restriction (e.g. jet lag, shift work). Analysis of 17 RCTs showed no evidence of adverse events of melatonin in short-term use (3 months or less).[20]

Melatonin has also been evaluated in children with insomnia and mental disorders. It has been found to advance the sleep–wake rhythm in children with idiopathic chronic sleep-onset insomnia.[21] In young patients with epilepsy, melatonin has been shown to reduce wake–sleep disorders[22] and to be of potential use as an adjunct to antiepileptic therapy in reducing oxidant stress.[23–25] In a systematic review of melatonin treatment in children with neurodevelopmental disabilities and sleep impairment, melatonin was found to significantly reduce time to sleep onset, but there was no significant effect on the other outcome measures of total sleep time, night-time awakenings and parental opinions on their children's sleep.[26]

Studies have also evaluated melatonin for potential benefit for sleep disorders in patients with dementia. Two studies have shown no evidence that melatonin is effective in improving sleep in patients with dementia.[27,28] A Cochrane review found some – albeit insufficient – evidence to support the use of melatonin in managing cognitive disturbances in people with dementia. However, there was some evidence of benefit on some behavioural symptoms.[29]

A prospective open-label study has evaluated the potential for melatonin to improve tinnitus, particularly in those with sleep disturbance caused by tinnitus. A total of 24 patients took 3 mg melatonin per day for 4 weeks, followed by 4 weeks of observation. Melatonin use was associated with improvement in tinnitus and sleep. There was an association between the amount of improvement in sleep and tinnitus. The impact of melatonin on sleep was greatest in those with the worst sleep quality, but its impact on tinnitus was not associated with the severity of tinnitus. The authors concluded that melatonin may be a safe treatment for patients with idiopathic tinnitus, especially those with sleep disturbance due to tinnitus.[30]

Cancer

A group of 80 patients with advanced solid tumours, all of whom refused chemotherapy or who did not respond to previous chemotherapy, were randomised to receive either interleukin 2 (IL-2) or IL-2 and melatonin (40 mg) starting 1 week before IL-2. Melatonin increased the anti-tumour activity of IL-2, resulting in accelerated tumour regression rate, increased progression-free survival and longer overall survival in these patients.[31]

In a small preliminary study involving 14 women with metastatic breast cancer, melatonin was shown to increase the effects of tamoxifen.[32]

In a controlled study, 50 patients with brain metastases caused by solid neoplasms were randomised to receive supportive care alone (steroids and anticonvulsants) or supportive care plus melatonin 20 mg daily. Survival at 1 year, free from brain progression, and mean survival time were significantly higher in the melatonin group.[33]

Another study randomised 80 patients with metastatic tumours to receive chemotherapy or chemotherapy plus melatonin (20 mg daily). Melatonin was associated with a significant reduction in frequency of thrombocytopenia, malaise and asthenia, and a non-significant trend towards less stomatitis and neuropathy compared with controls. However, melatonin had no effect on alopecia and vomiting.[34]

A systematic review of 10 RCTs of melatonin in the treatment of cancer found that melatonin reduced the risk of death at 1 year (RR 0.66; 95% CI, 0.59 to 0.73). Effects were consistent across melatonin dose and type of cancer. No adverse events were reported. The authors concluded that the reduction in risk of death and lack of adverse events suggest potential for melatonin in cancer management, but these effects must be confirmed by further good-quality RCTs.[35]

Blood pressure

The biological clock has been shown to be involved in autonomic cardiovascular regulation. Recent research has investigated the effect of enhancing the functioning of the biological clock by melatonin in blood pressure. A double-blind, crossover RCT in 16 men with untreated essential hypertension evaluated the influence of oral melatonin 2.5 mg daily, 1 hour before sleep, on 24-h ambulatory blood pressure and actigraphic estimates of sleep quality. Repeated melatonin intake over 3 weeks (but not an acute single dose) reduced systolic and diastolic blood pressure during sleep by 6 and 4 mmHg, respectively. The treatment did not affect heart rate. The day–night amplitudes of the rhythms in systolic and diastolic blood pressures were increased by 15% and 25% respectively. Repeated (but not acute) melatonin also improved sleep. The authors concluded that support of circadian pacemaker function may provide a new strategy in the treatment of essential hypertension.[36]

A further trial has found a similar effect in women. In a double-blind RCT 18 women (aged 47–63 years) with normal blood pressure ($n = 9$) or treated essential hypertension ($n = 9$) received a 3-week course of slow-release melatonin (3 mg) 1 h before going to bed. They were then crossed over for 3 weeks. In comparison with placebo, melatonin administration did not influence diurnal blood pressure but did significantly decrease nocturnal systolic (-3.77 ± 1.7 mmHg, $P = 0.04$) and diastolic (-3.63 ± 1.3 mmHg, $P = 0.013$) pressure without modifying heart rate. The effect was inversely related to the day–night difference in blood pressure, suggesting that prolonged administration may improve the day–night rhythm of blood pressure, particularly in women with a blunted nocturnal decline.[37]

Another RCT in young patients with type 1 diabetes also found that melatonin (5 mg daily) amplifies the nocturnal decline in blood pressure and suggested that melatonin should be considered in trials of prevention of hypertension in type 1 diabetes.[38]

Cognitive impairment

A number of studies suggest a relationship between decline of melatonin function and the symptoms of dementia. A Cochrane review of three RCTs designed to evaluate melatonin for sleep disorders associated with dementia found no evidence of efficacy for cognitive function, with evidence from a single small trial that there may be some benefit for behavioural problems.[39]

Miscellaneous

Melatonin has been evaluated in other disorders. Studies have shown insufficient evidence of benefit for melatonin in chronic fatigue syndrome[40] and in tardive dyskinesia.[41] However, supplemental melatonin has been associated with significant reduction in nocturia in men with benign prostatic enlargement,[42] and attenuation of abdominal pain and reduced rectal pain sensitivity in patients with IBS.[43] Animal models suggest that melatonin could be a candidate neuroprotective agent for human stroke.[44]

Conclusion

Melatonin has been promoted widely for the prevention and treatment of jet lag and sleep disorders. For jet lag, melatonin appears promising, but results from studies on supplements and sleep have been conflicting. Reduced secretion has also been associated with cancer, and preliminary research suggests that melatonin may reduce adverse effects associated with chemotherapy and increase survival time. Reduced secretion has also been linked with CVD, epilepsy and depression, but its role as a potential supplement in these conditions is unclear. There is preliminary evidence that melatonin may have a blood pressure lowering effect.

Precautions/contraindications

Caution in taking melatonin (as any other sleep therapy) for prolonged periods without medical assessment of the patient. Melatonin should be avoided in women wishing to conceive (large doses may inhibit ovulation); in children and in patients with mental illness, including depression.

Pregnancy and breast-feeding

Melatonin should be avoided in pregnancy.

Adverse effects

No known toxicity or serious side-effects, but the effects of long-term supplementation are unknown. However, there have been reports of headaches, abdominal cramp, inhibition of fertility and libido, gynaecomastia, exacerbation of symptoms of fibromyalgia and also sleep disturbance. In addition, there have been reports of increased seizures in children suffering from neurological disorders. Inhibition of ovulation has been observed with high doses, but melatonin should not be used as a contraceptive.

Interactions

No data are available, but in theory melatonin may be additive with medication that causes CNS depression. In addition, beta-blockers inhibit melatonin release, and this may be the mechanism by which beta-blockers cause sleep disturbance. Other drugs, including fluoxetine, ibuprofen and indomethacin, may also reduce nocturnal melatonin secretion. Melatonin may influence the effects of warfarin.

References

1   Arendt J, Aldhous M, Marks V. Alleviation of jet lag by melatonin: preliminary results of controlled double blind trial. *BMJ* 1986; 292: 1170.

2   Petrie K, Conaglen JV, Thompson L, Chamberlain K. Effect of melatonin on jet lag after long haul flights. *BMJ* 1989; 298: 705–707.

3   Petrie K, Dawson AG, Thompson L, *et al.* A double-blind trial of melatonin as a treatment for jet lag in international cabin crew. *Biol Psychiatry* 1993; 33; 526–530.

4   Spitzer RL, Terman M, Williams JBW, *et al.* Jet lag: clinical features, validation of a new syndrome-specific scale, and lack of response to melatonin in a randomised, double-blind trial. *Am J Psychiatry* 1999; 156: 1392–1396.

5   Hao H, Rivkees S. Melatonin does not shift circadian phase in baboons. *J Clin Endocrinol Metab* 2000; 85: 3618–3622.

6   Suhner A, Schlagenhauf P, Hofer I, *et al.* Effectiveness and tolerability of melatonin and zolpidem for the alleviation of jet lag. *Aviat Space Environ Med* 2001; 72: 638–646.

7   Beaumont M, Batejat D, Pierard C, *et al.* Caffeine or melatonin effects on sleep and sleepiness after rapid eastward transmeridian travel. *J Appl Physiol* 2004; 96: 50–58.

8   Herxheimer A, Petrie KJ. Melatonin for the prevention and treatment of jet lag. Cochrane database, issue 2, 2002. London: Macmillan.

9   Zhdanova IV, Wurtman RJ, Lynch HJ, *et al.* Sleep inducing effects of low doses of melatonin ingested in the evening. *Clin Pharmacol Ther* 1995; 57: 552–558.

10 Garfinkel D, Laudon M, Nof D, *et al.* Improvement of sleep quality in elderly people by controlled release melatonin. *Lancet* 1995; 346: 541–544.

11 Hughes RJ, Sack RJ, Lewy AJ. The role of melatonin and circadian phase in age-related sleep maintenance insomnia: assessment in a clinical trial of melatonin replacement. *Sleep* 1998; 21: 52–58.

12 Olde Rikkert MG, Rigaud AS. Melatonin in elderly patients with insomnia: a systematic review. *Z Gerontol Geriat* 2001; 34: 491–497.

13 Baskett JJ, Broad JB, Wood PC, *et al.* Does melatonin improve sleep in older people? A randomized crossover trial. *Age Ageing* 2003; 32: 123–124.

14 Almeida Montes LG, Ontiveros Uribe MP, Cortes Sotres J, Heinze Martin G. Treatment of primary insomnia with melatonin: a double-blind, placebo-controlled, crossover study. *J Psychiatr Neurosci* 2003; 28: 191–196.

15 Kunz D, Mahlberg R, Muller C, *et al.* Melatonin in patients with reduced REM sleep duration: two randomized controlled trials. *J Clin Endocrinol Metab* 2004; 89: 128–134.

16 Niederhofer H, Staffen W, Mair A, Pittschieler K. Brief report: melatonin facilitates sleep in individuals with mental retardation and insomnia. *J Autism Dev Disord* 2003; 33: 469–472.

17 Buscemi N, Vandermeer B, Pandya R, *et al.* Melatonin for Treatment of Sleep Disorders. Agency for Healthcare Research and Quality Evidence Report/Technology Assessment: Number 108. AHRQ Publications Number 05-E002–1. Available from http://www.ahrq.gov/ clinic/epcsums/melatsum.htm (accessed 6 November 2006). Rockville, MD: AHRQ, November 2004.

18 Buscemi N, Vandermeer B, Hooton N, *et al.* The efficacy and safety of exogenous melatonin for primary sleep disorders. A meta-analysis. *J Gen Intern Med* 2005; 20: 151–158.

19 Brzezinski A, Vangel MG, Wurtman RJ, *et al.* Effects of exogenous melatonin on sleep: a meta-analysis. *Sleep Med Rev* 2005; 9: 41–50.

20 Buscemi N, Vandermeer B, Hooton N, *et al.* Efficacy and safety of exogenous melatonin for secondary sleep disorders and sleep disorders accompanying sleep restriction: meta-analysis. *BMJ* 2006; 332: 385–393.

21 Smits MG, van Stel HF, van der Heijden K, *et al.* Melatonin improves health status and sleep in children with idiopathic chronic sleep-onset insomnia: a randomized placebo-controlled trial. *J Am Acad Child Adolesc Psychiatry* 2003; 42: 1286–1293.

22 Coppola G, Iervolino G, Mastrosimone M, *et al.* Melatonin in wake-sleep disorders in children, adolescents and young adults with mental retardation with or without epilepsy: a double-blind, cross-over, placebo-controlled trial. *Brain Dev* 2004; 26: 373–376.

23 Gupta M, Aneja S, Kohli K. Add-on melatonin improves quality of life in epileptic children on valproate monotherapy: a randomized, double-blind, placebo-controlled trial. *Epilepsy Behav* 2004; 5: 316–321.

24 Gupta M, Gupta YK, Agarwal S, *et al.* A randomized, double-blind, placebo-controlled trial of melatonin add-on therapy in epileptic children on valproate monotherapy: effect of glucose peroxidase and glutathione reductase enzymes. *Br J Clin Pharmacol* 2004; 58: 542–547.

25 Gupta M, Gupta YK, Agarwal S. Effects of add-on melatonin administration on antioxidant enzymes in children with epilepsy taking carbamazepine monotherapy: a randomized, double-blind, placebo-controlled trial. *Epilepsia* 2004; 45: 1636–1639.

26 Phillips L, Appleton RE. Systematic review of melatonin treatment in children with neurodevelopmental disabilities and sleep impairment. *Dev Med Child Neurol* 2004; 46: 771–775.

27 Serfaty M, Kennell-Webb S, Warner J, *et al.* Double blind randomized placebo controlled trial of low dose melatonin for sleep disorders in dementia. *Int J Geriatr Psychiatry* 2002; 17: 1120–1127.

28 Singer C, Tractenberg RE, Kaye J, *et al.* A multicenter, placebo-controlled trial of melatonin for sleep disturbance in Alzheimer's disease. *Sleep* 2003; 26: 893–901.

29 Jansen S, Forbes DA, Duncan V, Morgan DG. Melatonin for cognitive impairment. Cochrane database, issue 1, 2006. London: Macmillan.

30 Megwalu UC, Finnell JE, Piccirillo JF. The effects of melatonin on tinnitus and sleep. *Otolaryngol Head Neck Surg* 2006; 134: 210–213.

31 Lissoni P, Barni S, Tancini G, *et al.* A randomised study with subcutaneous low-dose interleukin 2 alone vs. interleukin 2 plus the pineal neurohormone melatonin in advanced solid neoplasms other than renal cancer and melanoma. *Br J Cancer* 1994; 69: 196–199.

32 Lissoni P, Barni S, Meregalli S, *et al.* Modulation of cancer endocrine therapy by melatonin: a phase II study of tamoxifen plus melatonin in metastatic breast cancer patients progressing under tamoxifen alone. *Br J Cancer* 1995; 71: 854–856.

33 Lissoni P, Barni S, Ardizzoia A, *et al.* A randomised study with the pineal hormone melatonin versus supportive care alone in patients with brain metastases due to solid neoplasms. *Cancer* 1994; 73: 699–701.

34 Lissoni P, Tancini G, Barni S, *et al.* Treatment of cancer chemotherapy-induced toxicity with the pineal hormone melatonin. *Support Care Cancer* 1997; 5: 126–129.

35 Mills E, Wu P, Seely D, Guyatt G. Melatonin in the treatment of cancer: a systematic review of randomized controlled trials and meta-analysis. *J Pineal Res* 2005; 39: 360–366.

36 Scheer FA, Van Montfrans GA, van Someren EJ, *et al.* Daily nighttime melatonin reduces blood pressure in male patients with essential hypertension. *Hypertension* 2004; 43: 192–197.

37 Cagnacci A, Cannoletta M, Renzi A, *et al.* Prolonged melatonin administration decreases nocturnal blood pressure in women. *Am J Hypertens* 2005; 18: 1614–1618.

38 Cavallo A, Daniels SR, Dolan LM, *et al.* Blood pressure response to melatonin in type 1 diabetes. *Pediatr Diabetes* 2004; 5: 26–31.

39 Jansen SL, Forbes DA, Duncan V, Morgan DG. Melatonin for cognitive impairment. Cochrane database, issue 1, 2006. London: Macmillan.

40 Williams G, Waterhouse J, Mugarza J, *et al.* Therapy of circadian rhythm disorders in chronic fatigue syndrome: no symptomatic improvement with melatonin or phototherapy. *Eur J Clin Invest* 2002; 32: 831–837.

41 Nelson LA, McGuire LM, Hausafus SM, *et al.* Melatonin for the treatment of tardive dyskinesia. *Ann Pharmacother* 2003; 37: 1128–1131.

42 Drake MJ, Mills IW, Noble JG. Melatonin pharmacotherapy for nocturia in men with benign prostatic enlargement. *J Urol* 2004; 171: 1199–1202.

43 Song GH, Leng PH, Gwee KA, *et al.* Melatonin improves abdominal pain in irritable bowel syndrome patients who have sleep disturbances: a randomized, double blind, placebo controlled study. *Gut* 2005; 54: 1402–1407.

44 Macleod MR, O'Collins T, Horky LL, *et al.* Systematic review and meta-analysis of the efficacy of melatonin in experimental stroke. *J Pineal Res* 2005; 38: 35–41.

Methylsulfonylmethane

Description

Methylsulfonylmethane (MSM) is an organic sulphur-containing compound. It is an oxidation product of the organic solvent, dimethyl sulfoxide (DMSO). DMSO has been used (although is of unproven efficacy) in the treatment of arthritis and connective tissue injuries.

Action

MSM is claimed by manufacturers to be an organic source of sulphur for synthetic processes. However, there is no evidence to support the need for this in humans. There are many other dietary sources of sulphur, including the sulphur-containing amino acids, cysteine and methionine, which are found in dietary protein.

Because cartilage has a high content of sulphur, and sulphur is needed for the formation of connective tissue, it has been suggested that MSM as a source of sulphur could be useful in the management of conditions such as osteoarthritis and joint injuries where there is degeneration or destruction of cartilage. Because MSM is a metabolite of DMSO, it has been suggested that some of the supposed benefits of DMSO (see above) could be attributed to MSM.

There is some very preliminary evidence that MSM reduces homocysteine levels and that it might reduce lipid peroxidation.[1]

Dietary sources

MSM is found naturally in a variety of fruits, vegetables, milk, meat, fish, coffee, tea and chocolate.

Possible uses

Extravagant claims for MSM have been made since the 1980s. Many of these claims have been made by manufacturers and marketers of supplements, and one website was warned by the US Food and Drug Administration (FDA) about making illegal claims. Claims and a rationale for taking MSM can be found on a website that describes two unpublished studies showing benefits of MSM on firstly arthritis, muscle and joint pain, and secondly, on muscle strain and other athletic injuries.[2]

There is some evidence from two small controlled trials that MSM, either in combination with glucosamine or alone, could improve symptoms of pain in arthritis. In one double-blind RCT, 188 patients with mild to moderate osteoarthritis were randomised to glucosamine 500 mg three times daily, MSM 500 mg three times daily or glucosamine 500 mg plus MSM 500 mg three times daily for 12 weeks. All three treatments produced an analgesic and anti-inflammatory effect. Compared with the individual agents, the combination of glucosamine and MSM produced more rapid onset of analgesia and was associated with better anti-inflammatory effect, better efficacy in reducing pain and swelling and better improvement in the functional ability of joints.[3]

A pilot clinical trial randomised 50 men and women with knee osteoarthritis pain to MSM 3 g twice daily or placebo twice daily for 12 weeks. MSM improved symptoms of pain and physical function, but did not reduce stiffness or a total aggregate of osteoarthritis symptom scores. The authors cautioned that the benefits and safety of MSM in managing osteoarthritis and long-term use cannot be confirmed with this pilot trial.[1]

Preliminary evidence from an open trial found that MSM 2600 mg daily for 30 days could relieve respiratory symptoms in seasonal allergic rhinitis with no adverse events. No significant changes were observed in plasma IgE or histamine levels. The authors concluded that the results merited further investigation in a larger controlled trial.[4]

MSM has also been used for snoring, scleroderma, fibromyalgia, SLE, repetitive stress injuries, HIV/AIDS, depression, breast and colon cancer, eye inflammation, insect bites and Alzheimer's disease. However there are no data from clinical trials in humans to support these uses.

> **Conclusion**
> MSM has been studied as a source of sulphur for the management of arthritic conditions. There is preliminary evidence from two small controlled trials that MSM could reduce pain and improve physical function in patients with osteoarthritis. Many extravagant claims have been made for the value of MSM in other conditions, but evidence is lacking and further trials are needed to confirm suggested benefits, including those in arthritis.

Precautions/contraindications

None reported.

Pregnancy and breast-feeding

No problems have been reported, but there have not been sufficient studies to guarantee the safety of MSM in pregnancy and breast-feeding.

Adverse effects

MSM is a component of foods and has not been reported to be toxic. No adverse effects were reported when rats were given 1–5 g/kg body weight for 3 months.[5] A 30-day study in humans revealed no side-effects with a 2600 mg daily dosage.[4]

Interactions

None reported.

Dose

The dose is not established. Supplements typically provide 1500–3000 mg in a daily dose.

References

1 Kim LS, Axelrod LJ, Howard P, *et al*. Efficacy of methylsulfonylmethane (MSM) in osteoarthritis pain of the knee: a pilot clinical trial. *Osteoarthritis Cartilage* 2006; 14: 286–294.
2 Fine Nutraceuticals Inc. http://www.msm.com (accessed 8 November 2006).
3 Usha PR, Naidu MUR. Randomised, double-blind, parallel, placebo-controlled study of oral glucosamine, methylsulfonylmethane and their combination in osteoarthritis. *Clin Drug Invest* 2004; 24: 353–363.
4 Barrager E, Veltmann JR Jr, Schauss AG, Schiller RN. A multicentered, open-label trial on the safety and efficacy of methylsulfonylmethane in the treatment of seasonal allergic rhinitis. *J Altern Complement Med* 2002; 8: 167–173.
5 Horvath K, Noker PE, Somfai-Relle S, *et al*. Toxicity of methylsulfonylmethane in rats. *Food Chem Toxicol* 2002; 40: 1459–1462.

Molybdenum

Description

Molybdenum is an essential ultratrace mineral.

Human requirements

No Reference Nutrient Intake or Estimated Average Requirement has been set for molybdenum in the UK but a safe and adequate daily intake is: for adults, 50–400 µg; infants, children and adolescents, 0.5–1.5 µg/kg. The UK Food Standards Agency has not set a safe upper level.

In the USA, daily adequate intakes (AIs) are: for infants, 0–6 months, 2 µg, 7–12 months, 3 µg. RDAs are: for children, 1–3 years, 17 µg, 4–8 years, 22 µg; for males and females, 9–13 years, 34 µg, 14–18 years, 43 µg, 19–70+ years, 45 µg; pregnancy and breast-feeding, 50 µg. The daily Tolerable Upper Intake Level from food, water and supplements is: for children 1–3 years, 300 µg, 4–8 years, 600 µg; 9–13 years, 1100 µg, 14–18 years, 1700 µg, 19–70+ years, 2000 µg, pregnancy, 1700 µg, breast-feeding 2000 µg.

Dietary intake

Average adult intakes of molybdenum are 120–140 µg daily (USA figures).

Action

Molybdenum functions as an essential co-factor for several enzymes, including aldehyde oxidase (oxidises and detoxifies various pyrimidines, purines and related compounds involved in DNA metabolism); xanthine oxidase/dehydrogenase (catalyses the formation of uric acid); sulphite oxidase (involved in sulphite metabolism).

Dietary sources

The richest sources of molybdenum include milk and milk products, dried beans and peas, wholegrain cereals and liver and kidney.

Metabolism

Absorption

Molybdenum is readily absorbed, but the mechanism of absorption is uncertain.

Distribution

Molybdenum is transported in the blood, loosely attached to erythrocytes, and binds specifically α_2-macroglobulin. The highest concentrations are found in the liver and kidney.

Elimination

Excretion of manganese is mainly via the kidneys, but significant amounts are eliminated in the bile.

Deficiency

A precise description of molybdenum deficiency in humans has not been clearly documented. Evidence so far has been limited to a single patient on long-term total parenteral nutrition, who developed hypermethioninaemia, decreased urinary excretion of sulphate and uric acid, and increased urinary excretion of sulphite and xanthine. In addition, the patient suffered irritability and mental disturbances that progressed into coma. Supplementation with molybdenum improved the clinical condition and normalised uric acid production.

Possible uses

None established.

Adverse effects

Molybdenum is a relatively non-toxic element. High dietary intakes (10–15 mg daily) have been associated with elevated uric acid concentrations in blood and an increased incidence of gout, and may also result in impaired bioavailability of copper and altered metabolism of nucleotides.

Interactions

None reported.

Dose

Molybdenum is available mainly in multivitamin and mineral supplements.

There is no established dose.

N-acetyl cysteine

Description

N-acetyl cysteine (NAC) is a derivative of the dietary amino acid, L-cysteine. It is a source of sulphydryl groups and, as such, can stimulate the synthesis of reduced glutathione (GSH), an endogenous antioxidant. It has been in clinical use for more than 30 years as a mucolytic agent for a variety of respiratory conditions, but is now available as a dietary supplement.

Action

By stimulating the production of glutathione, NAC acts as an antioxidant. It also helps to protect the liver from various toxicants and is used at high doses for the treatment of paracetamol-induced toxicity. NAC also chelates heavy metals such as cadmium, lead and mercury, and may be useful for the treatment of heavy metal toxicity.

Possible uses

NAC is promoted for influenza, bronchitis and the management of symptoms related to HIV and cancer.

Respiratory conditions

Oral NAC has been used since the 1960s for the treatment of bronchitis and it has also been advocated as a prophylactic in patients with chronic bronchitis. Various trials have also reported that supplementation may reduce the duration of bronchitic exacerbations.

In a study in nine patients for 4 weeks,[1] regular use of NAC 200 mg three times a day resulted in no significant differences in lung function, mucociliary clearance curves or sputum viscosity compared with placebo. In another study involving 181 patients randomised to receive either NAC 200 mg three times a day or placebo for 5 months in a double-blind manner, the number of exacerbations of bronchitis and the total number of days taking an antibiotic was reduced in the NAC group compared with placebo, but the differences were not significant.[2]

A further study in 526 patients suffering from chronic bronchitis found no significant differences between NAC and placebo in the number of exacerbations, but there was a significant reduction with NAC in the number of days patients were incapacitated.[3] Yet another double-blind, randomised, placebo-controlled trial found that NAC tablets 300 mg three times a day were associated with a significant reduction in the number of sick leave days after 4 months of treatment during the winter. After 6 months, the number of sick leave days and exacerbations of bronchitis remained lower in the NAC group, but the differences were not significant.[4]

An open randomised study involving 169 patients with COPD found that NAC 600 mg daily plus standard treatment compared with placebo plus standard treatment was associated with a reduction in the number of sick leave days and exacerbations.[5]

A meta-analysis of nine double-blind, placebo-controlled trials of oral NAC in chronic bronchopulmonary disease concluded that a prolonged course of NAC prevents acute exacerbations of chronic bronchitis, thus possibly reducing morbidity and healthcare costs.[6]

A quantitative systematic review of 11 trials published between 1976 and 1994 found that oral NAC reduces the risk of exacerbations and

219

improves symptoms in patients with chronic bronchitis compared with placebo, without increasing the risk of adverse effects. However, the question of whether this benefit is sufficient to justify the routine use of NAC in all patients with bronchitis should be addressed with further studies, the authors concluded.[7]

More recent trials have not demonstrated positive results. An NAC/vitamin C combination had no clinical benefit in chronic bronchitis.[8] In one RCT involving 523 patients in 50 centres, oral NAC 600 mg daily and placebo produced similar clinical outcomes (fall in vital capacity, number of exacerbations). However, amongst patients not taking inhaled corticosteroids, those on NAC had significantly fewer exacerbations.[9] Two further trials have found that NAC reduced the oxidative burden (as shown by reduced exhaled hydrogen peroxide) in airways of stable COPD patients.[10,11]

A multinational study in 155 patients with idiopathic pulmonary fibrosis found that mortality was no different between groups treated with NAC and placebo. However, the NAC group had 9% better vital capacity and improved carbon monoxide diffusing capacity. There was also a slightly lower rate of myelotoxicity in the NAC group.[12] An Italian trial evaluated the impact of oxygen treatment on oxidation free radicals and the effect of NAC in that process. Forty-five stable COPD patients were given oxygen along with placebo or NAC (1200 or 1800 mg daily). Oxygen therapy increased free radical production and disturbed redox balance, but this was prevented by NAC.[13]

Influenza

In a randomised, double-blind study, 262 subjects, 62% of whom had chronic but non-respiratory degenerative disease (e.g. CVD, diabetes, arthritis) received NAC 1200 mg daily or placebo for 6 months. In the NAC group, there was a significant reduction in influenza-like episodes, severity of illness and length of time confined to bed as compared with the placebo group.[14] However, NAC did not prevent subclinical influenza infection (as assessed by antibody response to A/H_1N_1 virus), but the

authors concluded that it reduced the incidence of clinically apparent disease.

Human immunodeficiency virus

In general, HIV-positive individuals have low levels of cysteine and GSH, and it has been suggested that NAC may benefit these patients by raising GSH levels,[15,16] but evidence for the value of NAC supplementation is equivocal.

In a double-blind, placebo-controlled trial, 45 HIV-positive patients on retroviral therapy were randomised to receive 800 mg NAC or placebo for 4 months. In the NAC group, cysteine levels increased from their low pretreatment levels, and TNF-α levels fell. In addition, the decline in CD4+ lymphocyte count found at the start of the study was less severe in the NAC group compared with placebo.[17] Another trial found that NAC was capable of raising CD4 cell count faster than a placebo.[18]

NAC has also been investigated in combination with trimethoprim-sulfamethoxazole in the prophylaxis of *Pneumocystis carinii* in HIV-positive patients.[19,20] It has been suggested that adverse reactions to the antibiotics are due to low GSH levels in these patients, which may be improved by NAC supplementation. However, NAC did not reduce the risk of adverse reactions to trimethoprim-sulfamethoxazole in either study.

A further 180-day RCT found that there were no measurable benefits of supplementing anti-retroviral therapy with NAC in terms of viral load, TNF-α and lymphocyte apoptosis. Baseline levels of GSH were not recovered.[21]

Cancer

Preliminary *in vitro* studies have indicated that NAC could have a role in the prevention and management of some forms of cancer. In a large randomised trial, 2592 patients (60% with head and neck cancer and 40% with lung cancer), most of whom were previous or current smokers, received either vitamin A (300 000 units daily for 1 year, followed by 150 000 units daily during the second year), NAC (600 mg daily for 2 years), both compounds, or placebo.[22] However, there was no benefit in terms of survival, event-free survival or second primary tumours with either vitamin A or NAC. A further small trial in smokers found that NAC has the potential to modulate certain cancer-associated biomarkers in specific organs, and could therefore impact upon tobacco smoke carcinogenicity in humans.[23]

Conclusion

NAC may be useful as prophylaxis in patients with chronic bronchitis and COPD. There is preliminary evidence from one study that it may also reduce symptoms of influenza in older people. Preliminary studies in HIV-positive patients suggest that NAC may improve the clinical picture in such patients, although further research is required. *In vitro* work has indicated that NAC could reduce the risk of cancer, although one large study has shown no significant benefits.

Precautions/contraindications

None reported.

Pregnancy and breast-feeding

No problems have been reported, but there have not been sufficient studies to guarantee the safety of NAC in pregnancy and breast-feeding.

Adverse effects

None reported, but there are no long-term studies assessing the safety of NAC. It has been used since the 1970s with few side-effects (e.g. mild gastrointestinal side-effects and skin rash). Such adverse effects that have been noted have occurred mainly with large oral doses of NAC given for paracetamol poisoning.

Interactions

None reported.

Dose

NAC is available in the form of tablets.

The dose is not established (for use as a supplement). Clinical trials have used 600–1200 mg daily.

References

1 Millar AB, Pavia D, Agnew JE, *et al*. Effect of oral N-acetylcysteine on mucus clearance. *Br J Dis Chest* 1985; 79: 262–266.

2 British Thoracic Society Research Committee. Oral N-acetylcysteine and exacerbation rates in patients with chronic bronchitis and severe airways obstruction. *Thorax* 1985; 40: 832–835.

3 Parr GD, Huitson A. Oral Fabrol (oral N-acetyl cysteine) in chronic bronchitis. *Br J Dis Chest* 1987; 81: 341–348.

4 Rasmussen JB, Glennow C. Reduction in days of illness after long-term treatment with N-acetylcysteine controlled-release tablets in patients with chronic bronchitis. *Eur Respir J* 1988; 1: 341–345.

5 Pela R, Calcagni AM, Subiaco S, *et al*. N-acetylcysteine reduces the exacerbation rate in patients with moderate to severe COPD. *Respiration* 1999; 66: 495–500.

6 Grandjean EM, Berthet P, Ruffmann R, Leuenberger P. Efficacy of oral long-term N-acetylcysteine in chronic bronchopulmonary disease: a meta-analysis of published double-blind, placebo-controlled clinical trials. *Clin Ther* 2000; 22: 209–221.

7 Stey C, Steurer J, Bachmann S, *et al*. The effect of N-acetylcysteine in chronic bronchitis: a quantitative systematic review. *Eur Respir J* 2000; 16: 253–262.

8 Lukas R, Scharling B, Schultze-Werninghaus G, Gillissen A. Antioxidant treatment with N-acetylcysteine and vitamin C in patients with chronic bronchitis. *Deutsch Med Wochenschr* 2005; 130: 563–567.

9 Decramer M, Rutten-van Molken M, Dekhuijzen PN, *et al*. Effects of N-acetylcysteine on outcomes in chronic obstructive pulmonary disease (Bronchitis Randomized NAC Cost-Utility Study, BRONCUS): a randomized placebo-controlled study. *Lancet* 2005; 365: 1552–1560.

10 De Benedetto F, Aceto A, Dragani B, *et al*. Long-term oral N-acetylcysteine reduces exhaled hydrogen peroxide in stable COPD. *Pulm Pharmacol Ther* 2005; 18: 41–47.

11 Kasielski M, Nowak D. Long-term administration of N-acetylcysteine decreases hydrogen peroxide exhalation in subjects with chronic obstructive airways disease. *Respir Med* 2001; 95: 448–456.

12 Demedts M, Behr J, Buhl R, *et al*. High dose acetylcysteine in idiopathic pulmonary fibrosis. *N Engl J Med* 2005; 353: 2229–2242.

13 Foschino Barbaro MP, Serviddio G, Resta O, *et al.* Oxygen therapy at low flow causes oxidative stress in chronic obstructive pulmonary disease. Prevention by *N*-acetylcysteine. *Free Radic Res* 2005; 39: 1111–1118.

14 De Flora S, Grassi C, Carati L. Attenuation of influenza-like symptomatology and improvement of cell-mediated immunity with long-term *N*-acetyl cysteine treatment. *Eur Respir J* 1997; 10: 1535–1541.

15 Herzenberg LA, De Rosa SC, Dubs JG, *et al.* Glutathione deficiency is associated with impaired survival in HIV disease. *Proc Natl Acad Sci USA* 1997; 94: 1967–1972.

16 De Rosa SC, Zaretsky MD, Dubs JG, *et al.* *N*-acetylcysteine replenishes glutathione in HIV infection. *Eur J Clin Invest* 2000; 30: 915–929.

17 Akerlund B, Jarstrand C, Lindeke B, *et al.* Effect of *N*-acetylcysteine (NAC) treatment on HIV-1 infection: a double-blind placebo-controlled trial. *Eur J Clin Pharmacol* 1996; 50: 457–461.

18 Spada C, Treitlinger A, Reis M, *et al.* The effect of *N*-acetylcysteine supplementation upon viral load, CD4, CD8 total lymphocyte count and haematrocrit in individuals undergoing antiretroviral treatment. *Clin Chem Lab Med* 2002; 40: 452–455.

19 Akerlund B, Tynell E, Bratt G, *et al. N*-acetylcysteine treatment and the risk of toxic reactions to trimethoprim-sulphamethoxazole in primary *Pneumocystis carinii* prophylaxis in HIV-infected patients. *J Infect* 1997; 35: 143–147.

20 Walmsley SL, Khorasheh S, Singer J, *et al.* A randomised trial of *N*-acetylcysteine for prevention of trimethoprim-sulphamethoxazole hypersensitivity reactions in *Pneumocystis carinii* pneumonia prophylaxis (CTN 057). Canadian HIV Trials Network 057 Study Group. *J Acquir Immune Defic Syndr Hum Retrovir* 1998; 19: 498–505.

21 Treitinger A, Spada C, Masokawa IY, *et al.* Effect of *N*-acetyl-L-cysteine on lymphocyte apoptosis, lymphocyte viability, TNF-alpha and IL-8 in HIV infected patients undergoing antiretroviral treatment. *Br J Infect Dis* 2004; 8: 363–371.

22 Van Zandwijk N, Dalesio O, Pastorino U, *et al.* EUROSCAN, a randomized trial of vitamin A and *N*-acetylcysteine in patients with head and neck cancer or lung cancer. For the European Organization for Research and Treatment of Cancer Head and Neck and Lung Cancer Cooperative Groups. *J Natl Cancer Inst* 2000; 92: 977–986.

23 Van Schooten FJ, Besaratinia A, De Flora S, *et al.* Effects of oral administration of *N*-acetyl-L-cysteine: a multi-biomarker study in smokers. *Cancer Epidemiol Biomarkers Prev* 2002; 11: 167–175.

Niacin

Description

Niacin is a water-soluble vitamin of the vitamin B complex.

Nomenclature

Niacin is a generic term used to describe the compounds that exhibit the biological properties of nicotinamide. It occurs in food as nicotinamide and nicotinic acid. It is sometimes known as niacinamide.

Units

Requirements and food values for niacin are the sum of the amounts of nicotinic acid and nicotinamide. Niacin is also obtained in the body from the amino acid tryptophan. On average, 60 mg tryptophan is equivalent to 1 mg niacin.

Niacin (mg equivalents) = nicotinic acid (mg) + nicotinamide (mg) + tryptophan (mg)/60

Human requirements

Niacin requirements depend on energy intake; values are therefore given as mg/1000 kcal and also as total values based on estimated average energy requirements for the majority of people in the UK (Table 1).

Dietary intake

In the UK, the average adult diet provides (niacin equivalents): for men, 44.7 mg daily; for women, 30.9 mg.

Action

Nutritional

As a vitamin, niacin functions as a component of two coenzymes, nicotinamide adenine dinucleotide (NAD) and nicotinamide adenine dinucleotide diphosphate (NADP). These coenzymes participate in many metabolic processes including glycolysis, tissue respiration, lipid, amino acid and purine metabolism.

Pharmacological

In doses in excess of nutritional requirements, nicotinic acid (but not nicotinamide) reduces serum cholesterol and triglycerides by inhibiting the synthesis of VLDLs, which are the precursors of LDLs. Nicotinic acid also causes direct peripheral vasodilatation.

Dietary sources

See Table 2 for dietary sources of niacin.

Metabolism

Absorption

Both nicotinamide and nicotinic acid are absorbed in the duodenum by facilitated diffusion (at low concentrations) and by passive diffusion (at high concentrations).

Distribution

Conversion of niacin to its coenzymes occurs in most tissues.

Table 1   Dietary Reference Values for niacin (nicotinic acid equivalent) (mg/day)

| | UK | | | | | USA | | FAO/WHO |
Age	LNRI[1]	EAR[1]	RNI[1]	RNI[2]	EVM	RDA[2]	TUL[2]	RNI[2]
							EU RDA $= 18$ mg	
0–6 months	4.4	5.5	6.6	3		2	–	2
7–12 months	4.4	5.5	6.6	5		3	–	4
1–3 years	4.4	5.5	6.6	8		6	10	6
4–6 years	4.4	5.5	6.6	11		–	–	9
4–8 years		–	–	–		8	15	–
7–10 years	4.4	5.5	6.6	12		–	–	12[a]
9–13 years	–	–	–	–		12	20	–
Males								
11–14 years	4.4	5.5	6.6	15		–	–	16[b]
15–18 years	4.4	5.5	6.6	18		–	–	16
14–18 years	–	–	–	–		16	30	–
19–50 years	4.4	5.5	6.6	17	17[3]	16	35	16
51–65+ years	–	–	–	–		–	–	16
51–70+ years	–	–	–	–		16	35	–
Females								
11–14 years	4.4	5.5	6.6	12		–	–	14[b]
15–18 years	4.4	5.5	6.6	14		–	–	14
14–18 years	–	–	–	–		14	30	–
19–50 years	4.4	5.5	6.6	13	17[3]	14	35	14
51–65+ years	–	–	–	–		–	–	14
51–70+ years	–	–	–	–		14	35	–
Pregnancy	*	*	*	–		18	35[4]	18
Lactation	*	*	+2.3	+2		17	35[4]	17

[a] 7–9 years.   [b] 10–14 years.
[1] mg/1000 kcal.   [2] mg/day.
[3] Likely safe daily intake of nicotinamide from supplements alone is 500 mg daily.   [4] Women <18 years = 30 mg daily.
EVM = Likely safe daily intake of nicotinic acid from supplements alone.
TUL = Tolerable Upper Intake Level.

Elimination

Elimination occurs mainly via the urine. Niacin appears in breast milk.

Bioavailability

Niacin is remarkably stable and can withstand reasonable periods of heating, cooking and storage with little loss. Bioavailability of niacin from cereals may be low, but much of the niacin in breakfast cereals comes from fully available synthetic niacin added to fortify such products.

Deficiency

Niacin deficiency (rare in the UK) may lead to pellagra. Early signs of deficiency are vague and non-specific and may include reduced appetite, weight loss, gastrointestinal discomfort, weakness, irritability and inability to concentrate. Signs of more advanced deficiency include sore

Table 2	Dietary sources of niacin

Food portion	Niacin content[1] (mg)
Breakfast cereals	
1 bowl All-Bran (45 g)	*6.5*
1 bowl Bran Flakes (45 g)	*7.5*
1 bowl Corn Flakes (30 g)	*5.0*
1 bowl muesli (95 g)	**8.0**
1 bowl Start (40 g)	**10.0**
2 pieces Shredded Wheat	*3.0*
2 Weetabix	*6.0*
Cereal products	
Bread, brown, 2 slices	*3.0*
white, 2 slices	*2.5*
wholemeal 2 slices	*4.0*
1 chapati	*2.5*
1 naan bread	*5.0*
1 white pitta bread	*2.5*
Pasta, brown, boiled (150 g)	*3.5*
white, boiled (150 g)	*2.0*
Rice, brown, boiled (160 g)	*3.0*
white, boiled (160 g)	*2.0*
2 heaped tablespoons wheatgerm	*1.5*
Milk and dairy products	
½ pint milk, whole, semi-skimmed, or skimmed	*2.5*
½ pint soya milk	*1.5*
1 pot yoghurt (150 g)	*1.5*
Cheese (50 g)	*1.5*
1 egg, size 2 (60 g)	*2.5*
Meat and fish	
Beef, roast (85 g)	**10.0**
Lamb, roast (85 g)	**10.0**
Pork, roast (85 g)	**10.0**
1 chicken leg portion	**16.0**
Liver, lambs, cooked (90 g)	**18.0**
Kidney, lambs, cooked (75 g)	**11.5**
Fish, cooked (150 g)	**10–15**
Vegetables	
Peas, boiled (100 g)	*2.5*
Potatoes, boiled (150 g)	*1.5*
1 small can baked beans (200 g)	*2.6*
Chickpeas, cooked (105 g)	*2.0*
Red kidney beans (105 g)	*2.0*
Dahl, lentil (150 g)	*1.5*
Nuts	
30 peanuts	*6.5*
Yeast	
Brewer's yeast (10 g)	*1.5*
Marmite, spread on 1 slice bread	*3.5*

Niacin equivalents (includes both pre-formed niacin and niacin obtained from tryptophan).
Excellent sources (**bold**); good sources (*italics*).

mouth, glossitis and stomatitis. The severe deficiency state of pellagra is characterised by dermatitis (predominantly in the areas of skin exposed to sunlight), dementia (associated with confusion, disorientation, seizures and hallucinations) and diarrhoea.

Possible uses

Despite claims made for niacin, it is of unproven value in arthritis, alcohol dependence, schizophrenia and other mental disorders unrelated to niacin deficiency. Nicotinic acid is prescribable on the NHS for hyperlipidaemia, but should not be sold as a supplement for this purpose.

Niacin (nicotinamide) is being evaluated in studies either alone or with statins for effect in cholesterol lowering. Some studies[1-3] and a meta-analysis[4] have demonstrated efficacy. However, doses used are high (500–1000 mg daily) and exceed the UK safe upper level, which makes this use unsuitable for dietary supplementation. In any case, further studies are required to confirm these findings.

Precautions/contraindications

Large doses of niacin are best avoided in gout (may increase uric acid levels); peptic ulcer (large doses may activate an ulcer); and liver disease (large doses cause deterioration). Large doses should also be used with caution in diabetes mellitus. However, studies suggest that lipid-modifying doses can safely be used in patients with diabetes.[5] Supplements containing nicotinic acid should not be used as a cholesterol-lowering agent without medical advice.

Pregnancy and breast-feeding

No problems reported.

Adverse effects

Both nicotinamide and nicotinic acid can be toxic in excessive amounts, but the effects are somewhat different.

Nicotinamide

In normal doses, nicotinamide is not toxic, but chronic administration at doses of 3 g daily for periods of more than 3 months may cause nausea, headaches, heartburn, fatigue, sore throat, dry hair, dry skin and blurred vision.

Nicotinic acid

Acute flushing (at doses of 100–200 mg, but reduced risk with sustained-release preparations), pounding headache, dizziness, nausea, vomiting, pruritis; occasionally decreased glucose tolerance and increased uric acid levels; rarely hepatic impairment (risk may be increased with sustained-release preparations) and hypertension.

Interactions

Drugs

Lipid-lowering drugs: increased risk of rhabdomyolysis and myopathy (combined therapy should include careful monitoring).

Nutrients

Adequate amounts of all B vitamins are required for optimal functioning; deficiency or excess of one B vitamin may lead to abnormalities in the metabolism of another.

Dose

Nicotinamide is available in the form of tablets, but is found mainly in multivitamin and mineral products.

Dietary supplements generally provide 30–50 mg daily.

References

1 Whitney EJ, Krasuski RA, Personius BE, *et al.* A randomized trial of a strategy for increasing high-density lipoprotein cholesterol levels: effects on progression of coronary heart disease and clinical events. *Ann Intern Med* 2005; 142: 95–104.

2 Taylor AJ, Sullenberger LE, Lee HJ, *et al.* Arterial Biology for the Investigation of the Treatment Effects of Reducing Cholesterol (ARBITER) 2: a double-blind atherosclerosis progression in secondary prevention patients treated with statins. *Circulation* 2004; 110: 3512–3517.

3 McKenney JM, McCormick LS, Schaefer EJ, *et al.* Effect of niacin and atorvastatin on lipoprotein subclasses in patients with atherogenic dyslipidaemia. *Am J Cardiol* 2001; 88: 270–274.

4 Goldberg AC. A meta-analysis of randomized controlled studies on the effects of extended-release niacin in women. *Am J Cardiol* 2004; 94: 121–124.

5 Elam MB, Hunninghake DB, Davis KB, *et al.* Effect of niacin on lipid and lipoprotein levels and glycemic control in patients with diabetes and peripheral arterial disease. *JAMA* 2000; 284: 1263–1270.

Nickel

Description

Nickel is a trace element. It can exist in oxidation states –I, 0, +I, +II, +III and +IV. State II is the most important in biological systems.[1] Nickel has not been shown to be essential in humans, but it is present in a few multivitamin/multimineral supplements in the UK.

Human requirements

Human requirements for nickel have not been established. There are no Dietary Reference Values. The Food Standards Agency Expert Vitamins and Minerals (EVM) group stated that UK dietary intake of nickel would not be expected to have any harmful effects but did not set a safe upper level or guidance level for adults for supplemental nickel intake.[2] The US Food and Nutrition Board set a Tolerable Upper Intake Level of 1 mg daily for adolescents and all adults.

Intake

Mean intake of dietary nickel in the UK is 130 μg daily, with an estimated maximum intake of 260 μg daily.[2]

Action

Nickel is an essential component in the enzymes of many plants, bacteria, algae and fungi. In humans, nickel influences iron absorption and metabolism and may be essential in red blood cell metabolism.[2]

Dietary sources

Nickel is present in a variety of foods, particularly pulses, grains (especially oats) and nuts. It is also present in drinking water.

Metabolism

Absorption

Dietary nickel is poorly absorbed. Absorption takes place in the small intestine via a carrier-mediated mechanism, but passive diffusion may also occur.

Distribution

The majority of nickel in human serum is bound to albumin, with some bound to nickeloplasmin, an α-macroglobulin, and some to amino acids, such as histidine, cysteine and aspartic acid.[1] It is distributed widely throughout the tissues with the highest concentrations in bone, lung, liver, kidney and endocrine glands. Nickel is also found in hair, nails, saliva and breast milk.

Elimination

Absorbed nickel is excreted predominantly in the urine, but some is also lost through sweat.

Bioavailability

Reported values of nickel absorption are < 1% when consumed with food, ascorbic acid, milk, tea, coffee and orange juice.[1] In a fasting state, 20–25% of nickel (from a nickel salt) may be absorbed.[2] Absorption is increased under conditions of low nickel and iron bioavailability.

Deficiency

Nickel deficiency has not been observed in humans. In animals, deficiency is associated with delayed sexual maturity, perinatal mortality, reduced growth and reduced haematopoiesis.

Possible uses

There are no known beneficial human health effects from consuming dietary nickel.

Precautions/contraindications

None reported.

Pregnancy and breast-feeding

There are no data in humans, but in animal studies, nickel toxicity is associated with perinatal mortality.

Adverse effects

Acute nickel exposure is associated with gastrointestinal disturbances, visual disturbance, headache, cough, wheezing and giddiness. Approximately 7–10% of the population (predominantly women) is affected by nickel-allergic dermatitis. Ingestion of nickel may exacerbate eczema due to nickel sensitivity. Iron deficiency may increase the risk of nickel sensitisation.[2]

Interactions

None reported.

Dose

The dose is not established. Supplements in the UK contain up to 5 µg in a daily dose.

References

1 Eckert C. Other trace elements. In: Shils ME, Shike M, Ross AC, *et al*, eds. *Modern Nutrition in Health and Disease*, 10th edn. London: Lippincott, Williams and Wilkins, 2006: 338–350.
2 Food Standards Agency. Risk assessment: nickel. http://www.eatwell.gov.uk/healthydiet/nutritionessentials/vitaminsandminerals/nickel (accessed 9 July 2006).

Octacosanol

Description

Octacosanol is the main component of policosanol, which is isolated from sugar cane wax. Octacosanol has also been isolated from *Eupolyphaga sinensis*, some *Euphorbia* species, *Acacia modeseta*, *Serenoa repens* and other plants, including whole grains, fruit and vegetables. It is a 28-carbon long-chain alcohol.

Action

Octacosanol appears to have a lipid-lowering effect, and there is some evidence (albeit limited) that octacosanol may improve muscle endurance. However, almost all of the studies conducted to date have emanated from a few research groups in Cuba and use one source of policosanol from Cuban cane sugar. The results from these groups have not been consistently replicated elsewhere.

Possible uses

It has been claimed that octacosanol is protective against CVD, can improve endurance in athletes, and is beneficial in patients with Parkinson's disease.

Cardiovascular disease
Animal studies have shown that policosanol reduces serum lipids,[1–3] platelet aggregation[4] and atherosclerosis,[5,6] and that it may help to protect against cerebral ischaemia.[7]

Platelet aggregation
In a double-blind, placebo-controlled study, 37 healthy volunteers were randomised to receive either placebo or policosanol 10 mg daily for 7 days, 20 mg daily for the next 7 days, then 40 mg daily for the next 7 days. Platelet aggregation (induced by ADP and epinephrine) reduced as the dose of policosanol increased, with significant effects observed after the second and third but not the first dose level. Coagulation time remained unchanged during the trial.[8]

In a further randomised, placebo-controlled, double-blind study involving healthy volunteers, policosanol (5, 10, 25 and 50 mg), administered orally, inhibited platelet aggregation (induced by ADP and epinephrine), and at a dose of 20 mg daily for 7 days the inhibition was significant. A modest effect on collagen-induced platelet aggregation was observed only at the highest dose (50 mg daily) while the lowest dose (5 mg daily) was ineffective. Policosanol did not affect coagulation time.[9] Further studies in healthy volunteers[10] and those with type II hypercholesterolaemia[11] have shown similar effects on platelet aggregation.

A randomised, double-blind, placebo-controlled study was carried out in 43 healthy volunteers to compare the effects of policosanol (20 mg daily), aspirin (100 mg daily) and combination therapy (policosanol 20 mg daily plus aspirin 100 mg daily) on platelet aggregation. With policosanol, platelet aggregation induced by ADP, epinephrine and collagen was significantly reduced. Aspirin reduced platelet aggregation induced by collagen and epinephrine but not by ADP. Combined therapy significantly inhibited platelet aggregation by all agonists. Coagulation time did not change during the trial. The authors concluded that policosanol (20 mg daily) was as effective as aspirin (100 mg daily), and that combination therapy showed some advantages over the respective monotherapies.[12]

A further double-blind RCT compared the antiplatelet effects of two doses of policosanol (20 and 40 mg daily) with placebo. Both doses significantly reduced platelet aggregation, compared with placebo, but no differences were observed in the effects produced by the two doses. Effects on platelet aggregation were similar in normal and hypercholesterolaemic patients. In addition, after 30 days, both 20 mg and 40 mg policosanol reduced LDL and total cholesterol and raised HDL cholesterol.[13]

Lipid lowering

A pilot single-blind, randomised, placebo-controlled trial was conducted in 23 middle-aged outpatients with well-documented chronic CHD and primary or marginal hyperlipidaemia. Twelve patients received 1 mg policosanol twice a day and 11 patients received placebo. The treated group showed a significant reduction in total (14.8%) and LDL (15.6%) cholesterol. The authors stated there was also a clinical tendency in five out of 12 of the treated patients towards improvement of CHD.[14]

In a 2-year, double-blind, randomised, placebo-controlled trial involving 69 patients with total and LDL cholesterol poorly controlled by diet, octacosanol 5 mg twice a day was associated with a 25% reduction in LDL cholesterol and an 18% reduction in total cholesterol. Ratios of LDL to HDL cholesterol were also reduced. All changes were significant and were maintained throughout the 2 years of the study.[15]

Another double-blind, placebo-controlled trial in 29 patients with non-insulin-dependent diabetes mellitus (NIDDM) and hypercholesterolaemia found that 10 mg policosanol daily significantly reduced total cholesterol by 17.5% and LDL cholesterol by 21.8%, non-significantly reduced triglycerides by 6.6%, and non-significantly raised HDL cholesterol by 11.3%. Glycaemic control was unaffected and no adverse effects were attributable to policosanol. The authors concluded that policosanol is safe and effective in patients with NIDDM and hypercholesterolaemia.[16]

A further double-blind, randomised study comparing the effect of policosanol (10 mg daily; 55 patients) with the two HMG-CoA reductase inhibitors, lovastatin (20 mg daily; 26 patients) or simvastatin (10 mg daily; 25 patients), showed that LDL cholesterol reduced by 24% with policosanol, 22% with lovastatin and 15% with simvastatin. HDL cholesterol was increased in the policosanol group but not in the two groups using the HMG-CoA reductase inhibitors.[17]

A similar study comparing policosanol (10 mg daily) with acipimox (750 mg daily), involving 63 patients, showed that policosanol reduced total cholesterol and LDL cholesterol by 15.8% and 21%, respectively, and lowered the ratio of LDL to HDL cholesterol by 15.8%. Acipimox reduced both total cholesterol and LDL cholesterol by 7.5%.[18]

A further study comparing policosanol (10 mg daily) and pravastatin (10 mg daily) showed reductions in total and LDL cholesterol with policosanol of 13.9% and 19.3%, respectively, and lowered the LDL:HDL cholesterol ratio by 28.3%. Pravastatin lowered total cholesterol by 11.8% and LDL cholesterol by 15.6%. Policosanol reduced platelet aggregation to a greater extent than pravastatin. The authors concluded that policosanol (10 mg daily) produces more favourable effects on serum lipids and platelet aggregation than pravastatin (10 mg daily).[19] A further study comparing policosanol (10 mg daily) with lovastatin (20 mg daily) in 53 patients showed similar effects on serum lipid levels.[20] A further study comparing policosanol 10 mg daily with lovastatin 20 mg daily found that policosanol was slightly more effective than lovastatin in reducing the LDL/HDL and total cholesterol/HDL ratios, in increasing HDL levels and preventing LDL oxidation.[21] A Russian study found that policosanol 10 mg daily was superior in lowering cholesterol to bezafibrate 400 mg daily.[22] In a study comparing policosanol 10 mg daily with atorvastatin 10 mg daily, policosanol was less effective than atorvastatin in reducing serum LDL and triglyceride levels in elderly patients with hypercholesterolaemia. Policosanol, but not atorvastatin, significantly increased serum HDL, while both reduced serum triglycerides and other measures of atherogenesis.[23]

Further studies have shown that policosanol reduced serum total and LDL cholesterol and raised HDL cholesterol in a study involving 437 individuals with type II hypercholesterolaemia and additional coronary risk factors,[24] and in a study involving 69 healthy subjects, policosanol decreased the susceptibility of LDL cholesterol to oxidation *in vitro*.[25] Similar influences on cholesterol with policosanol have been shown in a trial involving 244 post-menopausal women with hypercholesterolaemia.[26]

Newer studies have found that policosanol is effective, safe and well tolerated in older patients with hypercholesterolaemia and high coronary risk,[27] in post-menopausal women with hypercholesterolaemia,[28] and in older patients with hypertension and hypercholesterolaemia.[29] A dose of 40 mg policosanol was not found to offer any lipid-lowering advantage over a dose of 20 mg daily.[30] In a study comparing policosanol with mixtures of higher aliphatic primary alcohols, policosanol was found to reduce LDL cholesterol while the other mixtures did not.[31] A study evaluating the effect of policosanol with omega-3 fatty acids found that the combination lowered LDL and total cholesterol and triglycerides and raised HDL cholesterol.[32] Another study found that policosanol could provide additional benefits in lowering blood pressure in people taking beta-blockers.[33]

However, a Dutch study investigating policosanol from wheatgerm found that a dose of 20 mg daily had no beneficial effect on blood lipids.[34]

A recent meta-analysis[35] compared the effect of policosanol with plant sterols and stanols and found that policosanol is more effective for LDL cholesterol reduction and more favourably alters the lipid profile. A *Bandolier* review[36] concluded that policosanol from Cuban sugar cane reduces total and LDL cholesterol by an amount equivalent to statins and has fewer, less serious, adverse events. However, all the Cuban trials show exactly the same 10–15% reduction in total cholesterol regardless of patient characteristics, duration of study (although most were longer than 6 weeks) or dose of policosanol. The inter-subject variation in cholesterol lowering with statins is much greater, making the policosanol results appear quite strange.

A recent South African RCT investigated the effect of a policosanol supplement (20 mg daily) for 12 weeks on 19 subjects with hypercholesterolaemia (some of whom had familial hypercholesterolaemia). However, the supplement had no significant effect on total or LDL cholesterol compared with placebo.[37] A further trial has evaluated policosanol derived from Cuban sugar cane in lipid outpatient clinics and general practices in Germany. A total of 143 patients with hypercholesterolaemia or combined hyperlipidaemia were randomised to receive policosanol 10, 20, 40 or 80 mg daily or placebo. No statistically significant difference between policosanol and placebo was observed in lipid lowering.[38]

Intermittent claudication

The Cuban researchers have also investigated the effect of policosanol in patients with intermittent claudication. A 2-year study found that policosanol 10 mg twice daily was more effective in improving walking distance than placebo.[39] A further study comparing policosanol (10 mg daily) with lovastatin (20 mg daily) found that policosanol (not lovastatin) was effective in improving walking distance,[40] while another study found policosanol (10 mg twice a day) to be as effective as ticlopidine (now discontinued in the UK) (250 mg three times a day).[41]

Parkinson's disease

Octacosanol has been evaluated in patients with mild to moderate Parkinson's disease. In a double-blind crossover trial, 10 patients received either 5 mg octacosanol or placebo (both three times a day) for 6 weeks. Only three patients improved significantly at the study's end. Some responded slightly or had no disease progression during the study. Activities of daily living and mood improved, but physical endurance and parkinsonian symptoms did not. One patient experienced dizziness and another experienced exacerbation of dyskinesias. The authors concluded that octacosanol might be beneficial for patients with mild Parkinson's disease, but that the benefit is likely to be small and less than that exerted by existing treatments.[42]

Amyotrophic lateral sclerosis

Anecdotally, octacosanol has been claimed to improve symptoms of amyotrophic lateral sclerosis (AMS), but a placebo-controlled, double-blind, crossover trial in which patients received either 40 mg octacosanol or placebo for 3 months and were then crossed over showed no difference between octacosanol and placebo.[43]

Athletes

Octacosanol is now being widely advertised for enhancing performance in athletes, particularly in the USA and Australia. However, there are almost no supporting data.

One study in 33 male student athletes (20 controls, 13 supplemented) showed that supplementation with a pack containing 29 supplements including 2000 µg octacosanol was associated with a decrease in body fat and increase in muscle girth measurement, indicating the formation of lean body mass. However, the study was not blinded, the diet not controlled and the pack contained a variety if supplements in addition to octacosanol.[44]

Another study in 16 subjects (students and lecturers in physical education) measured grip strength, chest strength, and reaction time to both auditory and visual stimuli. Following supplementation with 1000 µg octacosanol for 8 weeks, only grip strength and reaction time to visual stimuli were improved.[45]

Conclusion

A number of human studies have now been conducted with policosanol and have shown benefits in lipid lowering and platelet aggregation compared with placebo. They have also shown similar effects to various lipid-lowering drugs. However, nearly all of the studies have been conducted by one research group in Havana, Cuba, and with policosanol from Cuban sugar cane. They have not been replicated outside Cuba or using policosanol from other sources. There is very little evidence that octacosanol is useful for athletes.

Precautions/contraindications

None reported.

Pregnancy and breast-feeding

No problems have been reported, but there have not been sufficient studies to guarantee the safety of octacosanol in pregnancy and breast-feeding. The effects are unknown, and octacosanol is best avoided.

Adverse effects

None reported, but there are no long-term studies assessing the safety of octacosanol. In a trial investigating the effects of placebo and policosanol, 5 mg, 10 mg and 20 mg daily, policosanol was said by the authors to be well tolerated with no disturbances of blood or clinical biochemistry. Adverse effects were found to be mild and transient with no differences between the groups.[46]

Interactions

None reported. A study in rats investigated the effect of adding policosanol to warfarin. Policosanol did not enhance the prolongation of bleeding time induced by warfarin alone.[47]

Dose

Octacosanol is available in the form of tablets and capsules.

The dose is not established. Doses used in studies have varied from 1 to 20 mg policosanol daily.

References

1 Arruzazabala ML, Carbajal D, Mas R, *et al*. Cholesterol-lowering effect of policosanol in rabbits. *Biol Res* 1994; 27: 205–208.

2 Menendez R, Amor AM, Gonzalez RM, *et al*. Effect of policosanol on the hepatic cholesterol biosynthesis of normocholesterolemic rats. *Biol Res* 1996; 29: 253–257.

3 Menendez R, Arruzazabala L, Mas R, *et al*. Cholesterol-lowering effect of policosanol on rabbits

with hypercholesterolaemia induced by a wheat starch-casein diet. *Br J Nutr* 1997; 77: 923–932.

4 Arruzazabala ML, Carbajal D, Mas R, *et al*. Effects of policosanol on platelet aggregation in rats. *Thromb Res* 1993; 69: 321–327.

5 Noa M, Mas R, de la Rosa MC, *et al*. Effect of policosanol on lipofundin-induced atherosclerotic lesions in rats. *J Pharm Pharmacol* 1995; 47: 289–291.

6 Arruzazabala ML, Noa M, Menendez R, *et al*. Protective effect of policosanol on atherosclerotic lesions in rabbits with exogenous hypercholesterolaemia. *Braz J Med Biol Res* 2000; 33: 835–840.

7 Molina V, Arruzazabala D, Carbajal D, *et al*. Effect of policosanol on cerebral ischemia in Mongolian gerbils. *Braz J Med Biol Res* 1999; 32: 1269–1276.

8 Arruzazabala ML, Valdes S, Mas R, *et al*. Effect of policosanol successive dose increases on platelet aggregation in healthy volunteers. *Phamacol Res* 1996; 34: 181–185.

9 Valdes S, Arruzazabala ML, Fernandez L, *et al*. Effect of policosanol on platelet aggregation in healthy volunteers. *Int J Clin Pharmacol Res* 1996; 16: 67–72.

10 Carbajal D, Arruzazabala ML, Valdes S, *et al*. Effect of policosanol on platelet aggregation and serum levels of arachidonic acid metabolites in healthy volunteers. *Prostaglandins Leukot Essent Fatty Acids* 1998; 58: 61–64.

11 Arruzazabala ML, Mas R, Molina V, *et al*. Effect of policosanol on platelet aggregation in type II hypercholesterolemic patients. *Int J Tissue React* 1998; 20: 119–124.

12 Arruzazabala ML, Valdes S, Mas R, *et al*. Comparative study of policosanol, aspirin and the combination therapy policosanol-aspirin on platelet aggregation in healthy volunteers. *Pharmacol Res* 1997; 36: 293–297.

13 Arruzazabala ML, Molina V, Mas R, *et al*. Antiplatelet effects of policosanol (20 and 40mg/day) in healthy volunteers and dyslipidaemic patients. *Clin Exp Pharmacol Physiol* 2002; 29: 891–897.

14 Batista J, Stusser R, Saez F, *et al*. Effect of policosanol on hyperlipidemia and coronary heart disease in middle-aged patients. A 14-month pilot study. *Int J Clin Phamacol Ther* 1996; 34: 134–137.

15 Canetti M, Moreira M, Mas R, *et al*. A two-year study on the efficacy and tolerability of policosanol in patients with type II hyperlipoproteinaemia. *Int J Clin Pharmacol Res* 1995; 15: 159–165.

16 Torres O, Agramonte AJ, Illnait J, *et al*. Treatment of hypercholesterolemia in NIDDM with policosanol. *Diabetes Care* 1995; 18: 393–397.

17 Prat H, Roman O, Pino E. Comparative effects of policosanol and two HMG-CoA reductase inhibitors on type II hypercholesterolemia. *Rec Med Chil* 1999; 127: 286–294.

18 Alcocer L, Fernandez L, Campos E, *et al*. A comparative study of policosanol versus acipimox in patients with type II hypercholesterolemia. *Int J Tissue React* 1999; 21: 85–92.

19 Castano G, Mas R, Arruzazabala ML, *et al*. Effect of policosanol and pravastatin on lipid profile, platelet aggregation and endothelemia in older hypercholesterolemic patients. *Int J Clin Pharmacol Res* 1999; 19: 105–116.

20 Crespo N, Illnait J, Mas R, *et al*. Comparative study of the efficacy and tolerability of policosanol and lovastatin in patients with hypercholesterolemia and noninsulin dependent diabetes mellitus. *Int J Clin Pharmacol Res* 1999; 19: 117–127.

21 Castano G, Menendez R, Mas R, *et al*. Effects of policosanol and lovastatin on lipid profile and lipid peroxidation in patients with dyslipidaemia associated with type 2 diabetes mellitus. *Int J Clin Pharmacol Res* 2002; 22: 89–99.

22 Nitkin IuP, Slepchenko NV, Gratsianskii NA, *et al*. Results of the multicenter controlled study of the hypolipidemic drug polycosanol in Russia. *Ter Arkh* 2000; 72: 7–10.

23 Castano G, Mas R, Fernandez L, *et al*. Comparison of the efficacy and tolerability of policosanol with atorvastatin in elderly patients with type II hypercholesterolaemia. *Drugs Aging* 2003; 20: 153–163.

24 Mas R, Castano G, Illnait J, *et al*. Effects of policosanol in patients with type II hypercholesterolemia and additional risk factors. *Clin Pharmacol Ther* 1999; 65: 439–447.

25 Menendez R, Mas R, Amor AM, *et al*. Effects of policosanol treatment on the susceptibility of low density lipoprotein (LDL) isolated from healthy volunteers to oxidative modification *in vitro*. *Br J Clin Pharmacol* 2000; 50: 255–262.

26 Castano G, Mas R, Fernandez L, *et al*. Effects of policosanol on postmenopausal women with type II hypercholesterolemia. *Gynecol Endocrinol* 2000; 14: 187–195.

27 Castano G, Mas R, Fernandez JC, *et al*. Effects of policosanol in older patients with type II hypercholesterolemia and high coronary risk. *J Gerontol A Biol Sci Med Sci* 2001; 56: M186–M192.

28 Mirkin A, Mas R, Martino M, *et al*. Efficacy and tolerability of policosanol in hypercholesterolaemic, postmenopausal women. *Int J Pharmacol Res* 2001; 21: 31–41.

29 Castano G, Mas R, Fernandez JC, *et al*. Effects of policosanol on older patients with hypertension and type II hypercholesterolaemia. *Drugs R D* 2002; 3: 159–172.

30 Castano G, Mas R, Fernandez L, *et al*. Effects of policosanol 20 versus 40 mg/day in the treatment of patients with type II hypercholesterolemia: a

6-month double-blind study. *Int J Clin Pharmacol Res* 2001; 21: 43–57.

31 Castano G, Fernandez L, Mas R, *et al.* Comparison of the efficacy, safety and tolerability of original policosanol versus other mixtures of higher aliphatic primary alcohols in patients with type II hypercholesterolemia. *Int J Pharmacol Res* 2002; 22: 55–66.

32 Castano G, Fernandez L, Mas R, *et al.* Effects of addition of policosanol to omega-3 fatty acids therapy on the lipid profile of patients with type II hypercholesterolaemia. *Drugs R D* 2005; 6: 207–219.

33 Castano G, Mas R, Gamez R, *et al.* Concomitant use of policosanol and beta-blockers in older patients. *Int J Clin Pharmacol Res* 2004; 24: 65–77.

34 Lin Y, Rudrum M, van der Wielen RP, *et al.* Wheat germ policosanol failed to lower plasma cholesterol in subjects with normal to mildly elevated cholesterol concentrations. *Metabolism* 2004; 53: 1309–1314.

35 Chen JT, Wesley R, Shanburek RD, *et al.* Meta-analysis of natural therapies for hyperlipidemia: plant sterols and stanols versus policosanol. *Pharmacotherapy* 2005; 25: 171–183.

36 Anonymous. Policosanol for lipid-lowering. *Bandolier* January 2005 (available from http://www. jr2.ox.ac.uk/bandolier/Extraforbando/Policosanol.pdf).

37 Greyling A, De Witt C, Oosthuizen W, Jerling JC. Effects of a policosanol supplement on serum lipid concentrations in hypercholesterolaemic and heterozygous familial hypercholesterolaemic subjects. *Br J Nutr* 2006; 95: 968–975.

38 Berthold HK, Unverdorben S, Degenhardt R, *et al.* Effect of policosanol on lipid levels among patients with hypercholesterolaemia or combined hyperlipidaemia. *JAMA* 2006; 295: 2262–2269.

39 Castano G, Mas Ferreiro R, Fernandez L, *et al.* A long-term study of policosanol in the treatment of intermittent claudication. *Angiology* 2001; 52: 115–125.

40 Castano G, Mas R, Fernandez L, *et al.* Effects of policosanol and lovastatin in patients with intermittent claudication: a double-blind comparative pilot study. *Angiology* 2003; 54: 25–38.

41 Castano G, Mas R, Gamez R, *et al.* Effects of policosanol and ticlodipidine in patients with intermittent claudication: a double-blinded pilot comparative study. *Angiology* 2004; 55: 361–371.

42 Snider SR. Octacosanol in Parkinsonism. *Ann Neurol* 1984; 16: 273 (letter).

43 Norris FH, Denys EH, Fallat RJ. Trial of octacosanol on amyotrophic lateral sclerosis. *Neurology* 1986; 36: 1263–1264.

44 Cockerill DL, Bucci LR. Increases in muscle girth and decreases in body fat associated with a nutritional supplement program. *Chiro Sports Med* 1987; 1: 73–76.

45 Saint-John M, McNaughton L. Octacosanol ingestion and its effects on metabolic responses to submaximal cycle ergometry, reaction time, and chest and grip strength. *Int Clin Nutr Rev* 1986; 6: 81–87.

46 Pons P, Rodriguez M, Robaina C, *et al.* Effects of successive dose increases of policosanol on the lipid profile of patients with type II hypercholesterolaemia and tolerability to treatment. *Int J Clin Pharmacol Res* 1994; 14: 27–33.

47 Carbajal D, Arruzazabala ML, Valdes S, *et al.* Interaction of policosanol-warfarin on bleeding time and thrombosis in rats. *Pharmacol Res* 1998; 38: 89–91.

Pangamic acid

Description and nomenclature

An alternative name for pangamic acid is vitamin B_{15}, but it is not an officially recognised vitamin. Pangamic acid is the name given to a product originally claimed to contain D-gluconodimethyl aminoacetic acid, which was obtained from apricot kernels and later from rice bran.

Constituents

The composition of supplements is undefined, but they may contain one or more of the following substances: calcium gluconate, glycine, N,N-dimethylglycine and N,N-diisopropylamine dichloroacetate (N,N-diisopropylamine dichloroacetate has pharmacological activity).

Dietary sources

Apricot kernels, brewer's yeast, liver, wheatgerm, bran and wholegrains.

Possible uses

Research by Soviet sports scientists focused attention on pangamic acid, but very little research has been done in other countries. Pangamic acid is claimed to enhance athletic performance and to be beneficial in CVD, asthma and diabetes mellitus. Scientific studies show no evidence of therapeutic efficacy for pangamic acid.

Precautions/contraindications

Pangamic acid should not be taken at all, by anyone.

Adverse effects

Pangamic acid may be mutagenic and thus potentially able to cause cancer. It may cause occasional transient flushing of the skin.

Interactions

None reported.

Dose

Pangamic acid should be avoided. Dietary supplements are rarely available in UK high-street outlets, but may be available on the Internet.

Pantothenic acid

Description

Pantothenic acid is a water-soluble B complex vitamin.

Human requirements

See Table 1 for Dietary Reference Values for pantothenic acid.

Dietary intake

In the UK, the average adult diet provides 5.1 mg daily.

Action

Pantothenic acid functions mainly as a component of coenzyme A and acyl carrier protein. Coenzyme A has a central role as a cofactor for enzymes involved in the metabolism of lipids, carbohydrates and proteins; it is also required for the synthesis of cholesterol, steroid hormones, acetylcholine and porphyrins. As a component of acyl carrier protein, pantothenic acid is involved in various transfer reactions and in the assembly of acetate units into longer-chain fatty acids.

Table 1 Dietary Reference Values for pantothenic acid (mg/day)

					EU RDA = 6 mg
Age	UK		USA		FAO/WHO RNI
	Safe intake	EVM	AI	TUL	
0–6 months	1.7		1.7	–	1.7
7–12 months	1.7		1.8	–	1.8
1–3 years	1.7		2.0	–	2.0
4–10 years	3–7		–	–	$3.0^1 4.0^2$
4–8 years				3.0	
9–13 years			4.0	–	
Males and females					
11–50+ years	3–7	200	–	5.0	
14–70+ years			5.0	–	–
Pregnancy	–		6.0	–	6.0
Lactation	–		7.0	–	7.0

[1] 4–6 years.   [2] 7–9 years.

EVM = Likely safe daily intake from supplements alone.

TUL = Tolerable Upper Intake Level (not determined for pantothenic acid).

Table 2   Dietary sources of pantothenic acid

Food portion	Pantothenic acid content (mg)
Breakfast cereals	
1 bowl All-Bran (45 g)	0.7
1 bowl Bran Flakes (45 g)	0.7
1 bowl Corn Flakes (30 g)	0.1
1 bowl muesli (95 g)	**1.1**
2 pieces Shredded Wheat	0.4
2 Weetabix	0.3
Cereal products	
Bread, brown, 2 slices	0.2
white, 2 slices	0.2
wholemeal, 2 slices	0.4
1 chapati	0.1
Milk and dairy products	
½ pint milk, whole, semi-skimmed or skimmed	0.8
1 pot yoghurt (150 g)	0.6
Cheese (50 g)	0.2
1 egg, size 2 (60 g)	**1.0**
Meat and fish	
Beef, roast (85 g)	0.5
Lamb, roast (85 g)	0.5
Pork, roast (85 g)	0.8
1 chicken leg portion	**1.5**
Liver, lambs, cooked (90 g)	**7.0**
Kidney, lambs, cooked (75 g)	**4.0**
Fish, cooked (150 g)	0.5
Vegetables	
1 small can baked beans (200 g)	0.4
Chickpeas, cooked (105 g)	0.3
Red kidney beans (105 g)	0.2
Peas, boiled (100 g)	0.1
Potatoes, boiled (150 g)	0.6
Green vegetables, average, boiled (100 g)	0.2
Fruit	
1 banana	0.5
1 orange	0.6
Nuts	
30 peanuts	0.7
Yeast	
Brewer's yeast (10 g)	**1.0**

Excellent sources (> 1 mg/portion) (**bold**).

Dietary sources

See Table 2 for dietary sources of pantothenic acid.

Metabolism

Absorption
Absorption occurs in the small intestine.

Distribution
Pantothenic acid is widely distributed in body tissues (particularly in the liver, adrenal glands, heart and kidneys), mainly as coenzyme A.

Elimination
About 70% is excreted unchanged via the urine and 30% in the faeces.

Bioavailability

Bioavailability may be reduced by some drugs (see Interactions) and a high fat intake, and increased by a diet high in protein.

Deficiency

Deficiency has not been clearly identified in humans consuming a mixed diet.

Possible uses

Pantothenic acid has been used for a wide range of disorders such as acne, alopecia, allergies, burning feet, asthma, grey hair, dandruff, cholesterol lowering, improving exercise performance, depression, osteoarthritis, rheumatoid arthritis, multiple sclerosis, stress, shingles, ageing and Parkinson's disease. It has been investigated in clinical trials for arthritis, cholesterol lowering and exercise performance.

Arthritis
In an uncontrolled trial, patients treated with pantothenate 12.5 mg twice a day showed a limited, variable improvement within 1–2 weeks of therapy, which ended upon discontinuation of therapy.[1] In a double-blind, placebo-controlled trial,[2] 94 patients with arthritis (of whom 27

had rheumatoid arthritis) were randomised to receive large doses of calcium pantothenate (titrated up from 500 mg daily to 2000 mg daily) or a placebo for 8 weeks. There was no significant reduction in either group in the duration of morning stiffness or disability, but both groups experienced significant relief from pain. When the subjects with rheumatoid arthritis were analysed separately, the group receiving pantothenate showed statistically significant reduction in morning stiffness, disability and pain compared with placebo.

Cholesterol lowering

A double-blind, placebo-controlled, crossover study in 29 patients with various types of dyslipidaemia found that 900 mg pantothenic acid daily reduced total and LDL cholesterol in type IIb hyperlipidaemia, with varying effects in type IV patients.[3]

Exercise performance

Two double-blind, placebo-controlled studies with pantothenic acid in runners[4] and cyclists[5] showed that pantothenic acid had no effect on exercise performance.

> **Conclusion**
> Research is too limited to be able to make recommendations for pantothenic acid.

Precautions/contraindications

None reported.

Pregnancy and breast-feeding

No problems reported.

Adverse effects

No adverse effects, except for occasional diarrhoea, have been reported in humans. High intake of pantothenic acid (and biotin and riboflavin) with low intake of calcium, folate, nicotinic acid, vitamin E, retinol and beta-carotene, has been associated with increased genome instability.[6]

Interactions

Drugs

Alcohol: excessive alcohol intake may increase requirement for pantothenic acid.
Oral contraceptives: may increase requirement for pantothenic acid.

Nutrients

Adequate amounts of all B vitamins are required for optimal functioning; deficiency or excess of one B vitamin may lead to abnormalities in the metabolism of another.

Dose

Pantothenic acid and calcium pantothenate are available in the form of tablets and capsules, but they are found mainly in multivitamin and mineral preparations.

The dose is not established. Dietary supplements contain up to 100 mg daily.

References

1 Annand J. Pantothenic acid and OA. *Lancet* 1963; 2: 1168.
2 General Practitioner Research Group. Calcium pantothenate in arthritic conditions. A report from the General Practitioner Research Group. *Practitioner* 1980; 224: 208–211.
3 Gaddi A, Descovich GC, Noseda G, *et al.* Controlled evaluation of pantethine, a natural hypolipemic compound, in patients with hyperlipidaemia. *Atherosclerosis* 1984; 50: 73–83.
4 Nice C, Reeves AG, Brinck-Johnsen T, *et al.* The effects of pantothenic acid on human exercise capacity. *J Sports Med Phys Fitness* 1984; 24: 26–29.
5 Webster MJ. Physiological and performance responses to supplementation with thiamin and pantothenic acid derivatives. *Eur J Appl Physiol* 1998; 77: 486–491.
6 Fenech M, Baghurst P, Luderer W, *et al.* Low intake of folate, nicotinic acid, vitamin E, retinol, beta-carotene, and high intake of pantothenic acid, biotin and riboflavin are significantly associated with increased genome instability – result from a dietary intake and micronutrients intake survey in South Australia. *Carcinogenesis* 2005; 26: 991–999.

Para-amino benzoic acid

Description and nomenclature

Para-amino benzoic acid (PABA) is a member of the vitamin B complex, but is not an officially recognised vitamin.

Dietary sources

Brewer's yeast, liver, wheatgerm, bran and wholegrains.

Possible uses

PABA is claimed to prevent greying hair and to be useful as an anti-ageing supplement. It has been used in digestive disorders, arthritis, insomnia and depression. There is no convincing scientific evidence available.

A derivative of PABA is used topically as a sunscreen agent; this is effective in the prevention of sunburn.

Adverse effects

Toxicity is low, but high doses ($>30\,$mg) may cause anorexia, nausea, vomiting, liver toxicity, fever, itching and skin rash.

Interactions

Sulphonamides: kill bacteria by mimicking PABA; supplements containing PABA should be avoided while taking these drugs.

Dose

PABA is available in the form of tablets and capsules.

There is no established dose. Supplements are not justified. Dietary supplements provide 100–500 mg per dose.

Phosphatidylserine

Description

Phosphatidylserine belongs to a class of fat-soluble compounds called phospholipids. Phospholipids are essential components of cell membranes, with high concentrations found in the brain. Phosphatidylserine is the most abundant phospholipid in the brain.

Action

Phosphatidylserine helps to ensure fluidity, flexibility and permeability in cell membranes. It stimulates the release of various transmitters, such as acetylcholine and dopamine, enhances ion transport and increases the number of neurotransmitter receptor sites in the brain.

Possible uses

Phosphatidyl serine is claimed to be useful in enhancing memory, treating depression and preventing age-related neurotransmitter defects.

Age-related cognitive decline

A double-blind, randomised, controlled study was conducted in 42 hospitalised demented patients, in which half the patients received 300 mg phosphatidylserine and the other half placebo. The trial lasted for 6 weeks. Two distinct rating scales were used: the Crighton Scale and the Peri Scale. Results showed a trend towards improvement in the treated patients and analysis of covariance showed a significant treatment effect on the Peri Scale. The results at the end of treatment were compared with results obtained 3 weeks later and there was still a significant difference on the Peri Scale,

indicating (according to the authors) a drug-related effect.[1]

The effects of phosphatidylserine on cognitive, affective and behavioural symptoms were studied in a group of elderly women with depressive disorders. The treatment was not blinded or randomised. Patients were treated with placebo for 15 days followed by phosphatidylserine (300 mg daily) for 30 days. Changes in depression, memory and general behaviour were measured according to four different scales before and after placebo, and after treatment. Depressive symptoms were marked before placebo, did not change after placebo, and were significantly reduced by phosphatidylserine treatment. There was also improvement in memory (recall, long-term retrieval), but there were no changes in plasma levels of various neurochemicals.[2]

In a double-blind, placebo-controlled study, 149 patients with age-associated memory impairment were treated with phosphatidylserine 300 mg or placebo for 12 weeks. The supplemented subjects improved relative to placebo on performance tests related to learning and memory tasks of daily life. Analysis of subgroups showed that subjects who performed at a relatively low level before treatment were most likely to respond to phosphatidylserine. The authors concluded that phosphatidylserine may be a promising candidate for treating memory loss in later life.[3]

In a double-blind, placebo-controlled study, 51 patients with probable Alzheimer's disease were treated with phosphatidylserine (300 mg daily) or placebo for 12 weeks. Two rating scales were used to assess the patients, and after 12 weeks, the treated group improved on three of the 12 variables on one scale and five of the 25 variables on the other scale. Family members rated significant improvements with phosphatidylserine after 6 and 9 weeks but not at 12 weeks. The authors stressed that phosphatidylserine could be helpful in patients with early-stage disease, but might have no effect in middle and later stages.[4]

In a double-blind, placebo-controlled, crossover study, 33 patients with mild primary degenerative dementia received either phosphatidylserine 300 mg daily or placebo for 8 weeks. Clinical global rating scales showed significantly more patients improving with phosphatidylserine than placebo. However, there were no significant improvements in dementia rating scale or psychometric tests.[5]

In a double-blind, placebo-controlled study 494 elderly patients (aged 65–93 years) with moderate to severe cognitive decline were randomised to receive either phosphatidylserine 300 mg daily or placebo for 6 months. Sixty-nine patients dropped out of the trial. Patients were examined before the study, and 3 and 6 months after. Statistically significant improvements in the treated group compared to placebo were observed in terms of both behavioural and cognitive parameters.[6]

Physical stress

In a double-blind trial, eight healthy men underwent three experiments with a bicycle ergometer. Before the exercise, each subject received intravenously 50 or 75 mg of phosphatidylserine or placebo. Blood samples were collected before and after the exercise and analysed for epinephrine, norepinephrine, dopamine, adrenocorticotrophin, cortisol, growth hormone, prolactin and glucose. Physical stress induced a clear-cut increase in plasma epinephrine, norepinephrine, adrenocorticotrophic hormone (ACTH), cortisol, growth hormone and prolactin, whereas no significant change was found in plasma dopamine and glucose. Pretreatment with both 50 mg and 75 mg phosphatidylserine significantly blunted the ACTH and cortisol responses to physical stress.[7]

In a study using the same exercise protocol in the same research centre, nine healthy men were treated for three 10-day periods with placebo, 400 mg and 800 mg phosphatidylserine daily.

Oral phosphatidylserine rather than the intravenous formulation was used. Phosphatidylserine 800 mg significantly blunted the ACTH and cortisol responses to physical exercise. The authors concluded that chronic oral administration of phosphatidylserine might counteract stress-induced activation of the hypothalamic-pituitary-adrenal axis in men.[8]

Psychological stress

Recent research has investigated the effects of phosphatidylserine on psychological stress. A study assigned four groups of 20 subjects to 400 mg, 600 mg or 800 mg phosphatidylserine complex (PAS) or placebo for 3 weeks, then exposed them to the Trier Social Stress Test. Treatment with 400 mg PAS resulted in a pronounced blunting of both serum ACTH and cortisol, but did not affect heart rate. The effect was not seen with the larger doses of PAS. After the test, the placebo group showed the expected increased distress while the 400 mg PAS group showed reduced distress. The authors concluded that this study provides initial evidence of a selective stress dampening effect of PAS on the pituitary-adrenal axis, suggesting the potential for PAS in the treatment of stress-related disorders.[9]

Conclusion
There is evidence from controlled trials that phosphatidylserine improves memory and other symptoms of cognitive decline in elderly patients. There is also some limited evidence that phosphatidylserine attenuates the cortisol response to exercise. However, this response is a natural phenomenon and interfering with it could delay recovery in athletes. Further research is required to ascertain whether phosphatidylserine is beneficial in athletes or not.

Precautions/contraindications

None reported.

Pregnancy and breast-feeding

No problems have been reported, but there have not been sufficient studies to guarantee the safety of phosphatidylserine in pregnancy and breast-feeding.

Adverse effects

No known toxicity or side-effects, but there are no long-term studies assessing the safety of phosphatidylserine. There have been concerns about phosphatidylserine supplements derived from bovine brain tissue, because of concerns about diseases such as bovine spongiform encephalopathy (BSE), and supplements based on soy have been developed. The two supplements are slightly different and there has been discussion about whether they have the same level of efficacy. Most research to date has been conducted with bovine-based supplements. Preliminary research in animals suggests that the effects are similar, but further work needs to be done in this area.

Interactions

None reported.

Dose

Phosphatidylserine is available in the form of tablets, capsules and powder.

The dose is not established. Doses used in studies have been 300 mg daily in investigations on cognitive function, and up to 800 mg daily in studies on physical stress. Supplements provide 100–800 mg daily.

References

1 Delwaide PJ, Gyselynck-Mambourg AM, Hurlet A, et al. Double-blind randomized controlled study of phosphatidyserine in senile demented patients. *Acta Neurol Scand* 1986; 73: 136–140.
2 Maggioni M, Picotti GB, Bondiolotti GP, et al. Effects of phosphatidylserine in geriatric patients with depressive disorders. *Acta Psychiatr Scand* 1990; 81: 265–270.
3 Crook TH, Tinklenberg, Yesavage J, et al. Effects of phosphatidylserine in age-associated memory impairment. *Neurology* 1991; 41: 644–649.
4 Crook T, Petrie W, Wells C, et al. Effects of phosphatidylserine in Alzheimer's disease. *Psychopharmacol Bull* 1992; 28: 61–66.
5 Cenacchi T, Bertoldin T, Farina C, et al. Cognitive decline in the elderly: a double-blind, placebo-controlled multicenter study on efficacy of phosphatidylserine administration. *Aging (Milano)* 1993; 5: 123–133.
6 Engel RR, Satzger W, Gunther W, et al. Double-blind, crossover study of phosphatidylserine versus placebo in patients with early dementia of the Alzheimer's type. *Eur Neuropsychopharmacol* 1992; 2: 149–155.
7 Monteleone P, Beinat L, Tanzillo C, et al. Effects of phosphatidylserine on the neuroendocrine response to physical stress in humans. *Neuroendocrinology* 1990; 52: 243–248.
8 Monteleone P, Maj M, Beinat L, et al. Blunting by chronic phosphatidylserine administration of the stress-induced activation of the hypothalamic-pituitary-adrenal axis in healthy men. *Eur J Clin Pharmacol* 1992; 42: 285–288.
9 Hellhammer J, Fries E, Buss C, et al. Effects of soy lecithin phosphatidic acid and phosphatidylserine complex (PAS) on the endocrine and psychological responses to mental stress. *Stress* 2004; 7: 119–126.

Phytosterols

Description

Phytosterols are plant compounds found naturally in the diet, with a similar chemical structure to cholesterol. They are also added to foods such as spreads, cream cheese, yoghurt, salad dressings, bread and drinks. A small, but increasing, number of food supplements in the form of tablets and capsules also contain them. Most phytosterols, like cholesterol, have a double bond in the steroid nucleus, but they contain an extra methyl or ethyl group in a side chain. Their role in plants is to stabilise the phospholipid bilayers in plant cell membranes, as cholesterol does in animal cell membranes.

Constituents

There are more than 100 different phytosterols, but the most abundant are the unsaturated compounds sitosterol, campesterol and stigmasterol, and the saturated compounds sitostanol and campestanol. Clinical studies generally focus on free phytosterols and phytosterol esters.[1] *Note*: the term phytosterol is used here to include both the saturated (stanols) and the unsaturated plant sterols.

Dietary intake

The daily dietary intake varies between 100 and 400 mg.[1,2] However, plant sterol intake would have been considerably higher 5–7 million years ago, up to 1 g/day (because the intake of fruit, vegetables and other plant foods was much higher than it is today).

Absorption

Absorption efficiency for plant sterols in humans is low, around 2–5%, which is considerably less than that of cholesterol, which is about 60%.[2] The saturated stanols are less well absorbed than the unsaturated sterols. Percent absorption of β-sitostanol is <1% while that of β-sitosterol is around 5%. However, the stanols are as effective as the unsaturated sterols in lowering serum cholesterol, but because absorption of the former is lower, there is less chance of adverse consequences.

Dietary sources

Phytosterols exist in all plant foods and are mainly associated with the cell wall as structural components. Vegetarians therefore consume more phytosterols than do omnivores. Plant foods with a high fat and/or fibre content (e.g. oils, nuts, seeds and grains) are the most concentrated dietary sources.[1] A US analysis of the phytosterol content of nuts and seeds found that sesame seeds and wheatgerm had the highest concentration (>400 mg/100 g), followed by pistachio nuts (279 mg/100 g), sunflower seeds (270 mg/100 g), with English walnuts and Brazil nuts having a lower content (113 mg/100 g and 95 mg/100 g, respectively). Peanut butter (smooth) contains 135 mg/100 g.[3]

Action

The cholesterol lowering effect of phytosterols is well documented.[1,2,4–10] At intakes of 2–2.5 g daily, products enriched with phytosterol esters lower plasma LDL cholesterol levels by 10–14%.[9] The phytosterol component of typical diets is generally considered to be too small to influence cholesterol absorption.

Phytosterols reduce blood levels of total cholesterol and LDL cholesterol through reduction of cholesterol absorption,[9] although they may also influence cellular cholesterol metabolism within intestinal enterocytes.[9] The reduction of cholesterol absorption by phytosterols leads to increased synthesis of hepatic cholesterol. However, a reduction in LDL cholesterol occurs because of up-regulation of LDL receptor synthesis. Generally, phytosterols have no effect on HDL cholesterol or triglycerides.[11]

Plant stanol esters have been suggested to be more effective in lowering cholesterol than sterol esters. However, evidence for a significant difference in efficacy between stanols and sterols when they are esterified is limited.[1] One trial did find that the cholesterol-lowering effect of plant sterol esters was attenuated between 1 and 2 months, while plant stanol esters maintained their cholesterol-lowering efficacy.[12] In this same study, the effect of plant sterol esters after 2 months was not significantly different from baseline. This was accompanied by an increase in plasma plant sterols and a reduction in bile acid synthesis, which results in attenuation of cholesterol-lowering efficacy.[13] One placebo-controlled trial in 10 subjects with normal lipid levels found that unesterified sitostanol is more effective in reducing LDL cholesterol than esterified sitostanol.[14]

Possible uses

Cholesterol lowering

Cholesterol lowering with free phytosterols and phytosterol esters has been studied in more than 60 human trials that have investigated subjects with normal lipid levels, hypercholesterolaemia, familial hypercholesterolaemia and diabetes mellitus. The mean reduction of LDL cholesterol with an average dose of 2.4 g daily is 9.9%.[1] A meta-analysis in familial hypercholesterolaemic subjects found that fat spreads enriched with 2.3 ± 0.5 g phytosterols daily reduced total cholesterol by 7–11% and LDL cholesterol by 10–15% in 6.5 ± 1.9 weeks compared to control treatment.[10]

Phytosterols seem to be effective against a background of both low- and high-fat diets, although some studies have found that they are more effective when cholesterol intake is high.[15]

Most studies have investigated the effect of phytosterols administered in a fat spread vehicle. A trial in an outpatient setting found that routine prescription of 25 g daily spread containing 2 g phytosterols is effective for management of hypercholesterolaemia in this setting.[16] However, giving phytosterols in other vehicles such as low-fat milk,[17–19] yoghurt,[18,20,21] low-fat cheese,[21] orange juice,[22] and in a lemon-flavoured drink or egg white has also been shown to reduce serum cholesterol.[23] However, other studies have suggested that phytosterols added to non-fat and low-fat beverages are not effective in modifying lipid levels.

Two trials have investigated the effect on LDL cholesterol of phytosterols in tablet form. A rapidly disintegrating stanol lecithin tablet (1.26 g stanols daily) produced a decrease in LDL cholesterol of 10.4% and a reduction in the ratio of LDL to HDL cholesterol of 11.4% in a trial involving 52 human subjects. On the other hand, slowly disintegrating tablets had no effect on any lipid parameter.[24] Another trial in 26 patients following the American Heart Association Heart Healthy Diet and on long-term statin therapy found that 1.8 g daily of dispersible soy stanols in tablet form reduced LDL cholesterol by a further 9.1% (beyond statins alone), providing evidence that stanol tablets could offer potential adjunctive therapy for patients who have not reached their target LDL cholesterol goal during statin therapy.[25]

Although phytosterols favourably influence total cholesterol and LDL cholesterol levels, their effects on other indicators of CVD risk have not been so intensively studied. One trial showed that phytosterols could attenuate exercise-induced beneficial increase in HDL cholesterol,[26] and another concluded that these compounds have no effect on CHD risk.[27]

Miscellaneous

Phytosterols have been studied *in vitro* and in animals for other activity, including anti-atherogenic activity, anti-cancer activity, antioxidant activity and anti-inflammatory activity. Results are promising but require confirmation in controlled clinical trials in humans.

> **Conclusion**
> The cholesterol-lowering effect of phyto-
> sterols is well documented. At intakes of
> 2–2.5 g daily products enriched with phy-
> tosterol esters lower plasma LDL cholesterol
> levels by 10–14%. The mean reduction in
> LDL cholesterol with an average dose of
> 2.4 g daily is 9.9%. Despite the cholesterol-
> lowering effect, the benefit of phytosterols
> in reducing cardiovascular risk remains to
> be proven. Whether stanol esters or sterol
> esters are the most beneficial is debatable
> and more evidence is required. Most studies
> have investigated the effect of phytosterols
> given in fat spreads. However, there is
> evidence that these compounds can also
> lower cholesterol if given in the form of
> milks, yoghurts, orange juice and low-fat
> cheese. Preliminary evidence from trials
> incorporating phytosterols in tablets have
> also demonstrated efficacy in cholesterol
> lowering, but the formulation must be well
> dispersible. There is preliminary evidence
> that phytosterols may have activity against
> cancer.

Precautions/contraindications

There are a few people with rare genetic defects such as phytosterolaemia, who are susceptible to high phytosterol intakes.[2] The impact of phytosterols in these people is unknown, but there is increased absorption of phytosterols, which may lead to increased atherosclerosis as cholesterol does and also to cell fragility. In addition, the larger number of people who are heterozygous for such conditions may also have some increased susceptibility to high phytosterol intakes.

There are no data in children under 5 years with normocholesterolaemia. It would seem prudent, pending such data, to caution against the use of phytosterols in children because of the potential risk of reduced absorption of fat-soluble nutrients. Phytosterols have the same cholesterol-lowering effect in hypercholes-terolaemic children as in hypercholesterolaemic adults.

Pregnancy and breast-feeding

There are no long-term data in pregnancy and breast-feeding.

Adverse effects

Within the range of intake that causes desirable reduction in blood levels of cholesterol and LDL cholesterol, phytosterols are thought to be clinically safe.[2] However, because phytosterols reduce the absorption of cholesterol it has been suggested that they might reduce the absorption of other lipid-soluble substances such as carotenoids (e.g. beta-carotene and lycopene) and vitamin E. The clinical evidence is controversial, with some studies showing that plant sterols do reduce blood levels of carotenoids and vitamin E, while other studies show no effect.[2] It would seem prudent to advise patients to consume five portions of fruit and vegetables daily and to include one carotenoid-rich source.

Interactions

Drugs
Statins: in theory, combination treatment of statins and phytosterols could have an additive effect on reduction of LDL cholesterol, because phytosterols and statins have different mechanisms of action. A review including five trials of combination therapy found that the addition of phytosterols reduced LDL cholesterol by a further 4.5% per gram of phytosterols.[1] A tablet containing stanols further reduced LDL cholesterol in patients taking statins by 9.1%.[25]

Nutrients
Lipid-soluble nutrients: in theory, phytosterols could reduce the absorption of lipid-soluble substances such as carotenoids and vitamin E, but evidence for this is conflicting.

Dose

Doses of phytosterols used in clinical studies have varied between 1 and 3 g daily (free sterol/stanol equivalent). In 2003, the Food and Drug Administration (FDA) stated that the science (as of January 2003) showed that the lowest effective daily intake of free phytosterols is 800 mg daily. The mean reduction of LDL cholesterol with an average dose of 2.4 g daily is 9.9%.[1] Few studies have looked at higher doses, but the reduction in cholesterol seems to plateau at doses >3 g daily. Further research is needed to identify the optimal dose of phytosterols, the relative efficacy of phytosterols in different populations, and the efficacy of these compounds when incorporated into different foods (other than fat spread) and tablet formulations.

References

1 Normen L, Holmes D, Frohlich J. Plant sterols and their role in combined use with statins for lipid lowering. *Curr Opin Investig Drugs* 2005; 6: 307–316.

2 Berger A, Jones PJ, Abumweis SS. Plant sterols: factors affecting their efficacy and safety as functional food ingredients. *Lipids Health Dis* 2004; 3: 5.

3 Phillips KM, Ruggio DM, Ashraf-Khorassani M. Phytosterol composition of nuts and seeds commonly consumed in the United States. *J Agric Food Chem* 2005; 53: 9436–9445.

4 Ling WH, Jones PJ. Dietary phytosterols: a review of metabolism, benefits and side effects. *Life Sci* 1995; 57: 195–206.

5 Jones PJ, MacDougall DE, Ntanios F, Vanstone CA. Dietary phytosterols as cholesterol-lowering agents in humans. *Can J Physiol Pharmacol* 1997; 75: 217–227.

6 Moghadasian MH, Frohlich JJ. Effects of dietary phytosterols on cholesterol metabolism and atherosclerosis: clinical and experimental evidence. *Am J Med* 1999; 107: 588–594.

7 Law M. Plant sterol and stanol margarines and health. *BMJ* 2000; 320: 861–864.

8 Katan MB, Grundy SM, Jones P, et al. Efficacy and safety of plant stanols and sterols in the management of blood cholesterol levels. *Mayo Clin Proc* 2003; 78: 965–978.

9 Plat J, Mensink RP. Plant stanol and sterol esters in the control of blood cholesterol levels: mechanism and safety aspects. *Am J Cardiol* 2005; 96(1A): D15–22.

10 Moruisi KG, Oosthuizen W, Opperman AM. Phytosterols/stanols lower cholesterol concentrations in familial hypercholesterolemic subjects: a systematic review with meta-analysis. *J Am Coll Nutr* 2006; 25: 41–48.

11 Plat J, Mensink RP. Effects of plant stanol esters on LDL receptor protein expression and on LDL receptor and HMG-CoA reductase mRNA expression in mononuclear blood cells of healthy men and women. *Faseb J* 2002; 16: 258–260.

12 O'Neill FH, Brynes A, Mandeno R, et al. Comparison of the effects of dietary plant sterol and stanol esters on lipid metabolism. *Nutr Metab Cardiovasc Dis* 2004; 14: 133–142.

13 O'Neill FH, Sanders TA, Thompson GR. Comparison of efficacy of plant stanol ester and sterol ester: short-term and longer-term studies. *Am J Cardiol* 2005; 96(1A): D29–36.

14 Sudhop T, Lutjohann D, Agna M, et al. Comparison of the effects of sitostanol, sitostanol acetate, and sitostanol oleate on the inhibition of cholesterol absorption in normolipemic healthy male volunteers. A placebo controlled randomized cross-over study. *Arzneimittelforschung* 2003; 53: 708–713.

15 Mussner MJ, Parhofer KG, Von Bergmann K, et al. Effects of phytosterol ester-enriched margarine on plasma lipoproteins in mild to moderate hypercholesterolemia are related to basal cholesterol and fat intake. *Metabolism* 2002; 51: 189–194.

16 Patch CS, Tapsell LC, Williams PG. Plant sterol/stanol prescription is an effective treatment strategy for managing hypercholesterolemia in outpatient clinical practice. *J Am Diet Assoc* 2005; 105: 46–52.

17 Clifton PM, Noakes M, Sullivan D, et al. Cholesterol-lowering effects of plant sterol esters differ in milk, yoghurt, bread and cereal. *Eur J Clin Nutr* 2004; 58: 503–509.

18 Noakes M, Clifton PM, Doornbos AM, Trautwein EA. Plant sterol ester-enriched milk and yoghurt effectively reduce serum cholesterol in modestly hypercholesterolemic subjects. *Eur J Nutr* 2005; 44: 214–222.

19 Thomsen AB, Hansen HB, Christiansen C, et al. Effect of free plant sterols in low-fat milk on serum lipid profile in hypercholesterolemic subjects. *Eur J Clin Nutr* 2004; 58: 860–870.

20 Mensink RP, Ebbing S, Lindhout M, et al. Effects of plant stanol esters supplied in low-fat yoghurt on serum lipids and lipoproteins, non-cholesterol sterols and fat soluble antioxidant concentrations. *Atherosclerosis* 2002; 160: 205–213.

21 Korpela R, Tuomilehto J, Hogstrom P, et al. Safety aspects and cholesterol-lowering efficacy of low fat dairy products containing plant sterols. *Eur J Clin Nutr* 2006; 60: 633–642.

22 Devaraj S, Jialal I, Vega-Lopez S. Plant sterol-fortified orange juice effectively lowers cholesterol levels in mildly hypercholesterolemic healthy individuals. *Arterioscler Thromb Vasc Biol* 2004; 24: e25–28.

23 Spilburg CA, Goldberg AC, McGill JB, et al. Fat-free foods supplemented with soy stanol-lecithin powder

reduce cholesterol absorption and LDL cholesterol. *J Am Diet Assoc* 2003; 103: 577–581.

24 McPherson TB, Ostlund RE, Goldberg AC, *et al.* Phytostanol tablets reduce human LDL-cholesterol. *J Pharm Pharmacol* 2005; 57: 889–896.

25 Goldberg AC, Ostlund RE Jr, Bateman JH, *et al.* Effect of plant stanol tablets on low-density lipoprotein cholesterol lowering in patients on statin drugs. *Am J Cardiol* 2006; 97: 376–379.

26 Alhassan S, Reese KA, Mahurin J, *et al.* Blood lipid responses to plant stanol ester supplementation and aerobic exercise training. *Metabolism* 2006; 55: 541–549.

27 Varady KA, St-Pierre AC, Lamarche B, Jones PJ. Effect of plant sterols and endurance training on LDL particle size and distribution in previously sedentary hypercholesterolemic adults. *Eur J Clin Nutr* 2005; 59: 518–525.

Potassium

Description

Potassium is an essential mineral.

Human requirements

See Table 1 for Dietary Reference Values for potassium.

Dietary intake

In the UK, the average adult diet provides: for men, 3279 mg daily; for women, 2562 mg.

Table 1 Dietary Reference Values for potassium (mg/day)

			EU RDA = none
Age	UK		USA minimum requirement[1]
	LRNI	RNI	
0–3 months	400	800	500
4–6 months	400	850	500
7–9 months	400	700	700
10–12 months	450	700	700
1–3 years	450	800	1000
4–6 years	600	1100	1400
7–10 years	950	2200	1600
11–14 years	1600	3100	2000
15–50+ years	2000	3500	2000
Pregnancy	*	*	*
Lactation	*	*	*

* No increment.
[1] Desirable intakes may exceed these values.
Note: No EAR has been derived for potassium.

Action

Potassium is the principal intracellular cation, and is fundamental to the regulation of acid–base and water balance. It contributes to transmission of nerve impulses, control of skeletal muscle contractility and maintenance of blood pressure.

Dietary sources

See Table 2 for dietary sources of potassium.

Metabolism

Absorption

Absorption occurs principally in the small intestine.

Elimination

Excretion is mainly via the urine (the capacity of the kidneys to conserve potassium is poor); unabsorbed and intestinally-secreted potassium is eliminated in the faeces; some is lost in saliva and sweat.

Deficiency

Potassium deficiency leads to hypokalaemia, symptoms of which include anorexia, nausea, abdominal distension, paralytic ileus; muscle weakness, reduced or absent reflexes, paralysis; listlessness, apprehension, drowsiness, irrational behaviour; respiratory failure; polydypsia, polyuria; and cardiac arrhythmias.

Possible uses

Hypertension

Potassium may lower blood pressure,[1,2] but there is evidence for a stronger relationship

Table 2 Dietary sources of potassium

Food portion	Potassium content (mg)	Food portion	Potassium content (mg)
Breakfast cereals		**Vegetables**	
1 bowl All-Bran (45 g)	450	Green vegetables, average, boiled (100g)	100–200
1 bowl Bran Flakes (45 g)	250	Potatoes, boiled (150 g)	450
1 bowl Corn Flakes (30 g)	30	baked (150 g)	950
1 bowl muesli (95 g)	500	1 small can baked beans (200 g)	600
2 pieces Shredded Wheat	150	Lentils, kidney beans or other pulses, cooked (105 g)	300
2 Weetabix	150	Soya beans, cooked (100 g)	500
Cereal products		Mixed vegetable curry (300 g)	1250
Bread, brown, 2 slices	100	**Fruit**	
white, 2 slices	70	1 apple	100
wholemeal, 2 slices	160	8 dried apricots	600
1 chapati	110	1 banana	350
Pasta, brown, boiled (150 g)	200	½ cantaloupe melon	750
white, boiled (150 g)	40	10 dates	300
Rice, brown, boiled (165 g)	150	4 figs	600
white, boiled (165 g)	80	1 orange	300
Milk and dairy products		1 handful raisins	350
½ pint milk, whole, semi-skimmed or skimmed	400	**Nuts**	
1 pot yoghurt (150 g)	370	20 almonds	150
Cheese (50 g)	50	10 Brazil nuts	200
1 egg, size 2 (60 g)	50	30 hazelnuts	250
Meat and fish		30 peanuts	200
Meat, cooked (100 g)	200–300	**Beverages**	
Liver, lambs, cooked (90 g)	300	1 mug hot chocolate	350
Kidney, lambs, cooked (75 g)	250	1 mug Build-Up	700
White fish, cooked (150 g)	400–500	1 mug Complan (sweet)	600
Herring or mackerel (110 g)	460	1 mug Horlicks	600
Pilchards, canned (105 g)	450	1 large glass grapefruit juice	200
Sardines, canned (70 g)	300	1 large glass orange juice	300
		1 large glass tomato juice	460

Good sources (italics).

of the sodium to potassium ratio to blood pressure than potassium alone.[3] Several other minerals (see Calcium and Magnesium) may affect blood pressure, and dietary measures to reduce blood pressure might be more effective if the intake of several minerals is changed simultaneously.

There is some evidence from double-blind, placebo-controlled trials that potassium supplementation (1500–3000 mg daily) can lower blood pressure in normotensive[4,5] and hypertensive[6] individuals, but another trial failed to show any benefit.[7]

Precautions/contraindications

Excessive doses are best avoided in patients with chronic renal failure (particularly in the elderly); gastrointestinal obstruction or ulceration;

peptic ulcer; Addison's disease; heart block; severe burns; and acute dehydration.

Pregnancy and breast-feeding

No data are available on potassium supplements in pregnancy. They should be avoided.

Adverse effects

Nausea, vomiting, diarrhoea and abdominal cramps may occur, particularly if potassium is taken on an empty stomach. Modified-release preparations may cause gastrointestinal ulceration. Hyperkalaemia is almost unknown with oral administration provided renal function is normal. Intakes exceeding 17 g daily (unlikely from oral supplements) would be required to cause toxicity.

Interactions

Drugs

ACE inhibitors: increased risk of hyperkalaemia.
Carbenoxolone: reduced serum potassium levels.
Corticosteroids: increased excretion of potassium.
Cyclosporin: increased risk of hyperkalaemia.
Laxatives: chronic use reduces absorption of potassium.
Loop diuretics: increased risk of hypokalaemia (but potassium supplements seldom necessary with small dose of diuretic).
NSAIDs: increased risk of hyperkalaemia.
Potassium-sparing diuretics: increased risk of hyperkalaemia.

Thiazide diuretics: increased risk of hypokalaemia (but potassium supplements seldom necessary with small dose of diuretic).

Dose

Mild deficiency, oral, 1500–4000 mg daily, with plenty of fluid (liquid preparations should be diluted well).

As a dietary supplement, no dose has been established.

References

1 Khaw KT, Thom S. Randomized double-blind crossover trial of potassium on blood pressure in normal subjects. *Lancet* 1982; ii: 1127–1129.
2 Cappuccio FP, MacGregor DA. Does potassium supplementation lower blood pressure? A meta-analysis of published trials. *J Hypertension* 1991; 9: 465–473.
3 Grobbee DE, Hofman A, Roelandt JT, *et al.* Sodium restriction and potassium supplementation in young people with mildly elevated blood pressure. *J Hypertension* 1987; 5: 115–119.
4 Sacks FM, Willett WC, Smith A, *et al.* Effect on blood pressure of potassium, calcium and magnesium in women with low habitual intake. *Hypertension* 1995; 26: 950–956.
5 Brancati FL, Appel LJ, Seidler AJ, *et al.* Effect of potassium supplementation on blood pressure in African Americans on a low-potassium diet. A randomized, double-blind, placebo-controlled trial. *Arch Intern Med* 1996; 156: 61–67.
6 Fotherby MD, Potter JF. Potassium supplementation reduces clinic and ambulatory blood pressure in elderly hypertensive patients. *J Hypertens* 1992; 10: 1403–1408.
7 Sacks FM, Brown LE, Appel L, *et al.* Combinations of potassium, calcium and magnesium supplements in hypertension. *Hypertension* 1995; 26: 950–956.

Probiotics and prebiotics

Description

A probiotic is a live microbial food supplement that beneficially affects the host animal by improving its intestinal microbial balance.[1,2] For human adult use, this includes fermented milk products and over-the-counter products, such as powders, tablets and capsules that contain lyophilised bacteria. The micro-organisms involved are usually producers of lactic acid, such as lactobacilli and bifidobacteria, which are widely used in yoghurt and dairy products. However, yeasts have also been used (Table 1).[3,4] These microbes are non-pathogenic and survive passage through the stomach and small bowel.

A prebiotic is a non-digestible food ingredient, which beneficially affects the host by selectively stimulating the growth, activity, or both, of one or a limited number of bacterial species already resident in the colon.[5] Prebiotics are not digested by intestinal enzymes, instead passing through the upper gastrointestinal tract to the colon where they are selectively used as fuel by beneficial bacteria.

Although any food residue entering the colon is a potential prebiotic candidate, it is the influence of the food residue on certain specific microbes that is important. Lactulose was used more than 40 years ago as a prebiotic infant formula food supplement to increase numbers of lactobacilli in the infant intestine,[6] but the specificity of this substrate for enhancing these micro-organisms has not been effectively proven scientifically. In humans, consumption of fructo-oligosaccharides increases the proportion of bifidobacteria in faeces.[7] Similar effects have been observed in rats fed with galacto-oligosaccharides and colonised with human faecal flora.[8]

Table 1 Examples of commonly used probiotics and prebiotics[4,5]

Probiotics	Prebiotics
Lactobacilli	Fructo-oligosaccharides
L. acidophilus	Galacto-oligosaccharides
L. casei	Inulin
L. delbrueckii subsp. bulgaricus	Lactulose
L. reuteri	Lactitol
L. brevis	
L. cellobiosus	
L. curvatus	
L. fermentium	
L.plantarum	
L. gasseri	
L. rhamnosus	
Gram-positive cocci	
Lactococcus lactis subsp. cremoris	
Streptococcus salivarius subsp. thermophilus	
Enterococcus faecium	
S. diacetylactis	
S. intermedius	
Bifidobacteria	
B. bifidum	
B. adolescentis	
B. animalis	
B. infantis	
B. longum	
B. thermophilum	
Yeasts	
Saccharomyces boulardii	
S. cerevisiae	

251

Possible uses

The possible benefits to health of probiotics and prebiotics are to:

- prevent and treat diarrhoea;
- alleviate lactose intolerance;
- prevent and treat vaginal infections;
- enhance the immune system;
- treat allergic conditions;
- lower serum cholesterol; and
- prevent cancer and tumour growth.

Acute diarrhoea

There is a relatively large volume of literature supporting the use of probiotics in diarrhoeal conditions, but it is only recently that the scientific basis for this has started to become established, with the publication of a number of respectable clinical studies. Probiotics have been examined for their effectiveness in the prevention and treatment of several types of diarrhoea, including antibiotic-associated diarrhoea, bacterial and viral diarrhoea (including travellers' diarrhoea), as well as that caused by lactose intolerance. The effects of probiotics, particularly with some bacterial strains and in some types of diarrhoea, appears promising, but the effects of prebiotics on diarrhoea are currently unknown.

Various mechanisms by which probiotics could be of benefit in diarrhoea have been proposed and summarised in two reviews.[9,10] These include reduction in gastrointestinal pH through stimulation of lactic acid-producing bacteria; a direct antagonistic action on gastrointestinal pathogens; competition with pathogens for binding and receptor sites; improved immune function and competition for limited nutrients.

A detailed review[11] of all placebo-controlled human studies supplementing *Lactobacillus acidophilus*, *Bifidobacterium longum*, *L. casei* GG and other selected micro-organisms from 1966 to 1995 concluded that: "these studies have shown that biotherapeutic agents have been used successfully to prevent antibiotic-associated diarrhoea, to prevent acute infantile diarrhoea, to treat recurrent *Clostridium difficile* disease, and to treat various other diarrhoeal illnesses." The authors also noted that many of the studies included small numbers of subjects.

A more recent systematic review concluded that available evidence does not support the administration of probiotics with antibiotics to prevent the development of *C. difficile* disease and is inadequate to justify its introduction as a treatment for *C. difficile* antibiotic-associated disease (at the McGill University Health Centre, where the study was conducted).[12] A meta-analysis of six RCTs found that the probiotic, *Saccharomyces boulardii*, significantly reduced the risk of *C. difficile* disease, but was the only probiotic that was effective.[13]

Evidence for a beneficial effect of probiotics in diarrhoea appears to be strongest for that caused by rotavirus. Rotavirus infection causes gastroenteritis, which is characterised by acute diarrhoea and vomiting. Gastroenteritis is a leading cause of morbidity and mortality among children worldwide. A review of studies that used *Lactobacillus*, *Bifidobacterium* and *Enterococcus* concluded that *Lactobacillus* GG (a *Lactobacillus* strain isolated from human intestine) consistently shortened the diarrhoeal phase of rotavirus by 1 day,[14] but that evidence was less strong for a role of *Lactobacillus* GG and other probiotics in the prevention of diarrhoea due to bacterial or other viral infections. A recent RCT showed no positive effect of *Lactobacillus* GG on the clinical course of watery diarrhoea in infants.[15]

A systematic review of 10 RCTs (treatment) and three RCTs (prevention) concluded that probiotics significantly reduced the duration of acute infectious diarrhoea in infants and children, especially diarrhoea caused by rotavirus. No conclusions could be reached about the use of probiotics in the prevention of diarrhoea, because of clinical and statistical heterogeneity among the studies.[16] A meta-analysis of 18 RCTs confirmed the efficacy of probiotic supplements in reducing duration of symptoms among children up to 5 years old with acute, non-bacterial diarrhoea. Probiotics, particularly lactobacilli, reduced the duration of an acute diarrhoeal episode in an infant or child by approximately 1 day.[17] A further meta-analysis involving nine trials that had used *Lactobacillus* in children with acute infectious diarrhoea found a reduction in diarrhoea duration of 0.7 days and a reduction in diarrhoea frequency of 1.6 stools on day 2 of treatment in participants receiving lactobacilli.[18]

The role of probiotic bacteria in the prevention of and treatment of paediatric diarrhoea is increasingly well established, but their role in adults has been less well investigated. However, an RCT involving 541 young men found a non-significant trend for reduction in the incidence of diarrhoea with yoghurt containing *L. casei* compared with placebo.[19]

A Cochrane review involving 23 studies found that probiotics reduced the risk of diarrhoea (in adults and children) at 3 days (RR 0.66; 95% CI, 0.55 to 0.77; 15 studies) and the mean duration of diarrhoea by 30.48 h (95% CI, 18.51 to 42.46; 12 studies). The authors concluded that probiotics appear to be a useful adjunct to rehydration therapy in treating acute infectious diarrhoea in adults and children and that more research is needed to identify the use of particular probiotic regimens in specific patient groups.[20]

Further trials have continued to show encouraging results. *L. rhamnosus* 19070-2 and *L. reuteri* DSM 12246 ameliorated acute diarrhoea in hospitalised children[21] and in children from day-care centres,[22] and reduced the period of rotavirus excretion. The beneficial effects were most prominent in children treated early in the diarrhoeal phase. *B. lactis* strain Bb12[23] or *B. breve* C50 with *S. thermophilus* 065[24] or *L. reuteri* with *B. lactis*,[25] added to an infant formula appear to have some protective effect against acute diarrhoea in healthy children. *S. boulardii* significantly reduced the duration of acute diarrhoea and the duration of hospital stay in children with acute diarrhoea.[26] The feeding of a cereal containing *S. thermophilus*, *B. lactis*, *L. acidophilus* and zinc reduced the severity and duration of acute gastroenteritis in young children, but whether the combination is better than either probiotics or zinc alone is unknown.[27] Administration of *L. rhamnosus* strains shortened the duration of rotaviral diarrhoea in children but not of diarrhoea of any aetiology.[28]

Travellers' diarrhoea

The prevention of travellers' diarrhoea by lactobacilli, bifidobacteria, enterococci and streptococci has been investigated in several studies, but results have been inconsistent. In a double-blind, placebo-controlled trial, 820 Finnish travellers to two holiday resorts in Turkey were randomised to receive either *Lactobacillus* GG or placebo.[29] The overall incidence of diarrhoea was 43.8%. Of the 331 sufferers, 178 (46.5%) were in the placebo group and 153 (41%) were in the *Lactobacillus* group, but the difference was not significant. However, in one of the resorts, the treatment significantly reduced the incidence of diarrhoea from 39.5% (30 out of 76) in the placebo group to 23.9% (17 out of 71) in the treatment group. In another study involving 245 travellers to developing countries, the risk of diarrhoea on any one day in travellers who took *Lactobacillus* GG was 3.9% compared with 7.4% in the control group.[30]

In another study, the incidence of diarrhoea was reduced from 71% to 43% in travellers to Egypt who were given capsules of *S. thermophilus*, *L. bulgaricus*, *L. acidophilus* and *B. bifidum*.[31] However, neither *L. acidophilus* nor *Enterococcus faecium* had any beneficial effects on diarrhoea in groups of Austrian tourists.[32] In addition, no effect of *L. acidophilus* or *L. fermentum* was observed in soldiers who were sent to Belize in Central America,[33] and it seems that the effect of probiotics on travellers' diarrhoea depends on the bacterial strain used and the destination of the traveller.[14]

Antibiotic-associated diarrhoea

Diarrhoea caused by the growth of pathogenic bacteria is the most common side-effect of antibiotic use, and *in vitro* studies have shown that some bacterial strains can inhibit this growth. *Lactobacillus* GG (in yoghurt) reduced the incidence and duration of diarrhoea in healthy men receiving erythromycin for 7 days,[34] and successfully eradicated *C. difficile* in five patients with relapsing colitis.[35] A recent meta-analysis of six trials evaluating the efficacy of *Lactobacillus* GG found that four of the trials were associated with a significant reduction in the risk of antibiotic-associated diarrhoea, one of the trials reduced the number of days of antibiotic-associated diarrhoea, while the sixth trial found no benefit with *Lactobacillus* GG.[36] *Lactobacillus* F19 had a limited effect on the emergence of resistant isolates during treatment with penicillin and quinolones.[37] *S. boulardii* has been shown to reduce the risk of antibiotic-associated diarrhoea in children.[38]

Enterococcus SF68 reduced the incidence of diarrhoea caused by antibiotics,[39] whereas studies with *L. acidophilus*[40,41] have provided no conclusive evidence of benefit with this strain in prevention of diarrhoea caused by antibiotics. A daily dose of *B. lactis* and *Streptococcus thermophilus* has been shown to prevent antibiotic-associated diarrhoea.[42]

A meta-analysis of nine RCTs suggested that probiotics can be used to prevent antibiotic-associated diarrhoea, and that both *S. boulardii* and lactobacilli have the potential for benefit in this situation. However, the meta-analysis also concluded that the efficacy of probiotics in treating antibiotic-associated diarrhoea remains unproven.[43] A further meta-analysis that included seven RCTs also suggested that probiotic supplements were associated with a significant decrease in the incidence of antibiotic-associated diarrhoea, while concluding that evidence of benefit is not conclusive, partly because of poor study design.[44] A further meta-analysis of five RCTs found that *S. boulardii* is moderately effective in preventing antibiotic-associated diarrhoea in children and adults treated with antibiotics for any reason (mainly respiratory tract infections). In this meta-analysis, for every 10 patients receiving daily *S. boulardii* with antibiotics, one fewer would develop antibiotic-associated diarrhoea.[45] A more recent meta-analysis including 25 RCTs found that probiotics significantly reduced the relative risk of antibiotic-associated diarrhoea (RR 0.43; 95% CI, 0.31 to 0.58, $P < 0.001$). Three types of probiotics were associated with this benefit: *S. boulardii*, *L. rhamnosus* GG and probiotic mixtures.[46]

Lactose intolerance

Lactose intolerance is a problem for a large proportion of the world's population for whom lactose acts like an osmotic non-digestible carbohydrate because they have a low amount of intestinal lactase. During fermentation of yoghurt and acidophilus milk, lactobacilli produce lactase that hydrolyses lactose to glucose and galactose. This pre-digestion of lactose could potentially reduce the symptoms associated with lactose intolerance in susceptible individuals, and probiotics have been shown to improve lactose digestion and intolerance in some studies[47,48] but not others.[49] A systematic review assessing the efficacy of oral probiotics in adults with lactose intolerance found that probiotics did not alleviate the signs and symptoms of this condition, but that specific strains, concentrations and preparations may be effective.[50] Further trials of specific strains and concentrations are necessary to clarify this potentially beneficial effect.

Vaginal infections

One of the claims frequently made for probiotics, specifically for *L. acidophilus*, is that they can prevent vaginal infections. The conclusions of a review were that there was evidence (albeit limited) for *L. acidophilus* in the prevention of candidal vaginitis.[51]

In a double-blind, controlled, crossover trial of 46 women with a history of vaginal infections, participants were randomised to receive either *L. acidophilus* yoghurt (150 ml daily) containing live organisms or pasteurised yoghurt (150 ml daily) for 2 months each with a 2-month washout period between interventions. However, only seven subjects completed the whole study, and the reason for the high drop-out rate was not explained. The yoghurt containing live organisms was associated with a significant reduction in episodes of bacterial vaginosis. Both yoghurts were associated with a decrease in candidal vaginitis, but there was no significant difference between the treatments.[52] A more recent RCT investigated the effect of *Lactobacillus* preparations taken orally or vaginally, or both, on vulvovaginitis following antibiotic treatment for a non-gynaecological infection. The study involved 235 Australian women aged 18–50 years. Overall 55/235 women developed post-antibiotic vulvovaginitis, but neither oral nor vaginal *Lactobacillus* treatment influenced the incidence of this condition compared with placebo.[53] At this time, the use of oral or vaginal forms of

Lactobacillus is not supported by evidence from RCTs.

Immunity

The colonic microflora affects systemic and mucosal immunity in the host. Probiotics are claimed to stimulate the immune system and preliminary evidence suggests that these substances could increase the immune response.[54–57] An RCT involving 136 university students under examination stress (which has been associated with a suppressed immune response) were given milk fermented with yoghurt cultures plus *L. casei* or a placebo of semi-skimmed milk for 3 weeks prior to and during the 3-week exam period. The fermented milk modulated the number of lymphocytes and CD56 cells, indicating an effect on the immune system.[58] In another human trial, a fermented product containing two probiotic strains (*L. gasser* CECT 5714, *L. coryniformis* CECT 5711) increased the proportion of phagocytic cells (monocytes and neutrophils) as well as their phagocytic activity, and increased the proportion of natural killer cells and IgA concentrations. The fermented product enhanced immunity to a greater extent than a standard yoghurt.[59] *L. casei* has been associated with positive effects on immune competence in middle-aged people.[60,61]

Allergic conditions

Recent research interest has focused on the potential role of probiotics in various conditions known to have an allergic component. There is evidence that *Lactobacillus* GG[62] and *Bifidobacterium* Bb-12[63] could improve symptoms in infants with atopic eczema. A combination of *L. rhamnosus* 19070–2 and *L. reuteri* DSM 122460[64] and supplementation with the probiotic *L. fermentum* VRI-033 PCC[65] has also been found to be effective in the management of atopic dermatitis. The benefits associated with *Lactobacillus* GG in atopic eczema/dermatitis have been observed to a greater extent in infants who are sensitised to immunoglobulin-E (Ig-E) than those who are non-IgE-sensitised.[66] Impairment of the intestinal mucosal barrier appears to be involved in the pathogenesis of atopic dermatitis and there is evidence that probiotic supplementation can stabilise the intestinal barrier function.[67]

Clinical studies also suggest that probiotics could be effective in the primary prevention of atopic disease. In infants at high risk of atopic disease, administration of probiotics to their mothers prenatally[68,69] and during breast-feeding[70] has been shown to prevent atopic disease, particularly eczema.

There is also preliminary evidence that fermented milk containing *L. paracasei* LP-33 can improve the quality of life of patients with allergic rhinitis and may serve as an alternative treatment.[71,72]

Cardiovascular disease

Probiotics have been evaluated for a potential effect on serum cholesterol and other cardiovascular risk factors. The influence of probiotics on serum cholesterol levels is the subject of controversy. Studies in the 1970s and 1980s frequently reported significant reductions in serum cholesterol with daily consumption of fermented milk, but these studies have been criticised on methodological grounds, including the fact that in most of the studies showing positive results, large volumes of yoghurt (0.5–8.4 L) were consumed.[73] Two controlled trials have shown that yoghurt (200 ml daily) containing live cultures of *L. acidophilus*[74] or yoghurt (375 ml daily) fermented with *L. acidophilus* with added fructo-oligosaccharides[75] (prebiotic) reduced serum cholesterol by 2.9% and 4.4%, respectively. Another study indicated that inulin (a prebiotic) may also lower cholesterol.[76] A further study found that the probiotic *B. longum* resulted in a significant reduction in serum total cholesterol in subjects with moderate hypercholesterolaemia,[77] while a yoghurt enriched with *L. acidophilus* and *B. longum*, and oligofructose (a synbiotic) increased serum HDL cholesterol and led to an improvement in the ratio of LDL:HDL cholesterol.[78]

However, a trial in post-menopausal women found that probiotic capsules containing bacteria *L. acidophilus* and *B. longum* had no effect on cholesterol either independently or in addition to soy.[79] A further trial in 80 volunteers with raised cholesterol found no effect of capsules containing freeze-dried *L. acidophilus* for 6 weeks on serum lipids.[80]

Probiotics have also been associated with a reduction in blood pressure[81,82] and other cardiovascular risk factors (e.g. fibrinogen, monocyte adhesion and pro-inflammatory markers).[81]

Helicobacter pylori infection

Probiotics are being investigated for potential benefit in reducing *H. pylori* colonisation and also in reducing the side-effects associated with *H. pylori* treatment. Ingestion of a product containing *Lactobacillus* La1[83] and in another study a yoghurt containing *Lactobacillus* and *Bifidobacterium*,[84] inhibited *H. pylori* colonisation. Supplementation with *L. casei*[85] and *S. boulardii*[86] conferred an enhanced therapeutic benefit on *H. pylori* eradication in subjects on triple therapy. A 4-week pretreatment with a yoghurt containing *Lactobacillus* and *Bifidobacterium* reduced *H. pylori* load, improving eradication rate with quadruple therapy, after triple therapy had failed.[87]

B. clausii reduced the incidence of the most common side-effects related to *H. pylori* antibiotic therapy.[88] *L. casei* supplementation has also been shown to reduce the side-effects of 10-day quadruple therapy and result in a slight improvement in eradicating *H. pylori*.[89] In another study, a range of probiotics (*Lactobacillus* GG, *S. boulardii*, a combination of *Lactobacillus* spp. and bifidobacteria) were found to be superior to placebo for side-effect prevention.[90] A further study also showed that a probiotic supplement improved tolerance to the eradication regimen.[91]

A systematic review concluded that regular intake of probiotics may be a useful alternative for populations at high risk of *H. pylori* colonisation.[92]

Irritable bowel syndrome

Recent research has investigated the potential benefit of probiotics in IBS. A double-blind RCT in 40 patients found that *L. plantarum* 299V was associated with resolution of abdominal pain and a trend towards normalisation of stool frequency in constipated patients.[93] In another study, however, the same probiotic had no apparent benefit in patients with IBS and no influence on colonic fermentation.[94] In a further study, short-term therapy with *L. plantarum* LP01 and *B. breve* BR03 or *L. plantarum* LP01 and *L. acidophilus* LA02 reduced the pain score and severity of characteristic IBS symptoms.[95] *B. infantis* 35624 was associated with a significant reduction in abdominal pain/discomfort, bloating/distension and bowel movement difficulty. This response was associated with normalisation of the ratio of an anti-inflammatory to a pro-inflammatory cytokine, suggesting an immune-modulating role for this organism in IBS.[96] *Lactobacillus* GG has been associated with a lower incidence of perceived abdominal distension (but no other symptomatic differences)[97] and a probiotic combination (VSL#3) with reduced flatulence and slower colonic transit in patients with IBS and bloating.[98] However, *L. reuteri* was not associated with significant improvement in IBS symptoms compared with placebo.[99] Two further controlled trials using probiotic mixtures[100,101] demonstrated reduction in IBS symptoms.

Crohn's disease

Human trial evidence for probiotics in Crohn's disease is generally not positive so far. Among five controlled trials to date,[102–106] only one has shown potentially positive effects of *S. boulardii* in the maintenance treatment of Crohn's disease.[102]

Ulcerative colitis

The evidence base for probiotics in ulcerative colitis is broader than that for Crohn's disease and generally more encouraging. Three placebo-controlled RCTs showed significant clinical improvement,[107–109] while other studies reported that probiotics (or prebiotics) were at least as effective as conventional treatment in reducing symptoms, obtaining remission and preventing relapse.[110–115]

Osteoporosis

There is some evidence that prebiotics (inulin and oligofructose) can improve calcium absorption,[116–118] and this effect could enhance BMD with a consequent reduction in the risk of osteoporosis. However, there are no human studies with prebiotics assessing the risk of osteoporosis.

Respiratory tract infections

Regular intake of probiotics may reduce nasal colonisation with pathogenic bacteria.[119] There is also evidence that intake of probiotic bacteria over at least 3 months shortens common cold episodes.[120]

Miscellaneous

Probiotics are being evaluated in a number of other conditions, including constipation, prevention of colorectal cancer, rheumatoid arthritis and other disorders of the immune system. Results from research are promising but await confirmation from controlled clinical trials.

Conclusion

The colonic microflora is important to health, and modification of the bacterial species inhabiting the large bowel – using probiotics and prebiotics – has been suggested to produce potential heath benefits. There are a growing number of published papers on the use of both probiotics and prebiotics, and although they show ability to alter the colonic microflora, evidence that they can reduce the risk of diseases is more limited. This may in part be because of differences in methodology, particularly the large number of different strains that have been used. The evidence for an effect of probiotics in acute diarrhoea appears to be greatest for rotavirus infection. Study results in travellers' diarrhoea have been inconsistent. Probiotics can be effective in preventing antibiotic-associated diarrhoea. There is also some evidence that probiotics can improve lactose intolerance, boost immunity, prevent vaginal infections and lower serum cholesterol, but further research is required. Moreover there is, as yet, no conclusive evidence that either prebiotics or probiotics can prevent cancer in humans.

Precautions/contraindications

None reported.

Pregnancy and breast-feeding

No known problems.

Adverse effects

Probiotics have a long history of apparently safe use.[121,122] However, they can exert potentially powerful immune effects so caution is required until more data are available. This may be relevant for probiotics added to infant formula or given to seriously immunocompromised patients, in whom there have been isolated cases of opportunistic infections from probiotic species.[121,122]

Interactions

None reported.

Dose

Probiotics are available in the form of tablets and capsules of *L. acidophilus*, often with other bacteria. They are also available in the form of yoghurts and various fermented milks. Many probiotics require refrigeration to maintain viability and like any other product should be used before the expiry date. Commercial products have not always been found to contain the bacterial strain listed on the label, and in some cases, the bacteria may not be viable.[42]

Prebiotics are available in the form of tablets, capsules and powders of fructo-oligosaccharides and inulin.

There is no established dose for any of these products.

References

1 Fuller R, ed. *Probiotics: The Scientific Basis*. London: Chapman & Hall, 1992.
2 Fuller R. A review: probiotics in man and animals. *J Appl Bacteriol* 1989; 66: 365–378.
3 Sadler MJ, Saltmarsh M, eds. *Functional Foods*. Cambridge: The Royal Society of Chemistry, 1998: 4–5.

4   Macfarlane GT, Cummings JH. Probiotics and prebiotics: can regulating the activities of intestinal bacteria benefit health? *BMJ* 1999; 318: 999–1003.

5   Gibson GR, Roberfroid MB. Dietary modulation of the human colonic microbiota: introducing the concept of prebiotics. *J Nutr* 1995; 125: 1401–1412.

6   MacGillivray PC, Finlay HVL, Binns TB. Use of lactulose to create a preponderance of lactobacilli in the intestine of bottle-fed infants. *Scott Med J* 1959; 4: 182–189.

7   Gibson GR, Beatty EB, Wang X, Cummings JH. Selective stimulation of bifidobacteria in the human colon by oligofructose and inulin. *Gastroenterology* 1995; 108: 975–982.

8   Rowland IR, Tanaka R. The effects of transgalactosylated oligosaccharides on gut flora metabolism in rats associated with human faecal microflora. *J Appl Bacteriol* 1993; 74: 667–674.

9   Collins MD, Gibson GR. Probiotics, prebiotics, and synbiotics: approaches for modulating the microbial ecology of the gut. *Am J Clin Nutr* 1999; 69: S1052–S1057.

10   Rolfe RD. The role of probiotic cultures in the control of gastrointestinal health. *J Nutr* 2000; 130: S396–S402.

11   Elmer GW, Surawicz CM, MacFarland LV. Biotherapeutic agents. A neglected modality for the treatment and prevention of selected intestinal and vaginal infections. *JAMA* 1996; 275: 870–876.

12   Dendukuri N, Costa V, McGregor M, Brophy J. *The Use of Probiotics in the Prevention and Treatment of Clostridium Difficile Diarrhea*. Montreal: Technology Assessment of the McGill Univesity Health Centre (MUHC), 2005: 37.

13   McFarland LV. Meta-analysis of probiotics for the prevention of antibiotic associated diarrhoea and the treatment of *Clostridium difficile* disease. *Am J Gastroenterol* 2006; 101: 812–822.

14   de Roos NM, Katan MB. Effects of probiotic bacteria on diarrhea, lipid metabolism, and carcinogenesis: a review of papers published between 1988 and 1998. *Am J Clin Nutr* 2000; 71: 405–411.

15   Salazar-Lindo E, Miranda-Langschwager P, Campos-Sanchez M, *et al*. *Lactobacillus casei* strain GG in the treatment of infants with acute watery diarrhoea: a randomized, double-blind, placebo-controlled clinical trial (ISRCTN67363048). *BMC Pediatr* 2004; 4: 18.

16   Szajewska H, Mrukowicz JZ. Probiotics in the treatment and prevention of acute infectious diarrhoea in infants and children: a systematic review of published, randomized, double-blind, placebo-controlled trials. *J Pediatr Gastroenterol Nutr* 2001; 33: S17–S25.

17   Huang JS, Bousvaros A, Lee JW, *et al*. Efficacy of probiotic use in acute diarrhoea in children: a meta-analysis. *Dig Dis Sci* 2002; 47: 2625–2634.

18   Van Niel CW, Feudtner C, Garrison MM, Christakis DA. Lactobacillus therapy for acute infectious diarrhea in children: a meta-analysis. *Pediatrics* 2002; 109: 678–684.

19   Pereg D, Kimhi O, Tirosh A, *et al*. The effect of fermented yogurt on the prevention of diarrhea in a healthy adult population. *Am J Infect Control* 2005; 33: 122–125.

20   Allen SJ, Okoko B, Martinez E, *et al*. Probiotics for treating infectious diarrhoea. Cochrane database, issue 4, 2003. London: Macmillan.

21   Rosenfeldt V, Michaelsen KF, Jakobsen M, *et al*. Effect of probiotic Lactobacillus strains in young children hospitalized with acute diarrhoea. *Pediatr Infect Dis J* 2002; 21: 411–416.

22   Rosenfeldt V, Michaelsen KF, Jakobsen M, *et al*. Effect of probiotic Lactobacillus strains on acute diarrhea in a cohort of nonhospitalized children in day-care centers. *Pediatr Infect Dis J* 2002; 21: 417–419.

23   Chouraqui JP, Van Egroo LD, Fichot MC. Acidified milk formula supplemented with *Bifidobacterium lactis*: impact on infant diarrhea in residential care settings. *J Pediatr Gastroenterol Nutr* 2004; 38: 288–292.

24   Thibault H, Aubert-Jacquin C, Goulet O. Effects of long-term consumption of a fermented infant formula (with *Bifidobacterium breve* c50 and *Streptococcus thermophilus* 065) on acute diarrhea in healthy infants. *J Pediatr Gastroenterol Nutr* 2004; 39: 147–152.

25   Weizman Z, Asli G, Alsheikh A. Effect of a probiotic infant formula on infections in child care centers: comparison of two probiotic agents. *Pediatrics* 2005; 115: 5–9.

26   Kurugol Z, Koturoglu G. Effects of *Saccharomyces boulardii* in children with acute diarrhoea. *Acta Paediatr* 2005; 94: 44–47.

27   Shamir R, Makhoul IR, Etzioni A, Shehadeh N. Evaluation of a diet containing probiotics and zinc for the treatment of mild diarrheal illness in children younger than one year of age. *J Am Coll Nutr* 2005; 24: 370–375.

28   Szymanski H, Pejez J, Jawien M, *et al*. Treatment of acute infectious diarrhoea in infants and children with a mixture of three *Lactobacillus rhamnosus* strains – a randomized, double-blind, placebo-controlled trial. *Aliment Pharmacol Ther* 2006; 23: 247–253.

29   Oksanen PJ, Salminen S, Saxelin M, *et al*. Prevention of travellers' diarrhoea by *Lactobacillus GG*. *Ann Med* 1990; 22: 53–56.

30   Hilton E, Kolakowski P, Singer C, Smith M. Efficacy of *Lactobacillus GG* as a diarrheal

preventive in travellers. *J Travel Med* 1997; 4: 41–43.

31 Black FT, Andersen PL, Orskov J, *et al.* Prophylactic efficacy of lactobacilli on travellers' diarrhoea. In: Steffen R, ed. *Travel Medicine. Conference on International Travel Medicine 1, Zurich, Switzerland.* Berlin: Springer, 1989: 333–335.

32 Kollaritsch H, Wiedermann G. Travellers' diarrhoea among Austrian tourists: epidemiology, clinical features and attempts at non-antibiotic drug prophylaxis. In: Pasini W, ed. *Proceedings of the Second International Conference on Tourist Health.* Rimini: World Health Organization, 1990: 74–82.

33 Katelaris PH, Salam I, Farthing MJG. Lactobacilli to prevent travellers' diarrhea? *N Engl J Med* 1995; 333: 1360–1361.

34 Siitonen S, Vapaatalo H, Salminen S, *et al.* Effect of *Lactobacillus GG* yoghurt in prevention of antibiotic associated diarrhoea. *Ann Med* 1990; 22: 57–59.

35 Gorbach SL, Chang TW, Goldin B. Successful treatment of relapsing *Clostridium difficile* colitis with *Lactobacillus GG. Lancet* 1987; 2: 1519 (letter).

36 Hawrelak JA, Whiten DL, Myers SP. Is *Lactobacillus rhamnosus* GG effective in preventing the onset of antibiotic-associated diarrhoea: a systematic review. *Digestion* 2005; 72: 51–56.

37 Sullivan A, Johansson A, Svenungsson B, Nord CE. Effect of *Lactobacillus F19* on the emergence of antibiotic-resistant microorganisms in the intestinal microflora. *J Antimicrob Chemother* 2004; 54: 791–797.

38 Kotowska M, Albrecht P, Szajewska H. *Saccharomyces boulardii* in the prevention of antibiotic-associated diarrhoea in children: a randomized double-blind placebo-controlled trial. *Aliment Pharmacol Ther* 2005; 21: 583–590.

39 Wunderlich PF, Braun L, Fumagalli I, *et al.* Double-blind report on the efficacy of lactic acid producing *Enterococcus SF68* in the prevention of antibiotic-associated diarrhoea in the treatment of acute diarrhoea. *J Int Med Res* 1989; 17: 333–338.

40 Tankanow RM, Ross MB, Ertel IJ, *et al.* A double-blind, placebo-controlled study of the efficacy of Lactinex in the prophylaxis of amoxicillin-induced diarrhoea. *Ann Pharmacol* 1990; 24: 382–384.

41 Black F, Einarsson K, Lidbeck A, *et al.* Effect of lactic acid producing bacteria on the human intestinal microflora during ampicillin treatment. *Scand J Infect Dis* 1991; 23: 247–254.

42 Correa NB, Perret Filho LA, Penna FJ, *et al.* A randomized formula controlled trial of *Bifidobacterium lactis* and *Streptococcus thermophilus* for prevention of antibiotic-associated diarrhea in infants. *J Clin Gastroenterol* 2005; 39: 385–389.

43 D'Souza AL, Rajkumar C, Cooke J, Bulpitt CJ. Probiotics in prevention of antibiotic-associated diarrhoea: meta-analysis. *BMJ* 2002; 324: 1361–1364.

44 Cremonini F, Di Caro S, Nista EC, *et al.* A meta-analysis: the effect of probiotic administration on antibiotic-associated diarrhoea. *Aliment Pharmacol Ther* 2002; 16: 1461–1467.

45 Szajeska H, Mrukowicz J. Meta-analysis: non-pathogenic yeast *Saccharomyces boulardii* in the prevention of antibiotic-associated diarrhoea. *Aliment Pharmacol Ther* 2005; 22: 365–372.

46 McFarland LV. Meta-analysis of probiotics for the prevention of antibiotic associated diarrhea and the treatment of *Clostridium difficile* disease. *Am J Gastroenterol* 2006; 101: 812–822.

47 Sanders ME. Summary of the conclusions from a consensus panel of experts on health attributes of lactic cultures: significance to fluid milk products containing cultures. *J Dairy Sci* 1993; 76: 1819–1828.

48 Mustapha A, Jiang T, Savaino DA. Improvement of lactose digestion by humans following ingestion of unfermented acidophilus milk: influence of bile sensitivity, lactose transport, and acid tolerance of *Lactobacilllus acidophilus. J Dairy Sci* 1997; 80: 1537–1545.

49 Saltzman JR, Russell RM, Golner B, *et al.* A randomized trial of *Lactobacillus acidophilus* BG2F04 to treat lactose intolerance. *Am J Clin Nutr* 1999; 69: 140–146.

50 Levri KM, Ketvertis K, Deramo M, *et al.* Do probiotics reduce adult lactose intolerance? A systematic review. *J Fam Pract* 2005; 54: 613–620.

51 Shalev E, Battino S, Weiner E, *et al.* Ingestion of yogurt containing *Lactobacillus acidophilus* compared with pasteurized yoghurt as prophylaxis for recurrent candidal vaginitis and bacterial vaginosis. *Arch Fam Med* 1996; 5: 593–596.

52 De Simone C, Ciardi A, Grassi A, *et al.* Effect of *Bifidobacterium bifidum* and *Lactobacillus acidophilus* on gut mucosa and peripheral blood B lymphocytes. *Immunopharmacol Immunotoxicol* 1992; 14: 331–340.

53 Pirotta M, Gunn J, Chondros P, *et al.* Effect of lactobacillus in preventing post-antibiotic vulvovaginal candidiasis: a randomised controlled trial. *BMJ* 2004; 329: 548.

54 Schiffrin EJ, Rochat F, Link-Amster H, *et al.* Immunomodulation of human blood cells following the ingestion of lactic acid bacteria. *J Dairy Sci* 1995; 78: 491–497.

55 Majaama M, Isolauri E. Probiotics: a novel approach in the management of food allergy. *J Allergy Clin Immunol* 1997; 99: 179–185.

56 Galdeano CM, Perdigon G. The probiotic bacterium *Lactobacillus casei* induces activation of

the gut mucosal immune system through innate immunity. *Clin Vaccine Immunol* 2006; 13: 219–226.

57 Kim YG, Ohta T, Takahashi T, *et al*. Probiotic *Lactobacillus casei* activates innate immunity via NF-kappB and p38 MAP kinase signalling pathways. *J Microbes Infect* 2006; 8: 994–1004.

58 Marcos A, Warnberg J, Nova E, *et al*. The effect of milk fermented by yogurt cultures plus *Lactobacillus casei* DN-11401 on the immune response of subjects under academic examination stress. *Eur J Nutr* 2004; 43: 381–389.

59 Olivares M, Diaz-Ropero MP, Gomez N, *et al*. The consumption of two new probiotic strains, *Lactobacillus gasseri* CECT 5714 and *Lactobacillus coryniformis* CECT 5711 boosts the immune system of healthy humans. *Int Microbiol* 2006; 9: 47–52.

60 Parra D, Morentin BM, Cobo JM, *et al*. Monocyte function in healthy middle-aged people receiving fermented milk containing *Lactobacillus casei*. *J Nutr Health Aging* 2004; 8: 208–211.

61 Parra MD, Martinez de Morentin BE, Cobo JM, *et al*. Daily ingestion of fermented milk containing *Lactobacillus casei* DN114001 improves innate defense capacity in healthy middle-aged people. *J Physiol Biochem* 2004; 60: 85–91.

62 Majaama M, Isolauri E. Probiotics: a novel approach in the management of food allergy. *J Allergy Clin Immunol* 1997; 99: 179–185.

63 Isolauri E, Arvola T, Sutas Y, *et al*. Probiotics in the management of atopic eczema. *Clin Exp Allergy* 2000; 30: 1604–1610.

64 Rosenfeldt V, Benfeldt E, Nielsen SD, *et al*. Effect of probiotic Lactobacillus strains in children with atopic dermatitis. *J Allergy Clin Immunol* 2003; 111: 389–395.

65 Weston S, Halbert A, Richmond P, Prescott SL. Effects of probiotics on atopic dermatitis: a randomized controlled trial. *Arch Dis Child* 2005; 892–897.

66 Viljanen M, Savilahti E, Haahtela T, *et al*. Probiotics in the treatment of atopic eczema/dermatitis syndrome in infants: a double-blind placebo-controlled trial. *Allergy* 2005; 60: 494–500.

67 Rosenfeldt V, Benfeldt E, Valerius NH, *et al*. Effect of probiotics on gastrointestinal symptoms and small intestinal permeability in children with atopic dermatitis. *J Pediatr* 2004; 145: 612–616.

68 Jackson TG, Taylor GRJ, Clohessy AM, Williams CM. The effects of the daily intake of inulin on fasting lipid, insulin and glucose concentrations in middle-aged men and women. *Br J Nutr* 1999; 89: 23–30.

69 Kalliomaki M, Salkminen S, Arvilommi H, *et al*. Probiotics in primary prevention of atopic disease: a randomized placebo-controlled trial. *Lancet* 2001; 357: 1076–1079.

70 Rautava S, Kalliomaki M, Isolauri E. Probiotics during pregnancy and breast-feeding might confer immunomodulatory protection against atopic disease in the infant. *J Allergy Clin Immunol* 2002; 109: 119–121.

71 Wang MF, Lin HC, Wang YY, Hus CH. Treatment of perennial allergic rhinitis with lactic acid bacteria. *Pediatr Allergy Immunol* 2004; 15: 152–158.

72 Peng GC, Hsu CH. The efficacy and safety of heat-killed *Lactobacillus paracasei* for treatment of perennial allergic rhinitis induced by house-dust mite. *Pediatr Allergy Immunol* 2005; 16: 433–438.

73 Anderson JW, Gillialand SE. Effect of fermented milk (yogurt) containing *Lactobacillus acidophilus* L1 on serum cholesterol by hypercholesterolemic humans. *J Am Coll Nutr* 1999; 18: 43–50.

74 Schaafsma G, Meuling WJ, van Dokkum W, Bouley C. Effects of a milk product, fermented by *Lactobacillus acidophilus* and with fructo-oligosaccharides added, on blood lipids in male volunteers. *Eur J Clin Nutr* 1998; 52: 436–440.

75 Davidson MH, Maki KC, Synecki C. Evaluation of the influence of dietary inulin on serum lipids in adults with hypercholesterolemia. *Nutrition* 1998; 18: 503–517.

76 Mital BK, Garg SK. Anticarcinogenic, hypocholesterolemic and antagonistic activities of *Lactobacillus acidophilus*. *Crit Rev Microbiol* 1995; 21: 175–214.

77 Xiao JZ, Kondo S, Takahashi N, *et al*. Effects of milk products fermented by *Bifidobacterium longum* on blood lipids in rats and healthy adult male volunteers. *J Dairy Sci* 2003; 86: 2452–2461.

78 Kiessling G, Schneider J, Jahreis G. Long-term consumption of fermented dairy products over 6 months increases HDL cholesterol. *Eur J Clin Nutr* 2002; 56: 843–849.

79 Greany KA, Nettleton JA, Wangen KE, *et al*. Probiotic consumption does not enhance the cholesterol lowering effect of soy in postmenopausal women. *J Nutr* 2004; 134: 3277–3283.

80 Lewis SJ, Burmeister S. A double-blind placebo-controlled study of the effects of *Lactobacillus acidophilus* on plasma lipids. *Eur J Clin Nutr* 2005; 59: 776–780.

81 Naruszewicz M, Johansson ML, Zapolska-Downar D, Bukowska H. Effect of *Lactobacillus plantarum* 299v on cardiovascular disease risk factors in smokers. *Am J Clin Nutr* 2002; 76: 1249–1255.

82 Aihara K, Kajimoto O, Hirata H, *et al*. Effect of powdered fermented milk with *Lactobacillus*

helveticus on subjects with high-normal blood pressure or mild hypertension. *J Am Coll Nutr* 2005; 24: 257–265.

83   Cruchet S, Obregon MC, Salazar G, *et al*. Effect of ingestion of a dietary product containing *Lactobacillus johnsonii* La1 on *Helicobacter pylori* colonization in children. *Nutrition* 2003; 19: 716–721.

84   Wang KY, Li SN, Liu CS, *et al*. Effects of ingesting Lactobacillus- and Bifidobacterium-containing yogurt in subjects with colonized *Helicobacter pylori*. *Am J Clin Nutr* 2004; 80: 737–741.

85   Sykora J, Valeckova K, Amlerova J, *et al*. Effects of a specially designed fermented milk product containing probiotic *Lactobacillus casei* DN-114001 and the eradication of *H. pylori* in children: a prospective double-blind study. *J Clin Gastroenterol* 2005; 39: 692–698.

86   Gotteland M, Poliak L, Cruchet S, Brunser O. Effect of regular ingestion of *Saccharomyces boulardii* plus inulin or *Lactobacillus acidophilus* LB in children colonized by *Helicobacter pylori*. *Acta Paediatr* 2005 94; 1747–1751.

87   Sheu B-S, Cheng H-C, Kao A-W, *et al*. Pretreatmemt with Lactobacillus and Bifidobacterium-containing yogurt can improve the efficacy of quadruple therapy in eradicating residual *Helicobacter pylori* infection after failed triple therapy. *Am J Clin Nutr* 2006; 83: 864–869.

88   Nista EC, Candelli M, Cremonini GF, *et al*. *Bacillus clausii* therapy to reduce side effects of anti-*Helicobacter pylori* treatment: randomized, double-blind, placebo-controlled trial. *Aliment Pharmacol Ther* 2004; 20: 1181–1188.

89   Tursi A, Barndimarte G, Giogetti GM, Modeo ME. Effect of *Lactobacillus casei* supplementation on the effectiveness and tolerability of a new second-line 10-day quadruple therapy after failure of a first attempt to cure *Helicobacter pylori* infection. *Med Sci Monit* 2004; 10: CR662–666.

90   Cremonini F, Di Caro S, Covino M, *et al*. Effect of different probiotic preparations on anti-*Helicobacter pylori* therapy-related side effects: a parallel group, triple blind, placebo-controlled strudy. *Am J Gastroenterol* 2002; 97: 2744–2749.

91   Myllyloma E, Veijola L, Ahlroos T, *et al*. Probiotic supplementation improves tolerance to *Helicobacter pylori* eradication therapy – a placebo-controlled, double-blind randomized pilot study. *Aliment Pharmacol Ther* 2005; 21: 1263–1272.

92   Gotteland M, Brunser O, Cruchet S. Systematic review: are probiotics useful in controlling gastric colonization by *Helicobacter pylori*? *Aliment Pharmacol Ther* 2006; 23: 1077–1086.

93   Niedzielin K, Kordecki H, Birkenfeld B. A controlled, double-blind, randomized study on the efficacy of *Lactobacillus plantarum* 299V in patients with irritable bowel syndrome. *Eur J Gastroenterol Hepatol* 2001; 13: 1143–1147.

94   Sen S, Mullan MM, Parker TJ, *et al*. Effect of *Lactobacillus plantarum* 299V on colonic fermentation and symptoms of irritable bowel syndrome. *Dig Dis Sci* 2002; 47: 2615–2620.

95   Saggioro A. Probiotics in the treatment of irritable bowel syndrome. *J Clin Gastroenterol* 2004; 38: S104–S106.

96   O'Mahony L, McCarthy J, Kelly P, *et al*. Lactobacillus and bifidobacterium in irritable bowel syndrome: symptom responses and relationship to cytokine profiles. *Gastroenterology* 2005; 128: 541–551.

97   Bausserman M, Michail S. The use of Lactobacillus GG in irritable bowel syndrome in children: a double-blind randomized control trial. *J Pediatr* 2005; 147: 197–201.

98   Kim HJ, Vazquez-Roque MI, Camilleri M, *et al*. A randomized controlled trial of a probiotic combination VSL#3 and placebo in irritable bowel syndrome with bloating. *Neurogastroenterol Motil* 2005; 17: 687–696.

99   Niv E, Naftali T, Hallak R, Vaisman N. The efficacy of *Lactobacillus reuteri* ATCC 55730 in the treatment of patients with irritable bowel syndrome – a double blind, placebo-controlled, randomized study. *Clin Nutr* 2005; 24: 925–931.

100 Bittner AC, Croffut RM, Stranahan MC. Prescript-Assist probiotic-prebiotic treatment for irritable bowel syndrome: a methodologically oriented, 2-week, randomized, placebo-controlled, double-blind clinical study. *Clin Ther* 2005; 27: 75–61.

101 Kajander K, Hatakka K, Poussa T, *et al*. A probiotic mixture alleviates symptoms in irritable bowel syndrome patients: a controlled 6-month intervention. *Aliment Pharmacol Ther* 2005; 22: 387–394.

102 Guslandi M, Mezzi G, Sorghi M, Testoni PA. *Saccharomyces boulardii* in maintenance treatment of Crohn's disease. *Dig Dis Sci* 2000; 45: 1462–1464.

103 Prantera C, Scribano ML, Flasco G, Andreoli A, Luzi C. Ineffectiveness of probiotics in preventing recurrence after curative resection for Crohn's disease: a randomised controlled trial with *Lactobacillus GG*. *Gut* 2002; 51: 405–409.

104 Schultz M, Timmer A, Herfarth HH, *et al*. *Lactobacillus GG* in inducing and maintaining remission of Crohn's disease. *BMC Gastroenterol* 2004; 4: 5.

105 Bousvaros A, Guandalini S, Baldassano RN, *et al*. A randomized, double-blind trial of *Lactobacillus GG* versus placebo in addition to standard maintenance therapy for children with Crohn's disease. *Inflamm Bowel Dis* 2005; 11: 833–839.

106 Marteau P, Lemann M, Seksik P, *et al*. Ineffectiveness of *Lactobacillus johnsonii* LA1 for prophylaxis of postoperative recurrence in Crohn's disease: a randomised, double-blind, placebo-controlled GETAID trial. *Gut* 2005; Dec 23 (Epub ahead of print).

107 Furrie E, Macfarlane S, Kennedy A, *et al*. Synbiotic therapy (*Bifidobacterium longum*/Synergy 1) initiates resolution of inflammation in patients with active ulcerative colitis: a randomised controlled pilot trial. *Gut* 2005; 54: 242–249.

108 Kato K, Misumo S, Umesaki Y, *et al*. Randomized placebo-controlled trial assessing the effect of bifidobacteria-fermented milk on active ulcerative colitis. *Aliment Pharmacol Ther* 2004; 20: 11333–11341.

109 Laake KO, Bjorneklett A, Aamodt G, *et al*. Outcome of four weeks' intervention with probiotics on symptoms and endoscopic appearance after surgical reconstruction with a J-configurated ileal-pouch-anal anastomosis in ulcerative colitis. *Scand J Gastroenterol* 2005; 40: 43–51.

110 Kruis W, Schutz E, Fric P, *et al*. Double-blind comparison of an oral *Escherichia coli* preparation and mesalazine in maintaining remission of ulcerative colitis. *Aliment Pharmacol Ther* 1997; 11: 853–858.

111 Kruis W, Fric P, Pokrotnieks J, *et al*. Maintaining remission of ulcerative colitis with the probiotic *Escherichia coli* Nissle 1917 is as effective as standard mesalazine. *Gut* 2004; 53: 1617–1623.

112 Tursi A, Brandimarte G, Giorgetti GM, *et al*. Low dose balsalazide plus a high-potency probiotic preparation is more effective than balsalazide alone or mesalazine in the treatment of acute mild to moderate ulcerative colitis. *Med Sci Monit* 2004; 10: P1126–1131.

113 Hanai H, Kanauchi O, Mitsuyama K, *et al*. Germinated barley foodstuff prolongs remission in patients with ulcerative colitis. *Int J Mol Med* 2004; 13: 643–647.

114 Ishikawa H, Akedo I, Umesaki Y, *et al*. Randomized controlled trial of the effect of bifidobacteria-fermented milk on ulcerative colitis. *J Am Coll Nutr* 2003; 22: 53–63.

115 Rembacken BJ, Snellin Am, Hawkey PM, *et al*. Non-pathogenic *Escherichia coli* versus mesalazine for the treatment of ulcerative colitis: a randomised trial. *Lancet* 1999; 354: 635–639.

116 Coudray C, Bellanger J, Catiglia-Delavaud C, *et al*. Effect of soluble and partly soluble dietary fibres supplementation on absorption and balance of calcium, magnesium, iron and zinc in healthy young men. *Eur J Clin Nutr* 1997; 51: 375–380.

117 van den Heuvel EGHM, Muys T, van Dokkum W, Schaafsma G. Oligofructose stimulates calcium absorption in adolescents. *Am J Clin Nutr* 1999; 69: 544–548.

118 Abrams SA, Griffin IJ, Hawthorne KM, *et al*. A combination of prebiotic short- and long-chain inulin-type fructans enhances calcium absorption and bone mineralization in young adolescents. *Am J Clin Nutr* 2005; 82: 471–476.

119 Gluck U, Gebbers JO. Ingested probiotics reduce nasal colonization with pathogenic bacteria (*Staphylococcus aureus*, *Streptococcus pneumoniae* and beta-hemolytic streptococci). *Am J Clin Nutr* 2003; 77: 517–520.

120 de Vrese M, Winkler P, Rautenberg P, *et al*. Effect of *Lactobacillus gasseri* PA 16/8, *Bifidobacterium longum* SP07/3, *B. bifidum* MF 20/5 on common cold episodes: a double-blind, randomized, controlled trial. *Clin Nutr* 2005; 24: 481–491.

121 Ezendam J, van Loveren H. Probiotics: immunomodulation and evaluation of safety and efficacy. *Nutr Rev* 2006; 64: 1–14.

122 Senok AC, Ismaeel AY, Botta GA. Probiotics: facts and myths. *Clin Microbiol Infect* 2005; 11: 958–966.

Psyllium

Description

Psyllium (ispaghula) is the mucilage obtained from the seed coat (husk or hull) of *Plantago ovata*. It is a rich source of dietary fibre.

Constituents

The main active ingredient in psyllium is a water-soluble, gel-forming polysaccharide, which appears chemically to be a highly branched arabinoxylan, with the main chain of 1,4-linked xylopyranose residues densely substituted with either single xylose units or trisaccharides. The arabinoxylan has been found to contain 74.1% xylose, 22.4% arabinose, 1.8% galactose and trace amounts of glucose, rhamnose and uronic acid.[1]

Action

The water-soluble polysaccharide in psyllium forms a viscous gel in the intestine. As a result of this gel formation, psyllium has several effects, acting to:

- stimulate peristalsis, reduce gastrointestinal transit time, increase stool weight and function as a bulk laxative;[2,3]
- lubricate the stools, so facilitating defecation;[4]
- increase the water-absorbing capacity and viscosity of the faeces, delaying gastric emptying time and improving the consistency of the faeces in both diarrhoea and constipation;[2,5]
- reduce the production of gastric acid;
- prolong gastrointestinal transit time in cases of diarrhoea, possibly by delaying the production of gaseous fermentation products;[5]

- reduce serum cholesterol by elimination of cholesterol in bile acids[6] and reducing absorption of dietary fats;[7,8]
- delay the rate of absorption of carbohydrates, which can reduce post-meal blood glucose levels in patients with diabetes mellitus.[9,10]

Psyllium, like other soluble fibres, appears to be partially fermented by the bacteria in the colon to produce short-chain fatty acids (e.g. butyrate).[5,11]

Possible uses

Psyllium has a long history of use as a dietary fibre supplement to promote the regulation of large bowel function and, more recently, has been shown to lower blood cholesterol levels.

Constipation
Psyllium is effective as a bulk laxative in the management of constipation,[2,4,12,13] and several commercial preparations of ispaghula husk are licensed and prescribable as bulk laxatives in the UK.

Diarrhoea
Psyllium has been shown to improve faecal consistency in patients with diarrhoea.[4,5] Studies in tube-fed patients have also shown an improvement in diarrhoea with psyllium.

Hypercholesterolaemia
Psyllium is effective in reducing serum cholesterol in people with hypercholesterolaemia. Psyllium 5.1 g twice a day for 8 weeks produced a modest but significant improvement in total cholesterol and LDL cholesterol in men and women on either high- or low-fat

diets.[14] In a further study, psyllium 3.4 g three times a day for 8 weeks reduced total and LDL cholesterol in men.[15] Another study with psyllium 6.7 g daily for 2 weeks and a low-fat diet reduced total, LDL, HDL and the LDL/HDL ratio with no effect on triglycerides.[8] Further studies have indicated that psyllium supplementation is effective in lowering LDL cholesterol, but has no or limited effect on HDL cholesterol and triglycerides.[16,17] Studies of 6 months' duration have demonstrated the potential for long-term benefit of psyllium in lowering LDL cholesterol.[18,19] There appear to be some advantages in combining psyllium with monounsaturated fat to further reduce the LDL to HDL cholesterol.[20] Trials of psyllium in children have also shown potential benefits in cholesterol lowering.[21,22] Meta-analyses have confirmed the cholesterol-lowering effect of psyllium in adults as an adjunct to a low-fat diet.[23,24] The maximum effect is seen when psyllium is consumed with food.

Psyllium supplementation in patients taking 10 mg simvastatin seems to be as effective in lowering cholesterol as 20 mg simvastatin alone.[25] A combination of psyllium and colestipol at half the usual doses lowered cholesterol as effectively as either psyllium or colestipol alone.[26] Addition of psyllium to colestyramine produced further reduction in total and LDL cholesterol levels and also helped to improve compliance by reducing the gastrointestinal side-effects of colestyramine.[27]

Diabetes
Preliminary evidence has indicated that psyllium has some influence on post-prandial blood glucose, glycated haemoglobin, insulin, total cholesterol and LDL cholesterol in patients with type 2 diabetes and hypercholesterolaemia.[9,10,28–32] However, studies are not totally consistent.

Irritable bowel syndrome
Studies evaluating the effect of psyllium in IBS have produced inconsistent results, with some showing no benefit[33] and others showing benefit.[34–36]

Ulcerative colitis
There is some evidence of benefit of psyllium in ulcerative colitis. It has been shown to be helpful in maintaining remission[37] and to be as effective as mesalazine in maintaining remission.[38] However, a trial of psyllium in juvenile ulcerative colitis patients found no influence on faecal bile acid excretion.[39]

Side-effects of orlistat
In one trial, psyllium has been shown to relieve the side-effects of orlistat (e.g. flatulence, diarrhoea, abdominal cramps, oily discharge).[40]

Conclusion
Psyllium has been well studied for its effect on bowel function, with studies generally showing an increase in stool weight and reduced gastrointestinal transit time in patients with constipation. Faecal consistency is also generally improved in patients with diarrhoea. Psyllium produces a modest reduction in total and LDL cholesterol in patients with hypercholesterolaemia and is effective as an adjunct to dietary management and possibly to drug management. It does not appear to influence HDL cholesterol or triglycerides. In patients with diabetes, psyllium has produced modest reductions in post-prandial blood glucose, glycated haemoglobin and insulin, but further research is needed to confirm these effects. There is conflicting evidence for the value of psyllium in IBS and ulcerative colitis.

Precautions/contraindications

Psyllium is contraindicated in people with conditions causing gastrointestinal obstruction, hypersensitivity to psyllium and swallowing disorders.

Psyllium may cause reduction in blood glucose levels. People with diabetes should be monitored.

Some psyllium preparations are sweetened with aspartame. These products should be avoided in people with phenylketonuria.

Pregnancy and breast-feeding

Psyllium is considered to be safe in pregnancy and breast-feeding, although studies in humans have not been conducted.

Adverse effects

Psyllium can cause flatulence, abdominal pain, bloating, diarrhoea, constipation and nausea. Starting with a dose and building up gradually can help to minimise gastrointestinal effects. Psyllium can also cause gastrointestinal obstruction, especially in patients with dysphagia and other swallowing disorders, but it can occur in anyone, unless it is consumed with plenty of water.

Allergic reactions (e.g. rhinitis, sneezing, headache, conjunctivitis, urticaria, itching, dyspnoea and flushing) can occur. Severe allergic reactions include wheezing, angio-oedema, asthma, cough, diarrhoea and anaphylactic shock

Interactions

Drugs

Anti-diabetic drugs: psyllium may lower blood glucose and have an additive effect with anti-diabetic drugs.
Aspirin: absorption may be reduced.
Carbamazepine: absorption may be reduced.
Digoxin: absorption may be reduced.
Lithium: absorption may be reduced.
Statins: psyllium may have an additive effect in reducing blood cholesterol.
Warfarin: theoretical risk of reduced absorption, but clinical studies have not demonstrated an effect.

Nutrients

Minerals and vitamins: psyllium may reduce the absorption of all nutrients (in particular minerals such as calcium, iron, zinc and magnesium).

Dose

Wide ranges of doses have been used in studies, but are not clearly established.

- In constipation, 7–40 g daily in two to three divided doses has been used.
- In cholesterol lowering, the most commonly used doses in adults have ranged from 10 to 20 g psyllium daily and in children 5–10 g daily, in two or three divided doses.
- In type 2 diabetes, up to 45 g daily has been given to lower blood glucose.
- For IBS, 6–30 g daily has been used.

For commercial licensed and prescribable preparations of ispaghula, doses can be found in the *British National Formulary*.

Psyllium should always be taken with plenty of fluid and doses avoided just before bedtime (to prevent gastrointestinal obstruction).

References

1 Fischer M, Nanxiong Y, Gray G, *et al*. The gel-forming polysaccharide of psyllium husk. *Carbohydr Res* 2004; 339; 2009–2017.
2 Ashraf W, Park F, Lof J, Quigley EM. Effects of psyllium therapy on stool characteristics, colon transit and anorectal function in chronic idiopathic constipation. *Aliment Pharmacol Ther* 1995; 9: 639–647.
3 Marteau P, Flourie B, Cherbut C, *et al*. Digestibility and bulking effect of ispaghula husks in healthy humans. *Gut* 1994; 35: 1747–1752.
4 Marlett JA, Kajs TM, Fischer MH. An unfermented gel component of psyllium seed husk promotes laxation as a lubricant in humans. *Am J Clin Nutr* 2000; 72: 784–789.
5 Washington N, Harris M, Mussellwhite A, Spiller RC. Moderation of lactulose-induced diarrhea by psyllium: effects on motility and fermentation. *Am J Clin Nutr* 1998; 67: 317–321.
6 Chaplin MF, Chaudhury S, Dettmar PW, *et al*. Effect of ispaghula husk on the faecal output of bile acids in healthy volunteers. *J Steroid Biochem Mol Biol* 2000; 72: 283–292.
7 Ganji V, Kies CV. Psyllium husk fibre supplementation to soybean and coconut oil diets of humans: effect on fat digestibility and faecal fatty acid excretion. *Eur J Clin Nutr* 1994; 48: 595–597.
8 Wolever TM, Jenkins DJ, Mueller S, *et al*. Psyllium reduces blood lipids in men and women

with hyperlipidemia. *Am J Med Sci* 1994; 307: 269–273.

9 Anderson JW, Allgood LD, Turner J, *et al*. Effects of psyllium on glucose and serum lipid responses in men with type 2 diabetes and hypercholesterolemia. *Am J Clin Nutr* 1999; 70: 466–473.

10 Wolever TM, Vuksan V, Eshuis H, *et al*. Effect of method of administration of psyllium on glycemic response and carbohydrate digestibility. *J Am Coll Nutr* 1991; 10: 364–371.

11 Wolever TM, Robb PA. Effect of guar, pectin, psyllium, soy polysaccharide, and cellulose on breath hydrogen and methane in healthy subjects. *Am J Gastroenterol* 1992; 87: 305–10.

12 Ashraf W, Pfeiffer RF, Park F, *et al*. Constipation in Parkinson's disease: objective assessment and response to psyllium. *Mov Disord* 1997; 12: 946–951.

13 Marlett JA, Li BU, Patrow CJ, Bass P. Comparative laxation of psyllium with and without senna in an ambulatory constipated population. *Am J Gastroenterol* 1987; 82: 333–337.

14 Sprecher DL, Harris BV, Goldberg AC, *et al*. Efficacy of psyllium in reducing serum cholesterol levels in hypercholesterolemic patients on high- or low-fat diets. *Ann Intern Med* 1993; 119 (7 Pt 1): 545–554.

15 Anderson JW, Zettwoch N, Feldman T, *et al*. Cholesterol-lowering effects of psyllium hydrophilic mucilloid for hypercholesterolemic men. *Arch Intern Med* 1988; 148: 292–296.

16 Anderson JW, Riddell-Mason S, Gustafson NJ, *et al*. Cholesterol-lowering effects of psyllium-enriched cereal as an adjunct to a prudent diet in the treatment of mild to moderate hypercholesterolemia. *Am J Clin Nutr* 1992; 56: 93–98.

17 Roberts DC, Truswell AS, Bencke A, *et al*. The cholesterol-lowering effect of a breakfast cereal containing psyllium fibre. *Med J Aust* 1994; 161: 660–664.

18 Davidson MH, Maki KC, Kong JC, *et al*. Long-term effects of consuming foods containing psyllium seed husk on serum lipids in subjects with hypercholesterolemia. *Am J Clin Nutr* 1998; 67: 367–376.

19 Anderson JW, Davidson MH, Blonde L, *et al*. Long-term cholesterol-lowering effects of psyllium as an adjunct to diet therapy in the treatment of hypercholesterolemia. *Am J Clin Nutr* 2000; 71: 1433–1438.

20 Jenkins DJ, Wolever TM, Vidgen E, *et al*. Effect of psyllium in hypercholesterolemia at two monounsaturated fatty acid intakes. *Am J Clin Nutr* 1997; 65: 1524–1533.

21 Dennison BA, Levine DM. Randomized, double-blind, placebo-controlled, two-period crossover clinical trial of psyllium fiber in children with hypercholesterolemia. *J Pediatr* 1993; 123: 24–29.

22 Davidson MH, Dugan LD, Burns JH, *et al*. A psyllium-enriched cereal for the treatment of hypercholesterolemia in children: a controlled, double-blind, crossover study. *Am J Clin Nutr* 1996; 63: 96–102.

23 Olson BH, Anderson SM, Becker MP, *et al*. Psyllium-enriched cereals lower blood total cholesterol and LDL cholesterol, but not HDL cholesterol, in hypercholesterolemic adults: results of a meta-analysis. *J Nutr* 1997; 127: 1973–1980.

24 Anderson JW, Allgood LD, Lawrence A, *et al*. Cholesterol-lowering effects of psyllium intake adjunctive to diet therapy in men and women with hypercholesterolemia: meta-analysis of 8 controlled trials. *Am J Clin Nutr* 2000; 71: 472–479.

25 Moreyra AE, Wilson AC, Koraym A. Effect of combining psyllium fiber with simvastatin in lowering cholesterol. *Arch Intern Med* 2005; 165: 1161–1166.

26 Spence JD, Huff MW, Heidenheim P, *et al*. Combination therapy with colestipol and psyllium mucilloid in patients with hyperlipidemia. *Ann Intern Med* 1995; 123: 493–499.

27 Maciejko JJ, Brazg R, Shah A, *et al*. Psyllium for the reduction of cholestyramine-associated gastrointestinal symptoms in the treatment of primary hypercholesterolemia. *Arch Fam Med* 1994; 3: 955–960.

28 Pastors JG, Blaisdell PW, Balm TK, *et al*. Psyllium fiber reduces rise in postprandial glucose and insulin concentrations in patients with non-insulin-dependent diabetes. *Am J Clin Nutr* 1991; 53: 1431–1435.

29 Frati Munari AC, Benitez Pinto W, Raul Ariza Andraca C, Casarrubias M. Lowering glycemic index of food by acarbose and Plantago psyllium mucilage. *Arch Med Res* 1998; 29: 137–41.

30 Rodriguez-Moran M, Guerrero-Romero F, Lazcano-Burciaga G. Lipid- and glucose-lowering efficacy of Plantago Psyllium in type II diabetes. *J Diabetes Complications* 1998; 12: 273–278.

31 Ziai SA, Larijani B, Akhoondzadeh S, *et al*. Psyllium decreased serum glucose and glycosylated hemoglobin significantly in diabetic outpatients. *J Ethnopharmacol* 2005; 102: 202–207.

32 Sierra M, Garcia JJ, Fernandez N, *et al*. Therapeutic effects of psyllium in type 2 diabetic patients. *Eur J Clin Nutr* 2002; 56: 830–842.

33 Longstreth GF, Fox DD, Youkeles L, *et al*. Psyllium therapy in the irritable bowel syndrome. A double-blind trial. *Ann Intern Med* 1981; 95: 53–56.

34 Prior A, Whorwell PJ. Double blind study of ispaghula in irritable bowel syndrome. *Gut* 1987; 28: 1510–1513.

35 Jalihal A, Kurian G. Ispaghula therapy in irritable bowel syndrome: improvement in overall

well-being is related to reduction in bowel dissatisfaction. *J Gastroenterol Hepatol* 1990; 5: 507–513.

36 Misra SP, Thorat VK, Sachdev GK, Anand BS. Long-term treatment of irritable bowel syndrome: results of a randomized controlled trial. *Q J Med* 1989; 73: 931–939.

37 Hallert C, Kaldma M, Petersson BG. Ispaghula husk may relieve gastrointestinal symptoms in ulcerative colitis in remission. *Scand J Gastroenterol* 1991; 26: 747–750.

38 Fernandez-Banares F, Hinojosa J, Sanchez-Lombrana JL, *et al*. Randomized clinical trial of Plantago ovata seeds (dietary fiber) as compared with mesalamine in maintaining remission in ulcerative colitis. Spanish Group for the Study of Crohn's Disease and Ulcerative Colitis (GETECCU). *Am J Gastroenterol* 1999; 94: 427–433.

39 Ejderhamn J, Hedenborg G, Strandvik B. Long-term double-blind study on the influence of dietary fibres on faecal bile acid excretion in juvenile ulcerative colitis. *Scand J Clin Lab Invest* 1992; 52: 697–706.

40 Cavaliere H, Floriano I, Medeiros-Neto G. Gastrointestinal side effects of orlistat may be prevented by concomitant prescription of natural fibers (psyllium mucilloid). *Int J Obes Relat Metab Disord* 2001; 25: 1095–1099.

Pycnogenol

Description

Pycnogenol is a registered trade name for a specific standardised extract of procyanidins (a category of flavonoids) from the bark of the French maritime pine (*Pinus pinaster* ssp. *atlantica*), which is grown in the Bay of Biscay in south-west France. The term pycnogenol was originally intended to serve as a scientific name for this category of flavonoids and was therefore applied to any preparation consisting of procyanidins.

Constituents

Pycnogenol is a mixture of monomeric and polymeric procyanidins. Catechin is the main monomeric procyanidin, while epicatechin is present in trace amounts. Catechin and epicatechin units are linked together to form bipolymers and larger procyanidin units. Other constituents of pycnogenol include another flavonoid, taxifolin, and a range of phenolic acids such as *p*-hydroxybenzoic acid, protocatechic acid, vanillic acid, gallic acid, caffeic acid, ferulic acid and *p*-coumaric acid. Calcium, copper, iron, manganese, potassium and zinc are also present.[1,2]

Action

Pycnogenol stimulates production of nitric oxide *in vitro* and *in vivo* from the natural substrate L-arginine.[1] Nitric oxide prevents platelet aggregation and causes the release of cyclic guanosine monophosphate in smooth muscle cells, leading to vasodilatation. By virtue of these effects, pycnogenol has a range of pharmacological activities on the vascular system including:

- inhibition of platelet aggregation and vasodilation; pycnogenol also appears to improve the efficacy of acetylsalicylic acid in inhibition of platelet function;[3]
- inhibition of ACE with reduction in blood pressure;[1,4]
- improved endothelial function;[5]
- improved lipid profiles;[6]
- enhanced capillary integrity and stabilisation of cell membranes;[7]
- improved erectile function.[8]

Other effects that have been demonstrated *in vitro* and in animals include:

- antioxidant and free radical activity;[2,6,7]
- inhibition of nuclear factor kappa B (NF-κB), various interleukins and other factors centrally involved in inflammatory processes;[9]
- inhibition of histamine realease;[1]
- stimulation of the immune system (e.g. enhanced phagocytosis and natural killer cell activity);[10]
- lowering of blood glucose;[11]
- inhibition of cyclooxygenase (COX) 1 and 2 activity.[12]

Possible uses

A variety of claims have been made for pycnogenol and there is enormous research interest in this substance. Traditionally, pycnogenol was used in the treatment of scurvy and wound healing. Today it is marketed mainly for its supposed effects on the circulation, and its antioxidant, free radical and anti-inflammatory activity.

Cardiovascular function

Pycnogenol supplementation of 60 patients with CVD has been shown to increase vasodilatation and reduce the incidence of cardiovascular events.[1] Inhibition of platelet aggregation has been demonstrated in smokers and in cardiovascular patients.[1] A double-blind crossover study in 11 patients with mild hypertension found that supplementation with 200 mg pycnogenol normalised blood pressure and lowered thromboxane levels.[1] A further double-blind placebo-controlled trial involved 58 patients on the calcium channel blocker nifedipine. Supplementation with 100 mg pycnogenol allowed a reduction in the dosage of nifedipine used in the management of hypertension with a reduction in plasma concentration of endothelin-1 and increase in prostacyclin.[5]

In another study involving 25 subjects, pycnogenol 150 mg daily significantly reduced LDL cholesterol levels and raised HDL cholesterol.[6] Two further small studies also found that supplementation with pycnogenol significantly lowered total cholesterol and LDL.[8,13]

Pycnogenol has been associated with significant reduction in symptoms of chronic venous insufficiency (CVI).[1] A prospective trial in 86 patients with chronic CVI, ankle swelling and previous history of venous ulceration compared pycnogenol 150 mg or 300 mg daily for 8 weeks with a combination of diosmin and hersperidin (Daflon) 1000 mg daily. Clinical improvement in the pycnogenol group was significantly greater than in the Daflon group.[14] Pycnogenol has also been demonstrated to be more efficacious in CVI than a commercial horse chestnut extract (a remedy for CVI).[13]

Pycnogenol has also been shown to prevent deep vein thrombosis (DVT) after long-haul flights.[15]

Analgesic activity

Clinical trials have examined the effect of pycnogenol in pain. A study in 47 patients with menstrual pain found that pycnogenol 30 mg twice a day through three menstrual cycles was associated with significant abdominal and back pain relief during the second and third cycles.[16] A further study found that pycnogenol prevents cramps, muscular pain at rest and pain after/during exercise in healthy subjects, athletes prone to cramps, patients with venous disease, patients with intermittent claudication and patients with diabetic microangiopathy.[17]

Diabetes

Two clinical trials have provided evidence that pycnogenol could be beneficial in type 2 diabetes. An open, controlled trial in 18 men and 12 women found that pycnogenol lowered postprandial glucose, HBA_{1c} and endothelin 1.[11] This finding was confirmed in a double-blind, placebo-controlled study in 77 patients.[18]

Sexual function

Supplementation with pycnogenol has been found to improve erectile function.[8,19] Pycnogenol has also been associated with improvement in sperm quality and function.[20]

Attention deficit hyperactivity disorder (ADHD)

There have been anecdotal reports of benefit of pycnogenol in ADHD. A randomised, placebo-controlled, double-blind trial involving 61 children (mostly boys) supplemented with 1 mg/kg/day pycnogenol or placebo over 4 weeks found improvements in some ADHD scores in the treatment compared with placebo group, but not all aspects of the condition improved. Scores measured a month after stopping treatment returned to baseline. Based on these results, the authors suggested that pycnogenol has some activity in relieving ADHD symptoms in children.[21]

Miscellaneous

Pycnogenol has been found to improve lung function in asthma,[22] minimise gingival bleeding and plaque accumulation,[23] and reduce inflammation in SLE.[24]

Conclusion

Trials have shown pycnogenol to have beneficial effects in cardiovascular conditions, pain, diabetes, sexual function, ADHD, asthma, gingivitis and SLE. However, these trials should be treated with circumspection as some have been open-label, and those that have been placebo-controlled have been small, short-term studies. However, the benefits observed justify further larger controlled trials.

Precautions/contraindications

None reported.

Pregnancy and breast-feeding

No teratogenic effects have been observed, but pycnogenol should be avoided as a general precaution.

Adverse effects

No serious side-effects reported. Mild side-effects such as gastrointestinal problems, nausea, headache, dizziness and skin sensitisation are rare and transient in most cases.

Interactions

None reported.

Dose

The dose is not established. Clinical trials have used 40–100 mg pycnogenol daily or 1 mg/kg body weight daily.

References

1 Rohdewald P. A review of the French maritime pine bark extract (Pycnogenol), a herbal medication with a diverse clinical pharmacology. *Int J Clin Pharmacol Ther* 2002; 40: 158–168.

2 Packer L, Rimbach G, Virgili F. Antioxidant activity and biologic properties of a procyanidin-rich extract from pine (Pinus maritima) bark, pycnogenol. *Free Radic Biol Med* 1999; 27: 704–724.

3 Golanski J, Muchova J, Golanski R, *et al*. Does pycnogenol intensify the efficacy of acetylsalicylic acid in the inhibition of platelet function? In vitro experience. *Postepy Hig Med Dosw* (Online) 2006; 60: 316–321.

4 Hosseini S, Lee J, Sepulveda RT, *et al*. A randomized, double-blind, placebo-controlled, prospective 16 week crossover study to determine the role of Pycnogenol in modifying blood pressure in mildly hypertensive patients. *Nutr Res* 2001; 21: 1251–1260.

5 Liu X, Wei J, Tan F, Zhou S, *et al*. Pycnogenol, French maritime pine bark extract, improves endothelial function of hypertensive patients. *Life Sci* 2004; 74: 855–862.

6 Devaraj S, Vega-Lopez S, Kaul N, *et al*. Supplementation with a pine bark extract rich in polyphenols increases plasma antioxidant capacity and alters the plasma lipoprotein profile. *Lipids* 2002; 37: 931–934.

7 Grimm T, Schafer A, Hogger P. Antioxidant activity and inhibition of matrix metalloproteinases by metabolites of maritime pine bark extract (pycnogenol). *Free Radic Biol Med* 2004; 36: 811–822.

8 Durackova Z, Trebaticky B, Novotny V, *et al*. Lipid metabolism and erectile function improvement by Pcynogenol R extract from the bark of Pinus pinaster in patients suffering from erectile dysfunction - a pilot study. *Nutr Res* 2003; 23: 1189–1198.

9 Grimm T, Chovanova Z, Muchova J, *et al*. Inhibition of NF-kappaB activation and MMP-9 secretion by plasma of human volunteers after ingestion of maritime pine bark extract (Pycnogenol). *J Inflamm (Lond)* 2006; 3: 1.

10 Kim HC, Healey JM. Effects of pine bark extract administered to immunosuppressed adult mice infected with Cryptosporidium parvum. *Am J Chin Med* 2001; 29: 469–475.

11 Liu X, Zhou HJ, Rohdewald P. French maritime pine bark extract Pycnogenol dose-dependently lowers glucose in type 2 diabetic patients. *Diabetes Care* 2004; 27: 839.

12 Schafer A, Chovanova Z, Muchova J, *et al*. Inhibition of COX-1 and COX-2 activity by plasma of human volunteers after ingestion of French maritime pine bark extract (Pycnogenol). *Biomed Pharmacother* 2006; 60: 5–9.

13 Koch R. Comparative study of Venostatin and Pycnogenol in chronic venous insufficiency. *Phytother Res* 2002: Suppl 1: S1–5.

14 Cesarone MR, Belcaro G, Rohdewald P, *et al*. Comparison of Pycnogenol and Daflon in treating chronic venous insufficiency: a prospective,

controlled study. *Clin Appl Thromb Hemost* 2006; 12: 205–212.

15 Belcaro G, Cesarone MR, Rohdewald P, *et al*. Prevention of venous thrombosis and thrombophlebitis in long-haul flights with pycnogenol. *Clin Appl Thromb Hemost* 2004; 10: 373–377.

16 Kohama T, Suzuki N, Ohno S, Inoue M. Analgesic efficacy of French maritime pine bark extract in dysmenorrhea: an open clinical trial. *J Reprod Med* 2004; 49: 828–832.

17 Vinciguerra G, Belcaro G, Cesarone MR, *et al*. Cramps and muscular pain: prevention with pycnogenol in normal subjects, venous patients, athletes, claudicants and in diabetic microangiopathy. *Angiology* 2006; 57: 331–339.

18 Liu X, Wei J, Tan F, *et al*. Antidiabetic effect of Pycnogenol French maritime pine bark extract in patients with diabetes type II. *Life Sci* 2004; 75: 2505–2513.

19 Stanislavov R, Nikolova V. Treatment of erectile dysfunction with Pycnogenol and L-arginine. *J Sexual Marital Ther* 2003; 29: 207–213.

20 Roseff SJ. Improvement in sperm quality and function with French maritime pine tree bark extract. *J Reprod Med* 2002; 47: 821–824.

21 Trebaticka J, Kopasova S, Hradecna Z, *et al*. Treatment of ADHD with French maritime pine bark extract, Pycnogenol((R)). *Eur Child Adolesc Psychiatry* 2006. 15: 329–335.

22 Lau BH, Riesen SK, Truong KP, *et al*. Pycnogenol as an adjunct in the management of childhood asthma. *J Asthma* 2004; 41: 825–832.

23 Kimbrough C, Chun M, de la Roca G, Lau BH. PYCNOGENOL chewing gum minimizes gingival bleeding and plaque formation. *Phytomedicine* 2002; 9: 410–413.

24 Stefanescu M, Matache C, Onu A, *et al*. Pycnogenol efficacy in the treatment of systemic lupus erythematosus patients. *Phytother Res* 2001; 15: 698–704.

Quercetin

Description

Quercetin (3,3′,4′,5,7-pentahydroxyflavone)[1] is a flavonoid that forms the chemical backbone for other flavonoids such as hesperidin, naringin, rutin and tangeritin. Rutin is the most common flavonoid containing the quercetin backbone, in which quercetin is attached to a glucose-rhamnose moiety. Quercetin is also found bound to one or two glucose molecules (monoglycoside and diglycoside forms).[2]

Dietary sources

Quercetin is one of the most abundant dietary flavonoids. It is found in apples; black, green and buckwheat tea; onions (particularly the outer rings); raspberries; red wine; red grapes; cherries; citrus fruits; broccoli and other green leafy vegetables.[3] Preliminary work by the University of Queensland, Australia, suggests that quercetin is also found in varieties of honey such as that derived from eucalyptus and tea tree. Quercetin is also found in ginkgo biloba and St John's wort.

Dietary intake

Estimated dietary intake is 25–50 mg daily.[4]

Action

Quercetin has a range of activities. It has been shown *in vitro* to:

- act as an antioxidant;[5]
- inhibit LDL oxidation;[4,6,7]
- inhibit the nitric oxide pathway;[8,9]
- have anti-inflammatory activity, possibly due to an influence on the production of eicosanoids, including leukotrienes and prostaglandins,[4] and also cytokines;[10]
- have potential as an anti-cancer agent through interaction with type II oestrogen-binding sites,[11] inhibition of tyrosine kinase,[12] up-regulation of tumour suppressor genes,[13,14] induction of apoptosis,[15,16] and inhibition of tumour necrosis factor-alpha;[17]
- have antihistamine activity.[18]

Possible uses

Quercetin offers several potential therapeutic uses in the prevention of CVD, cancer, cataract, schizophrenia and prostatitis. However, there are few clinical trials in humans to date.

Cardiovascular disease

Quercetin may have a role in the prevention of CVD, but there are no data from controlled clinical trials. An epidemiological study suggested that high intakes of dietary flavonoids, particularly quercetin, are associated with a reduced risk of CVD in older men.[19] This protective effect is thought to be due to a variety of quercetin's activities, such as its antioxidant capacity,[4] including inhibition of LDL oxidation,[6] nitric oxide inhibition,[8] inhibition of tissue factor (the cellular receptor that initiates blood coagulation),[20] platelet aggregation,[21] and a range of anti-inflammatory activities. However, quercetin supplementation does not appear to reduce total and LDL cholesterol or to increase HDL cholesterol.[21,22]

Cancer

In vitro studies have shown quercetin to have various properties that could give it anti-cancer activity (e.g. cell cycle regulation, interaction with type II oestrogen-binding sites, inhibition of tyrosine kinase and reduction in the number of aberrant crypt foci;[23] inhibition of tyrosine kinase,[12] inhibition of tumour necrosis factor-alpha[17] and inhibition of tumour angiogenesis.[1])

Quercetin has been shown *in vitro* to inhibit growth of colorectal cancer cells,[14,24,25] possibly by up-regulation in the expression of tumour suppressor genes[14] and modulation of cell-cycle related and apoptosis genes.[25]

It has also been shown to have potential activity against prostate cancer. It can attenuate the function of the androgen receptor (AR), inhibiting AR-mediated expression of prostate-specific antigen (PSA),[26] up-regulating tumour suppressor genes while down-regulating oncogenes and cell cycle genes,[13] and inhibit other receptors involved in growth and metastasis of prostate cancer.[27]

Quercetin has also been shown *in vitro* to have activity against leukaemia cells[15,16] and pancreatic tumour cells.[28] Other preliminary studies suggest that quercetin could have inhibitory effects on other cancer types, including breast, ovary, endometrial, non-small-cell lung, gastric and squamous cell.[29]

Cataract

One study in rats has shown that quercetin could have a possible role in reducing the incidence of cataracts, by inhibiting oxidative damage in the lens. Quercetin was converted to its metabolite 3-O-methyl quercetin by catechol-O-methyltransferase (COMT) in the rat lens, and both compounds were found to inhibit hydrogen peroxide-induced opacification.[30]

Autoimmune disease

Quercetin was found in one study to ameliorate experimental allergic encephalomyelitis by blocking IL-12 signalling and Th1 differentiation, suggesting that it may be effective in treating multiple sclerosis and other Th1-cell-mediated autoimmune diseases.[31]

Schizophrenia

Evidence from one study suggests that quercetin (in combination with other antioxidants) might benefit patients with schizophrenia.[32]

Miscellaneous

Preliminary evidence suggests that quercetin may be of benefit in allergic rhinitis and against various viruses, including herpes simplex and respiratory syncytial viruses.[4]

Conclusion
Quercetin is the subject of intense research on the basis of its antioxidant, anti-inflammatory and anti-cancer activities. *In vitro* studies have demonstrated that quercetin offers potential in preventing CVD and cancer, and possibly cataract. However, controlled clinical trials in humans are needed before any conclusions can be drawn about the value of quercetin supplementation.

Precautions/contraindications

None reported.

Pregnancy and breast-feeding

No problems have been reported, but there have not been sufficient studies to guarantee the safety of quercetin in pregnancy and breast-feeding.

Adverse effects

Orally, quercetin may cause headache and tingling of the extremities.

Interactions

None reported.

Dose

The dose is not established. Typical oral doses range from 400 to 500 mg three times daily.

Quercetin is administered by injection (but this is not a dietary supplement use).

References

1   Igura K, Ohta T, Kuroda Y, Kaji K. Resveratrol and quercetin inhibit angiogenesis in vitro. *Cancer Lett* 2001; 171: 11–16.

2 Erlund I, Kosonen T, Alfthan G, *et al.* Pharmaco-kinetics of quercetin from quercetin aglycone and rutin in healthy volunteers. *Eur J Clin Pharmacol* 2000; 56: 545–553.

3 Hertog MG, Hollman PC. Potential health effects of the dietary flavonol quercetin. *Eur J Clin Nutr* 1996; 50: 63–71.

4 Formica JV, Regelson W. Review of the biology of Quercetin and related bioflavonoids. *Food Chem Toxicol* 1995; 33: 1061–1080.

5 Filipe P, Haigle J, Silva JN, *et al.* Anti- and pro-oxidant effects of quercetin in copper-induced low density lipoprotein oxidation. Quercetin as an effective antioxidant against pro-oxidant effects of urate. *Eur J Biochem* 2004; 271: 1991–1999.

6 Janisch KM, Williamson G, Needs P, Plumb GW. Properties of quercetin conjugates: modulation of LDL oxidation and binding to human serum albumin. *Free Radic Res* 2004; 38: 877–884.

7 Yamamoto N, Moon JH, Tsushida T, *et al.* Inhibitory effect of quercetin metabolites and their related derivatives on copper ion-induced lipid peroxidation in human low-density lipoprotein. *Arch Biochem Biophys* 1999; 372: 347–354.

8 Chan MM, Mattiacci JA, Hwang HS, *et al.* Synergy between ethanol and grape polyphenols, quercetin, and resveratrol, in the inhibition of the inducible nitric oxide synthase pathway. *Biochem Pharmacol* 2000; 60: 1539–1548.

9 Mu MM, Chakravortty D, Sugiyama T, *et al.* The inhibitory action of quercetin on lipopolysaccharide-induced nitric oxide production in RAW 264.7 macrophage cells. *J Endotoxin Res* 2001; 7: 431–438.

10 Wadsworth TL, Koop DR. Effects of the wine polyphenolics quercetin and resveratrol on pro-inflammatory cytokine expression in RAW 264.7 macrophages. *Biochem Pharmacol* 1999; 57: 941–949.

11 Shenouda NS, Zhou C, Browning JD, *et al.* Phyto-estrogens in common herbs regulate prostate cancer cell growth in vitro. *Nutr Cancer* 2004; 49: 200–208.

12 Huang YT, Hwang JJ, Lee PP, *et al.* Effects of luteolin and quercetin, inhibitors of tyrosine kinase, on cell growth and metastasis-associated properties in A431 cells overexpressing epidermal growth factor receptor. *Br J Pharmacol* 1999; 128: 999–1010.

13 Nair HK, Rao KV, Aalinkeel R, *et al.* Inhibition of prostate cancer cell colony formation by the flavonoid quercetin correlates with modulation of specific regulatory genes. *Clin Diagn Lab Immunol* 2004; 11: 63–69.

14 van Erk MJ, Roepman P, van der Lende TR, *et al.* Integrated assessment by multiple gene expression analysis of quercetin bioactivity on anticancer-related mechanisms in colon cancer cells in vitro. *Eur J Nutr* 2005; 44: 143–156.

15 Mertens-Talcott SU, Talcott ST, Percival SS. Low concentrations of quercetin and ellagic acid synergistically influence proliferation, cytotoxicity and apoptosis in MOLT-4 human leukemia cells. *J Nutr* 2003; 133: 2669–2674.

16 Mertens-Talcott SU, Percival SS. Ellagic acid and quercetin interact synergistically with resveratrol in the induction of apoptosis and cause transient cell cycle arrest in human leukemia cells. *Cancer Lett* 2005; 218: 141–151.

17 Wadsworth TL, McDonald TL, Koop DR. Effects of Ginkgo biloba extract (EGb 761) and quercetin on lipopolysaccharide-induced signaling pathways involved in the release of tumor necrosis factor-alpha. *Biochem Pharmacol* 2001; 62: 963–974.

18 Marozzi FJ Jr, Kocialski AB, Malone MH. Studies on the antihistaminic effects of thymoquinone, thymohydroquinone and quercetin. *Arzneimittelforschung* 1970; 20: 1574–1577.

19 Hertog MG, Feskens EJ, Hollman PC, *et al.* Dietary antioxidant flavonoids and risk of coronary heart disease: the Zutphen Elderly Study. *Lancet* 1993; 342: 1007–1011.

20 Di Santo A, Mezzetti A, Napoleone E, *et al.* Resveratrol and quercetin down-regulate tissue factor expression by human stimulated vascular cells. *J Thromb Haemost* 2003; 1: 1089–1095.

21 Janssen K, Mensink RP, Cox FJ, *et al.* Effects of the flavonoids quercetin and apigenin on hemostasis in healthy volunteers: results from an in vitro and a dietary supplement study. *Am J Clin Nutr* 1998; 67: 255–262.

22 Conquer JA, Maiani G, Azzini E, *et al.* Supplementation with quercetin markedly increases plasma quercetin concentration without effect on selected risk factors for heart disease in healthy subjects. *J Nutr* 1998; 128: 593–597.

23 Lamson DW, Brignall MS. Antioxidants and cancer, part 3: quercetin. *Altern Med Rev* 2000; 5: 196–208.

24 Richter M, Ebermann R, Marian B. Quercetin-induced apoptosis in colorectal tumor cells: possible role of EGF receptor signaling. *Nutr Cancer* 1999; 34: 88–99.

25 Murtaza I, Marra G, Schlapbach R, *et al.* A preliminary investigation demonstrating the effect of quercetin on the expression of genes related to cell-cycle arrest, apoptosis and xenobiotic metabolism in human CO115 colon-adenocarcinoma cells using DNA microarray. *Biotechnol Appl Biochem* 2006; 45 (Pt 1): 29–36.

26 Xing N, Chen Y, Mitchell SH, Young CY. Quercetin inhibits the expression and function of the androgen receptor in LNCaP prostate cancer cells. *Carcinogenesis* 2001; 22: 409–414.

27 Huynh H, Nguyen TT, Chan E, Tran E. Inhibition of ErbB-2 and ErbB-3 expression by quercetin prevents transforming growth factor alpha (TGF-alpha)- and epidermal growth factor (EGF)-induced human PC-3 prostate cancer cell proliferation. *Int J Oncol* 2003; 23: 821–829.

28 Lee LT, Huang YT, Hwang JJ, *et al*. Blockade of the epidermal growth factor receptor tyrosine kinase activity by quercetin and luteolin leads to growth inhibition and apoptosis of pancreatic tumor cells. *Anticancer Res* 2002; 22: 1615–1627.

29 ElAttar TM, Virji AS. Modulating effect of resveratrol and quercetin on oral cancer cell growth and proliferation. *Anticancer Drugs* 1999; 10: 187–193.

30 Cornish KM, Williamson G, Sanderson J. Quercetin metabolism in the lens: role in inhibition of hydrogen peroxide induced cataract. *Free Radic Biol Med* 2002; 33: 63–70.

31 Muthian G, Bright JJ. Quercetin, a flavonoid phytoestrogen, ameliorates experimental allergic encephalomyelitis by blocking IL-12 signaling through JAK-STAT pathway in T lymphocyte. *J Clin Immunol* 2004; 24: 542–552.

32 Rachkauskas GS. The efficacy of enterosorption and a combination of antioxidants in schizophrenics. *Lik Sprava* 1998; 4: 122–124 (in Russian).

Resveratrol

Description

Resveratrol is a polyphenol, more specifically a phytoalexin (3,5,4′-trihydroxy-trans-stilbene), which exists as cis- and trans-stereoisomers.[1] It is produced by plants as a defence against infection by pathogenic micro-organisms such as fungi.

Dietary sources

The most abundant sources of resveratrol are the wine-making grapes *Vitis vinifera*, Labrusca and Muscatine. It occurs in the vines, roots, seeds and stalks, but the skin of the grape contains the highest concentration (50–100 µg per gram). The resveratrol content of red wine is much higher than that of white wine. This is largely because, apart from the type of grapes used, in red wine production the skins and seeds are used, while white wine is prepared mainly from the juice, the skins being removed earlier in the process. The skins and seeds of grapes contain, in addition to resveratrol, a variety of other polyphenols including proanthocyanidins, quercetin, catechins and gallocatechins.

The resveratrol content of red wine varies considerably depending on the grapes and length of time the skins are present during the fermentation process. Red wines with the highest resveratrol content are Pinot Noir and Cabernet Sauvignon, produced in cold, humid climates (e.g. Bordeaux and Canada) rather than hot, dry climates. This is because fungal infections are more common in cooler climates, and resveratrol is produced in response to fungal infections in plants. Unfermented grape juice does not contain significant quantities of resveratrol.

Smaller amounts of resveratrol are found in mulberries and peanuts, and in other plants such as eucalyptus, lily and spruce. Resveratrol is also found in significant amounts in the dried roots and stems of the plant *Polygonium cuspidatum*, also known as Japanese knotweed. The dried root and stem of this plant are used in traditional Chinese and Japanese remedies (known as Hu Zhang, Hu Chang, tiger cane, kojo-kon and hadori-kon) for circulatory problems.[2]

Action

Knowledge of the potential benefits of resveratrol has developed partly from an appreciation of the beneficial effects of red wine on cardiovascular health.

Mechanisms for protection of the cardiovascular system that have been identified include:[3,4]

- antioxidant;[5]
- inhibition of cholesterol synthesis;
- inhibition of atherosclerosis;
- inhibition of LDL oxidation;
- protection and maintenance of endothelial tissue;
- suppression of platelet aggregation;[6–11]
- promotion of vasodilatation;
- defence against ischaemic reperfusion injury;
- oestrogenic activity.

Resveratrol has also been shown to have anti-cancer properties,[12] inhibiting activation of carcinogenic compounds and suppressing tumour progression.[13] *In vitro* studies have shown a number of protective mechanisms in relation to cancer, including inhibition of carcinogen activation, suppression of tumour initiation by inhibiting cyclooxygenase 1 (COX-1), inhibition of cellular-signalling cascades and influence on apoptosis.[14]

Resveratrol has also been shown to reduce cell proliferation in a human retinal epithelium cell line and may therefore have the ability to protect against ARMD.[15]

Possible uses

In vitro studies have clearly demonstrated potential mechanisms for benefit of resveratrol in the prevention of CVD and cancer. However, these studies have been short-term and there have been very few studies in humans. Two small studies (both from the same research group in China) found that resveratrol inhibited platelet aggregation in rabbits and humans.[8,9] However, it would be premature to recommend resveratrol as a food supplement, despite the industry's claims that resveratrol is the component in red wine responsible for the beneficial effects on CVD.

Conclusion

Resveratrol is the subject of much interest as a food supplement, mainly because it is claimed to be the component in red wine responsible for its beneficial effects in CVD. *In vitro* studies have demonstrated mechanisms by which resveratrol could reduce the risk of CVD and cancer, but there have been no intervention trials in humans. The main dietary source is red wine, and care should be taken not to encourage high intake of any alcoholic drink.

Precautions/contraindications

The main dietary source of resveratrol is red wine. Recommending increased consumption of red wine to increase resveratrol intake is not necessarily responsible given the health risks, including liver damage, physical addiction and social implications of any alcoholic beverage if consumed in more than moderate amounts.

Pregnancy and breast-feeding

No problems reported, but resveratrol may be oestrogenic. Alcohol should not be consumed during pregnancy.

Adverse effects

Resveratrol is similar in structure to diethylstilbestrol (a synthetic oestrogen) and it could have the potential to stimulate breast cancer.[16] More studies are needed.

Interactions

None reported.

Dose

The dose is not established.

References

1 Fremont L. Biological effects of resveratrol. *Life Sci* 2000; 66: 663–673.
2 Soleas GJ, Diamandis EP, Goldberg DM. Resveratrol: a molecule whose time has come? And gone? *Clin Biochem* 1997; 30: 91–113.
3 Hao HD, He LR. Mechanisms of cardiovascular protection by resveratrol. *J Med Food* 2004; 7: 290–298.
4 Wu JM, Wang ZR, Hsieh TC, *et al*. Mechanism of cardioprotection by resveratrol, a phenolic antioxidant present in red wine (Review). *Int J Mol Med* 2001; 8: 3–17.
5 O'Brien NM, Carpenter R, O'Callaghan YC, *et al*. Modulatory effects of resveratrol, citroflavan-3-ol, and plant-derived extracts on oxidative stress in U937 cells. *J Med Food* 2006; 9: 187–195.
6 Pace-Asciak CR, Hahn S, Diamandis EP, *et al*. The red wine phenolics trans-resveratrol and quercetin block human platelet aggregation and eicosanoid synthesis: implications for protection against coronary heart disease. *Clin Chim Acta* 1995; 235: 207–219.
7 Bertelli AA, Giovannini L, Giannessi D, *et al*. Antiplatelet activity of synthetic and natural resveratrol in red wine. *Int J Tissue React* 1995; 17: 1–3.
8 Wang Z, Huang Y, Zou J, *et al*. Effects of red wine and wine polyphenol resveratrol on platelet aggregation in vivo and in vitro. *Int J Mol Med* 2002; 9: 77–79.

9 Wang Z, Zou J, Huang Y, *et al*. Effect of resveratrol on platelet aggregation in vivo and in vitro. *Chin Med J (Engl)* 2002; 115: 378–380.

10 Olas B, Wachowicz B. Resveratrol, a phenolic antioxidant with effects on blood platelet functions. *Platelets* 2005; 16: 251–260.

11 Pace-Asciak CR, Rounova O, Hahn SE, *et al*. Wines and grape juices as modulators of platelet aggregation in healthy human subjects. *Clin Chim Acta* 1996; 246: 163–182.

12 Soleas GJ, Grass L, Josephy PD, *et al*. A comparison of the anticarcinogenic properties of four red wine polyphenols. *Clin Biochem* 2006; 39: 492–497.

13 Gusman J, Malonne H, Atassi G. A reappraisal of the potential chemopreventive and chemotherapeutic properties of resveratrol. *Carcinogenesis* 2001; 22: 1111–1117.

14 Gescher AJ, Steward WP. Relationship between mechanisms, bioavailibility, and preclinical chemopreventive efficacy of resveratrol: a conundrum. *Cancer Epidemiol Biomarkers Prev* 2003; 12: 953–957.

15 King RE, Kent KD, Bomser JA. Resveratrol reduces oxidation and proliferation of human retinal pigment epithelial cells via extracellular signal-regulated kinase inhibition. *Chem Biol Interact* 2005; 151: 143–149.

16 Gehm H. Resveratrol, a polyphenolic compound found in grapes and wine, is an agonist for the estrogen receptor. *Proc Natl Acad Sci* 1997; 94: 557–562.

Riboflavin

Description

Riboflavin is a water-soluble vitamin of the vitamin B complex.

Nomenclature

Riboflavin is the British Approved Name for use on pharmaceutical labels. It is known also as vitamin B_2.

Human requirements

See Table 1 for Dietary Reference Values for riboflavin.

Dietary intake

In the UK, the average adult diet provides: for men, 2.11 mg daily; for women, 1.60 mg.

Action

Riboflavin functions as a component of two flavin coenzymes – flavin mononucleotide (FMN) and flavin adenine dinucleotide (FAD). It participates in oxidation–reduction reactions in numerous metabolic pathways and in energy production. Examples include the oxidation of glucose, certain amino acids and fatty acids; reactions with several intermediaries of the Krebs cycle; conversion of pyridoxine to its active coenzyme; and conversion of tryptophan to niacin.

Riboflavin has a role as an antioxidant. It may be involved in maintaining the integrity of erythrocytes.

Dietary sources

See Table 2 for dietary sources of riboflavin.

Metabolism

Absorption

Riboflavin is readily absorbed by a saturable active transport system (principally in the duodenum).

Distribution

Some circulating riboflavin is loosely associated with plasma albumin, but significant amounts complex with other proteins. Conversion of riboflavin to its coenzymes occurs in most tissues (particularly in the liver, heart and kidney).

Elimination

Riboflavin is excreted primarily in the urine (mostly as metabolites); excess amounts are excreted unchanged. Riboflavin crosses the placenta and is excreted in breast milk.

Bioavailability

Riboflavin is remarkably stable during processing that involves heat, such as canning, dehydration, evaporation and pasteurisation. Boiling in water results in leaching of the vitamin into the water, which should then be used for soups and sauces. Considerable losses occur if food is exposed to light; exposure of milk in glass bottles will result in loss of riboflavin. Animal sources of riboflavin are better absorbed and hence more available than vegetable sources.

Deficiency

Deficiency of riboflavin isolated from other B vitamin deficiencies is rare. Early symptoms

Table 1 Dietary Reference Values for riboflavin (mg/day)

							EU RDA = 1.6 mg
Age	UK				USA		FAO/WHO RNI
	LNRI	EAR	RNI	EVM	RDA	TUL	
0–6 months	0.2	0.3	0.4		0.3	–	0.3
7–12 months	0.2	0.3	0.4		0.4	–	0.4
1–3 years	0.3	0.5	0.6		0.5	–	0.5
4–6 years	0.4	0.6	0.8		–	–	0.6
4–8 years	–	–	–		0.6	–	–
7–10 years	0.5	0.8	1.0		1.2	–	0.9[a]
9–13 years	–	–	–		0.9	–	–
Males							
11–14 years	0.8	1.0	1.2		–	–	1.2[b]
15–18 years	0.8	1.0	1.3		–	–	1.2
19–50+ years	0.8	1.0	1.3		–	–	1.3
14–70+ years				100	1.3	–	–
Females							
11–14 years	0.8	0.9	1.1		–	–	1.0[b]
14–18 years					1.0	–	1.0
15–50+ years	0.8	0.9	1.1		–	–	1.1
19–70+ years	–	–	–	100	1.1	–	–
Pregnancy	*	*	+0.3		1.4		1.4
Lactation	–	–	+0.5		1.6	–	1.6

* No increment.
[a] 7–9 years.   [b] 10–14 years.
EVM = Likely safe daily intake from supplements alone.
TUL = Tolerable Upper Intake Level (not determined for riboflavin).

include soreness of the mouth and throat, burning and itching of the eyes, and personality deterioration. Advanced deficiency may lead to cheilosis, angular stomatitis, glossitis (red, beefy tongue), corneal vascularisation, seborrhoeic dermatitis (of the face, trunk and extremities), normochromic normocytic anaemia, leucopenia and thrombocytopenia.

Possible uses

Supplements may be required by vegans (strict vegetarians who consume no milk or dairy produce).

Migraine

Riboflavin has been investigated for a possible role in migraine. In an open pilot study in 49 migraine patients, 26 patients were given oral riboflavin 400 mg daily or the same plus aspirin 75 mg daily for 3–5 months. The number of migraine days reduced from 8.7 ± 1.5 to 2.9 ± 1.2. There were no significant differences between the two groups.[1]

In a randomised, double-blind, placebo-controlled trial, 55 patients with a history of migraine for at least 1 year (with two to eight attacks monthly) were randomised to receive riboflavin 400 mg or placebo daily. Migraine attack frequency and duration was significantly

Table 2 Dietary sources of riboflavin

Food portion	Riboflavin content (mg)
Breakfast cereals	
1 bowl All-Bran (45 g)	*0.5*
1 bowl Bran Flakes (45 g)	*0.6*
1 bowl Corn Flakes (30 g)	*0.4*
1 bowl muesli (95 g)	*0.6*
1 bowl Shreddies (50 g)	**1.1**
1 bowl Start (40 g)	**0.8**
2 Weetabix	*0.6*
Milk and dairy products	
½ pint milk, whole, semi-skimmed or skimmed	*0.5*
½ pint soya milk	**0.7**
1 pot yoghurt (150 g)	*0.4*
Cheese (50 g)	*0.2*
1 egg, size 2 (60 g)	*0.3*
Meat and fish	
Beef, roast (85 g)	*0.2*
Lamb, roast (85 g)	*0.3*
Pork, roast (85 g)	*0.2*
1 chicken leg portion	*0.2*
Liver, lambs, cooked (90 g)	**3.0**
Kidney, lambs, cooked (75 g)	**1.6**
Fish, cooked (150 g)	*0.2*
Yeast	
Brewer's yeast (10 g)	*0.4*
Marmite, spread on 1 slice bread	*0.5*

Excellent sources (**bold**); good sources (*italics*).

reduced in the riboflavin group compared with placebo.[2]

A further randomised, double-blind, placebo-controlled trial evaluated the effect of a supplement providing a daily dose of riboflavin 400 mg, magnesium 300 mg and feverfew 100 mg. The placebo contained 25 mg riboflavin. Forty-nine patients completed the 3-month trial. For the primary outcome measure, a 50% or greater reduction in migraines, there was no difference between the treatment and placebo groups, achieved by 10 (42%) and 11 (44%) individuals, respectively. There were no differences in the mean number of migraines, migraine days, migraine index or triptan doses. Compared to baseline, both groups showed a significant reduction in number of migraines, migraine days and migraine index. This effect exceeds that reported for placebo agents in previous migraine trials, suggesting that riboflavin 25 mg may be an active comparator.[3]

Miscellaneous

A case report demonstrated successful therapy with riboflavin 50 mg daily in a patient with documented riboflavin deficiency and carpal tunnel syndrome.[4] Riboflavin has also been used successfully in the treatment of lactic acidosis induced by antiretroviral therapy in patients with AIDS.[5,6] Homocysteine metabolism is dependent on riboflavin and riboflavin has been investigated for a role in homocysteine lowering. However, studies to date have not demonstrated any clear benefit of riboflavin in lowering homocysteine. Moreover, riboflavin is of unproven value for acne, mouth ulcers or muscle cramps. At present, there is no convincing scientific data to support its use in human cancer.

Conclusion
At normal doses there is no good evidence for the use of riboflavin for any indication other than riboflavin deficiency. Preliminary evidence exists that higher doses may be useful in migraine and in lactic acidosis induced by antiretroviral therapy.

Precautions/contraindications

None reported.

Pregnancy and breast-feeding

No problems reported.

Adverse effects

Riboflavin toxicity is unknown in humans. Large doses may cause yellow discoloration of the urine.

Interactions

Drugs

Alcohol: excessive alcohol intake induces riboflavin deficiency.

Barbiturates: prolonged use may induce riboflavin deficiency.

Oral contraceptives: prolonged use may induce riboflavin deficiency.

Phenothiazines: may increase the requirement for riboflavin.

Probenecid: reduces gastrointestinal absorption and urinary excretion of riboflavin.

Tricyclic antidepressants: may increase the requirement for riboflavin.

Nutrients

Adequate amounts of all B vitamins are required for optimal functioning; deficiency or excess of one B vitamin may lead to abnormalities in the metabolism of another.

Iron: deficiency of riboflavin may impair iron metabolism and produce anaemia.

Dose

Riboflavin is available in the form of tablets and capsules, but is mainly found as a constituent of multivitamin and mineral preparations.

Dietary supplements provide 1–3 mg daily.

References

1 Schoenen J, Lenaerts M, Bastings E. High-dose riboflavin as a prophylactic treatment of migraine: results of an open pilot study. *Cephalgia* 1994; 14: 328–329.

2 Schoenen J, Jacquy J, Lenaerts M. Effectiveness of high-dose riboflavin in migraine prophylaxis: a randomized controlled trial. *Neurology* 1998; 50: 466–470.

3 Maizels M, Blumenfeld A, Burchette R. A combination of riboflavin, magnesium and feverfew for migraine prophylaxis: a randomized trial. *Headache* 2004; 44: 885–890.

4 Folkers K, Wolaniuk A, Vadhanavikit S. Enzymology of the response of the carpal tunnel syndrome to riboflavin and to combined riboflavin and pyridoxine. *Proc Natl Acad Sci* 1984; 81: 7076–7078.

5 Fouty B, Frerman F, Reves R. Riboflavin to treat nucleoside analogue-induced lactic acidosis. *Lancet* 1998; 352: 291–292.

6 Luzzati R, DelBravo P, DiPerri G, *et al*. Riboflavine and severe lactic acidosis. *Lancet* 1999; 353: 901–902.

Royal jelly

Description

Royal jelly is a yellow-white liquid secreted by the hypopharyngeal glands of 'nurse' worker bees from the 6th to the 12th day of their adult lives. It is an essential food for the queen bee.

Constituents

See Table 1 for the claimed nutrient composition of royal jelly.

Action

Royal jelly may have some pharmacological effects, but the only available evidence comes from *in vitro* studies and animal studies. It appears to have anti-tumour effects;[1] improve the efficiency of insulin;[2] have vasodilator activity;[3] and exhibit anti-microbial activity.[4]

Possible uses

Published papers on the effects of royal jelly in humans are relatively few, and many of these are single case histories and not clinical trials.

Royal jelly has been claimed to be beneficial in anorexia, fatigue and headaches;[5] and hypercholesterolaemia.[6,7]

A systematic review and meta-analysis[7] examined the effect of royal jelly in 17 animal studies and nine human studies. In the animal studies, royal jelly significantly reduced serum cholesterol and total lipid levels in rats and rabbits, and slowed the progress of atheromas in rabbits fed a high-fat diet. Meta-analysis of the controlled human trials showed that royal jelly (30–100 mg daily for 3–6 weeks) resulted in a significant reduction in total serum lipids and

Table 1 Claimed nutrient composition in a typical daily dose (500 mg) of royal jelly

Nutrient	Amount	% RNI[1]
Water (mg)	350	–
Carbohydrate (mg)	60	–
Protein (mg)	60	–
Lipids (mg)	25	–
Thiamine (µg)	2	0.2
Riboflavin (µg)	7	0.6
Niacin (µg)	20	0.1
Vitamin B$_6$ (µg)	3	0.2
Folic acid (ng)	15	0.08
Biotin (µg)	1	–
Pantothenic acid (µg)	3	–
Calcium (µg)	130	0.02
Magnesium (µg)	150	0.07
Potassium (mg)	2.5	0.07
Iron (µg)	25	0.2
Zinc (µg)	15	0.2

Reference Nutrient Intake for men aged 19–50 years.

cholesterol and normalisation of LDL and HDL cholesterol in subjects with hyperlipidaemia.

Royal jelly has been investigated in hay fever. A placebo-controlled, double-blind RCT in 80 children (aged 5–16 years) evaluated the effect of royal jelly administered 3–6 months before and throughout the pollen season. Sixty-four children completed the study. All of the patients in both groups developed hay fever symptoms during the pollen season. The severity of symptoms and need for additional hay fever treatment was similar in both groups, suggesting that royal jelly has no benefit on hay fever symptoms during the pollen season.[8]

Claims for the value of royal jelly in arthritis, depression, diabetes mellitus, dysmenorrhoea, eczema, morning sickness, multiple sclerosis, muscular dystrophy, myalgic encephalomyelitis (ME) and PMS are purely anecdotal and there is no evidence for any of these claims.

Conclusion

Anecdotally, royal jelly is thought to be beneficial in a wide range of conditions. However, there is no sound evidence to support its use.

Precautions/contraindications

Royal jelly should be avoided in asthma (adverse effects reported).

Pregnancy and breast-feeding

No problems reported, but there have not been sufficient studies to guarantee the safety of royal jelly in pregnancy and breast-feeding. Royal jelly is probably best avoided.

Adverse effects

Allergic reactions, which can be severe. Life-threatening bronchospasm has occurred in patients with asthma after ingestion of royal jelly.[9–12] Royal jelly has been responsible for IgE-mediated anaphylaxis,[13] leading to death in at least one individual.[14] One report of haemorrhagic colitis occurred in a 53-year-old woman after taking royal jelly for 25 days.[15]

Interactions

None reported.

Dose

Royal jelly is available in the form of tablets and capsules.

The dose is not established. Dietary supplements provide 250–500 mg daily.

References

1   Tamura T, Fujii A, Kuboyama N. Antitumour effects of royal jelly. *Nippon Yakurigaku Zasshi* 1987; 89: 73–80.
2   Kramer KJ, Tager HS, Childs CN, Spiers RD. Insulin-like hypoglycaemic and immunological activities in honey bee royal jelly. *J Insect Physiol* 1977; 23: 293–296.
3   Shinoda M, Nakajin S, Oikawa T, *et al*. Biochemical studies on vasodilator factor of royal jelly. *Yakugaku Zasshi* 1978; 98: 139–145.
4   Fujiwara S, Imaj J, Fujiwara M, *et al*. A potent antibacterial protein in royal jelly. Purification and determination of the primary structure of royalisin. *J Biol Chem* 1990; 265: 11333–11337.
5   Tamura T. Royal jelly from the standpoint of clinical pharmacology. *Honeybee Sci* 1985; 6: 117–124.
6   Cho YT. Studies on royal jelly and abnormal cholesterol and triglycerides. *Am Bee J* 1977; 117: 36–38.
7   Vittek J. Effect of royal jelly on serum lipids in experimental animals and humans with atherosclerosis. *Experientia* 1995; 51: 927–935.
8   Andersen AH, Mortensen S, Agertoft L, Pedersen S. Double-blind randomized trial of the effect of Bidro on hay fever in children. *Ugeskr Laeger* 2005; 167: 3591–3594.
9   Leung R, Thien FCK, Baldo BA, *et al*. Royal jelly induced asthma and anaphylaxis: clinical characteristics and immunologic correlations. *J Allergy Clin Immunol* 1995; 96: 1004–1007.
10 Peacock S, Murray V, Turton C. Respiratory distress and royal jelly. *BMJ* 1995; 311: 1472.
11 Larporte JR, Ibaanez L, Vendrell L, *et al*. Bronchospasm induced by royal jelly. *Allergy* 1996; 51: 440.
12 Harwood M, Harding S, Beasley R, *et al*. Asthma following royal jelly. *NZ Med J* 1996; 109: 325.
13 Thien FC, Leung R, Baldo BA, *et al*. Asthma and anaphylaxis induced by royal jelly. *Clin Exp Allergy* 1996; 26: 216–222.
14 Bullock RJ, Rohan A, Straatmans JA. Fatal royal jelly induced asthma. *Med J Aust* 1994; 160: 44.
15 Yonei Y, Shibagaki K, Tsukada N, *et al*. Case report: hemorrhagic colitis associated with royal jelly intake. *J Gastroenterol Hepatol* 1997; 12: 495–499.

S-adenosyl methionine

Description

S-adenosyl methionine (SAMe) is synthesised in the body from the essential amino acid methionine.

Action

SAMe is involved in several biochemical pathways. It functions mainly as a methyl donor in synthetic pathways that lead to the production of DNA and RNA, neurotransmitters and phospholipids. Its involvement in phospholipid synthesis may mean that it has a role in membrane fluidity. SAMe is also involved in transulphuration reactions, regulating the formation of sulphur-containing amino acids, cysteine, glutathione (GSH) and taurine. GSH is an antioxidant, so SAMe is proposed to have antioxidant activity.

Possible uses

SAMe is being investigated for its effects on a number of conditions, such as depression, osteoarthritis, fibromyalgia and CVD.

Depression

SAMe may be of potential use as an antidepressant. Its mechanism of action for this indication is still a matter of speculation, although there is some evidence that it may raise dopamine levels.[1] Initially it was used for this purpose by parenteral administration. However, in an uncontrolled study[2] in 20 outpatients with major depression, the group as a whole improved with oral SAMe.

In a randomised, double-blind, placebo-controlled trial involving 15 inpatients with major depression, oral SAMe was found to improve symptoms of depression. However, it induced mania in one patient with no history of the condition.[3]

The efficacy of oral SAMe was assessed in the treatment of 80 depressed post-menopausal women (aged 45–59 years). The 30-day, double-blind, placebo-controlled randomised trial found a significantly greater improvement in depressive symptoms in the group treated with 1600 mg daily of SAMe from day 10 of the study.[4]

A meta-analysis of the effect of SAMe on depression compared with placebo or tricyclic antidepressants showed a greater response rate with SAMe than placebo and an antidepressant effect comparable with tricyclic antidepressants.[5]

An in-depth literature review, which included RCTs, controlled clinical trials, meta-analyses and systematic reviews, evaluated evidence on the use of SAMe for the treatment of depression (and also osteoarthritis and liver disease). Compared to placebo, SAMe was associated with a clinically significant improvement of depression. Compared with conventional antidepressant therapy, SAMe was not associated with a statistically significant difference in outcomes.[6]

A more recent multicentre trial found that the efficacy of 1600 mg SAMe daily taken orally[7] and 400 mg SAMe daily[7,8] intramuscularly is comparable with that of imipramine 150 mg daily, but SAMe is better tolerated.

Osteoarthritis

SAMe appears to possess analgesic activity, and in joints there is some evidence that it stimulates the synthesis of proteoglycans by the articular chondrocytes.[9]

In a range of double-blind randomised trials, all reported in one issue of one journal, oral SAMe was found to exert the same analgesic activity as a range of NSAIDs. In one study with 734 subjects, SAMe 1200 mg daily was as effective as naproxen 750 mg daily.[10] Another study in 45 patients showed that SAMe 1200 mg daily was as effective as piroxicam (20 mg daily) in osteoarthritis of the knee.[11] Two further studies in each of 36 patients over 4 weeks, showed that SAMe 1200 mg daily was as effective as indometacin (150 mg daily)[12] or ibuprofen (1200 mg daily).[13] A 16-week study in 56 patients diagnosed with osteoarthritis of the knee found that SAMe (1200 mg daily) has a slower onset of action, but is as effective as celecoxib (200 mg daily) in the management of symptoms of knee osteoarthritis.[14]

In an uncontrolled study lasting 24 months, 108 patients received 600 mg SAMe daily for 2 weeks, then 400 mg daily thereafter. Clinical symptoms, such as morning stiffness, pain at rest and pain on movement, improved during the period of SAMe administration.[15]

Fibromyalgia

Intravenous SAMe has been shown to reduce pain in patients with fibromyalgia.[16] In a double-blind, placebo-controlled trial lasting 6 weeks and involving 44 patients, oral SAMe (800 mg) produced significant improvement in clinical disease activity, pain suffered during the last week, and fatigue. SAMe was associated with an improvement in mood on the Face Scale but not on the Beck Depression Inventory.[17]

Cardiovascular disease

Elevation of homocysteine is an independent risk factor for CVD, and SAMe controls enzymes in homocysteine metabolism. Whole-blood SAMe has been found to be lower in patients with CHD than in controls, suggesting that low levels of SAMe might be a risk factor for the development of CHD.[18] A study with oral SAMe (400 mg in a single dose) in healthy subjects showed that SAMe did not inhibit the enzyme (5,10-methylene tetrahydrofolate reductase). This is the enzyme that catalyses the formation of 5-methyltetrahydrofolate, which is the active form of folate involved in the remethylation of homocysteine to methionine. However, there were no changes in plasma homocysteine levels.[19]

> ### Conclusion
> Research suggests there is some evidence that SAMe has value in depression and osteoarthritis, and that it may have an influence in the metabolism of homocysteine.

Precautions/contraindications

SAMe should be used with caution in individuals with a history of bleeding or haemostatic disorders. SAMe has been reported to block platelet aggregation *in vitro*.[20]

Pregnancy and breast-feeding

No problems reported, but there have not been sufficient studies to guarantee the safety of SAMe in pregnancy and breast-feeding. SAMe is best avoided.

Adverse effects

Minor side-effects, including nausea, dry mouth and restlessness, have been occasionally reported.

Interactions

None reported, but in theory SAMe could potentiate the activity of antidepressants, anticoagulants and anti-platelet drugs.

Dose

SAMe is available in the form of tablets and capsules. A review of 13 US products found that six failed testing for content. Among those failing, the amount of SAMe was, on average, less than half of that declared on the labels.[21]

The dose is not established. Studies have used doses of 400–1600 mg daily.

References

1   Fava M, Rosenbaum JF, MacLaughlin JR, *et al*. Neuroendocrine effects of S-adenosyl-L-methionine, a novel putative antidepressant. *J Psychiatr Res* 1990; 24: 177–184.

2   Rosenbaum JF, Fava M, Falk WE, *et al*. The antidepressant potential of oral S-adenosylmethionine. *Acta Psychiatr Scand* 1990; 81: 432–436.

3   Kagan BL, Sultzer DL, Rosenlicht N, *et al*. Oral S-adenosyl methionine in depression: a randomised, double-blind, placebo-controlled trial. *Am J Psychiatry* 1990; 147: 591–595.

4   Salmaggi P, Bressa GM, Nicchia G, *et al*. Double-blind, placebo-controlled study of S-adenosyl-L-methionine in depressed postmenopausal women. *Psychother Psychosom* 1993; 59: 34–40.

5   Bressa GM. S-adenosyl-L-methionine (SAMe) as antidepressant: meta-analysis of clinical studies. *Acta Neurol Scand Suppl* 1994; 154: 7–14.

6   Agency for Healthcare Research and Evaluation. *S-Adenosyl-L-Methionine for Treatment of Depression, Osteoarthritis and Liver Disease*. Evidence Report/Technology Assessment: Number 64. AHRQ Publication Number 02-E033. Available from http://www.ahrq.gov/clinic/epcsums/samesum.htm (accessed 6 November 2006). Rockville, MD: AHRQ, August 2002.

7   Delle Chiaie R, Pancheri P, Scapicchio P. Efficacy and tolerability of oral and intramuscular S-adenosyl-L-methionine 1,4-butanedisulfonate (SAMe) in the treatment of major depression: comparison with imipramine in 2 multicenter studies. *Am J Clin Nutr* 2002; 76: S1172–S1176.

8   Pancheri P, Scapicchio P, Chiaie RD. A double-blind, randomized parallel-group, efficacy and safety study of intramuscular S-adenosyl-L-methionine 1,4-butanedisulphonate (SAMe) versus imipramine in patients with major depressive disorder. *Int J Neuropsychopharmacol* 2002; 5: 287–294.

9   di Padova C. S-adenosylmethionine in the treatment of osteoarthritis. Review of clinical studies. *Am J Med* 1987; 83(5A): 60–65.

10 Caruso I, Pietrogrande V. Italian double-blind multicenter study comparing S-adenosylmethionine, naproxen, and placebo in the treatment of degenerative joint disease. *Am J Med* 1987; 83(5A): 66–71.

11 Maccagno A, Di Giorgio EE, Caston OL, *et al*. Double-blind controlled clinical trial of oral S-adenosylmethionine versus piroxicam in knee osteoarthritis. *Am J Med* 1987; 83(5A): 72–77.

12 Vetter G. Double-blind comparative clinical trial with S-adenosylmethionine and indomethacin in the treatment of osteoarthritis. *Am J Med* 1987; 83(5A): 78–80.

13 Muller-Fassbender H. Double-blind clinical trial of S-adenosylmethionine versus ibuprofen in the treatment of osteoarthitis. *Am J Med* 1987; 83(5A); 81–83.

14 Najm WI, Reinsch S, Hoehler F, *et al*. S-adenosyl methionine (SAMe) versus celecoxib for the treatment of osteoarthritis symptoms: a double-blind crossover trial. [ISRCTN362334950]. *BMC Musculoskelet Disord* 2004; 26: 5–6.

15 Konig B. A long-term (two years) clinical trial with S-adenosylmethionine for the treatmemt of osteoarthritis. *Am J Med* 1987; 83(5A): 89–94.

16 Volkmann H, Norregaard J, Jacobsen S, *et al*. Double-blind, placebo-controlled cross-over study of intravenous S-adenosyl-L-methionine in patients with fibromyalgia. *Scand J Rheumatol* 1997; 26: 206–211.

17 Jacobsen S, Danneskiold-Samsoe B, Andersen RB. Oral S-adenosylmethionine in primary fibromyalgia. Double-blind clinical evaluation. *Scand J Rheumatol* 1991; 20: 294–302.

18 Loehrer FM, Angst CP, Haefeli WE, *et al*. Low whole-blood S-adenosylmethionine and correlation between 5-methyltetrahydrofolate and homocysteine in coronary artery disease. *Arterioscler Thromb Vasc Biol* 1996; 16: 727–733.

19 Loehrer FM, Schwab R, Angst CP, *et al*. Influence of oral S-adenosylmethionine on plasma 5-methyltetrahydrofolate, S-adenosylhomocysteine, homocysteine and methionine in healthy humans. *J Pharmacol Exp Ther* 1997; 282: 845–850.

20 De La Cruz JP, Merida M, Gonzalez-Correa JA, *et al*. Effects of S-adenosyl-L-methionine on platelet thromboxane and vascular prostacyclin. *Biochem Pharmacol* 1997; 53: 1761–1763.

21 Consumerlab. Product review. SAMe. http://www.consumerlab.com (accessed 13 November 2006).

Selenium

Description

Selenium is an essential trace element.

Human requirements

See Table 1 for Dietary Reference Values for selenium.

Dietary intake

In the UK, the average adult diet provides 39 µg daily.[1] Selenium enters the food chain through plants, which take it up from the soil. Selenium intake is low in parts of the world where soil selenium content is low, and human dietary intakes therefore vary from high to low according to geography. Selenium intakes in most parts of Europe (including the UK) are considerably lower than in the USA, European soils being a poorer source of selenium. Current UK intakes are about half the Reference Nutrient Intake, having declined considerably over the past 25 years, and this may have implications for disease risk.

Action

Selenium functions as an integral part of the enzyme glutathione peroxidase and other seleno-proteins. Glutathione peroxidase prevents the generation of oxygen free radicals that cause the destruction of polyunsaturated fatty acids in cell membranes. Selenium spares the requirement for vitamin E and vice versa. Selenium has additional effects, particularly in relation to the immune response and cancer prevention, which are not entirely due to these enzymic functions.

Dietary sources

See Table 2 for dietary sources of selenium.

Metabolism

Absorption

Little is known about the intestinal absorption of selenium, but it appears to be easily absorbed.

Distribution

Selenium is stored in red cells, liver, spleen, heart, nails, tooth enamel, testes and sperm. It is incorporated into the enzyme glutathione peroxidase, the metabolically active form of selenium.

Elimination

Selenium is excreted mainly in the urine.

Deficiency

Deficiency has been associated with muscle pain and tenderness; some cases of cardiomyopathy have occurred in patients on total parenteral nutrition with low selenium status. Keshan disease (seen mainly in China) is a syndrome of endemic cardiomyopathy that is alleviated by selenium supplementation.

There is evidence that less overt selenium deficiency can have adverse consequences for health. Low selenium status has been linked to loss of immunocompetence,[2] the development of virulence and progression of some viral infections,[3] miscarriage,[4] male infertility,[5] depressed mood,[6] senility and Alzheimer's disease[6] and poor thyroid function.[7]

Table 1   Dietary Reference Values for selenium (µg/day)

Age	UK			USA			FAO/WHO
						EU RDA = none	
	LRNI	RNI	EVM	RDA	AI	TUL	RNI
0–3 months	4	10		–	15	45	6
4–6 months	5	13		–	15	45	6
7–9 months	5	10		–	20	45	10
10–12 months	6	10		–	20	45	10
1–3 years	7	15		20		90	17
4–6 years	10	20			–	–	22
4–8 years	–	–	–	30		150	–
7–10 years	16	30		–		–	21[a]
Males							
11–14 years	25	45		40		400	32[b]
15–18 years	40	70		50		400	32
19–50+ years	40	75	200	70		400	34[1]
Females							
11–14 years	25	45		45		400	26[b]
15–18 years	40	60		50		400	26
19–50+ years	40	60	200	55		400	26[2]
Pregnancy	*	*		65		400	28–30
Lactation	+15	+15		75		400	35–42

* No increment.

[a] 7–9 years.   [b] 10–14 years.

[1] > 65 years, 33 µg.

[2] 51–65 years, 26 µg, > 65 years, 25 µg.

EVM = Safe upper level from supplements alone.

TUL = Tolerable Upper Intake Level from diet and supplements.

Selenium deficiency has also been associated with CVD, although results from epidemiological studies have been mixed. Thus, a two- to three-fold increase in cardiovascular mortality was found in individuals with serum selenium concentrations below 45 µg/L compared with individuals above that concentration at baseline.[8] A Danish study[9] showed that middle-aged and elderly men with serum selenium below 70 µg/L had a significantly increased risk of ischaemic heart disease. The 10-centre EURAMIC study[10] found an inverse relationship between toenail selenium levels and risk of myocardial infarction, but only in the centre with the lowest selenium (Germany).

However, other studies have shown no such links.

Low selenium intake has been linked to cancer mortality. In one study,[11] dietary intake of selenium in 27 countries was found to correlate inversely with total age-adjusted cancer mortality, and low selenium status has been linked with an increased risk of cancer incidence and mortality.[12,13] A nested case-control study within a cohort of 9000 Finnish individuals showed the adjusted relative risk of lung cancer between the highest and lowest tertiles of serum selenium to be 0.41.[14] In a study looking at the association between selenium intake and prostate cancer involving 34 000 men, those

Table 2   Dietary sources of selenium

Food portion	Selenium content (µg)
Cereals[1]	
2 slices bread	**30**
Milk and dairy products	
½ pint milk	3–30
1 egg	3–25
Meat and fish	
Beef, cooked (100 g)	3
Lamb, cooked (100 g)	1
Pork, cooked (100 g)	*15*
Chicken, cooked (100 g)	8
Liver (90 g)	*20*
Fish, cooked (150 g)	**30–50**
Vegetables	
1 small can baked beans (200 g)	4
Lentils, red kidney beans or other pulses, cooked (105 g)	5
Green vegetables, average, boiled (100 g)	1–3
Fruit	
1 banana	2
1 orange	2
Nuts	
20 almonds	1
10 Brazil nuts	**200**
30 peanuts	1

[1] Cereals are important sources of selenium, but the content reflects the selenium content of the soils on which they are grown and is therefore highly variable.
Excellent sources (**bold**); good sources (*italics*).

in the lowest quintile of selenium status were found to have three times the likelihood of developing advanced prostate cancer as those in the highest quintile.[15]

Possible uses

Cancer (prevention)
Studies have shown that selenium supplementation may reduce the risk of certain cancers (e.g. colon, gastric, lung and prostate), but not others (breast, oesophageal and skin).

The US Nutritional Prevention of Cancer (NPC) trial[16] was the first double-blind, placebo-controlled trial in a Western population designed to test the hypothesis that selenium supplementation could reduce the risk of cancer. A total of 1312 individuals with a history of non-melanoma skin cancer were randomised to placebo or 200 µg selenium a day (as selenium yeast) for an average treatment period of 4.5 years with a total follow-up of 6.4 years. There were no statistically significant differences in incidence of basal cell carcinoma or squamous cell carcinoma. However, total cancer incidence was 37% lower in the selenium group, with 63% fewer cancers of the prostate, 58% fewer cancers of the colon, and 46% fewer cancers of the lung. There were more cases of breast cancer and leukaemia-lymphoma in the selenium group, but these differences were not statistically significant. Further analysis of the trial data across the entire treatment period, which ended 3 years after the first analysis was conducted, continued to demonstrate that selenium supplementation was ineffective at preventing basal cell carcinoma, but that it increases the risk of squamous cell carcinoma and total non-melanoma skin cancer.[17] Yet further analysis of the entire treatment period of this trial continued to show a significant protective effect of selenium on the overall incidence of prostate cancer, although the effect was restricted to those with lower baseline prostate-specific antigen (PSA) levels and plasma selenium concentrations.[18]

A systematic review and meta-analysis of 16 studies concluded that selenium may reduce the risk of prostate cancer.[19] Further large randomised trials, which are ongoing, will help to throw more light on this issue.

Supplements of dietary antioxidants (including selenium), reduced the incidence of oesophageal and gastric cancer and total cancer in a study in 30 000 adults in Linxian, China,[20] an area where the incidence of oesophageal and stomach cancer is high, and the intake of certain nutrients is low. There is also some evidence that selenium may protect against colorectal cancer[21] and lung cancer.[22]

Selenium has been studied for a link with breast cancer. A number of case-control studies have explored this link, but no significant associations have been found. The evidence has been summarised by Attract.[23] Low selenium status seems not to be an important factor in the development of breast cancer.

Cardiovascular disease

Selenium may have a role in the prevention of CVD, but evidence for the benefit of supplementation is limited. In a double-blind, placebo-controlled study,[24] 81 patients received either selenium-rich yeast (100 µg daily) or placebo for a 6-month period. During the study period there were four cardiac deaths in the placebo group but none in the selenium group. There were two non-fatal reinfarctions in the placebo group, and one in the selenium group.

In a further trial, 504 participants (free of CVD) were randomised to selenium 200 µg daily and 500 participants (free of CVD) to placebo. Selenium supplementation was not significantly associated with any of the CVD end points or all CVD mortality during 7.6 years of follow-up. The authors concluded that there was no overall effect of selenium supplementation on the primary prevention of CVD in this population.[25]

Infertility

Selenium supplementation (selenomethionine 100 µg daily) increased sperm motility in a study involving 64 subfertile men.[26] Sperm count was unchanged after supplementation for 3 months, but sperm motility increased in 56% of the men. By the time of publication, 11% of the selenium-supplemented men had confirmed paternity, but none of the placebo group had. A further study found beneficial effects of selenium (with vitamin E) on semen quality.[27] However, another trial found a decrease in sperm motility with selenium, suggesting caution and the need for further studies to assess this potential effect.[28]

Rheumatoid arthritis

Selenium may be useful as an adjunct in the treatment of recent-onset rheumatoid arthritis. In a study, 15 women with rheumatoid arthritis of less than 5 years' duration who had been treated with NSAIDs and/or with other anti-rheumatic drugs received selenium (200 µg daily from selenium-rich yeast) supplementation for 3 months.[29] This led to improvement in subjective pain and clinical assessment of joint involvement in six out of eight of the treated subjects but none of the controls, and improvements disappeared 3 months after therapy was withdrawn, even though indicators of selenium status remained elevated. However, selenium (256 µg daily from selenium-rich yeast) was not effective in a trial of 40 men and women with an average arthritis duration of 13.5 years.[30] A further trial in 55 patients with moderate rheumatoid arthritis did not show any clinical benefit with selenium (selenium-rich yeast 200 µg daily).[31]

Miscellaneous

Selenium has been found to improve mood in some studies but not others.[32] There is some evidence that selenium may be of benefit in asthma,[33] immune function,[34] and the management of HIV infection.[35]

> **Conclusion**
> Epidemiological research and evidence from a large controlled intervention trial suggest that selenium may reduce cancer risk. The role of selenium in heart disease is unclear and controlled clinical trials are required to identify any benefits of supplementation. Results from studies of selenium in rheumatoid arthritis are conflicting.

Precautions/contraindications

Yeast-containing selenium products should be avoided by patients taking monoamine oxidase inhibitors.

Pregnancy and breast-feeding

No problems with normal intakes.

Adverse effects

There is a narrow margin of safety for selenium. Adverse effects include hair loss, nail changes, skin lesions, nausea, diarrhoea, irritability, metallic taste, garlic-smelling breath, fatigue and peripheral neuropathy.

Interactions

There is some evidence that clozapine may reduce selenium levels and that this could be important in the pathogenesis of cardiac side-effects with clozapine.[36]

Dose

Selenium is available mainly in 'antioxidant' supplements with vitamin E and vitamin A, and is also an ingredient in multivitamin supplements.

The dose is not established; 50–100 µg daily is considered to be safe.

References

1   Ministry of Agriculture, Fisheries and Food. *1997 Total Diet Study – Aluminium, Arsenic, Cadmium, Chromium, Copper, Lead, Mercury, Nickel, Selenium, Tin and Zinc.* London: MAFF, 1999.

2   Spallholz JE, Boylan LM, Larsen HS, *et al.* Advances in understanding selenium's role in the immune system. *Ann NY Acad Sci* 1990; 587: 129–139.

3   Taylor EW, Nadimpalli RG, Ramanathan CS, *et al.* Genomic structures of viral agents in relation to the biosynthesis of selenoproteins. *Biol Trace Elem Res* 1997; 56: 63–91.

4   Barrington JW, Taylor M, Smith S, Bowen-Simpkins P. Selenium and recurrent miscarriage. *J Obstet Gynaecol* 1997; 17: 199–200.

5   Oldereid NB, Thomassen Y, Purvis K, *et al.* Selenium in human male reproductive organs. *Hum Reprod* 1998; 13: 2172–2176.

6   Hawkes WC, Hornbostel L. Effects of dietary selenium on mood in healthy men living in a metabolic research unit. *Biol Psychiatry* 1996; 39: 121–128.

7   Olivieri O, Girelli D, Azzini M, *et al.* Low selenium status in the elderly influences thyroid hormones. *Clin Sci* 1995; 89: 637–642.

8   Salonen JT, Alfhthan G, Pikkarainen J, *et al.* Association between cardiovascular death and myocardial infarction and serum selenium in a matched pair longitudinal study. *Lancet* 1982; ii: 175–179.

9   Virtamo J, Valkiela E, Alfhthan G, *et al.* Serum selenium and the risk of coronary heart disease and stroke. *Am J Epidemiol* 1985; 122: 276–282.

10 Kardinaal AFM, Kok FJ, Kohlmeier L, *et al.* Association between toenail selenium and risk of myocardial infarction in European men: the EURAMIC study. *Am J Epidemiol* 1997; 145: 373–379.

11 Schrauzer GN, White DA, Schneider CJ, *et al.* Cancer mortality correlation studies. III. Statistical association with dietary selenium intakes. *Bioinorg Chem* 1977; 7: 35–36.

12 Combs GF Jr, Gray WP. Chemopreventive agents: selenium. *Pharmacol Ther* 1998; 79: 179–182.

13 Kok FJ, de Bruin AM, Hofman A, *et al.* Is serum selenium a risk factor for cancer in men only? *Am J Epidemiol* 1987; 125: 12–16.

14 Knekt P, Marniemi J, Teppo L, *et al.* Is low selenium status a risk factor for lung cancer? *Am J Epidemiol* 1998; 148: 975–982.

15 Yoshizawa K, Willett WC, Morris SJ, *et al.* Study of prediagnostic selenium level in toenails and the risk of advanced prostate cancer. *J Natl Cancer Inst* 1998; 90: 1219–1224.

16 Clark LC, Combs Jr GF, Turnbill BW. Effects of selenium supplementation for cancer prevention in patients with carcinoma of the skin: a randomized controlled trial: Nutritional Prevention of Cancer Study Group. *JAMA* 1996; 276: 1957–1963.

17 Duffield-Lillico AJ, Slate EH, Reid ME, *et al.* Selenium supplementation and secondary prevention of nonmelanoma skin cancer in a randomized trial. *J Natl Cancer Inst* 2003; 95: 1477–1481.

18 Duffield-Lillico AJ, Dalkin BL, Reid ME, *et al.* Selenium supplementation, baseline plasma selenium status and incidence of prostate cancer: an analysis of the complete treatment period of the Nutritional Prevention of Cancer Trial. *BJU Int* 2003; 91: 608–612.

19 Etminan M, FitzGerald JM, Gleave M, Chambers K. Intake of selenium in the prevention of prostate cancer: a systematic review and meta-analysis. *Cancer Causes Control* 2005; 16: 1125–1131.

20 Blot WJ, Li J-Y, Taylor PR, *et al.* Nutrition intervention trial in Linxian, China: supplementation with specific vitamin/mineral combinations, cancer incidence and disease-specific mortality in the general population. *J Natl Cancer Inst* 1993; 85: 1483–1492.

21 Jacobs ET, Jiang R, Alberts DS, *et al.* Selenium and colorectal adenoma: results of a pooled analysis. *J Natl Cancer Inst* 2004; 96: 1669–1675.

22 Zhuo H, Smith AH, Steinmaus C. Selenium and lung cancer: a quantitative analysis of heterogeneity in the current epidemiological literature. *Cancer Epidemiol Biomarkers Prev* 2004; 13: 771–778.

23 Is there any evidence to suggest selenium supplementation is effective in the prevention of breastcancer? ATTRACT15/10/02. http://www.attract.wales.nhs.uk/question_answers.cfm?question_id=930 (accessed 3 March 2006).

24 Korpela H, Kumpulainen J, Jussila E. Effect of selenium supplementation after acute myocardial infarction. *Res Commun Pathol Pharmacol* 1989; 65: 249–252.

25 Stranges S, Marshall JR, Trevisan M, *et al.* Effects of selenium supplementation on cardiovascular disease

incidence and mortality: secondary analyses in a randomised clinical trial. *Am J Epidemiol* 2006; 163: 694–699.

26 Scott R, MacPherson A, Yates RWS, *et al*. The effect of oral selenium supplementation on human sperm motility. *Br J Urol* 1998; 82: 76–80.

27 Keskes-Ammar L, Feki-Chakroun N, Rebai T, *et al*. Sperm oxidative stress and the effect of oral vitamin E and selenium supplement on semen quality in infertile men. *Arch Androl* 2003; 49: 83–84.

28 Hawkes WC, Turek PJ. Effects of dietary selenium on sperm motility in healthy men. *J Androl* 2001; 22: 764–772.

29 Peretz A, Neve J, Duchateau J, *et al*. Adjuvant treatment of recent onset rheumatoid arthritis by selenium supplementation. *Br J Rheumatol* 1992; 31: 281–282.

30 Tarp U, Overvad K, Thorling EB, *et al*. Selenium treatment in rheumatoid arthritis. *Scand J Rheumatol* 1985; 14: 364–368.

31 Peretz A, Siderova V, Neve J. Selenium supplementation in rheumatoid arthritis investigated in a double-blind, placebo-controlled trial. *Scand J Rheumatol* 2001; 30: 208–212.

32 Rayman M, Thompson A, Warren-Perry M, *et al*. Impact of selenium on mood and quality of life. *Biol Psychiatry* 2006; 59: 147–154.

33 Allam MF, Lucane RA. Selenium supplementation for asthma. Cochrane database, issue 2, 2004. London: Macmillan.

34 Broome CS, McArdle F, Kyle JA, *et al*. An increase in selenium intake improves immune function and poliovirus handling in adults with marginal selenium status. *Am J Clin Nutr* 2004; 80: 154–162.

35 Burbano X, Miguez-Barbano MJ, McCollister K, *et al*. Impact of a selenium chemoprevention clinical trial on hospital admissions of HIV-infected participants. *HIV Clin Trials* 2002; 3: 483–491.

36 Vaddadi KS, Soosai E, Vaddadi G. Low blood selenium concentrations in schizophrenic patients on clozapine. *Br J Clin Pharmacol* 2003; 55: 307–309.

Shark cartilage

Description

Cartilage obtained from various types of shark.

Constituents

Cartilage tissue contains a mixture of glycosaminoglycans, one of which is chondroitin sulphate. Shark cartilage is also thought to contain compounds known as anti-angiogenesis factors, including sphyrnastatin 1 and 2.[1] These are factors that inhibit the growth of new blood vessels, typically seen in malignant tumours, and this mechanism could, in theory, be helpful in human cancer.

Action

It has been suggested that shark cartilage may prevent tumour growth. The proposed mechanism is that the anti-angiogenesis factors prevent tumours from developing the network of blood vessels they need to supply them with nutrients. This supposedly starves tumours and causes them to shrink. The popularity of this anti-cancer theory increased as a result of a popular book, *Sharks Don't Get Cancer*.[2]

Possible uses

Shark cartilage has been proposed as a supplement for the treatment of cancer and (because of its chondroitin content) for the treatment of osteoarthritis.

Cancer

Various *in vitro*,[2-4] animal[5] and human[6] studies have shown that shark cartilage has anti-angiogenic properties. However, there is no evidence from controlled trials that shark cartilage cures cancer in humans.

In a study of cancer patients taking shark cartilage either rectally or orally, 10 of the 20 patients reported an improved quality of life, including increased appetite and reduced pain, after 8 weeks. In addition, four of the 20 patients showed partial or complete response (50–100% reduction in tumour mass). However, information on patient selection criteria, cartilage dose and concomitant cytotoxic therapy was not provided.[7]

A 12-week open clinical trial on 60 patients with advanced cancer assessed the efficacy and safety of shark cartilage at a dose of 1 g/kg daily. No complete or partial positive responses were found, and the authors concluded that shark cartilage had no anti-cancer activity and no effect on quality of life.[8]

> ### Conclusion
> There is currently no evidence from clinical trials that shark cartilage helps to cure cancer in humans.

Precautions/contraindications

Avoid in patients with hepatic disease. There has been a single case report of hepatitis attributed to shark cartilage.[9]

Pregnancy and breast-feeding

There are no available data. Shark cartilage should be avoided.

Adverse effects

Hepatitis and various gastrointestinal effects (e.g. nausea, vomiting constipation) have been reported. A case study has found that shark cartilage dust can be a cause of asthma. A 38-year-old man reported chest symptoms at work in association with exposure to shark cartilage dust and was diagnosed with asthma. Six months later he complained of shortness of breath and died from autopsy-confirmed asthma.[10]

Interactions

None reported.

Dose

Shark cartilage is available in the form of tablets, capsules and powder.

The dose is not established. There is no proven value of shark cartilage supplements.

References

1 McGuire TR, Kazakoff PW, Hoie EB, *et al*. Antiproliferative activity of shark cartilage with and without tumor necrosis factor-alpha in human umbilical vein endothelium. *Pharmacotherapy* 1996; 16: 237–244.

2 Lane IW. *Sharks Don't Get Cancer*. Garden City Park, New York: Avery Publishing Group, 1992: 107–118.

3 Sheu JR, Fu CC, Tsai ML, *et al*. Effect of U-995, a potent shark cartilage-derived angiogenesis inhibitor, on anti-angiogenesis and anti-tumour activities. *Anticancer Res* 1998; 18: 4435–4441.

4 Dupont E, Savard PE, Jourdain C, *et al*. Antiangiogenic properties of a novel shark cartilage extract: potential role in the treatment of psoriasis. *J Cutan Med Surg* 1998; 2: 146–152.

5 Horsman MR, Alsner J, Overgaard J. The effect of shark cartilage extracts on the growth and metastatic spread of the SCCVII carcinoma. *Acta Oncol* 1998; 37: 441–445.

6 Berbari P, Thibodeau A, Germain L, *et al*. Antiangiogenic effect of the oral administration of liquid cartilage extract in humans. *J Surg Res* 1999; 87: 108–113.

7 Mathews J. Media feeds frenzy over shark cartilage as cancer cancer treatment. *J Natl Cancer Inst* 1993; 85: 1190–1191.

8 Miller DR, Anderson GT, Stark JJ, *et al*. Phase I/II trial of the safety and efficacy of shark cartilage in the treatment of advanced cancer. *J Clin Oncol* 1998; 16: 3649–3655.

9 Ahsar B, Vargo E. Shark-cartilage induced hepatitis. *Ann Intern Med* 1996; 125: 780–781.

10 Ortega HG, Kreiss K, Schill DP, Weissman DN. Fatal asthma from powdering shark cartilage and review of fatal occupational asthma literature. *Am J Ind Med* 2002; 42: 50–54.

Silicon

Description

Silicon is a non-metallic element found in plants, animals and most living organisms. The term silica is used to refer to naturally-occurring materials composed principally of silicon dioxide (SiO_2). It is thought to be essential for human beings.

Human requirements

Although silicon is thought to be essential, human requirements for silicon have not been established. There are no Dietary Reference Values.

Intake

The intake of dietary silicon in the UK is unknown. Intakes in the USA range from 20 to 50 mg daily.[1]

Action

Silicon is involved in the formation of bone and connective tissues. The precise mechanism is uncertain. However, it has been suggested that silicon could facilitate the formation of glycosaminoglycan and collagen components of the bone matrix through its role as a constituent of the enzyme prolyhydrolase. Alternatively, it may have a structural role in glycosaminoglycans and linking different polysaccharides in the bone matrix.[2] Silicon also appears to have a role in reducing the absorption of aluminium.[3]

Dietary sources

Silicon is found principally in foods derived from plants, particularly grains such as oats, barley and rice. Animal foods contain lower concentrations. Beer is also a rich source of silicon.[4] Silicon is also found in drinking water as orthosilicic acid. Consumption of 2 L a day of drinking water could result in consumption of 10 mg silicon.[2]

Metabolism

Absorption

Silicon in the form of silicic acid is readily absorbed by human beings, and absorption is increased by dietary fibre.

Distribution

Silica is freely transported in the blood and is freely diffusible into tissues from the plasma. High levels are present in bone, nails, tendons and the walls of the aorta. Lower levels are present in red blood cells and serum. Silicon has also been found in the liver, kidneys, lungs and spleen.

Elimination

Silicon is readily excreted in the urine with smaller amounts being excreted in the faeces. Silicon excretion increases as dietary intake is increased.

Bioavailability

Silicon bioavailability depends on the solubility of the silicon compounds in question. It is thought that silicic acid is the form absorbed in the gastrointestinal tract. Absorption of silicic acid from the gut has been reported to be 20–75%.

Deficiency

Silicon deficiency has not been observed in humans. In rats and chickens, silicon deficiency produces deformities of the skull and peripheral bones.[1] In silicon-deficient animals, glycosaminoglycan and collagen concentrations in bone are reduced. The concentration of other minerals in bone such as calcium, magnesium, zinc, sodium, iron, potassium and manganese may also be decreased in silicon-deficient animals.

Possible uses

Silicon has been claimed to have various benefits such as reducing the risk of osteoporosis and osteoarthritis, and preventing CHD and hypertension. Silicon has been shown to have an inhibitory effect on bone mass loss and stimulation of bone formation in rats.[5,6] It may have a role in reducing the risk of Alzheimer's disease, because it may reduce the absorption of aluminium.[3] It is also claimed to improve hair growth and have benefits for the skin. However, no clinical trials in humans have been identified.

Precautions/contraindications

No at-risk groups or situations have been documented.

Pregnancy and breast-feeding

No problems have been reported, but there have not been sufficient studies to guarantee the safety of silicon in pregnancy and breast-feeding.

Adverse effects

There are few data on the oral toxicity of silicon in humans. In humans, adverse effects are primarily limited to silicosis, a lung disease resulting from the inhalation of silica particles.

Interactions

Nutrients

Silicon has been reported to interact with a number of minerals, including aluminium, copper and zinc.

Drugs

None reported.

Dose

The dose is not established. Dietary supplements in the UK provide doses of up to 500 mg daily.

Upper safety levels

The Food Standards Agency Expert Vitamins and Minerals (EVM) group set a safe upper level for adults for total silicon intake (from foods and supplements) of 760 mg daily.[1]

References

1   Eckert C. Other trace elements. In: Shils ME, Shike M, Ross AC, Caballero B, Cousins RJ, eds. *Modern Nutrition in Health and Disease*, 10th edn. London: Lippincott, Williams and Wilkins, 2006: 338–350.
2   Food Standards Agency. Risk assessment. Silicon. http://www.eatwell.gov.uk/healthydiet/nutritionessentials/vitaminsandminerals/silicon (accessed 8 July 2006).
3   Edwardson JA, Moore PB, Ferrier IN, *et al.* Effect of silicon on gastrointestinal absorption of aluminium. *Lancet* 1993; 342: 211–212.
4   Bellia JP, Birchall JD, Roberts NB. Beer: a dietary source of silicon. *Lancet* 1994; 343: 235.
5   Rico H, Gallego-Lago JL, Hernandez ER, *et al.* Effect of silicon supplement on osteopenia induced by ovariectomy in rats. *Calcif Tissue Int* 2000; 66: 53–55.
6   Calomme M, Geusens P, Demeester N, *et al.* Partial prevention of long-term femoral bone loss in aged ovariectomized rats supplemented with choline-stabilized orthosilicic acid. *Calcif Tissue Int* 2006; 78: 227–232.

Spirulina

Description

Spirulina is a blue-green microscopic alga; it grows in freshwater ponds and lakes, thriving in warm and alkaline environments.

Constituents

See Table 1 for the claimed nutrient content of spirulina.

Action

Spirulina consists of approximately 65–70% crude protein, high concentration of B vitamins, phenylalanine, iron and other minerals. However all the B vitamins (including B_{12}) are thought to be in the form of analogues and nutritionally insignificant. The iron is believed to be highly bioavailable with 1.5–2 mg being absorbed from a 10-g dose of spirulina.

Possible uses

Lipid lowering

Various pilot studies have shown that spirulina may have a lipid-lowering and hypoglycaemic effect in patients with non-insulin-dependent diabetes mellitus (NIDDM). One study[1] looked at the long-term effect of spirulina supplementation (2 g daily) on blood sugar levels, serum lipid profile and glycated serum protein levels in 15 NIDDM patients. Supplementation for 2 months resulted in a significant reduction in triglycerides and total cholesterol, as well as a reduction in blood sugar and glycated serum protein levels. Levels of HDL increased, while those of LDL fell.

Table 1 Claimed[1] nutrient content of spirulina

Nutrient	per 100 g	per typical dose (10 g)	% RNI[2]
Protein (g)	70	7	–
Fat (g)	7	0.7	–
Carbohydrate (g)	15	1.5	–
Beta-carotene (mg)	170	17	–
Thiamine (mg)	5.5	0.5	55
Riboflavin (mg)	4.0	0.4	33
Niacin (mg)	11.8	1.2	8
Pyridoxine (mg)	0.3	0.03	2.5
Vitamin B_{12} (µg)	200	20	1333
Folic acid (µg)	50	5	2.5
Pantothenic acid (mg)	1.1	0.1	–
Biotin (µg)	40	4	–
Vitamin E (mg)	19	0.2	–
Inositol (mg)	35	3.5	–
Calcium (mg)	132	13	2
Magnesium (mg)	192	19	6
Potassium (mg)	1540	154	4
Phosphorus (mg)	894	89	16
Iron (mg)	58	5.8	48
Zinc (mg)	4	0.4	6
Manganese (mg)	2.5	0.2	–
Selenium (µg)	40	4	2

[1] Reported on a product label.
[2] Reference Nutrient Intake for males aged 19–50 years.

Miscellaneous

Spirulina has been shown *in vitro* to have antiviral activity.[2,3] It may also modulate inflammatory compounds in allergic conditions. A recent double-blind crossover study investigated the effect of spirulina 1000 mg or 2000 mg daily for 12 weeks in individuals with allergic rhinitis. A dose of 2000 mg daily inhibited the production of interleukin-4 (a type of cytokine), which could be protective against allergic rhinitis.[4]

Spirulina is claimed to act as a tonic and be beneficial in Alzheimer's disease; peptic ulcer; increasing stamina in athletes; and retarding ageing. There is no evidence for any of these claims. When spirulina was introduced into the USA in 1979 as a slimming aid, the Food and Drug Administration could find no evidence to support these claimed benefits.

> **Conclusion**
> There is preliminary evidence that spirulina could lower lipids and have an anti-viral and anti-allergic effect. However, controlled trials are required to confirm these effects.

Precautions/contraindications

Spirulina may be contaminated with mercury.

Pregnancy and breast-feeding

Avoid (contaminants – see Precautions).

Adverse effects

Effects not known (contaminants – see Precautions).

Interactions

None known.

Dose

Spirulina is available in the form of tablets, capsules and powders.

The dose is not established. There is no proven benefit of spirulina. Dietary supplements provide 6–10 g per daily dose.

References

1   Mani UV, Desai S, Iyer U. Studies on the long term effect of spirulina supplementation on serum lipid profile and glycated proteins in NIDDM patients. *J Nutraceut Funct Med Foods* 2000; 2: 25–32.
2   Hayashi K, Hayashi T, Kojima I. A natural sulfated polysaccharide, calcium spirulan, isolated from *Spirulina platensis*: *in vitro* and *ex vivo* evaluation of anti-herpes simplex virus and anti-human immunodeficiency virus activities. *AIDS Res Hum Retroviruses* 1996; 12: 1463–1471.
3   Hayashi T, Hayashi K, Maeda M, *et al.* Calcium spirulan, an inhibitor of enveloped virus replication, from blue-green algae *Spirulina platensis*. *J Nat Prod* 1996; 59: 83–87.
4   Mao TK, Van de Water J, Gershwin ME. Effects of a Spirulina-based dietary supplement on cytokine production from allergic rhinitis patients. *J Med Food* 2005; 8: 27–30.

Superoxide dismutase

Description

Superoxide dismutase (SOD) is a group of enzymes that is widely distributed in the body; several different forms exist with varying metal content. Copper-containing SOD is extracellular and present in high concentrations in the lungs, thyroid and uterus and in small amounts in plasma. SOD containing copper and zinc is present within the cells and found in high concentrations in brain, erythrocytes, kidney, liver, pituitary and thyroid.

Action

SOD enzymes act as scavengers of superoxide radicals, and protect against oxidative damage (by catalysing conversion of superoxide radicals to peroxide).

Possible uses

SOD is claimed to be useful for prevention of CVD, cancer and retardation of ageing. Such claims are partly based on studies that have used SOD by injection in clinical management. SOD is not absorbed from an oral dose and dietary supplements are therefore likely to be ineffective.

Precautions/contraindications

None reported.

Pregnancy and breast-feeding

No problems reported, but there have been insufficient studies to guarantee the safety of SOD in pregnancy and breast-feeding.

Adverse effects

None reported from oral doses.

Interactions

None reported.

Dose

SOD is available in the form of tablets and capsules. However, products may not have any of the stated activity because they are acid-labile and break down before absorption.

The dose is not established. Not recommended as a dietary supplement (probably ineffective).

Thiamine

Description

Thiamine is a water-soluble vitamin of the vitamin B complex.

Nomenclature

Thiamine is the British Approved Name for use on pharmaceutical labels. Thiamin is used to describe the vitamin present in food. It is known also as vitamin B_1 and aneurine.

Human requirements

Thiamine requirements depend on energy intake; values are therefore often given as mg/1000 kcal and also as total values based on estimated average energy requirements for the majority of people in the UK (Table 1).

Dietary intake

In the UK, the average adult diet provides: for men, 2.0 mg daily; for women, 1.54 mg.

Action

Thiamine functions as a coenzyme in the oxidative decarboxylation of alpha-ketoacids (involved in energy production) and in the transketolase reaction of the pentose phosphate pathway (involved in carbohydrate metabolism). Thiamine is also important in nerve transmission (independently of coenzyme function).

Dietary sources

See Table 2 for dietary sources of thiamine.

Metabolism

Absorption

Absorption occurs mainly in the jejunum and ileum by both active transport and passive diffusion.

Distribution

Thiamine is transported in the plasma bound to albumin, and stored in the heart, liver, muscle, kidneys and brain. Only small amounts are stored and turnover is relatively high, so continuous intake is necessary. Thiamine is rapidly converted to its biologically active form, thiamine pyrophosphate (TPP).

Elimination

Thiamine is eliminated mainly in the urine (as metabolites). Excess beyond requirements is excreted as free thiamine. Thiamine crosses the placenta and is excreted in breast milk.

Bioavailability

Bioavailability may be reduced by alcohol. Requirements are increased by increasing carbohydrate intake. Thiamine is unstable above pH 7, and the addition of sodium bicarbonate to peas or green beans (to retain the green colour) can lead to large losses of thiamine. It is also destroyed by heat and by processing foods at alkaline pHs, high temperature and in the presence of oxygen or other oxidants. Freezing does not affect thiamine.

Thiamine antagonists (thiaminases) in coffee, tea, raw fish, betel nuts and some vegetables can lead to thiamine destruction in foods during food processing or in the gut after ingestion.

301

Table 1 Dietary Reference Values for thiamine (mg/day)

Age	UK					USA		FAO/WHO
							EU RDA = 1.6 mg	
	LNRI[1]	EAR[1]	RNI[1]	RNI[2]	EVM	RDA[2]	TUL	RNI[2]
0–6 months	0.2	0.23	0.3	0.2		0.2	–	0.2
7–12 months	0.2	0.23	0.3	0.3		0.3	–	0.3
1–3 years	0.23	0.3	0.4	0.5		0.5	–	0.5
4–6 years	0.23	0.3	0.4	0.7		0.7	–	0.6
4–8 years						0.6		
7–10 years	0.23	0.3	0.4	0.7		–	0.9[a]	
9–13 years				0.9	–	–		
Males								
11–14 years	0.23	0.3	0.4	0.9			–	1.2[b]
15–50 years	0.23	0.3	0.4	0.9	100[2]		–	1.2
14–70+ years					1.2			
Females								
11–14 years	0.23	0.3	0.4	0.7			–	1.1[b]
14–18 years						1.0	–	–
15–50+ years	0.23	0.3	0.4	0.8	100[2]		–	1.1
19–70+ years						1.1	–	–
Pregnancy	0.23	0.3	0.4	+0.1[3]		1.4	–	+0.1
Lactation	0.23	0.3	0.4	+0.2		1.5–	–	+0.2

[a] 7–9 years.   [b] 10–14 years.
[1] mg/1000 kcal.   [2] mg/day.   [3] Last trimester only.
EVM = Likely safe daily intake from supplements alone.
TUL = Tolerable Upper Intake Level (not determined for thiamine).

Deficiency

Thiamine deficiency may lead to beri-beri (rare in the UK). Deficiency is associated with abnormalities of carbohydrate metabolism. Early signs of deficiency (including subclinical deficiency) are anorexia, irritability and weight loss; later features include headache, weakness, tachycardia and peripheral neuropathy.

Advanced deficiency is characterised by involvement of two major organ systems: the cardiovascular system (wet beri-beri) and the nervous system (dry beri-beri, Wernicke's encephalopathy and Korsakoff's psychosis). The Wernicke–Korsakoff syndrome may be associated with a genetic variant of transketolase, which requires a higher than normal concentration of thiamine diphosphate for activity.[1] This would suggest that there may be a group of the population who have a higher than average requirement for thiamine, but the evidence is not convincing. Signs of wet beri-beri include enlarged heart with normal sinus rhythm (usually tachycardia), and peripheral oedema. Signs of dry beri-beri include mental confusion, anorexia, muscle weakness and wasting, ataxia and ophthalmoplegia.

Thiamine deficiency has been observed in HIV-positive patients,[2] those with chronic fatigue syndrome,[3] hospitalised elderly patients,[4] and patients on emergency admission to hospital.[5]

Table 2 Dietary sources of thiamine

Food portion	Thiamine content (mg)
Breakfast cereals	
1 bowl All-Bran (45 g)	**0.4**
1 bowl Bran Flakes (45 g)	**0.5**
1 bowl Corn Flakes (30 g)	**0.3**
1 bowl muesli (95 g)	**0.4**
1 bowl porridge (160 g)	0.1
2 pieces Shredded Wheat	*0.15*
1 bowl Shreddies (50 g)	**0.6**
1 bowl Start (40 g)	**0.6**
2 Weetabix	**0.4**
Cereal products	
Bread, brown, 2 slices	*0.2*
white, 2 slices	*0.15*
wholemeal, 2 slices	*0.2*
1 chapati	*0.15*
1 naan bread	**0.3**
1 white pitta bread	*0.15*
Pasta, brown, boiled (150 g)	**0.3**
white, boiled (150 g)	0.01
Rice, brown, boiled (160 g)	*0.2*
white, boiled (160 g)	0.01
2 heaped tablespoons wheatgerm	**0.3**
Milk and dairy products	
½ pint milk, whole, semi-skimmed, or skimmed	0.1
½ pint soya milk	*0.15*
Cheese, 50 g	*0.15*
Meat and fish	
3 rashers bacon, back, grilled	**0.3**
Beef, roast (85 g)	0.07
Lamb, roast (85 g)	0.12
Pork, roast (85 g)	**0.55**
1 pork chop, grilled (135 g)	**0.7**
2 slices ham	**0.3**
1 gammon rasher, grilled (120 g)	**1.1**
1 chicken leg portion	0.1
Liver, lambs, cooked (90 g)	*0.2*
Kidney, lambs, cooked (75 g)	**0.4**
Fish, cooked (150 g)	*0.15*
Vegetables	
Peas, boiled (100 g)	**0.3**
Potatoes, boiled (150 g)	**0.3**
1 small can baked beans (200 g)	*0.2*
Chickpeas, cooked (105 g)	0.1
Red kidney beans (105 g)	*0.2*
Dahl, lentil (150 g)	0.1
Fruit	
1 apple, banana, or pear	0.04
1 orange	*0.2*
Nuts	
10 Brazil nuts	**0.3**
30 hazelnuts	0.1
30 peanuts	**0.3**
1 tablespoon sunflower seeds	0.1
Yeast	
Brewer's yeast (10 g)	**1.6**
Marmite, spread on 1 slice bread	*0.15*

Excellent sources (**bold**); good sources (*italics*).

Long-term furosemide use may be associated with thiamine deficiency through urinary loss, contributing to cardiac insufficiency in patients with CHF. It has been suggested that thiamine supplementation could improve left ventricular function. However, study results are controversial. One review suggested that, pending further studies, thiamine administration could be considered in patients receiving very large doses of diuretics and others at risk for thiamine deficiency (elderly, malnourished, alcoholic).[6]

There is also a form of diabetes that is dependent on thiamine (thiamine-responsive megaloblastic anaemia syndrome (TRMA)), which is the association of diabetes mellitus, anaemia and deafness, caused by mutations in a gene encoding a thiamine transporter protein. This syndrome responds to thiamine initially, but most patients become fully insulin-dependent after puberty.[7]

Possible uses

Supplementary thiamine may be beneficial in older people (> 65 years), people who consume quantities of alcohol in excess of two units daily, smokers and in HIV-positive patients. However, deficiency of one B vitamin is often associated with deficiencies in other B vitamins and a multivitamin supplement is often more appropriate.

A double-blind, placebo-controlled trial in 76 elderly people found that thiamine 10 mg daily for 3 months significantly improved quality of life, and reduced blood pressure and weight in comparison with placebo, but only in subjects with low thiamine status. There was also a non-significant trend to improvements in sleep and energy levels with supplementary thiamine, and the authors concluded that older people could benefit from increasing thiamine intake from supplements or diet.[8]

Thiamine has been considered of value in various conditions such as Alzheimer's disease and mouth ulcers.

Alzheimer's disease

Preclinical and laboratory studies show an effect of thiamine on the release and breakdown of acetylcholine. Some intellectual functions, including attention and memory, are influenced by neurons that release acetylcholine. Cholinergic function is impaired in Alzheimer's disease. It has therefore been hypothesised that thiamine many be beneficial in Alzheimer's disease. Biochemical abnormalities have been found in the brains of patients with Alzheimer's disease. One double-blind, placebo-controlled trial found that 3000 mg thiamine daily improved global cognitive scores compared with a niacinamide placebo, but had no effect on behavioural ratings or clinician's subjective judgement of symptoms.[9] Another small, double-blind, placebo-controlled trial using 3000 mg thiamine found no benefits of thiamine over placebo in slowing the development of Alzheimer's disease.[10] A more complex placebo-controlled trial in patients with Alzheimer's disease, designed with two phases, used doses of 3000 mg thiamine in the first phase, which lasted 1 month, and then doses of 4000–8000 mg daily over 5–13 months. In the second phase, high-dose thiamine improved scores on various neuropsychological tests, but the authors advised caution in interpretation of the results, to prevent hopes being unrealistically raised.[11] A Cochrane review[12] of three RCTs concluded that the detail in the results was insufficient to combine the results. The review therefore found no evidence of the efficacy of thiamine in people with Alzheimer's disease.

Mouth ulcers

Low erythrocyte thiamine has been found in people with recurrent mouth ulcers,[13] and replacement of B vitamins (thiamine, riboflavine and pyridoxine) led to improvement in clinical symptoms in individuals who were deficient in one or more of these vitamins.[14]

Insect repellent

Anecdotally, thiamine has been found to be of value as an insect repellent, but studies have shown it to be ineffective.[15,16] Thiamine should not be relied upon as an insect repellent in areas where malaria is endemic.

Miscellaneous

Higher doses of thiamine (25–50 mg daily) have been found to be beneficial in diabetic

neuropathy,[17] HIV,[18] erectile dysfunction,[19] and periodontal wound healing,[20] but usually only in those with poor thiamine status. Studies have sometimes used other B vitamins as well, so it is difficult to attribute any benefits to thiamine supplementation alone. One RCT has shown that thiamine (100 mg daily) could be an effective treatment for dysmenorrhoea.[21]

> **Conclusion**
> There is some evidence that the elderly could benefit from increased thiamine intake, but evidence for a benefit of thiamine supplementation in Alzheimer's disease is equivocal, and studies have used very high doses (3000–7000 mg daily). Preliminary evidence suggests that thiamine deficiency could be associated with mouth ulcers, but further research is required to find out whether supplements can improve the condition.

Precautions/contraindications

Known hypersensitivity to thiamine.

Pregnancy and breast-feeding

No problems reported.

Adverse effects

There appear to be no toxic effects (except possibly gastric upset) with high oral doses. Large parenteral doses are generally well tolerated, but there have been rare reports of anaphylactic reactions (coughing, difficulty in breathing and swallowing, flushing, skin rash, swelling of face, lips and eyelids).

Interactions

Drugs

Alcohol: excessive alcohol intake induces thiamine deficiency.
Furosemide: may increase urinary loss of thiamine;[22] prolonged furosemide therapy may induce thiamine deficiency;[23,24] thiamine

supplementation (200 mg daily) has been shown to improve left ventricular function in patients with CHF receiving furosemide therapy.[25]

Nutrients

Adequate amounts of all B vitamins are required for optimal functioning; deficiency or excess of one B vitamin may lead to abnormalities in the metabolism of another.

Dose

Thiamine is available in the form of tablets and capsules. It is also found in multivitamins and in brewer's yeast supplements.

No benefit of a dose beyond the RDA (as a food supplement) has been established.

Doses for mild and severe deficiency can be found in the *British National Formulary*. The dose for prophylaxis or treatment of Wernicke–Korsakoff syndrome caused by alcohol abuse, and the length of time that thiamine should be given after drinking has ceased, has not been clarified.[26]

Upper safety levels

The UK Expert Group on Vitamins and Minerals (EVM) has identified a likely safe total intake of thiamine for adults from supplements alone of 100 mg daily.

References

1 Bender DA. Optimum nutrition: thiamin, biotin and pantothenate. *Proc Nutr Soc* 1999; 58: 427–433.
2 Muri RM, Von Overbeck J, Furrer J, Ballmer PE. Thiamin deficiency in HIV-positive patients: evaluation by erythrocyte transketolase activity and thiamin pyrophosphate effect. *Clin Nutr* 1999; 18: 375–378.
3 Heap LC, Peters TJ, Wessely S. Vitamin B status in patients with chronic fatigue syndrome. *J R Soc Med* 1999; 92: 183–185.
4 Pepersack T, Garbusinski J, Robberecht J, *et al.* Clinical relevance of thiamine status amongst hospitalized elderly patients. *Gerontology* 1999; 45: 96–101.
5 Jamieson CP, Obeid OA, Powell Tuck J. The thiamin, riboflavin and pyridoxine status of patients on emergency admission to hospital. *Clin Nutr* 1999; 18: 87–91.
6 Blanc P, Boussuges A. Is thiamine supplementation necessary in patients with cardiac insufficiency? *Ann Cardiol Angeiol (Paris)* 2001; 50: 160–168.
7 Ricketts CJ, Minton JA, Samuel J, *et al.* Thiamine-responsive megaloblastic anaemia syndrome: long-term follow-up and mutation analysis of seven families. *Acta Paediatr* 2006; 95: 99–104.
8 Wilkinson TJ, Hanger HC, Elmslie J, *et al.* The response to treatment of subclinical thiamine deficiency in the elderly. *Am J Clin Nutr* 1997; 66: 925–928.
9 Blass JP, Gleason P, Brush D, *et al.* Thiamine and Alzheimer's disease. A pilot study. *Arch Neurol* 1988; 45: 833–835.
10 Nolan KA, Black RS, Sheu KF, *et al.* A trial of thiamine in Alzheimer's disease. *Arch Neurol* 1991; 48: 81–83.
11 Meador K, Loring D, Nichols M, *et al.* Preliminary findings of high-dose thiamine in dementia of Alzheimer's type. *J Geriatr Psychiatry Neurol* 1993; 6: 222–229.
12 Rodriguez-Martin JL, Qizilbash N, Lopez-Arrieta JM. Thiamine for Alzheimer's disease. Cochrane database, issue 2, 2001. London: Macmillan.
13 Haisreili-Shalish M, Livneh A, Katz J, *et al.* Recurrent aphthous stomatitis and thiamine deficiency. *Oral Surg Oral Med Oral Pathol Oral Radiol Endod* 1996; 82: 634–636.
14 Nolan A, McIntosh WB, Allam BF, *et al.* Recurrent aphthous ulceration: vitamin B1, B2 and B6 status and response to replacement therapy. *J Oral Pathol Med* 1991; 20: 389–391.
15 Holzer RB. Malaria prevention without drugs. *Schweiz Rundsch Med Prax* 1993; 82: 139–143.
16 Holzer RB. Protection against biting mosquitoes. *Ther Umsch* 2001; 58: 341–346.
17 Abbas ZG, Swai ABM. Evaluation of the efficacy of thiamine and pyridoxine in the treatment of diabetic peripheral neuropathy. *East Afr Med J* 1997; 74: 803–808.
18 Tang AM, Graham NMH, Saah AJ. Effects of multinutrient intake on survival in human immunodeficiency type 1 infection. *Am J Epidemiol* 1996; 143: 1244–1256.
19 Tjandra BS, Jangknegt RA. Neurogenic impotence and lower urinary tract symptoms due to vitamin B1 deficiency in chronic alcoholism. *J Urol* 1997; 157: 954–955.
20 Neiva RF, Al-Shammari K, Nociti FH, *et al.* Effects of vitamin-B complex supplementation on periodontal wound healing. *J Periodontol* 2005; 76: 1084–1091.
21 Proctor ML, Murphy PA. Herbal and dietary therapies for primary and secondary dysmenorrhoea. Cochrane database, issue 2, 2001. London: Macmillan.

22 Rieck J, Halkin H, Almog S, *et al*. Urinary loss of thiamine is increased by low doses of furosemide in healthy volunteers. *J Lab Clin Med* 1999; 134: 238–243.

23 Brady JA, Rock CL, Horneffer MR. Thiamin status, diuretic medications, and the management of congestive heart failure. *J Am Dietet Ass* 1995; 95: 541–544.

24 Seligmann H, Halkin H, Rauchfleish S, *et al*. Thiamin deficiency in patients with congestive heart failure receiving long-term furosemide therapy: a pilot study. *Am J Med* 1991; 91: 151–155.

25 Shimon I, Almog S, Vered Z, *et al*. Improved ventricular function after thiamine supplementation in patients with congestive heart failure receiving long-term furosemide therapy. *Am J Med* 1995; 98: 485–490.

26 Day E, Bentham P, Callaghan R, *et al*. Thiamine for Wernicke–Korsakoff Syndrome in people at risk from over-consumption of alcohol. Cochrane database, issue 4, 2003. London: Macmillan.

Tin

Description

Tin is a metallic element usually found in the form of the dioxide (SnO_2). It has oxidation states of II and IV. Tin has not been shown to be essential in humans, but it is present in a few multivitamin/multimineral supplements in the UK.

Human requirements

Human requirements for tin have not been established. There are no Dietary Reference Values. The Food Standards Agency Expert Vitamins and Minerals (EVM) group stated that intake of tin of up to 0.22 mg/kg body weight per day (equivalent to 13 mg tin daily in a 60-kg adult) would not be expected to have any harmful effects but did not set a safe upper level or guidance level for adults for supplemental tin intake.[1]

Intake

Mean intake of dietary tin in the UK is 1.8 mg daily, with an estimated maximum intake of 6.3 mg daily.[1]

Action

The actions of dietary tin are not known. However, it is thought that it may function as part of metalloenzymes.

Dietary sources

Tin intake is essentially dependent on food stored in tin cans. The main dietary sources of tin are canned vegetables and fruit products. The presence of tin in fresh food is highly dependent on the soil concentration of tin. Stannous chloride is a permitted food additive (E512).

Metabolism

Absorption
Tin is poorly absorbed from the gastrointestinal tract.

Distribution
Tin is concentrated principally in bone, lymph nodes, liver, kidney, lung, ovary and testis.

Elimination
The majority of ingested tin is eliminated in the faeces, with the remainder in the urine.

Bioavailability

Bioavailability varies and depends on the oxidation state of the tin salt.

Deficiency

Tin deficiency has not been observed in humans or animals.

Possible uses

No beneficial human health effects from consuming dietary tin are known. Tin has been claimed to have immune-enhancing properties in animals, but there is no evidence that tin has these effects in humans.

Precautions/contraindications

None reported.

Pregnancy and breast-feeding

No problems have been reported, but there have not been sufficient studies to guarantee the safety of tin in pregnancy and breast-feeding.

Adverse effects

Acute tin poisoning (from food or drinks) is associated with gastrointestinal effects (cramps, vomiting, nausea and diarrhoea), headaches and chills.

Interactions

None reported.

Dose

The dose is not established. Supplements in the UK contain up to 10 µg in a daily dose.

References

1 Food Standards Agency. Risk assessment. Tin. http://www.eatwell.gov.uk/healthydiet/nutritionessentials/vitaminsandminerals/tin (accessed 8 July 2006).

Vanadium

Description

Vanadium is a trace element. It is debatable whether or not it is an essential element in the diet of human beings. It exists in at least six different oxidation states. The tetravalent and pentavalent forms are the most important in higher animals.

Human requirements

Human requirements for vanadium have not been established. There are no Dietary Reference Values. It is thought that 10 µg daily is adequate. The US Food and Nutrition Board set a Tolerable Upper Intake level of 1.8 mg daily in adult men and women from the age of 19 years.

Dietary intake

The intake of dietary vanadium in the UK averages 13 µg daily.[1] Intakes in the USA range from 10 to 60 µg daily.[2]

Action

Vanadium does not have a defined function in human beings. Vanadate ions inhibit the sodium/potassium-ATPase pump and phosphate-dependent enzymes (e.g. glucose-6-phosphatase, alkaline phosphatase).

Dietary sources

Grains and grain products are significant sources of dietary vanadium. Marine organisms, brown algae, lichen, parsley, oysters, spinach and mushrooms are rich sources of vanadium.[1,3]

Metabolism

Absorption

Vanadium is poorly absorbed. Absorption occurs in the duodenum and upper gastrointestinal tract. The vanadate ion enters cells through non-specific anion channels and is reduced by glutathione.

Distribution

Vanadium is rapidly cleared from plasma and accumulates in kidney, liver, testes, bone and spleen. The vanadate ion binds to the iron-binding proteins lactoferrin, transferrin and ferritin. Tissues with the highest concentrations include lung, thyroid, teeth and bone. The quadrivalent form of vanadium is most common intracellularly, while the pentavalent form is the most common extracellularly.[2]

Elimination

Vanadium is excreted primarily through the kidney, with a small amount through the bile.

Bioavailability

Only about 5% of ingested vanadium is absorbed.

Deficiency

No cases of human vanadium deficiency have been reported, but deficiency has been suggested to be associated with CVD.[1] Vanadium deficiency in goats leads to an increase in abortion, convulsions, bone malformations and early death. In rats, vanadium deficiency increases thyroid weight and decreases growth.

Possible uses

Diabetes mellitus

Vanadium appears to potentiate the effects of insulin and may have benefits in diabetes. *In vitro* and animal studies indicate that vanadium and other vanadium compounds increase glucose transport activity and improve glucose metabolism.

A few small human studies have investigated the effects of vanadium in diabetes. The earliest human trial involved five patients with type 1 diabetes and five patients with type 2 diabetes who were studied before and after 2 weeks of oral sodium metavanadate (125 mg daily). Glucose metabolism was not improved by vanadate therapy. There was a significant decrease in insulin requirements in the patients with type 1 diabetes, cholesterol levels decreased in both groups and there was an increase in mitogen-activated protein and S6 kinase activities in mononuclear cells from patients in both groups that mimicked the effects of insulin stimulation in controls.[4]

A further trial in six subjects with type 2 diabetes found that 3-week treatment with oral vanadyl sulphate improved hepatic and peripheral insulin sensitivity in insulin-resistant type 2 diabetics.[5] Another part of the same trial conducted by the same research group found that oral vanadyl sulphate improved hepatic and skeletal muscle insulin sensitivity in type 2 diabetics in part by enhancing insulin's inhibitory effect on lipolysis.[6]

Another trial in eight patients with type 2 diabetes found that oral vanadyl sulphate (50 mg twice daily for 4 weeks) was associated with a 20% decrease in fasting plasma glucose and a decrease in hepatic glucose output during hyperinsulinaemia (a reduction in hepatic insulin resistance).[7]

A later study investigated the effect of vanadyl sulphate at three doses in 16 type 2 diabetic patients. Fasting glucose and haemoglobin A1c decreased significantly in the 150- and 300-mg vanadyl sulphate groups, but the mechanism on insulin action was not clear from this study.[8]

A more recent study in 11 type 2 diabetic subjects found that vanadyl sulphate 150 mg daily for 6 weeks significantly improved hepatic and muscle insulin sensitivity and improved glycaemic control, reducing fasting plasma glucose and haemoglobin A1c, while decreasing total and LDL cholesterol.[9]

Ergogenics

Vanadium has been promoted as an ergogenic aid in sports. However, a 12-week, double-blind, placebo-controlled trial of vanadyl sulphate (0.5 mg/kg/day) in 31 weight-training subjects found no benefit of vanadium in improving performance.[10]

> **Conclusion**
> Vanadium is a trace element for which there is no evidence of dietary essentiality in humans. However, pharmacological doses appear to have a role in insulin and glucose metabolism. Human trials in diabetic subjects have shown beneficial effects in glycaemic control and insulin sensitivity, but they have involved small numbers of subjects. There is no evidence that vanadium supplements have a role in sports performance.

Precautions/contraindications

See Adverse effects.

Pregnancy and breast-feeding

No problems reported, but safety studies have not been conducted.

Adverse effects

Vanadium causes abdominal cramps, diarrhoea, haemolysis, increased blood pressure and fatigue. The primary toxic effect in humans occurs from inhaling vanadium dust in industrial settings. This is characterised by rhinitis, wheezing, conjunctivitis, cough, sore throat and chest pain.[2]

Interactions

None reported.

Dose

The dose is not established. Food supplements in the UK provide up to 25 µg in a daily dose.

References

1 Food Standards Agency. Risk assessment. Vanadium. http://www.eatwell.gov.uk/healthydiet/nutritionessentials/vitaminsandminerals/vanadium (accessed 8 July 2006).

2 Barceloux DG. Vanadium. *J Toxicol Clin Toxicol* 1999; 37: 265–278.

3 Eckert C. Other trace elements. In: Shils ME, Shike M, Ross AC, Caballero B, Cousins RJ, eds. *Modern Nutrition in Health and Disease*, 10th edn. London: Lippincott, Williams and Wilkins, 2006: 338–350.

4 Goldfine AB, Simonson DC, Folli F, *et al*. Metabolic effects of sodium metavanadate in humans with insulin-dependent and noninsulin-dependent diabetes mellitus in vivo and in vitro studies. *J Clin Endocrinol Metab* 1995; 80: 3311–3320.

5 Cohen N, Halberstam M, Shlimovich P, *et al*. Oral vanadyl sulfate improves hepatic and peripheral insulin sensitivity in patients with non-insulin-dependent diabetes mellitus. *J Clin Invest* 1995; 95: 2501–2509.

6 Halberstam M, Cohen N, Shlimovich P, *et al*. Oral vanadyl sulfate improves insulin sensitivity in NIDDM but not in obese nondiabetic subjects. *Diabetes* 1996; 45: 659–666.

7 Boden G, Chen X, Ruiz J, *et al*. Effects of vanadyl sulfate on carbohydrate and lipid metabolism in patients with non-insulin-dependent diabetes mellitus. *Metabolism* 1996; 45: 1130–1135.

8 Goldfine AB, Patti ME, Zuberi L, *et al*. Metabolic effects of vanadyl sulfate in humans with non-insulin-dependent diabetes mellitus: in vivo and in vitro studies. *Metabolism* 2000; 49: 400–410.

9 Cusi K, Cukier S, DeFronzo RA, *et al*. Vanadyl sulfate improves hepatic and muscle insulin sensitivity in type 2 diabetes. *J Clin Endocrinol Metab* 2001; 86: 1410–1417.

10 Fawcett JP, Farquhar SJ, Walker RJ, *et al*. The effect of oral vanadyl sulfate on body composition and performance in weight-training athletes. *Int J Sport Nutr* 1996; 6: 382–390.

Vitamin A

Description

Vitamin A is a fat-soluble vitamin.

Nomenclature

Vitamin A is a generic term used to describe compounds that exhibit the biological activity of retinol. The two main components of Vitamin A in foods are retinol and the carotenoids (see Carotenoids).

The term 'retinoid' refers to the chemical entity retinol or other closely related naturally-occurring derivatives. These include:

- retinal (retinaldehyde);
- retinoic acid;
- retinyl esters (e.g. retinyl acetate, retinyl palmitate, retinyl propionate).

Retinoids also include structurally related synthetic analogues that may or may not have retinol-like (vitamin A) activity.

Units

The UK Dietary Reference Values express the requirement for vitamin A in terms of retinol equivalents:

$$\text{Retinol equivalents (µg)} = \text{retinol (µg)} + \frac{\text{beta-carotene equivalents (µg)}}{6}$$

The system of International Units for Vitamin A was discontinued in 1954, but continues to be widely used (particularly on dietary supplement labels):

1 retinol equivalent (µg) = 3.3 units

One unit is equal to:

- 0.3 retinol equivalents (µg)
- 0.3 µg retinol
- 0.3 µg retinol acetate
- 0.5 µg retinol palmitate
- 0.4 µg retinol propionate.

Human requirements

See Table 1 for Dietary Reference Values for vitamin A.

Dietary intake

In the UK, the average adult diet provides (retinol equivalents): for men, 911 µg daily; for women, 671 µg.

Action

Vitamin A (in the form of retinal) is essential for normal function of the retina, particularly for visual adaptation to darkness. Other forms (retinol, retinoic acid) are necessary to maintain the structural and functional integrity of epithelial tissue and the immune system, cellular differentiation and proliferation, bone growth, testicular and ovarian function and embryonic development. Vitamin A may act as a cofactor in biochemical reactions.

Dietary sources

See Table 2 for dietary sources of vitamin A.

Metabolism

Absorption

Vitamin A is readily absorbed from the upper gastrointestinal tract (duodenum and jejunum) by a carrier-mediated process. Absorption

Table 1   Dietary Reference Values for vitamin A (µg retinol equivalent/day)

| Age | UK | | | | USA | | FAO/WHO |
	LNRI	EAR	RNI	EVM	RDA	TUL	RNI
						EU RDA = 800 µg	
0–6 months	150	250	350		400[1]	600	375
7–12 months	150	250	350		500[1]	600	400
1–3 years	200	300	400		300	600	400
4–6 years	200	300	400		–	–	450
4–8 years	–	–	–		400	900	–
7–10 years	250	350	500		–	–	500[a]
9–13 years	–	–	–		600	1700	–
Males							
11–14 years	250	400	600		–	–	600[b]
14–18 years	–	–	–		900	2800	600
15–50+ years	300	500	700	1500	–	–	600
19–70+ years	–	–	–		900	3000	–
Females							
11–14 years	250	400	600	1500	–	–	600[b]
14–18 years	–	–	–		700	2800	600
15–50+ years	250	400	250		700	3000	500
19–70+ years	–	–	–		700		
Pregnancy		+100			770[2]	3000[3]	800
Lactation		+350			1300[4]	3000[4]	850
Elderly 65+							600

* No increment.
[a] 7–9 years.   [b] 10–14 years.
[1] Adequate Intakes (AIs).   [2] aged <18 years, 750 µg.   [3] aged >18 years, 2800 µg.   [4] aged <18 years, 1200 µg.
EVM = Likely safe daily intake from supplements alone.
TUL = Tolerable Upper Intake Level from foods and supplements.

requires the presence of gastric juice, bile salts, pancreatic and intestinal lipase, protein and dietary fat.

Distribution

The liver contains at least 90% of body stores (approximately 2 years' adult requirements). Small amounts are stored in the kidney and lungs. Vitamin A is transported in the blood in association with a carrier, retinol binding protein (RBP).

Elimination

Vitamin A is eliminated in the bile or urine (as metabolites). It appears in the breast milk.

Bioavailability

Absorption of vitamin A is markedly reduced if the intake of dietary fat is < 5 g daily (extremely rare) and by the presence of peroxidised fat and other oxidising agents in food. Deficiencies of protein (extremely rare in the UK), vitamin E and zinc, and excessive amounts of alcohol, adversely affect vitamin A transport, storage and utilisation.

Deficiency

Vitamin A deficiency is widespread in young children in developing countries and is associated with general malnutrition in these

Table 2 Dietary sources of vitamin A

Food portion	Retinol (µg)
Cereals	
Breads, grains, cereals	0
Milk and dairy products	
½ pint whole milk	*150*
½ pint semi-skimmed milk	55
½ pint skimmed milk	2
½ pint skimmed milk, fortified	100–150 (various brands)
2 tablespoons dried skimmed milk, fortified (30 g)	120
Single cream (35 g)	100
Whipping cream (35 g)	*190*
Double cream (35 g)	*200*
Hard cheese (e.g. cheddar), 50 g	*160*
Hard cheese, reduced fat (50 g)	80
Brie cheese (50 g)	*140*
Cream cheese (30 g)	*130*
1 carton yoghurt, low fat (150 g)	10
1 carton yoghurt, whole milk (150 g)	45
Ice cream, dairy (75 g)	90
Ice cream, non-dairy (75 g)	1
1 egg, size 2 (60 g)	*110*
Fats and oils	
Butter, on 1 slice bread (10 g)	80
Margarine, on 1 slice bread (10 g)	80
Low-fat spread, on 1 slice bread (10 g)	92
2 tablespoons ghee (30 g)	*210*
2 teaspoons cod liver oil (10 ml)	1800
Meat and fish	
Bacon, beef, lamb, pork, poultry	Trace
Kidney, lambs, cooked (75 g)	80
Liver, lambs, cooked (90 g)	**20 000**
Liver, calf, cooked (90 g)	**36 000**
Liver, ox, cooked (90 g)	**18 000**
Liver, pigs, cooked (90 g)	**21 000**
Liver paté (60 g)	**4400**
4 slices liver sausage (35 g)	**870**
White fish	Trace
2 fillets herring, cooked (110 g)	60
2 fillets kipper, cooked (130 g)	40
2 fillets mackerel, cooked (110 g)	55

Note: For dietary sources of beta-carotene, see Carotenoids monograph.
Excellent sources (**bold**); good sources (*italics*).

countries. In the UK, deficiency is relatively rare (especially in adults), but marginal intakes may occur in children.

Symptoms of deficiency include night blindness (due to decreased sensitivity of rod receptors in the retina); xerophthalmia (can be irreversible), characterised by conjunctival and corneal xerosis, ulceration and liquefaction; ultimately severe visual impairment and blindness; dryness of the skin and papular eruptions (not a unique indicator of vitamin A deficiency because other nutrient deficiencies cause similar disorders); metaplasia and keratinisation of the cells of the respiratory tract and other organs; increased susceptibility to respiratory and urinary tract infections; occasionally diarrhoea and loss of appetite.

Possible uses

Children

The Department of Health advises that most children from the age of 6 months to 5 years should receive supplements of vitamins A and D, unless the adequacy of their diet can be assured.[1]

Cancer

A large number of studies have assessed the association between vitamin A and cancer, but not all of them distinguish between retinol (preformed vitamin A) and carotenoids. Some case-control studies reporting on the association between preformed vitamin A and breast cancer have found modest decreases in risk with higher intake,[2–4] but others[5,6] have found no association. Prospective data are compatible with a modest protective effect of preformed vitamin A.[7–9]

There is some preliminary evidence that preformed vitamin A may be modestly protective against colon cancer in both men[10] and women.[11] In a nested case-control study,[12] subjects in the highest quintile of serum retinol were at reduced risk of colon cancer for up to 9 years of follow-up. However, another study[13] failed to find any association between colon cancer and vitamin A intake.

Most data suggest that preformed vitamin A does not protect against prostate cancer, and an initial study[14] suggesting an adverse effect has not been confirmed. However, the possibility that higher intakes of vitamin A increase the risk of prostate cancer requires further investigation.

The risk of lung cancer may be related to dietary carotene intake rather than retinol, and studies have shown no benefit of vitamin A in prevention of lung cancer.[15–17]

There is some evidence that people taking vitamin A-containing supplements have a lower risk of gastric cancer than non-users.[18]

Miscellaneous

There is no evidence of any value of vitamin A in eye problems, or prevention and treatment of infections unrelated to vitamin A deficiency. Vitamin A supplements in normal safe doses have no proven benefits in skin problems (e.g. acne), but synthetic retinoids may be prescribed for this purpose.

Single case studies have appeared periodically in the literature indicating that vitamin A may be beneficial in PMS, but these effects have not been confirmed in randomised trials.

> ### Conclusion
> The Department of Health recommends a supplement containing vitamin A (and vitamin D) in children aged 6 months to 5 years, unless a good diet can be assured. There is very little evidence for any benefit of vitamin A supplements except for cases of deficiency. Evidence for a role of preformed vitamin A in cancer is limited. Such evidence as exists relates more to carotenoids.

Pregnancy and breast-feeding

Excessive doses of vitamin A have been shown to be teratogenic,[19,20] although the level at which this occurs has not been firmly established. No teratogenic effects were observed in 1203 women receiving 6000 units daily at least from 1 month prior to conception until the 12th week of pregnancy,[21] and an apparent threshold of 10 000 units daily has been identified.[22] Other studies[23,24] suggest low risk with intakes up to 30 000 units daily.

The Department of Health has recommended that women who are (or may become) pregnant should not take dietary supplements that contain vitamin A (including fish liver oil), except on the advice of a doctor or antenatal clinic, and should also avoid liver and products containing liver (e.g. liver pate and liver sausage).

Adverse effects

Acute toxicity

Acute toxicity may be induced by single doses of 300 mg retinol (1 million units) in adults, 60 mg retinol (200 000 units) in children or 30 mg retinol (100 000 units) in infants.

Signs and symptoms are usually transient (usually occurring about 6 h after ingestion of acute dose and disappearing after 36 h) and include severe headache (due to raised intracranial pressure), sore mouth, bleeding gums, dizziness, vomiting, blurred vision, hepatomegaly, irritability and (in infants) bulging of the fontanelle.

Chronic toxicity

Signs of chronic toxicity may appear when daily intake is >15 mg retinol (50 000 units) in adults and 6 mg (20 000 units) in infants and young children.

Signs may include dryness of the skin, pruritis, dermatitis, skin desquamation, skin erythema, skin rash, skin scaliness, papilloedema, disturbed hair growth, fissure of the lips, bone and joint pain, hyperostosis, headache, fatigue, irritability, insomnia, anorexia, nausea, vomiting, diarrhoea, weight loss, hepatomegaly, hepatotoxicity, raised intracranial pressure, bulging fontanelle (in infants), and hypercalcaemia (due to increase in activity of alkaline phosphatase activity).

Not all signs appear in all patients, and relative severity varies widely among different individuals. Most signs and symptoms disappear within a week, but skin and bone changes may remain evident for several months.

Osteoporosis

Excessive vitamin A intake is thought to have a detrimental effect on bone and increase the risk of osteoporosis and fracture. Two Swedish studies – a cross-sectional study involving 175 women aged 28–74 years and a nested case-control study in 247 women aged 40–76 years – found that retinol intake was negatively associated with BMD.[25] A prospective analysis begun in 1980 with 18 years' follow-up within the Nurses' Health Study, and involving 72 337 post-menopausal women aged 34–77 years, found that women in the highest quintile of vitamin A intake ($\geq$3000 µg daily of retinol equivalents) had a significantly elevated risk of hip fracture compared with women in the lowest quintile of intake (< 1250 µg daily). This increased risk was attributable to retinol, not to beta-carotene, and was attenuated among women using post-menopausal oestrogens.[26] A longitudinal study in 2322 men aged 49–51 years found that the highest risk of fracture was found in men with the highest levels of serum retinol.[27] However, other studies in men,[28] perimenopausal women,[29] post-menopausal women,[30] and elderly women[31] have not found detrimental effects on bone. A review concluded that patients should be made aware of the potential risks of consuming vitamin A in amounts exceeding the RDA.[32]

Interactions

Drugs

Anticoagulants: large doses of vitamin A (>750 µg; 2500 units) may induce a hypoprothrombinaemic response.

Colestyramine and colestipol: may reduce intestinal absorption of vitamin A.

Colchicine: may reduce intestinal absorption of vitamin A.

Liquid paraffin: may reduce intestinal absorption of vitamin A.

Neomycin: may reduce intestinal absorption of vitamin A.

Retinoids (acitrecin, etreninate, isotretinoin, tretinoin): concurrent administration of vitamin A may result in additive toxic effects.

Statins: prolonged therapy with statins may increase serum vitamin A levels.

Sucralfate: may reduce intestinal absorption of vitamin A.

Nutrients

Iron: in vitamin A deficiency, plasma iron levels fall.

Vitamin C: under conditions of hypervitaminosis A, tissue levels of vitamin C may be reduced and urinary excretion of vitamin C increased; vitamin C may ameliorate the toxic effects of vitamin A.

Vitamin E: large doses of vitamin A increase the need for vitamin E; vitamin E protects against the oxidative destruction of vitamin A.

Vitamin K: under conditions of hypervitaminosis A, hypothrombinaemia may occur; it can be corrected by administration of vitamin K.

Dose

Vitamin A supplementation is not normally required in the UK.

Therapeutic doses may be given but only under medical supervision. For example, in cystic fibrosis, doses of 1200–3300 µg (4000–10 000 units) daily may be given.

Upper safety levels

The UK Expert Group on Vitamins and Minerals (EVM) has identified a likely safe total intake of vitamin A (retinol equivalents) for adults from supplements alone of 1500 µg daily.

References

1 Department of Health. Weaning and the weaning diet: Report of the Working Group on the Weaning Diet of the Committee on Medical Aspects of Food Policy. Report on Health and Social Subjects No 45. London: HMSO, 1994.

2 London SJ, Stein EA, Henderson IC. Carotenoids, retinol and vitamin E and risk of proliferative benign breast disease and breast cancer. *Cancer Causes Control* 1992; 3: 503–512.

3 Longnecker M, Newcomb P, Mittendorf PR, *et al*. Intake of carrots, spinach and supplements containing vitamin A in relation to the risk of breast cancer. *Cancer Epidemiol Biomarkers Prev* 1997; 6: 887–892.

4 Zaridze D, Lifanova Y, Maximovitch D, *et al*. Diet, alcohol consumption and reproductive factors in a case-control study of breast cancer in Moscow. *Int J Cancer* 1991; 48: 493–501.

5   Ingram DM, Nottage E, Roberts T. The role of diet in the development of breast cancer: a case-control study of patients with breast cancer, benign epithelial hyperplasia and fibrocystic disease of the breast. *Br J Cancer* 1991; 64: 187–191.

6   La Vecchia C, Decarli A, Franceschi S, *et al*. Dietary factors and the risk of breast cancer. *Nutr Cancer* 1987; 10: 205–214.

7   Graham S, Zielezny M, Marshall J. Diet in the epidemiology of breast cancer in the New York state cohort. *Am J Epidemiol* 1992; 136: 1327–1337.

8   Hunter DJ, Mason JE, Colditz GA. A prospective study of the intake of vitamins C, E and A and risk of breast cancer. *N Engl J Med* 1993; 329: 324–340.

9   Rohan TE, Howe GR, Friedenreich CM, *et al*. Dietary fiber, vitamins A, C and E, and risk of breast cancer: a cohort study. *Cancer Causes Control* 1993; 4: 29–37.

10 Graham S, Marshall B, Haughey B. Dietary epidemiology of cancer of colon in western New York. *Am J Epidemiol* 1986; 128: 490–503.

11 Heilbrun LK, Nomura A, Hankin JH, Stemmerman GN. Diet and colorectal cancer with special reference to fiber intake. *Int J Cancer* 1989; 44: 1–6.

12 Comstock GW, Helzlsouer KJ, Bush TL. Prediagnostic serum levels of carotenoids and vitamin E as related to subsequent cancer in Washington County, Maryland. *Am J Clin Nutr* 1991; 53: S260–264.

13 Potter JD, McMichael AJ. Diet and cancer of the colon and rectum: a case-control study. *J Natl Cancer Inst* 1986; 76: 557–569.

14 Graham S, Haughey B, Marshall J. Diet in the epidemiology of carcinoma of the prostate gland. *J Natl Cancer Inst* 1983: 70: 687–692.

15 Omenn GS, Goodman GE, Thornquist MD, *et al*. Effects of a combination of betacarotene and vitamin A on lung cancer and cardiovascular disease. *N Engl J Med* 1996; 334: 1150–1155.

16 De Klerk N, Musk W, Ambrosini G, *et al*. Vitamin A and cancer prevention II: comparison of the effects of vitamin A and betacarotene. *Int J Cancer* 1998; 75: 362–367.

17 Musk W, De Klerk N, Ambrosini G, *et al*. Vitamin A and cancer prevention I: observations in workers previously exposed to asbestos at Wittnoom, western Australia. *Int J Cancer* 1998; 75: 355–361.

18 Botterweck AA, van Den Brandt PA, Goldbohm RA. Vitamins, carotenoids, dietary fiber, and the risk of gastric carcinoma: Results from a prospective study after 6.3 years of follow-up. *Cancer* 2000; 88: 737–748.

19 Pinnock CB, Alderman CP. The potential for teratogenicity of vitamin A and its congeners. *Med J Aust* 1992; 157: 804–809.

20 Underwood BA. Teratogenicity of vitamin A. *Int J Vit Nutr Res* 1989; 30 (Suppl): 42–55.

21 Dudas I, Czeizel AE. Use of 6,000 IU vitamin A during early pregnancy without teratogenic effect (letter). *Teratology* 1992; 45: 335–336.

22 Rothman KJ, Moore LL, Singer MR, *et al*. Teratogenicity of high vitamin A intake. *N Engl J Med* 1995; 333: 1369–1373.

23 Mastroiacovo P, Mazzone T, Addis A, *et al*. High vitamin A intake in early pregnancy and major malformations: a multicenter prospective controlled study. *Teratology* 1999; 59: 7–11.

24 Miller RK, Hendrickx AG, Mils JL, *et al*. Periconceptual vitamin A use: how much is teratogenic? *Reprod Toxicol* 1998; 12: 75–88.

25 Melhus H, Michaelsson K, Kindmark A, *et al*. Excessive dietary intake of vitamin A is associated with reduced bone mineral density and increased risk for hip fracture. *Ann Intern Med* 1998; 129: 770–778.

26 Feskanich D, Singh V, Willet WC, Colditz GA. Vitamin A intake and hip fractures among postmenopausal women. *JAMA* 2002; 287: 47–54.

27 Michaelsson K, Lithell H, Vessby B, Melhus H. Serum retinol levels and the risk of fracture. *N Engl J Med* 2003; 348: 287–294.

28 Kawahara TN, Krieger DC, Engelke JA, *et al*. Short-term vitamin A supplementation does not affect bone turnover in men. *J Nutr* 2002; 132: 1169–1172.

29 Lim LS, Harnack LJ, Lazovich D, Folsom AR. Vitamin A intake and the risk of hip fracture in postmenopausal women: the Iowa Women's Health Study. *Osteoporosis Int* 2004; 15: 552–559.

30 Rejnmark L, Vestergaard P, Charles P, *et al*. No effect of vitamin A intake on bone mineral density and fracture risk in perimenopausal women. *Osteoporosis Int* 2004; 165: 872–880.

31 Barker ME, McCloskey E, Saha S, *et al*. Serum retinoids and beta-carotene as predictors of hip and other fractures in elderly women. *J Bone Miner Res* 2005; 20: 913–920.

32 Jackson HA, Sheehan HA. Effect of vitamin A on fracture risk. *Ann Pharmacother* 2005; 39: 2086–2090.

Vitamin B$_6$

Description

Vitamin B$_6$ is a water-soluble member of the vitamin B complex.

Nomenclature

Vitamin B$_6$ is a generic term used to describe compounds that exhibit the biological activity of pyridoxine. It occurs in food as pyridoxine, pyridoxal and pyridoxamine. Thus the term 'pyridoxine' is not synonymous with the generic term 'vitamin B$_6$'.

Human requirements

Vitamin B$_6$ requirements depend on protein intake; values are therefore given as µg/g protein and also as total values (Table 1).

Dietary intake

In the UK, the average adult daily diet provides: for men, 2.9 mg; for women, 2.0 mg.

Action

Vitamin B$_6$ is converted in erythrocytes to pyridoxal phosphate and, to a lesser extent, pyridoxamine phosphate. It acts as a cofactor for enzymes that are involved in more than 100 reactions affecting protein, lipid and carbohydrate metabolism. Pyridoxal phosphate is also involved in the synthesis of several neurotransmitters; the metabolism of several vitamins (e.g. the conversion of tryptophan to niacin); and haemoglobin and sphingosine formation.

Dietary sources

See Table 2 for dietary sources of vitamin B$_6$.

Metabolism

Absorption

Absorption occurs mainly by a non-saturable process (absorption is greatest in the jejunum).

Distribution

Vitamin B$_6$ is stored in the liver, muscle and brain. Pyridoxal phosphate is transported in the plasma (bound to albumin) and in erythrocytes (in association with haemoglobin).

Elimination

Primarily in the urine (mainly as metabolites), but excess amounts are excreted largely unchanged. It also appears in breast milk.

Bioavailability

Bioavailability of vitamin B$_6$ is affected by food processing and storage. The vitamin is sensitive to light, especially in acid or neutral solutions.

Deficiency

Deficiency of vitamin B$_6$ does not produce a characteristic syndrome, but as with deficiency of the other B vitamins, symptoms such as dermatitis, cheilosis, glossitis and angular stomatitis may occur. Advanced deficiency may produce weakness, irritability, depression, dizziness, peripheral neuropathy and seizures; diarrhoea, anaemia and seizures are particular characteristics of deficiency in infants and children. Chronic deficiency may lead to secondary hyperoxaluria (increased risk of kidney stone

Table 1 Dietary Reference Values for vitamin B$_6$ (mg/day)

								EU RDA = 2 mg
Age	UK					USA		FAO/WHO
	LNRI[1]	EAR[1]	RNI[1]	RNI[2]	EVM	RDA[2]	TUL[2]	RNI[2]
0–6 months	3.5	6	8	0.2		0.1[3]	–	0.1
7–9 months	6	8	10	0.3		0.3[3]	–	0.3
10–12 months	8	10	13	0.4		0.3	–	0.3
1–3 years	8	10	13	0.7		0.5	30	0.5
4–6 years	8	10	13	0.9		–	–	0.6
4–8 years	–	–	–	–		0.6	40	–
7–10 years	8	10	13	1.0		–	–	1.0[a]
9–13 years						1.0	60	–
Males								
11–14 years	11	13	15	1.2		–	–	1.3[b]
14–18 years						1.3	80	1.3
15–18 years	11	13	15	1.4				–
19–50+ years	11	13	15	1.4	10	1.3	100	1.3
51–70+ years	–	–	–	–	10	1.7	100	1.7
Females								
11–14 years	11	13	15	1.0		–	–	1.2[b]
14–18 years	–	–	–	–		1.2	80	1.2
15–18 years	11	13	15	1.2		–	–	–
19–50+ years	11	13	15	1.2	10	1.3	100	1.3
51–70+ years	–	–	–	–	10	1.5	100	1.5
Pregnancy	*	*	*	*		1.9	100[4]	1.9
Lactation	*	*	*	*		2.0	100[4]	2.0

*no increment.

[a] 7–9 years.   [b] 10–14 years.

[1] µg/g protein.   [2] mg/day.   [3] Adequate Intakes (AIs).   [4] ≤18 years = 80 mg.

EVM = Likely safe daily intake from supplements alone.

TUL = Tolerable Upper Intake Level from food and supplements.

formation) and to hypochromic, microcytic anaemia.

Possible uses

Vitamin B$_6$ has been investigated for a range of conditions, including carpal tunnel syndrome, PMS, asthma, diabetic neuropathy, CVD and autism.

Carpal tunnel syndrome

Idiopathic carpal tunnel syndrome, with swelling of the synovia and compression of the median nerve by the transverse carpal ligament, has been attributed to pyridoxine deficiency.[1,2] Several uncontrolled studies in the 1980s demonstrated the efficacy of vitamin B$_6$ treatment.[3–5] However, another study showed no consistent improvement in patients with carpal tunnel syndrome and normal vitamin B$_6$ status.[6] These findings led to the suggestion[7] that clinical improvement in some patients with carpal tunnel syndrome may be due to correction of unrecognised peripheral neuropathy, which could compound symptoms of the

Table 2 Dietary sources of vitamin B$_6$

Food portion	Vitamin B$_6$ content (mg)
Breakfast cereals	
1 bowl All-Bran (45 g)	**0.6**
1 bowl Bran Flakes (45 g)	**0.8**
1 bowl Corn Flakes (30 g)	**0.6**
1 bowl muesli (95 g)	**1.5**
1 bowl Start (40 g)	**1.1**
2 Weetabix	**0.4**
Milk and dairy products	
½ pint milk, whole, semi-skimmed or skimmed	0.15
½ pint soya milk	0.15
Meat and fish	
Beef, roast (85 g)	0.3
Lamb, roast (85 g)	0.2
Pork, roast (85 g)	0.3
2 slices ham	0.3
1 chicken leg portion	0.3
Liver, lambs, cooked (90 g)	**0.4**
Kidney, lambs, cooked (75 g)	0.2
Fish, cooked (150 g)	**0.5**
Vegetables	
Potatoes, boiled (150 g)	**0.5**
1 small can baked beans (200 g)	0.3
Fruit	
½ an avocado pear	**0.4**
1 banana	0.3
Nuts	
30 peanuts	0.2
Yeast	
Brewer's yeast (10 g)	0.2

Excellent sources (**bold**); good sources (*italics*).

syndrome. A review article concluded that studies have not provided sufficient evidence for the use of vitamin B$_6$ as the sole treatment for carpal tunnel syndrome, but that it could be of some benefit as adjunct therapy because of its potential benefit on pain perception and increasing pain threshold.[8]

Premenstrual syndrome

Pyridoxine has been reported to be of benefit in PMS,[9–11] but some researchers have found no significant benefit.[12–14] Doses of pyridoxine that have shown beneficial effects have been relatively high (500 mg daily) and these high doses should not be recommended because of the risk of toxicity. However, a good response has been reported with a dose of 50 mg daily.[15] Studies are complicated by the subjective nature of symptoms in PMS, and conclusions are limited by the low quality of many of the trials. Nevertheless, a systematic review[16] of nine published trials representing 940 patients with premenstrual syndrome suggests that doses of vitamin B$_6$ up to 100 mg daily are likely to be of benefit in treating premenstrual symptoms and premenstrual depression.

Asthma

Low vitamin B$_6$ status has been reported in adults with asthma,[17,18] and in asthmatic children.[19] This may in part be due to use of theophylline (which was more commonly used in the USA at the time of the studies), which reduces vitamin B status.[20,21] A supplement of 15 mg of pyridoxine per day reduced side-effects of theophylline related to nervous system function.[22]

Vitamin B$_6$ supplementation (50 mg daily) reduced the severity and frequency of asthma attacks,[18] and pyridoxine (200 mg daily) reduced the need for asthma medication in children.[23] However, a dose of 300 mg daily failed to improve asthma in patients requiring steroids.[24]

Diabetic neuropathy

Peripheral neuropathy in patients with diabetes has been suggested to be associated with pyridoxine deficiency. Diabetic patients with symptoms of neuropathy and low vitamin B$_6$ status were given 150 mg of vitamin B$_6$ daily for 6 weeks.[25] Neuropathic symptoms were eliminated in all subjects. The same dose of pyridoxine gradually improved pain in patients with painful neuropathy.[26] In diabetic patients whose vitamin B$_6$ status was normal, pyridoxine supplementation resulted in no improvement in neuropathic symptoms.[27] Further studies are required to investigate the possible benefits of vitamin B$_6$ in diabetic neuropathy.

Coronary heart disease

A raised level of plasma homocysteine is associated with an increased risk of CHD. This in turn has been linked with low intake and low level of folic acid and other B vitamins, including vitamin B$_6$. However, whether vitamin B$_6$ has an influence independent of folic acid is uncertain. In the Framingham Heart Study,[28] folic acid, vitamin B$_6$ and vitamin B$_{12}$ were determinants of homocysteine levels, with folic acid showing the strongest association. In the Nurse's Health Study,[29] those with the highest vitamin B$_6$ intake had a 33% lower risk of heart disease than those with the lowest intake, while in those with the highest intake of both vitamin B$_6$ and folate, the risk of heart disease was reduced by 45%. In a prospective, case-cohort study, heart disease was negatively associated with plasma vitamin B$_6$ in both men and women, and after correcting for a large number of risk factors, the association with pyridoxine still held, pointing to the possibility that vitamin B$_6$ offers independent protection.[30] However, two meta-analyses[31,32] concluded that although folic acid reduced plasma homocysteine, vitamin B$_6$ had no additional effect. In a recent Swiss RCT, 553 patients who had undergone percutaneous coronary intervention were randomised to receive a combination of vitamin B$_6$ (10 mg daily), vitamin B$_{12}$ (400 µg daily) and folic acid 1 mg daily. This vitamin combination was found to significantly reduce the incidence of major adverse events after percutaneous coronary intervention.[33]

Miscellaneous

Pyridoxine has also been reported to be effective in treating pregnancy sickness[34,35] and hypertension.[36] Some studies have shown it to be effective for depression,[37,38] but a systematic review concluded that meaningful benefit was not apparent.[39]

Autism has also been shown to respond to vitamin therapy, including vitamin B$_6$, but a review of 12 studies using vitamin B$_6$ and magnesium concluded that although results were favourable, studies suffered from methodological problems of poor design, small numbers of subjects and lack of long-term follow-up.[40] A Cochrane review investigated the effect of vitamin B$_6$ and magnesium in autism but due to the small number of studies, the methodological quality and small sample sizes, the review

concluded that no recommendation could be made regarding the use of vitamin B$_6$ and magnesium for autism.[41]

Vitamin B$_6$ has also been investigated for a possible role in cognitive function, on the basis of its possible homocysteine lowering effect. Homocysteine is a risk factor for cerebrovascular disease. However, a Cochrane review found no evidence from vitamin B$_6$ in improving cognitive function or mood.[42]

Conclusion

The role of vitamin B$_6$ supplements in carpal tunnel syndrome, PMS and asthma is controversial, although supplements may help some individuals. Low vitamin B$_6$ status has been linked with high plasma homocysteine levels and increased risk of CHD, but whether vitamin B$_6$ has an effect independent of folic acid and vitamin B$_{12}$ is not yet clear. Further properly controlled clinical trials are needed to assess the benefit of vitamin B$_6$ supplements for all these purposes, as well as for autism, depression and pregnancy sickness.

Precautions/contraindications

Hypersensitivity to pyridoxine.

Pregnancy and breast-feeding

No problems reported with normal intakes. Large doses may result in pyridoxine dependency in infants. There has been one report of amelia of the leg at the knee in an infant whose mother had taken 50 mg pyridoxine daily during pregnancy.

Adverse effects

Peripheral neuropathy; unsteady gait; numbness and tingling in feet and hands; loss of limb reflexes; impaired or absent tendon reflexes; photosensitivity on exposure to sun; dizziness; nausea; breast tenderness; exacerbation of acne.

Adverse effects usually occur with large doses only. Doses of 100–150 mg daily over 5–10 years have not generally been associated with toxicity. However, doses averaging 117 mg daily have been associated with neurological symptoms (e.g. numbness, tingling, bone pain) in 60% of women taking supplements for 3 years, but this study has been severely criticised. Moreover, symptoms were reversed 6 months after patients stopped taking the supplement.[43] Another paper reported that women taking 500–5000 mg daily for PMS developed peripheral neuropathy over a 1- to 3-year period.[44]

Interactions

Drugs

Alcohol: increases turnover of pyridoxine.
Cycloserine: may cause anaemia or peripheral neuritis by acting as pyridoxine antagonist.
Hydralazine: may cause anaemia or peripheral neuritis by acting as pyridoxine antagonist.
Isoniazid: may cause anaemia or peripheral neuritis by acting as pyridoxine antagonist.
Levodopa: effects of levodopa are reversed by pyridoxine (even doses as low as 5 mg daily); vitamin B$_6$ supplements should be avoided; interaction does not occur with co-beneldopa or co-careldopa.
Oestrogens: (including oral contraceptives) may increase requirement for vitamin B$_6$.
Penicillamine: may cause anaemia or peripheral neuritis by acting as pyridoxine antagonist.
Theophylline: may increase requirement for vitamin B$_6$.

Nutrients

Adequate amounts of all B vitamins are required for optimal functioning; deficiency or excess of one B vitamin may lead to abnormalities in the metabolism of another.
Vitamin C: deficiency of vitamin B$_6$ may lead to vitamin C deficiency.

Dose

As a dietary supplement, 2–5 mg daily.

References

1 Ellis J, Azuma J, Watanebe T, *et al*. Survey and new data on treatment with pyridoxine of patients having a clinical syndrome including carpal tunnel and other defects. *Res Commun Chem Pathol Pharmacol* 1977; 17: 165–177.

2 Fuhr JE, Farrow A, Nelson HS Jr. Vitamin B6 levels in patients with carpal tunnel syndrome. *Arch Surg* 1989; 124: 1329–1330.

3 Driskell JA, Wesley RL, Hess IE. Effectiveness of pyridoxine hydrochloride treatment on carpal tunnel syndrome patients. *Nutr Rep Int* 1986; 34: 1031–1040.

4 Ellis J, Folkers K, Levy M, *et al*. Therapy with vitamin B6 with and without surgery for treatment of patients having the idiopathic carpal tunnel syndrome. *Res Commun Chem Pathol Pharmacol* 1981; 33: 331–344.

5 Ellis J, Folkers K, Watanebe T, *et al*. Clinical results of a crossover treatment with pyridoxine and placebo of the carpal tunnel syndrome. *Am J Clin Nutr* 1979; 32: 2040–2046.

6 Smith GP, Rudge PJ, Peters TJ. Biochemical studies of pyridoxal and pyridoxal phosphate status and therapeutic trial of pyridoxine in patients with carpal tunnel syndrome. *Ann Neurol* 1984; 15: 104–107.

7 Byers CM, DeLisa JA, Frankel DL, Kraft GH. Pyridoxine metabolism in carpal tunnel syndrome with and without peripheral neuropathy. *Arch Phys Med Rehabil* 1984; 65: 712–716.

8 Jacobson MD, Plancher KD, Kleinman WB. Vitamin B$_6$ (pyridoxine) therapy for carpal tunnel syndrome. *Hand Clin* 1996; 12: 253–257.

9 Barr W. Pyridoxine supplements in the premenstrual syndrome. *Practitioner* 1984; 228: 425–427.

10 Day JB. Clinical trials in the premenstrual syndrome. *Curr Med Res Opin* 1979; 6: 40–45.

11 Kerr GD. The management of premenstrual syndrome. *Curr Med Res Opin* 1977; 4: 29–34.

12 Hagen I, Neshmein BI, Tuntlund T. No effect of vitamin B6 against premenstrual tension. *Acta Obstet Gynecol Scand* 1985; 64: 667–670.

13 Malmgren R, Collins A, Nilsson CG. Platelet serotonin uptake and effects of vitamin B6 treatment in premenstrual tension. *Neurophysiology* 1987; 18: 83–88.

14 Smallwood J, Ah-Kye D, Taylor I. Vitamin B6 in the treatment of pre-menstrual mastalgia. *Br J Clin Pract* 1986; 40: 532–533.

15 Mattes JA, Martin D. Pyridoxine in premenstrual depression. *Hum Nutr Appl Nutr* 1982; 36A: 131–133.

16 Wyatt KM, Dimmock PW, Jones PW, *et al*. Efficacy of vitamin B6 in the treatment of premenstrual syndrome. *BMJ* 1999; 318: 1375–1381.

17 Delport R, Ubbink JB, Serfontein WJ, *et al*. Vitamin B6 nutritional status in asthma: the effect of theophylline therapy on plasma pyridoxal-5'-phosphate and pyridoxal levels. *Int J Vit Nutr Res* 1988; 58: 67–72.

18 Reynolds RD, Natta CL. Depressed plasma pyridoxal phosphate concentrations in adult asthmatics. *Am J Clin Nutr* 1985; 41: 684–688.

19 Hall MA, Thom H, Russell G. Erythrocyte aspartate aminotransferase activity in asthmatic and non-asthmatic children and its enhancement by vitamin B6. *Ann Allergy* 1985; 47: 464–466.

20 Ubbink JB, Vermaak WJH, Delport R, *et al.* The relationship between vitamin B6 metabolism, asthma and theophylline therapy. *Ann NY Acad Sci* 1990; 585: 285–294.

21 Shimizu T, Maesda S, Arakawa H, *et al.* Relation between theophylline and circulating levels in children with asthma. *Pharmacology* 1996; 53: 384–389.

22 Bartel PR, Ubbink JB, Delport R, *et al.* Vitamin B6 supplementation and theophylline-related effects in humans. *Am J Clin Nutr* 1994; 60: 93–99.

23 Collipp PJ, Goldzier S, Weiss N, *et al.* Pyridoxine treatment in childhood bronchial asthma. *Ann Allergy* 1977; 35: 93–97.

24 Sur S, Camara M, Buchmeier A, *et al.* Double-blind trial of pyridoxine (vitamin B6) in the treatment of steroid-dependent asthma. *Ann Allergy* 1993; 70: 147–152.

25 Jones CL, Gonzalez V. Pyridoxine deficiency: a new factor in diabetic neuropathy. *J Am Podiatr Ass* 1978; 68: 646–653.

26 Bernstein AL, Lobitz CZ. A clinical and electrophysiologic study of the treatment of painful diabetic neuropathies with pyridoxine. In: Leklem JE, Reynolds RD, eds. *Clinical and Physiological Applications of Vitamin B$_6$.* New York: Alan R Liss, 1988: 415–423.

27 Levin ER, Hanscomb TA, Fisher M, *et al.* The influence of pyridoxine in diabetic neuropathy. *Diabetes Care* 1981; 4: 606–609.

28 Selhub J, Jaques PF, Wilson PWF, *et al.* Vitamin status and intake as primary determinants of homocystinaemia in an elderly population. *JAMA* 1993; 270: 2693–2698.

29 Rimm EB, Willett WC, Hu FB, *et al.* Folate and vitamin B$_6$ from diet and supplements in relation to risk of coronary heart disease among women. *JAMA* 1998; 279: 359–364.

30 Folsom AR, Nieto FJ, McGovern PG, *et al.* Prospective study of coronary heart disease incidence in relation to fasting total homocysteine, related genetic polymorphisms, and B vitamins: the Atherosclerosis Risk in Communities (ARIC) study. *Circulation* 1998; 98: 204–210.

31 Homocysteine Lowering Trialists' Collaboration. Lowering blood homocysteine with folic acid based supplements; meta-analysis of randomised trials. *BMJ* 1998; 316: 894–898.

32 Homocysteine Lowering Trialists' Collaboration. Dose-dependent effects of folic acid on blood concentrations of homocysteine: a meta-analysis of the randomized trials. *Am J Clin Nutr* 2005; 82: 806–812.

33 Schynder G, Roffi M, Flammer Y, *et al.* Effect of homocysteine-lowering therapy with folic acid, vitamin B12, and vitamin B6 on clinical outcome after percutaneous coronary intervention: the Swiss Heart Study: a randomized controlled trial. *JAMA* 2002; 288: 973–979.

34 Sahakian V, Rouse D, Sipes S. Vitamin B$_6$ is effective therapy for nausea and vomiting of pregnancy: a randomised, double-blind, placebo controlled study. *Obstet Gynecol* 1991; 78: 33–36.

35 Vutyavenich T, Wongra-ngan S, Ruangsvi R. Pyridoxine for nausea and vomiting of pregnancy: a randomised, double-blind, placebo-controlled trial. *Am J Obstet Gynecol* 1995; 173: 881–884.

36 Ayback M, Sermet A, Ayyildiz MO. Effect of oral pyridoxine hydrochloride supplementation on arterial blood pressure in patients with essential hypertension. *Arzneimittelforschung* 1995; 45: 1271–1273.

37 Bell IR, Edman JS, Marrow FD. B complex vitamin patterns in geriatric and young adult inpatients with major depression. *J Am Geriatr Soc* 1991; 39: 252–257.

38 Russ CS, Hendricks TA, Chrisley BM. Vitamin B6 status of depressed and obsessive-compulsive patients. *Nutr Rep Int* 1983; 27: 867–873.

39 Williams AL, Cotter A, Sabina A, *et al.* The role of vitamin B6 as treatment for depression: a systematic review. *Fam Pract* 2005; 22: 532–537.

40 Pfeiffer SI, Norton J, Nelson L, *et al.* Efficacy of vitamin B$_6$ and magnesium in the treatment of autism. *J Autism Dev Disord* 1995; 25: 481–483.

41 Nye C, Brice A. Combined vitamin B6-magnesium treatment in autism spectrum disorder. Cochrane database, issue 4, 2005. London: Macmillan.

42 Malouf R, Grimley Evans J. Vitamin B6 for cognition. Cochrane database, issue 2, 2003. London: Macmillan.

43 Dalton K, Dalton MJ. Characteristics of pyridoxine overdose neuropathy syndrome. *Acta Neurol Scand* 1987; 76: 8–11.

44 Bernstein AL. Vitamin B$_6$ in clinical neurology. *Ann NY Acad Sci* 1990; 585: 250–260.

Vitamin B$_{12}$

Description

Vitamin B$_{12}$ is a water-soluble member of the vitamin B complex.

Nomenclature

Vitamin B$_{12}$ is the generic term used to describe compounds that exhibit the biological activity of cyanocobalamin. It includes a range of cobalt-containing compounds, known as cobalamins. Cyanocobalamin and hydroxocobalamin are the two principal forms in clinical use.

Human requirements

See Table 1 for Dietary Reference Values for vitamin B$_{12}$.

Dietary intake

In the UK, the average adult daily diet provides: for men, 6.5 µg; for women, 4.8 µg.

Action

Vitamin B$_{12}$ is involved in the recycling of folate coenzymes and the degradation of valine. It is also required for nerve myelination, cell replication, haematopoiesis and nucleoprotein synthesis.

Dietary sources

See Table 2 for dietary sources of vitamin B$_{12}$.

Metabolism

Absorption

Absorption occurs almost exclusively in the terminal ileum by an active saturable process, but large amounts (>30 µg) may also be absorbed by passive diffusion (a maximum of 1.5 µg may be absorbed from oral doses of 5–50 µg). For normal absorption, the vitamin must bind to salivary haptocorrin and then to 'intrinsic factor', a highly specific glycoprotein secreted by the parietal cells of the stomach.

Distribution

Vitamin B$_{12}$ is stored mainly in the liver. In the blood, it is bound to specific plasma proteins (transcobalamins).

Elimination

Elimination is via the urinary, biliary and faecal routes. Enterohepatic recycling serves to conserve B$_{12}$. Vitamin B$_{12}$ appears in breast milk.

Deficiency

Deficiency of vitamin B$_{12}$ leads to macrocytic, megaloblastic anaemia. Symptoms include neurological manifestations (due to demyelination of the spinal cord, brain, and optic and peripheral nerves), and less specific symptoms such as weakness, sore tongue, constipation and postural hypotension. Neuropsychiatric manifestations of deficiency may occur in the absence of anaemia (particularly in the elderly).

Pernicious anaemia is a specific form of anaemia caused by lack of intrinsic factor (not lack of vitamin B$_{12}$ in the diet).

Individuals with a reduced ability to absorb vitamin B$_{12}$ develop deficiency within 2–3 years.

Table 1   Dietary Reference Values for vitamin B$_{12}$ (µg/day)

							EU RDA = 1 µg
Age	UK				USA		FAO/WHO
	LNRI	EAR	RNI	EVM	RDA	TUL	RNI
0–6 months	0.1	0.25	0.3		0.4	–	0.4
7–12 months	0.25	0.35	0.4		0.5	–	0.5
1–3 years	0.3	0.4	0.5		0.9	–	0.9
4–6 years	0.5	0.7	0.8			–	1.2
4–8 years					1.2	–	–
7–10 years	0.6	0.8	1.0		–	–	1.8[a]
9–13 years					1.8	–	–
Males							
11–14 years	0.8	1.0	1.2		–	–	2.4[b]
15–50+ years	1.0	1.25	1.5	1000	–	–	2.4
14–70+ years					2.4	–	–
Females							
11–14 years	0.8	1.0	1.2		–	–	2.4[b]
15–50+ years	1.0	1.25	1.5	1000	–	–	2.4
14–70+ years					2.4	–	–
Pregnancy		*			2.6	–	2.6
Lactation		+0.5			2.8	–	2.8

* No increment.
[a] 7–9 years.   [b] 10–14 years.
EVM = Likely safe daily intake from supplements alone.
TUL = Tolerable Upper Intake Level from food and supplements.

Strict vegetarians (at risk of dietary deficiency, but with normal absorptive efficiency) may not show signs and symptoms for 20–30 years.

Possible uses

Vegans
Vitamin B$_{12}$ is found only in animal products and certain foods fortified with the vitamin (see Table 2). If vegans do not regularly consume a source of vitamin B$_{12}$, they will require a supplement. This applies particularly to vegan women during pregnancy, as the infant may suffer deficiency. Breast-fed infants whose mothers do not take a source of B$_{12}$ should be supplemented.

The elderly
Prevalence of vitamin B$_{12}$ deficiency increases with age,[1,2] especially over the age of 65 years, and elderly people should be advised to take a supplement or obtain their requirements from fortified foods (e.g. breakfast cereals, yeast spreads). Poor vitamin B$_{12}$ (and folate) status may be associated with age-related hearing dysfunction[3] and tinnitus.[4]

Cognition
Supplementation has been used with some success in reversing impaired mental function due to low vitamin B$_{12}$ status. Several studies have shown that the best responders are those with impaired memory of <6 months' duration. In one study in 18 subjects, only those with

Table 2 Dietary sources of vitamin B$_{12}$

Food portion	Vitamin B$_{12}$ content (μg)
Breakfast cereals	
1 bowl All-Bran (45 g)	*0.5*
1 bowl Bran Flakes (45 g)	**0.8**
1 bowl Corn Flakes (30 g)	*0.5*
1 bowl Start (40 g)	**1.0**
Milk and dairy products	
½ pint milk, whole, semi-skimmed or skimmed	**1.0**
Soya milk	
Gold, ½ pint	**1.5**
Plamil, diluted, ½ pint	**3.2**
1 pot yoghurt (150 g)	*0.3*
Cheese, 50 g	**1.0**
1 egg, size 2 (60 g)	*0.4*
Fats and oils	
Butter, margarine, spreads, oils	Trace
Fortified margarine (vegetarian), 10 g	**0.5**
Meat and fish	
Meat, roast (85 g)	**1.6**
Liver, lambs, cooked (90 g)	**70.0**
Kidney, lambs, cooked (75 g)	**55.0**
White fish, cooked (150 g)	**1.5–4.0**
2 fillets herring, cooked (110 g)	**9.0**
2 fillets kipper, cooked (130 g)	**8.0**
2 fillets mackerel, cooked (110 g)	**15.0**
Pilchards, canned (100 g)	**12.0**
Sardines, canned (70 g)	**10.0**
Tuna, canned (95 g)	**4.0**
Vegetable protein mixes	
Protoveg Burgamix, 100 g	**3.6**
Protoveg Sosmix, 100 g	**1.8**
Yeast extracts	
Marmite, spread on 1 slice bread	*0.4*
Natex, spread on 1 slice bread	*0.4*
Vecon, spread on 1 slice bread	*0.6*

Note: Plant foods (unless fortified commercially) are devoid of vitamin B$_{12}$, except for the adventitious inclusion of microbiologically-formed B$_{12}$ from water or soil.
*Excellent sources (**bold**); good sources (italics).*

symptoms of <12 months' duration showed improvement with supplementation.[5]

In addition, vitamin B$_{12}$ deficiency appears to be common in patients with Alzheimer's disease.[6,7] Two Cochrane analyses[8,9] have found no evidence for vitamin B$_{12}$ for cognition and dementia.

Neural tube defects

Studies have suggested that deficiency of vitamin B$_{12}$ may be a risk factor for neural tube defects (NTDs). One study[10] showed that in affected pregnancies both plasma B$_{12}$ and folate influenced the maternal red cell folate concentration and were independent risk factors for neural defects. A systematic review of 17 case-control studies concluded that there is a moderate association between low maternal vitamin B$_{12}$ status and the risk of foetal NTDs, but that study design limited the conclusions.[11] More evidence is required before a definite recommendation can be made.

Multiple sclerosis

Vitamin B$_{12}$ has been used to treat multiple sclerosis because it was thought that it might have a role in the formation of myelin, the fatty substance that coats nerve cell axons. However, results of early studies in the 1950s and 1960s were inconclusive and interest in vitamin B$_{12}$ as a treatment for multiple sclerosis declined. Case reports[12,13] have described an association between vitamin B$_{12}$ and multiple sclerosis or clinical syndromes resembling multiple sclerosis, and it is possible that vitamin B$_{12}$ deficiency may exacerbate the disease.[14] However, other researchers have concluded that serum B$_{12}$ deficiency is uncommon in multiple sclerosis.[15] Further studies into the metabolism of vitamin B$_{12}$ in multiple sclerosis are warranted.

Sleep disorders

Results from studies investigating vitamin B$_{12}$ for sleep disorders have been equivocal. One study[16] showed that 3 mg vitamin B$_{12}$ was associated with a reduction in daytime melatonin production, improved sleep quality, and improved concentration and feelings of being refreshed the next day. Another study using the same dose of vitamin B$_{12}$ found no change in mood or daytime drowsiness or night sleep compared with placebo.[17]

Cardiovascular disease

Vitamin B$_{12}$, together with folic acid, has been found to reduce plasma homocysteine levels,[18–22] and is therefore thought to have the potential to reduce the risk of CVD.

However, low B$_{12}$ and low folate were not found to increase the risk of fatal CVD in an Australian cohort study.[23] Two large RCTs (the Heart Outcomes Prevention Evaluation[24] and the NORVIT Trial[25]) found that B$_{12}$, folic acid and B$_6$ in combination reduced plasma homocysteine, but did not reduce the risk of major cardiovascular events in patients with CVD,[24] and did not lower the risk of recurrent CVD after acute myocardial infarction.[25]

Miscellaneous

Vitamin B$_{12}$ has been used with some success in patients with diabetic neuropathy[26,27] and mouth ulcers.[28] Low serum levels of vitamin B$_{12}$ have been found in patients with HIV,[29] and have also been associated with a faster progress towards AIDS.[30] A Japanese study in patients with stroke found that vitamin B$_{12}$ may also reduce the risk of hip fractures.[31]

Conclusion

Vitamin B$_{12}$ deficiency is a risk in elderly people and can progress to produce symptoms of dementia. The role of supplements in dementia caused by B$_{12}$ deficiency seems to depend on the duration of the symptoms, and there is no good evidence that supplements help to delay the progress of Alzheimer's disease unrelated to vitamin B$_{12}$ deficiency. Vitamin B$_{12}$ (with folic acid) reduces plasma homocysteine, but studies investigating its effects in CVD have produced conflicting results. There is some evidence that supplementation can improve symptoms of diabetic neuropathy, but the role of vitamin B$_{12}$ in multiple sclerosis is unclear. Further research is needed to confirm the benefits of vitamin B$_{12}$ for any indication other than deficiency or marginal deficiency.

Precautions/contraindications

Vitamin B$_{12}$ should not be given for treatment of deficiency until the diagnosis is fully established (administration of > 10 µg daily may produce a haematological response in patients with folate deficiency).

Pregnancy and breast-feeding

No problems reported with normal intakes.

Adverse effects

Vitamin B$_{12}$ may occasionally cause diarrhoea and itching skin. Signs of polycythaemia vera may be unmasked. Megadoses may exacerbate acne.

Interactions

Drugs

Alcohol: excessive intake may reduce the absorption of vitamin B$_{12}$.
Aminoglycosides: may reduce the absorption of vitamin B$_{12}$.
Aminosalicylates: may reduce the absorption of vitamin B$_{12}$.
Antibiotics: may interfere with microbiological assay for serum and erythrocyte vitamin B$_{12}$ (false low results).
Chloramphenicol: may reduce the absorption of vitamin B$_{12}$.
Colestyramine: may reduce the absorption of vitamin B$_{12}$.
Colchicine: may reduce the absorption of vitamin B$_{12}$.
Histamine H$_2$-receptor antagonists: may reduce the absorption of vitamin B$_{12}$.
Metformin: may reduce the absorption of vitamin B$_{12}$.
Methyldopa: may reduce the absorption of vitamin B$_{12}$.
Nitrous oxide: prolonged nitrous oxide anaesthesia inactivates vitamin B$_{12}$.
Oral contraceptives: may reduce blood levels of vitamin B$_{12}$.
Potassium chloride (modified release): prolonged administration may reduce the absorption of vitamin B$_{12}$.
Proton-pump inhibitors: long-term therapy may reduce serum vitamin B$_{12}$ levels.

Nutrients

Folic acid: large doses given continuously may reduce vitamin B$_{12}$ in blood.

Vitamin C: may destroy vitamin B$_{12}$ (avoid large doses of vitamin C within 1 h of oral vitamin B$_{12}$).

Dose

Vitamin B$_{12}$ is available in the form of tablets and capsules, and is also found in many multi-vitamin supplements. Deficiency of vitamin B$_{12}$ due to lack of intrinsic factor is generally treated with parenteral cobalamin, but one study showed that 2 mg daily given orally was as efficient as 1 mg given intramuscularly each month.

In cases of deficiency, 2–25 µg daily are needed.

References

1 Sabler SP, Lindenbaum J, Allen RH. Vitamin B-12 deficiency in the elderly: current dilemmas. *Am J Clin Nutr* 1997; 66: 741–749.

2 Baik HW, Russell RM. Vitamin B12 deficiency in the elderly. *Ann Rev Nutr* 1999; 19: 357–377.

3 Houston DK, Johnson MA, Nozza RJ, *et al*. Age-related hearing loss, vitamin B-12, and folate in elderly women. *Am J Clin Nutr* 1999; 69: 564–571.

4 Shemesh Z, Attias J, Ornana M, *et al*. Vitamin B$_{12}$ deficiency in patients with chronic tinnitus and noise induced hearing loss. *Am J Otolaryngol* 1993; 14: 94–99.

5 Martin DC, Francis J, Protetch J, *et al*. Time dependency of cognitive recovery with cobalamin replacement: a report of a pilot study. *J Am Geriatr Soc* 1992; 40: 168–172.

6 Abalan F, Delile JM. B12 deficiency in presenile dementia. *Biol Psychiatr* 1985; 20: 1251.

7 Levitt AJ, Karlinsky H. Folate, vitamin B12 and cognitive impairment in patients with Alzheimer's disease. *Acta Psychiatr Scand* 1992; 86: 301–305.

8 Malouf R, Areosa Sastre A. Vitamin B12 for cognition. Cochrane database, issue 3, 2003. London: Macmillan.

9 Malouf R, Grimley Evans J, Sastre A. Folic acid with or without vitamin B12 for cognition and dementia. Cochrane database, issue 4, 2003. London: Macmillan.

10 Kirke PM, Molly AM, Daly LE, *et al*. Maternal plasma folate and vitamin B12 are independent risk factors for neural tube defects. *Q J Med* 1993; 86: 703–708.

11 Ray JG, Blom HJ. Vitamin B12 insufficiency and the risk of fetal neural tube defects. *Q J Med* 2003; 96: 289–295.

12 Ransohoff RM, Jacobsen DW, Green R. Vitamin B12 deficiency and multiple sclerosis. *Lancet* 1990; 1: 1285–1286.

13 Reynolds EH, Linnell JC. Vitamin B12 deficiency, demyelination and multiple sclerosis. *Lancet* 1987; 2: 920.

14 Reynolds E. Multiple sclerosis and vitamin B12 metabolism. *J Neuroimmunol* 1992; 40: 225–230.

15 Sandyk R, Awerbuch G. Vitamin B12 and its relationship to age of onset to multiple sclerosis. *Int J Neurosci* 1993; 71: 93–99.

16 Mayer G, Krozer M, Meier-Ewert K. Effects of vitamin B$_{12}$ on performance and circadian rhythm in normal subjects. *Neuropsychopharmacology* 1996; 15: 456–464.

17 Okawa M, Takahashi K, Egashira K, *et al*. Vitamin B$_{12}$ treatment for delayed sleep phase syndrome: a multi-center double-blind study. *Psychiatry Clin Neurosci* 1997; 51: 275–279.

18 Schynder G, Roffi M, Flammer Y, *et al*. Effect of homocysteine-lowering therapy with folic acid, vitamin B12, and vitamin B6 on clinical outcome after percutaneous coronary intervention: the Swiss Heart Study: a randomized controlled trial. *JAMA* 2002; 288: 973–979.

19 Lee BJ, Huang MC, Chung LJ, *et al*. Folic acid and vitamin B12 are more effective than vitamin B6 in lowering fasting plasma homocysteine concentration in patients with coronary artery disease. *Eur J Clin Nutr* 2004; 58: 481–487.

20 Homocysteine Lowering Trialists' Collaboration. Dose-dependent effects of folic acid on blood concentrations of homocysteine: a meta-analysis of the randomized trials. *Am J Clin Nutr* 2005; 82: 806–812.

21 Spence JD, Bang H, Chambless LE, Stampfer MJ. Vitamin Intervention for Stroke Prevention Trial: an efficacy analysis. *Stroke* 2005; 36: 2404–2409.

22 Flicker L, Vasikaran SD, Thomas J, *et al*. Efficacy of B vitamins in lowering homocysteine in older men: maximal effects for those with B12 deficiency and hyperhomocysteinemia. *Stroke* 2006; 37: 547–549.

23 Hung J, Beilby JP, Knuimaqn MW, Divitini M. Folate and vitamin B12 and risk of fatal cardiovascular disease: cohort study from Busselton, Western Australia. *BMJ* 2003; 326: 131.

24 The Heart Outcomes Prevention Evaluation (HOPE) 2 Investigators. Homocysteine lowering with folic acid and B vitamins in vascular disease. *N Engl J Med* 2006; 354: 1567–1577.

25 Bonaa KH, Njolstad I, Ueland PM, *et al* for the NORVIT Trial Investigators. Homocysteine

lowering and cardiovascular events after acute myocardial infarction. *N Engl J Med* 2006; 354: 1578–1588.

26 Yaqub BA, Siddique A, Sulimani R. Effects of methylcobalamin on diabetic neuropathy. *Clin Neurol Neurosurg* 1992; 94: 105–111.

27 Sun Y, Lai MS, Lu CJ. Effectiveness of vitamin B12 on diabetic neuropathy: systematic review of clinical controlled trials. *Acta Neurol Taiwan* 2005; 14: 48–54.

28 Weusten BL, van de Wile A. Aphthous ulcers and vitamin B12 deficiency. *Neth J Med* 1998; 53: 172–175.

29 Paltiel O, Falutz J, Veilleux M, *et al*. Clinical correlates of subnormal vitamin B$_{12}$ levels in patient infected with human immunodeficiency virus. *Am J Hematol* 1995; 49: 318–322.

30 Tang AM, Graham NM, Chandra RK, *et al*. Low serum vitamin B-12 concentrations are associated with faster human immunodeficiency virus type 1 (HIV-1) disease progression. *J Nutr* 1997; 127: 345–351.

31 Sato Y, Honda Y, Iwamoto J, *et al*. Effect of folate and mecobalamin on hip fractures in patients with stroke: a randomized controlled trial. *JAMA* 2005; 293: 1082–1088.

Vitamin C

Description
Vitamin C is a water-soluble vitamin.

Nomenclature
Vitamin C is a generic term used to describe compounds that exhibit the biological activity of ascorbic acid. These include L-ascorbic acid (ascorbic acid) and L-dehydroascorbic acid (dehydroascorbic acid).

Human requirements
See Table 1 for Dietary Reference Values for Vitamin C.

Dietary intake
In the UK, the average adult daily diet provides: for men, 83.4 mg; for women, 81.0 mg.

Action
The functions of vitamin C are based mainly on its properties as a reducing agent. It is required for:

- the formation of collagen and other organic constituents of the intercellular matrix in bone, teeth and capillaries; and
- the optimal activity of several enzymes – it activates certain liver-detoxifying enzyme systems (including drug-metabolising enzymes) and is involved in the synthesis of carnitine and noradrenaline and the metabolism of folic acid, histamine, phenylalanine, tryptophan and tyrosine.

Vitamin C also acts:

- as an antioxidant (reacting directly with aqueous free radicals), which is important in the protection of cellular function; and
- to enhance the intestinal absorption of non-haem iron.

Dietary sources
See Table 2 for dietary sources of vitamin C.

Metabolism
Absorption
Vitamin C is absorbed by passive and active transport mechanisms, predominantly in the distal portion of the small intestine (jejunum) and to a lesser extent in the mouth, stomach and proximal intestine. Some 70–90% of the dietary intake is absorbed, but absorption falls to 50% with a dose of 1.5 g.

Distribution
It is transported in the free form (higher concentrations in leukocytes and platelets than red blood cells and plasma), and is readily taken up by body tissues (highest concentration in glandular tissue, e.g. adrenals and pituitary); body stores are generally about 1.5 g.

Elimination
The urine is the main route of elimination, but very little is excreted unchanged (unless plasma concentration >1.4 mg/100 ml). Vitamin C crosses the placenta and is excreted in breast milk.

Table 1   Dietary Reference Values for vitamin C (mg/day)

	UK				USA				FAO/WHO
								EU RDA (for labelling purposes) = 60 mg	
Age	LNRI	EAR	RNI	EVM	EAR	RDA	AI	TUL	RNI
0–6 months	6	15	25		–	–	40	–	25
7–12 months	6	15	25		–	–	50	–	30
1–3 years	8	20	30		13	–	–	400	30
4–6 years	8	20	30		–	–	–	–	30
4–8 years	–	–	–		22	25	–	–	650
7–10 years	8	20	30		–	–	–	–	35[a]
9–13 years	–	–	–		39	45	–	1200	40
Males									
11–14 years	9	22	35		–	–	–	–	40[b]
14–18 years	–	–	–		63	75	–	1800	40
15–50+ years	10	25	40	1000	–	–	–	–	–
19–70+ years	–	–	–		75	90	–	2000	45
Females									
11–14 years	9	22	35		–	–	–	–	40[b]
14–18 years	–	–	–		56	65	–	1800	40
15–50+ years	10	25	40	1000	–	–	–	–	45
19–70+ years	–	–	–		60	75	–	2000	45
Pregnancy	–	–	+10		$66^1/70^2$	$80^1/85^2$		$1800^1/2000^2$	55
Lactation	–	–	+30		$96^1/100^2$	$115^1/120^2$	$1800^1/2000^2$	70	

[a] 7–9 years.   [b] 10–14 years.
^{1} Up to the age of 18 years ^{2} 19–50 years.
EVM = Likely safe daily intake from supplements alone.
TUL = Tolerable Upper Intake Level from diet and supplements.

Bioavailability

Storage and cooking lead to loss of vitamin C through oxidation, and boiling results in leaching of the vitamin into the cooking water (cooking water should be consumed in gravies and soups). Microwaving and stir-frying are the best cooking methods for preserving vitamin C.

Deficiency

Vitamin C deficiency may lead to scurvy. Subclinical deficiency has been associated with poor wound healing and ulceration. Early signs of deficiency may be non-specific and include general weakness, lethargy, fatigue, shortness of breath and aching of the limbs. As the disease progresses, petechiae are often prominent and may appear over the arms after application of a sphygmomanometer.

Signs of advanced deficiency include perifollicular haemorrhages (particularly about the hair follicles); swollen, bleeding gums; pallor and anaemia (the result of prolonged bleeding or associated folic acid deficiency); joints, muscles and subcutaneous tissue may become sites of haemorrhage. In children, disturbances of growth occur and bones, teeth and blood vessels develop abnormally; gum signs are only found in the presence of erupted teeth.

Groups at risk of low vitamin C status include smokers, the elderly, patients in hospitals and other institutions, and patients with diabetes.

Possible uses

Many health claims have been made for megadose intakes of vitamin C (i.e. 250–10 000 mg

Table 2   Dietary sources of vitamin C

Food portion	Vitamin C (mg)	Food portion	Vitamin C (mg)
Bread and cereals[1]	0	Blackberries, stewed (100 g)	10
Milk and dairy products	0	**Blackcurrants, stewed (100 g)**	115
Meat and fish[2]	0	12 cherries	10
Vegetables		Fruit salad	
Broccoli, boiled (100 g)	44	canned (130 g)	4
Brussels sprouts, boiled (100 g)	60	fresh (130 g)	20
Cabbage, raw (100 g)	49	**½ grapefruit**	54
Cabbage, boiled (100 g)	20	Grapes (100 g)	3
Carrots, boiled (100 g)	2	**Guava (100 g)**	230
Cauliflower, boiled (100 g)	43	**1 kiwi fruit**	60
Courgette, stir-fried (100 g)	15	**Lychees (100 g)**	45
Cucumber, raw (30 g)	2	**1 mango**	50
Kale, boiled (100 g)	71	**½ melon, cantaloupe**	60
Lettuce (30 g)	2	*1 slice melon, honeydew*	18
Mangetout peas, boiled (50 g)	14	1 slice watermelon	20
stir-fried (50 g)	26	1 orange	90
Peas, boiled (100 g)	16	4 passion fruits	20
Peppers, green, raw (50 g)	120	1 slice pawpaw	90
Peppers, red, raw (50 g)	140	1 peach	30
Potatoes		*1 pear*	9
chips (250 g)	27	*1 slice pineapple*	15
new, boiled (150 g)	15	3 plums	6
old, boiled (150 g)	9	**Raspberries (100 g)**	32
sweet, boiled (150 g)	23	**Strawberries (100 g)**	77
Spinach, boiled (100 g)	8	**1 tangerine**	22
Tomatoes, raw, two (150 g)	25	*Beverages*	
Watercress (20 g)	12	1 large glass apple juice	28
Fruit		1 large glass grapefruit juice	60
1 apple	15	1 large glass orange juice	80
1 banana	16	*1 large glass tomato juice*	16
		1 large glass Ribena (diluted)	120

[1] A few breakfast cereals have added vitamin C (average 10 mg/portion).
[2] Liver contains approx. 15 mg/100 g.
Excellent sources (**bold**); good sources (*italics*).

daily), including the prevention and treatment of colds, infections, stress, cancer, hypercholesterolaemia and atherosclerosis.

Respiratory conditions

Since Linus Pauling's claims about the beneficial effects of vitamin C on preventing colds and reducing their symptoms, many studies have investigated the effects of vitamin C on the common cold. A summary of 27 trials conducted between 1970 and 1986[1] concluded that vitamin C did not prevent colds, but could have a small therapeutic effect. Of these 27 trials, five were intervention trials of vitamin C or placebo given at the start of cold symptoms and for a few days, all of which found no benefit. The other 22 were double-blind controlled trials giving daily vitamin C or placebo before and during colds. Of these, 12 showed no preventive effect and no reduction in duration or severity of symptoms, five showed no prevention and only slight non-significant lessening of severity, and the other five reported no prevention and a small but significant reduction in the duration of colds.

One review of several studies indicated that vitamin C alleviates common cold symptoms,[2] although the magnitude of benefit appears to vary depending on the population group studied and the dose. A Cochrane review of 30 trials[3] concluded that long-term daily supplementation with large doses of vitamin C does not appear to prevent colds, but there appears to be a modest benefit in terms of reducing duration of cold symptoms from ingestion of high doses. The review also concluded that the relation of dose to therapeutic benefit needs further exploration. An update of this review in 2004 confirmed that vitamin C does not reduce the incidence of colds in the general population, but that it could be justified in people exposed to brief periods of severe physical exercise and/or cold environments. There was also a small benefit on duration and severity of colds for those using regular vitamin C prophylaxis. The trials in which vitamin C was introduced at the onset of colds as therapy did not show any benefit in doses up to 4 g daily, but one large trial reported equivocal benefit from an 8-g therapeutic dose at the onset of symptoms.

Vitamin C has also been evaluated in asthma. A Cochrane review[4] concluded that evidence to date from RCTs is insufficient to recommend a specific role for vitamin C in the treatment of asthma, and that further methodologically strong and large-scale trials are needed.

Cancer

It has been suggested that vitamin C may be useful in the prevention of cancer.[5] Possible mechanisms for this protective effect may be that vitamin C acts as an antioxidant, blocks formation of nitrosamines and faecal mutagens, enhances immune system response and accelerates detoxifying liver enzymes.

Many epidemiological studies have shown an inverse correlation between vitamin C intake and cancer incidence, but the evidence is largely indirect because it is based on the consumption of fruits and vegetables known to contain vitamin C and other nutrients such as beta-carotene and folate. The strongest evidence

for a protective effect seems to be for stomach cancer.[6–9] The evidence for oesophageal cancer is not as strong. Findings are contradictory for cancers of the lung, breast, colon and rectum.

There is some evidence that vitamin C supplements may help to prevent stomach cancer,[8] reduce pre-cancerous changes in colon cancer,[10] and help to manage prostate cancer.[11] However, subjects with advanced colorectal cancer responded no better than placebo to vitamin C supplementation.[12] Vitamin C may also benefit cancer patients undergoing radiation treatment, by enabling them to withstand larger doses of radiation with fewer side-effects.[13]

Cardiovascular disease

Epidemiological studies have shown associations between low vitamin C intakes and CVD risk.[14] However, two other epidemiological studies of about 87 000 female nurses and 4000 male health professionals found no effect of vitamin C intakes from diets or supplements on cardiovascular risk.[15,16]

An association between vitamin C and atherosclerosis has been suggested in studies investigating the relationship between vitamin C and cholesterol. When 1 g of vitamin C was given to healthy young people, cholesterol levels tended to fall,[17] but in older people no significant pattern of serum cholesterol change was found. Leukocyte levels were found to be lower in patients with CHD than in patients without CHD.[18] Vitamin C may also have beneficial effects on blood pressure[19] and on stroke.[20]

Vitamin C has been shown to reduce blood pressure in mildly hypertensive patients when given for short periods of time,[21] but not when given in the long term.[22] When given in combination with polyphenols, vitamin C has been found to be associated with raised blood pressure in hypertensive people.[23] The link between vitamin C and other cardiovascular risk factors has also been evaluated. Vitamin C has been found to protect against lipid-induced endothelial damage,[24–27] reduce early recurrence of atrial fibrillation and associated inflammation after atrial electrical remodelling,[28] and potentially reduce triglycerides[29,30] and apo B lipoprotein.[29]

Positive effects on cardiovascular risk factors have also been shown in people with diabetes. One study found that vitamin C 500 mg daily for 1 month reduced arterial blood pressure and improved arterial stiffness.[31] A further study found that vitamin C improved thrombotic markers.[32] However, another study found no effect of vitamin C on microvascular reactivity, inflammatory cytokines and oxidised LDL cholesterol.[33] Yet another study found no significant effect of vitamin C (1.5 g daily) for 3 weeks on oxidative stress, blood pressure or endothelial function in patients with type 2 diabetes.[34]

Cataracts

Patients with cataracts have been found to have lower levels of vitamin C in the lens than patients with no cataracts,[35] and as cataracts develop, the vitamin C content of the lens declines.[36] In a retrospective study, a lower incidence of cataract was found in subjects whose ascorbic acid intake was in the highest quintile compared with those in the lowest quintile.[37] There is some evidence that long-term supplementation of vitamin C (>10 years) may reduce the development of age-related opacities.[38,39]

Wound healing

Reductions in blood ascorbic acid levels have been reported in post-operative patients.[40,41] Some researchers suggest that this reduction represents increased need, while others suggest that ascorbic acid is redistributed to the tissues. Tissue ascorbic acid concentration at the site of a wound has been found to increase.[42] Studies have shown accelerated wound healing with vitamin C supplements.[42,43]

Periodontal disease

There is evidence that vitamin C status is related to periodontal disease. Vitamin C depletion in humans has been associated with significantly increased gum bleeding even though no clinical symptoms of scurvy were observed in any subject.[44] The degree of gingival inflammation was directly related to ascorbic acid status, and a reduction in bleeding was observed with vitamin C supplementation.

Smoking

Vitamin C requirements are higher in smokers than non-smokers,[45] and supplemental vitamin C may help to restore plasma vitamin C concentration in smokers. Beneficial effects of vitamin C on atherosclerotic plaque,[46] platelet aggregation,[47] oxidative stress,[48] and endothelial dysfunction[49] have been found in smokers. However, one study found no such effects in smokers.[50]

Sports

Vitamin C supplementation has been investigated in sports people. One study showed that vitamin C supplementation did not counter oxidative changes during or after a marathon.[51] Two further studies concluded that vitamin C supplements could attenuate antioxidant defence.[52,53]

Miscellaneous

Vitamin C (500 mg daily) has been found to reduce serum uric acid, suggesting that vitamin C might be beneficial in the prevention and management of gout.[54] The vitamin may protect against gastric mucosal atrophy in patients with chronic gastritis.[55] It has also been found to palliate response to acute stress, lowering blood pressure and cortisol,[56] and to reduce oxidative stress in patients with schizophrenia on atypical antipsychotics.[57]

Vitamin C has been thought to reduce the risk of pregnancy complications such as pre-eclampsia, intrauterine growth restriction and maternal anaemia. A Cochrane analysis concluded that the data are too few to say if vitamin C supplementation (alone or combined with other supplements) is beneficial during pregnancy, and it may result in increased risk of pre-term birth.[58] A recent trial involving 1877 women (935 women assigned to daily supplementation with 1000 mg of vitamin C and 400 units of vitamin E and 942 to placebo) found that there was no difference between the two groups in the risk of pre-eclampsia, intrauterine growth restriction or the risk of death or serious outcomes in the infants.[59]

Conclusion
Various groups of the population are at risk of vitamin C deficiency, particularly the elderly and smokers. Vitamin C may reduce the duration of the common cold and also the severity of symptoms such as sneezing and coughing, particularly if it is taken immediately the symptoms start. Preventive effects of vitamin C supplementation appear to be limited mainly to people with low dietary intake, while therapeutic effects may occur in wider population groups. Epidemiological studies have shown a link between low blood vitamin C concentrations and CVD, cancer and cataracts. However, further controlled clinical trials are needed to confirm the value of vitamin C supplements for these conditions.

Precautions/contraindications

Vitamin C supplements should be used with caution in diabetes mellitus (because of possible interference with glucose determinations); glucose-6-phosphate dehydrogenase (G6PD) deficiency (risk of haemolytic anaemia); haemochromatosis; sickle cell anaemia (risk of precipitating a crisis); sideroblastic anaemia; and thalassaemia. Prolonged administration of large doses (>1 g daily) of vitamin C in pregnancy may result in increased requirements and scurvy in the neonate.

Because ascorbic acid is a strong reducing agent it interferes with all diagnostic tests based on oxidation–reduction reactions. Vitamin C administration (megadoses only: >1 g daily) may interfere with tests for:

- blood glucose (false negative); and
- urinary glucose (false positive with analyses using cupric sulphate, e.g. Clinitest; false negative with analyses using glucose oxidase, e.g. Clinistix).

Adverse effects

Vitamin C is considered to be one of the safest of all the vitamins. There appear to be no serious health risks with doses up to 10 g daily, but doses of >1 g daily are associated with osmotic diarrhoea (due to large amounts of unabsorbed ascorbic acid in the intestine), gastric discomfort and mild increase in urination.

Oxalic acid is a major metabolite of vitamin C, and there has been concern about an increased risk of renal oxalate stones with high doses. Doses of 2 g and above are associated with an increased risk of oxalate stones.[60,61]

There have been occasional reports that vitamin C destroys vitamin B_{12} in the tissues and of rebound scurvy after administration of vitamin C is stopped, but such reports remain unsubstantiated.

Prolonged use of chewable vitamin C products may cause dental erosion and increased incidence of caries.

Interactions

Drugs

Vitamin C is important for the optimal activity of some of the drug-metabolising enzymes, including the hepatic cytochrome P450 mixed-function oxidase system. Large doses (>1 g daily) of ascorbic acid (but not ascorbates) may lower urinary pH, leading to increased renal tubular re-absorption of acidic drugs and increased excretion of alkaline drugs.

Aspirin: prolonged administration may reduce blood levels of ascorbic acid.

Anticoagulants: occasional reports that vitamin C reduces the activity of warfarin.

Anticonvulsants: administration of barbiturates or primidone may increase urinary excretion of ascorbic acid.

Desferrioxamine: iron excretion induced by desferrioxamine is enhanced by administration of vitamin C.

Disulfiram: prolonged administration of large doses (>1 g daily) of vitamin C may interfere with the alcohol–disulfiram reaction.

Mexiletine: large doses (>1 g daily) of ascorbic acid may accelerate excretion of mexiletine.

Oral contraceptives (containing oestrogens): may reduce blood levels of ascorbic acid; large doses (>1 g) of vitamin C may increase plasma oestrogen levels (possibly converting low-dose oral contraceptive to high-dose oral contraceptive); possibly breakthrough bleeding associated with withdrawal of high-dose vitamin C.

Tetracyclines: prolonged administration may reduce blood levels of ascorbic acid.

Nutrients

Copper: high doses of vitamin C (>1 g daily) may reduce copper retention.

Iron: vitamin C increases absorption of non-haem iron, but not haem iron. For maximal iron absorption from a non-meat meal, a source of vitamin C providing 50–100 mg should be ingested. Vitamin C supplements appear to have no deleterious effect on iron status in patients with iron overload. Iron administration reduces blood levels of ascorbic acid (ascorbic acid is oxidised).

Vitamin A: vitamin C may reduce the toxic effects of vitamin A.

Vitamin B_6: deficiency of vitamin C may increase urinary excretion of pyridoxine.

Vitamin B_{12}: excess vitamin C has been claimed to destroy vitamin B_{12}, but this does not appear to occur under physiological conditions.

Vitamin E: vitamin C can spare vitamin E, and vice versa.

Heavy metals

Vitamin C may reduce tissue and plasma levels of cadmium, lead, mercury, nickel and vanadium.

Dose

Vitamin C is available in the form of tablets, chewable tablets, capsules and powders. It is found in most multivitamin preparations. A review of 26 US vitamin C products found that three of the products failed to pass the tests for labelled content of vitamin C and one failed on disintegration.[62]

Dietary supplements contain between 25 and 1500 mg per daily dose.

References

1 Truswell AS. Ascorbic acid (letter). *N Engl J Med* 1986; 315: 709.

2 Hemila H. Vitamin C supplementation and common cold symptoms: factors affecting the magnitude of benefit. *Med Hypotheses* 1999; 52: 171–178.

3 Douglas RM, Hemila H, Chalker EB, . Vitamin C for preventing and treating the common cold. Cochrane database, issue 4, 2004. London: Macmillan.

4 Ram FSF, Rowe BH, Kaur B. Vitamin C supplementation for asthma. Cochrane database, issue 3, 2004. London: Macmillan.

5 Blocke G, Menkes M. Ascorbic acid in cancer prevention. In: Moon TE, Micozzi MS, eds. *Nutrition and Cancer Prevention. Investigating the Role of Micronutrients*. New York: Marcel Dekker, 1989: 341–348.

6 Bjelke E. Dietary factors and the epidemiology of cancer of the stomach and the large bowel. *Klin Prax Suppl* 1978; 2: 10–17.

7 Correa P, Malcom E, Schmidt B, *et al*. Antioxidant micronutrients and gastric cancer. *Aliment Pharmacol Ther* 1998; 12 (Suppl. 1): 73–82.

8 Risch HA, Jain M, Choi NW, *et al*. Dietary factors and the incidence of cancer of the stomach. *Am J Epidemiol* 1985; 122: 947–949.

9 You WC, Blot WJ, Chang YS, *et al*. Diet and high risk of stomach cancer in Shandong, China. *Cancer Res* 1988; 48: 3518–3523.

10 Waring AJ, Drake IM, Schorah CJ, *et al*. Ascorbic acid and total vitamin C concentrations in plasma, gastric juice and gastrointestinal mucosa: effects of gastritis and oral supplementation. *Gut* 1996; 38: 171–176.

11 Paganelli GM, Biasco G, Brandi G, *et al*. Effect of vitamin A, C, and E supplementation on rectal cell proliferation in patients with colorectal adenomas. *J Natl Cancer Inst* 1992; 84: 47–51.

12 Moertal CG, Fleming TR, Geegen ET. High dose vitamin C versus placebo in the treatment of patients with advanced cancer who have had no prior chemotherapy: a randomised double-blind comparison. *N Engl J Med* 1985; 312: 137–141.

13 Okunieff P. Interactions between ascorbic acid and the radiation of bone marrow, skin and tumour. *Am J Clin Nutr* 1991; 54: S1281–1283.

14 Gaby SK, Singh VN. Vitamin C. In: Gaby SK, Bendich A, Sing VN, Machlin LJ, eds. *Vitamin Intake and Health: A Scientific Review*. New York: Marcel Dekker, 1991: 103–161.

15 Rimm EB, Stampfer MJ, Ascherio A, *et al*. Vitamin E consumption and the risk of coronary heart disease in men. *N Engl J Med* 1993; 328: 1450–1456.

16 Stampfer MJ, Hennekens CH, Manson JE, *et al*. Vitamin E consumption and the risk of coronary heart disease in women. *N Engl J Med* 1993; 328; 1444–1449.

17 Spittle CR. Atherosclerosis and vitamin C. *Lancet* 1972; i: 798.

18 Ramirez J, Flowers NC. Leucocyte ascorbic acid and its relationship to coronary artery disease in man. *Am J Clin Nutr* 1980; 33: 2079–2087.

19 Ness AR, Chee D, Elliot P, *et al*. Vitamin C and blood pressure – an overview. *J Hum Hypertens* 1997; 11: 343–350.

20 Gale CR, Martyn CN, Winter PD, *et al*. Vitamin C and risk of death from stroke and coronary heart disease in cohorts of elderly people. *BMJ* 1995; 310: 1563–1566.

21 Hajjar IM, George V, Sasse EA, *et al*. A randomized, double-blind, controlled trial of vitamin C in the management of hypertension and lipids. *Am J Ther* 2003; 10: 234–235.

22 Kim MK, Sasaki S, Sasazuki S, *et al*. Lack of long-term effect of vitamin C supplementation on blood pressure. *Hypertension* 2002; 40: 789–791.

23 Ward NC, Hodgson JM, Croft KD, *et al*. The combination of vitamin C and grape-seed polyphenols increases blood pressure: a randomized, double-blind, placebo-controlled trial. *J Hypertens* 2005; 23: 427–434.

24 Pleiner J, Schaller G, Mittermayer F, *et al*. A-induced endothelial dysfunction can be corrected by vitamin C. *J Clin Endocrinol Metab* 2002; 87: 2913–2917.

25 Morel O, Jesel L, Hugel B, *et al*. Protective effects of vitamin C on endothelium damage and platelet activation during myocardial infarction in patients with sustained generation of circulating microparticles. *J Thromb Haemost* 2003; 1: 171–177.

26 Woolard KJ, Loryman CJ, Meredith E, *et al*. Effects of oral vitamin C on monocyte:endothelial cell adhesion in healthy subjects. *Biochem Biophys Res Commun* 2002; 294: 1161–1168.

27 Bayerle-Eder M, Pleiner J, Mitermayer F, *et al*. Effect of systemic vitamin C on free fatty acid-induced lipid peroxidation. *Diabetes Metab* 2004; 30: 433–439.

28 Shidfar F, Keshavarz A, Jallali M, *et al*. Comparison of the effects of simultaneous administration of vitamin C and omega-3 fatty acids on lipoproteins, apo A-1, apo B, and malondialdehyde in hyperlipidemic patients. *Int J Vitamin Nutr Res* 2003; 73: 163–170.

29 Korantzopoulos P, Kolettis TM, Kountouris E, *et al*. Oral vitamin C administration reduces early recurrence rates after electrical cardioversion of persistent atrial fibrillation and attenuates associated inflammation. *Int J Cardiol* 2005; 102: 361–362.

30 Kim MK, Sasaki S, Sasazuki S, *et al*. Long-term vitamin C supplementation has no markedly favourable effect on serum lipids in middle-aged Japanese subjects. *Br J Nutr* 2004; 91: 81–90.

31 Mullan BA, Young IS, Fee H, *et al*. Ascorbic acid reduces blood pressure and arterial stiffness in type 2 diabetes. *Hypertension* 2002; 40: 804–809.

32 Tousoulis D, Antoniades C, Tountas C, *et al*. Vitamin C affects thrombosis/fibrinolysis system and reactive hyperemia in patients with type 2 diabetes and coronary artery disease. *Diabetes Care* 2003; 26: 2749–2753.

33 Lu Q, Bjorkhem I, Wretlind B, *et al*. Effect of ascorbic acid on microcirculation in patients with Type II diabetes: a randomized placebo-controlled cross-over study. *Clin Sci* 2005; 108: 507–513.

34 Darko D, Dornhorst A, Kelly FJ, *et al*. Lack of effect of oral vitamin C on blood pressure, oxidative stress and endothelial function in Type II diabetes. *Clin Sci* 2002; 103: 339–344.

35 Chandra DB, Varma R, Ahmad S, Varma SD. Vitamin C in the human aqueous humour and cataracts. *Int J Vit Nutr Res* 1986; 56: 165–168.

36 Lohmann W. Ascorbic acid and cataract. *Ann NY Acad Sci* 1987; 498: 307–311.

37 Jaques PF, Phillips J, Chylack LT, *et al*. Vitamin intake and senile cataract. *J Am Coll Nutr* 1987; 6: 435.

38 Chasan-Taber L, Willett WC, Seddon JM, *et al*. A prospective study of vitamin supplement intake and cataract extraction among US women. *Epidemiology* 1999; 10: 679–684.

39 Jaques PF, Taylor A, Hankinson SE, *et al*. Long-term vitamin C supplement use and prevalence of early age-related lens opacities. *Am J Clin Nutr* 1997; 66: 911–916.

40 Irvin TT, Chattopadhyay DK, Smythe A. Ascorbic acid requirements in postoperative patients. *Surg Gynaecol Obstet* 1978; 147: 49–55.

41 Shukla SP. Plasma and urinary ascorbic acid levels in the post-operative period. *Experientia* 1969; 25: 704.

42 Crandon JH, Lennihan R Jr, Mikal S, Reif AE. Ascorbic acid economy in surgical patients. *Ann NY Acad Sci* 1961; 92: 246–267.

43 Ringsdorf WM Jr, Cheraskin E. Vitamin C and human wound healing. *Oral Surg* 1982; 53: 231–236.

44 Leggott PJ, Robertson PB, Rothman DL, *et al*. The effect of controlled ascorbic acid depletion and supplementation on periodontal health. *J Periodontol* 1986; 57: 480–485.

45 Lykkesfeldt J, Christen S, Wallock LM, *et al*. Ascorbate is depleted by smoking and repleted by moderate supplementation: a study in male smokers and nonsmokers with matched dietary antioxidant intakes. *Am J Clin Nutr* 2000; 71: 530–536.

46 Weber C, Erl W, Weber K, Weber PC. Increased adhesiveness of isolated monocytes to endothelium is prevented by vitamin C intake in smokers. *Circulation* 1996; 93: 1488–1492.

47 Schindler TH, Lewandowski E, Olschewski M, *et al*. Effect of vitamin C on platelet aggregation in smokers and nonsmokers. *Med Klin* 2002; 97: 263–269.

48 Dietrich M, Block G, Benowitz NL, *et al*. Vitamin C supplementation decreases oxidative stress biomarker f2-isoprostanes in plasma of nonsmokers exposed to environmental tobacco smoke. *Nutr Cancer* 2003; 45: 176–184.

49 Stamatelopoulos KS, Lekakis JP, Papamichael CM, *et al*. Oral administration of ascorbic acid attenuates endothelial dysfunction after short-term cigarette smoking. *Int J Vitamin Nutr Res* 2003; 73: 417–422.

50 Van Hoydonck PG, Schouten EG, Manuel-Y-Keenoy B, *et al*. Does vitamin C supplementation influence the levels of circulating oxidized LDL, sICAM-1, sVCAM-1 and vWF-antigen in healthy male smokers? *Eur J Clin Nutr* 2004; 58: 1587–1593.

51 Nieman DC, Henson DA, McAnulty SR, *et al*. Influence of vitamin C supplementation on oxidative and immune changes after an ultramarathon. *J Appl Physiol* 2002; 92: 1970–1977.

52 Khassaf M, McArdle A, Esanu C, *et al*. Effect of vitamin C supplements on antioxidant defence and stress proteins in human lymphocytes and skeletal muscle. *J Physiol* 2003; 549(pt2): 645–652.

53 Goldfarb AH, Patrick SW, Bryer S, *et al*. Vitamin C supplementation affects oxidative-stress blood markers in response to a 30-minute run at 75% VO2max. *Int J Sport Nutr Exerc Metab* 2005; 15: 279–290.

54 Huang HY, Appel LJ, Choi MJ, *et al*. The effects of vitamin C supplementation on serum concentrations of uric acid: results of a randomized controlled trial. *Arthritis Rheum* 2005; 52: 1843–1847.

55 Sasazuki S, Sasaki S, Tsubono Y, *et al*. The effect of 5-year vitamin C supplementation on serum pepsinogen level and *Helicobacter pylori* infection. *Cancer Sci* 2003; 94: 378–382.

56 Brody S, Preut R, Schommer K, *et al*. A randomized controlled trial of high dose ascorbic acid for reduction of blood pressure, cortisol, and subjective responses to psychological stress. *Psychopharmacology* 2002; 159: 319–324.

57 Dakhale GN, Khanzode SD, Khanzode SS, *et al*. Supplementation of vitamin C with atypical antipsychotics reduces oxidative stress and improves the outcome of schizophrenia. *Psychopharmacology* 2005; 182: 494–498.

58 Rumbold A, Crowther CA. Vitamin C supplementation in pregnancy. Cochrane database, issue 1, 2005. London: Macmillan.

59 Rumbold AR, Crowther CA, Haslam RR, *et al*. Vitamin C and E and the risks of pre-eclampsia and perinatal complications. *N Engl J Med* 2006; 354: 1796–1806.

60 Traxer O, Huet B, Poindexter J, *et al*. Effect of ascorbic acid consumption on urinary stone risk factors. *J Urol* 2003; 170 (2 Pt 1): 402–403.

61 Massey LK, Liebman M, Kynast-Gales SA. Ascorbate increases human oxaluria and kidney stone risk. *J Nutr* 2005; 135: 1673–1677.

62 Consumerlab. Product review. Vitamin C. http:// www.consumerlab.com (accessed 13 November 2006).

Vitamin D

Description

Vitamin D is a fat-soluble vitamin.

Nomenclature

Vitamin D is a generic term used to describe all sterols that exhibit the biological activity of cholecalciferol. These include:

- vitamin D_1 (calciferol)
- vitamin D_2 (ergocalciferol)
- vitamin D_3 (colecalciferol, cholecalciferol)
- $1(OH)D_3$ (1-hydroxycholecalciferol; alfacalcidol)
- $25(OH)D_3$ (25-hydroxycholecalciferol; calcifediol)
- $1,25(OH)_2D_3$ (1,25-dihydroxycholecalciferol; calcitriol)
- $24,25(OH)_2D_3$ (24,25-dihydroxycholecalciferol)
- dihydrotachysterol.

Vitamin D_2 is the form most commonly added to foods and dietary supplements.

Units

One International Unit of vitamin D is defined as the activity of 0.025 µg of cholecalciferol. Thus: 1 µg vitamin D = 40 units vitamin D and: 1 unit vitamin D = 0.025 µg vitamin D

Human requirements

See Table 1 for Dietary Reference Values for vitamin D.

Table 1 Dietary Reference Values for vitamin D (µg/day)

Age	UK		USA		FAO/ WHO
	RNI	EVM	AI	TUL	RNI
Males and females					
0–6 months	8.5		5	25	5
7–12 months	7.0		5	25	5
1–3 years	7.0		5	50	5
4–18 years	0[1]		5	50	5
19–50 years	0[1]	25	5	50	5
51–65 years	–		–	–	10
65+ years	10	25	–	–	2.5
51–70+ years	–	25	10	50	–
>65 years	–	–	–	–	15
>70 years	–	–	15	50	–
Pregnancy and lactation	10	–	5	50	10

EU RDA = 5 µg

[1] If skin is exposed to adequate sunlight.
EVM = Likely safe daily intake from supplements alone.
TUL = Tolerable upper intake level from diet and supplements.

Dietary intake

In the UK, the average adult daily diet provides: for men, 3.7 µg, for women, 2.8 µg.

Cutaneous synthesis

Exposure of the skin to ultraviolet (UV) rays results in the synthesis of cholecalciferol (vitamin D_3); this is the major source of vitamin D. The amount obtained depends on length of

339

exposure, area of skin exposed, wavelength of UV light, pollution, skin pigmentation (higher melanin concentration requires longer exposure to achieve same degree of synthesis) and age (the elderly may have approximately half the capacity for synthesis of younger people).

Brief, casual exposure of face, arms and hands to sunlight is thought to be equivalent to the ingestion of 5 µg (200 units) of vitamin D.[1] The use of sunscreens may affect vitamin D production; application of a sunscreen with a sun protection factor of 8 can completely prevent the cutaneous production of cholecalciferol. However, this should not discourage the use of sunscreens.

Action

Vitamin D is essential for promoting the absorption and utilisation of calcium and phosphorus and normal calcification of the skeleton. Along with parathyroid hormone and calcitonin, it regulates serum calcium concentration by altering serum calcium and phosphate blood levels as needed, and mobilising calcium from bone. It maintains neuromuscular function and various other cellular processes, including the immune system and insulin production.

Dietary sources

See Table 2 for dietary sources of vitamin D.

Metabolism

Absorption (dietary source)

Vitamin D is absorbed with the aid of bile salts from the small intestine via the lymphatic system and its associated chylomicrons. The efficiency of absorption is estimated to be about 50%.

Distribution

Vitamin D is converted by hydroxylation (predominantly in the liver) to $25(OH)D_3$; this is the major circulating form of vitamin D. From the liver, $25(OH)D_3$ is transported to the kidney and converted by further hydroxylation to $1,25(OH)_2D_3$, the metabolically active form, and to $24,25(OH)_2D_3$.

Table 2   Table 2 Dietary sources of vitamin D

Food portion	Vitamin D content (µg)
Breakfast cereals	
1 bowl All-Bran (45 g)	0.8
1 bowl Bran Flakes (45 g)	1.0
1 bowl Corn Flakes (25 g)	0.5
1 bowl Frosties (45 g)	1.0
1 bowl Rice Krispies (35 g)	0.7
1 bowl Special K (35 g)	0.9
Muesli, porridge, Shredded Wheat, Sugar Puffs, Weetabix	0
Bread	0
Milk and dairy products	
½ pint whole milk	0.1
½ pint semi-skimmed milk	0.03
½ pint skimmed milk	0
½ pint skimmed milk, fortified	0.2–0.5 (various brands)
2 tablespoons dried skimmed milk, fortified (30 g)	1.0
Hard cheese (50 g)	0.1
Feta cheese (50 g)	0.25
1 carton whole-milk yoghurt (150 g)	0.06
1 carton low-fat yoghurt (150 g)	0.01
1 egg, size 2 (60 g)	1.0
Fats and oils	
Butter, on 1 slice bread (10 g)	0.25
Margarine, on 1 slice bread (10 g)	*2.5*
Low-fat spread, on 1 slice bread (10 g)	*2.5*
2 tablespoons ghee (30 g)	0.6
2 teaspoons cod liver oil (10 ml)	**21.0**
Meat and fish	
Liver, lambs, cooked (90 g)	0.5
Liver, calf, cooked (90 g)	0.3
Liver, ox, cooked (90 g)	1.0
Liver, pig, cooked (90 g)	1.0
White fish	Trace
Sardines (70 g)	**5.6**
Tinned salmon (100 g)	**12.5**
Tinned pilchards (100 g)	**8.0**
Tinned tuna (100 g)	**5.0**
2 fillets herring, cooked (110 g)	**20.0**
2 fillets kipper, cooked (130 g)	**20.0**
2 fillets mackerel, cooked (110 g)	**21.0**
Beverages	
1 mug Ovaltine[1] (300 ml)	0.7
1 mug Horlicks[1] (300 ml)	0.7
1 mug Build-Up[1] (300 ml)	3.0
1 mug Complan[2] (300 ml)	*1.5*

[1] Made with milk (whole or skimmed).
[2] Made with water.
Excellent sources (> 5 µg/portion) (**bold**); good sources (> 1.5 µg/portion) (*italics*).

Synthesis is regulated mainly by circulating levels of $1,25(OH)_2D_3$. When levels of $1,25(OH)_2D_3$ are high, synthesis is low and vice versa. Synthesis is also stimulated by hypocalcaemia, hypophosphataemia and parathyroid hormone (PTH) and inhibited by hypercalcaemia. A second metabolite of vitamin D, $24,25(OH)_2D_3$, is produced in the kidney. Both $1,25(OH)_2D_3$ and $24,25(OH)_2D_3$ may be required for the biological activity of vitamin D.

Vitamin D is transported in the plasma bound to a specific vitamin D-binding protein, which is its main storage form. Small amounts are stored in the liver, and also in adipose tissue, which may cause a relative deficiency in obese people. Some vitamin D derivatives are excreted in breast milk.

Deficiency

Deficiency of vitamin D results in inadequate intestinal absorption of calcium and phosphate; hypocalcaemia, hypophosphataemia and increase in serum alkaline phosphatase activity; and hyperparathyroidism. Demineralisation of bone leads to rickets in children and osteomalacia in adults. Infants may develop convulsions and tetany.

Possible uses

Requirements may be increased and/or supplements necessary in:

- Infants who are breast-fed without supplemental vitamin D or who have minimal exposure to sunlight (the Department of Health[2] advises that all children from the age of 1–5 years should receive supplements of vitamins A and D).
- Pregnancy – women who have low intake of vitamin D during pregnancy have been shown to produce low birth weight infants.[3] Maternal vitamin D insufficiency during pregnancy has been associated with reduced bone-mineral accrual in the offspring during childhood.[4]
- Breast-feeding (particularly with babies born in the autumn).

- The elderly, whose exposure to sunlight may be reduced because of poor mobility.
- Individuals with dark skins.
- Strict vegetarians and vegans.
- Those who do not get much exposure to sunlight.
- Patients with malabsorption conditions (e.g. coeliac disease, cystic fibrosis, Crohn's disease, short bowel syndrome).

Lack of vitamin D has been associated with a range of different conditions, such as osteoporosis, cancer, CVD, diabetes mellitus and poor immune function.

Osteoporosis

Vitamin D (independently of calcium) may be useful in the prevention of osteoporosis. Some research has shown that women with hip fractures have lower levels of plasma vitamin D.[5] People with a certain type of vitamin D receptor may be more susceptible to osteoporosis, and women with different types of vitamin D receptor seem to respond differently to vitamin D supplements.[6]

There is some evidence that vitamin D supplementation helps to reduce bone loss[7–9] and fracture risk[10,11] and, in combination with calcium,[12] may enhance the effect of HRT. However, other studies have not shown any reduction in rates of fracture with vitamin D supplementation. A Dutch study involving 2500 healthy men and women over the age of 70 showed that a daily dose of 400 units of vitamin D had no effect on fracture rates.[13]

Differences in effects may be due to differences in populations studied, study designs and doses of vitamin D. A recent meta-analysis of four RCTs, each of which used a dose of 20 µg (800 units) vitamin D daily, found that this dose prevents approximately 30% of hip or non-vertebral fractures compared with placebo in adults over the age of 65 years, and concluded that lower intakes are not effective.[14] Another recent meta-analysis, which included five RCTs for hip fracture and seven RCTs for non-vertebral fracture risk, concluded that oral vitamin D supplementation between 700 and 800 units daily appears to reduce the risk of hip and any non-vertebral fractures in ambulatory or institutionalised elderly persons, but that an oral vitamin D dose of 400 units daily is not effective.[15] Indeed, a trial published after this meta-analysis found that a dose of calcium 1000 mg daily with vitamin D 400 units did not significantly reduce hip fracture.[16] However, a trial in a primary care setting involving 3314 women aged over 70 with one or more risk factors for hip fracture found that calcium 1000 mg daily and vitamin D 800 units did not reduce the risk of clinical fractures overall.[17]

Whether vitamin D or vitamin D analogues have a different effect on fracture incidence is unclear. With regard to post-menopausal osteoporosis, there is evidence that vitamin D analogues – rather than plain vitamin D – may have bone-sparing actions. This may be because the type of vitamin D deficiency is a reflection of $1,25(OH)_2D_3$ deficiency or resistance and plain vitamin D will have no effect. Thus, a vitamin D analogue (e.g. calcitriol) could reduce bone loss as a result of a pharmacological action rather than replenishing a deficiency.

A meta-analysis found that the vitamin D analogues, alfacalcidol and calcitriol, were superior to plain vitamin D in preventing spinal fractures.[18] A Cochrane review found no evidence for this and also concluded that vitamin D alone had no significant effect on hip fracture, vertebral fracture or any new fracture, while vitamin D given with calcium was associated with fewer hip and other non-vertebral fractures.[19] The anti-fracture effect of vitamin D and calcium is likely to be due to their effect on BMD, although again the results of controlled trials are inconsistent.

Vitamin D may also improve neuromuscular coordination, preserve muscle function and as a consequence decrease the risk of falling and falling-related fractures.[20,21] A meta-analysis of five RCTs involving 1237 participants found that vitamin D reduced the risk of falls among both ambulatory and institutionalised older people by 2%.[22] A trial published more recently found that supplementation with both colecalciferol (700 units daily) and calcium (500 mg daily) over a 3-year period reduced the risk of falling in ambulatory older women by 46% and in less active women by 65%, but supplements had no effect in men.[23]

Cancer

Evidence from epidemiological studies suggests that enhanced sunlight exposure is associated with reduced death rates from certain common cancers, including cancer of the colon, breast, prostate and ovary.[24,25] Prospective studies show relative risks for colon cancer of 0.33 to 0.74 with higher vitamin D intake or concentrations of $25(OH)D_3$ above 65 nmol/L.[26] Supplemental vitamin D and calcium has been associated with reduced recurrence of colorectal adenomas, although the association was weak.[27] However, an RCT involving 36 282 post-menopausal women found that daily supplementation for 7 years with calcium 1000 mg daily and vitamin D 400 units daily had no effect on the incidence of colorectal cancer.[28] Prostate cancer risk has been found to be higher in men with low serum $25(OH)D_3$ concentrations, but this protective role seems to be strongest in younger men when serum androgen levels are higher.[29] A recent prospective study in men found an inverse association between low vitamin D levels and risk of total cancer and mortality, particularly for cancers of the digestive system.[30]

Cardiovascular disease and diabetes

Epidemiological studies have demonstrated a weak inverse relationship between serum $25(OH)D_3$ levels and blood pressure, while some clinical trials have shown that administration of vitamin D, 1-α vitamin D or exposure to ultraviolet B can reduce blood pressure in people with hypertension. There is also evidence that poor vitamin D status is associated with high concentrations of various inflammatory markers (e.g. tumour necrosis factor and interleukin-6) that contribute to the development of atherosclerosis, and that vitamin D supplementation can improve the profile of these markers.[31] Reduced vitamin D status is also associated with a higher incidence of both type 1 and type 2 diabetes mellitus, insulin resistance, low insulin concentrations, and in some studies, high blood glucose levels.

Miscellaneous

Vitamin D has an important role in the immune system. There is growing evidence for an involvement of vitamin D in infections, particularly in tuberculosis, and also in various autoimmune and inflammatory conditions such as rheumatoid arthritis, multiple sclerosis and inflammatory bowel diseases, including ulcerative colitis and Crohn's disease. Vitamin D supplementation has been shown to improve symptoms of rheumatoid arthritis and multiple sclerosis.[31]

> **Conclusion**
> Vitamin D is important for bone health, and some research has shown that supplementation with vitamin D may reduce the risk of osteoporosis and fracture. It is unclear whether most benefit is achieved from vitamin D alone or from vitamin D with calcium, and what the appropriate doses are. Epidemiological studies have found a link between colon cancer and low vitamin D, but whether supplements can reduce the risk of cancer is unknown.

Precautions/contraindications

Vitamin D should be avoided in hypercalcaemia; and renal osteodystrophy with hyperphosphataemia (risk of metastatic calcification).

Vegetarians

Supplements containing vitamin D_3 (cholecalciferol) are obtained from animal sources (usually as a by-product of wool fat) and are not suitable for strict vegetarians (vegans). Vitamin D_2 (ergocalciferol) is obtained from plant sources and can be recommended.

Pregnancy and breast-feeding

No problems reported with normal intakes. There is a risk of hypercalcaemic tetany in breast fed infants whose mothers take excessive doses of vitamin D.

Adverse effects

Vitamin D is the most likely of all the vitamins to cause toxicity; the margin of safety is very narrow. There is a wide variation in tolerance to vitamin D, but doses of 250 µg (10 000 units) daily for 6 months may result in toxicity. Infants and children are generally more susceptible than adults; prolonged administration of 45 µg (1800 units) daily may arrest growth in children. Some infants seem to be hyper-reactive to small doses. There is no risk of vitamin D toxicity from prolonged exposure to sunlight.

Excessive intake leads to hypercalcaemia and its associated effects. These include apathy, anorexia, constipation, diarrhoea, dry mouth, fatigue, headache, nausea and vomiting, thirst and weakness.

Later symptoms are often associated with calcification of soft tissues and include bone pain, cardiac arrhythmias, hypertension, renal damage (increased urinary frequency, decreased urinary concentrating ability; nocturia, proteinuria), psychosis (rare) and weight loss.

Interactions

Drugs

Anticonvulsants (phenytoin, barbiturates or primidone): may reduce effect of vitamin D by accelerating its metabolism; patients on long-term anticonvulsant therapy may require vitamin D supplementation to prevent osteomalacia.

Calcitonin: effect of calcitonin may be antagonised by vitamin D.

Colestyramine, colestipol: may reduce intestinal absorption of vitamin D.

Digoxin: caution because hypercalcaemia caused by vitamin D may potentiate effects of digoxin, resulting in cardiac arrhythmias.

Liquid paraffin: may reduce intestinal absorption of vitamin D (avoid long-term administration of liquid paraffin).

Sucralfate: may reduce intestinal absorption of vitamin D.

Thiazide diuretics: may increase risk of hypercalcaemia.

Vitamin D analogues (alfacalcidol, calcitriol, dihydrotachysterol): increased risk of toxicity with vitamin D supplements.

Nutrients

Calcium: may increase risk of hypercalcaemia.

Dose

Vitamin D is available in the form of tablets and capsules, as well as in multivitamin preparations and fish oils.

A suitable dose of vitamin D in most cases is 10 µg (400 units) daily.

For prevention of fracture in older people, there is evidence that a higher dose of 20 µg (800 units) with calcium 1200 mg daily is required.

Upper safety levels

The UK Expert Group on Vitamins and Minerals (EVM) has identified a likely safe total intake of vitamin D for adults from supplements alone of 25 µg daily.

References

1 Haddad J. Vitamin D – solar rays, the milky way, or both? *N Engl J Med* 1992; 326: 1213–1215.
2 Department of Health. *Weaning and the weaning diet: Report of the Working Group on the Weaning Diet of the Committee on Medical Aspects of Food Policy.* Report on Health and Social Subjects No 45. London: HMSO, 1994.
3 Mannion CA, Gray-Donald K, Koski KG. Association of low intake of milk and vitamin D during pregnancy with decreased birthweight. *Can Med Assoc J* 2006; 174: 1273–1277.
4 Javaid MK, Crozier SR, Harvey NC, et al. Maternal vitamin D status during pregnancy and childhood bone mass at age 9 years: a longitudinal study. *Lancet* 2006; 367: 36–43.
5 LeBoff MS, Kohlmeier L, Hurwitz S, et al. Occult vitamin D deficiency in postmenopausal US women with acute hip fracture. *JAMA* 1999; 281: 1505–1511.
6 Graafmans WC, Lips P, Ooms ME, et al. The effect of vitamin D supplementation on the bone mineral density of the femoral neck is associated with vitamin D receptor genotype. *J Bone Miner Res* 1997; 12: 1241–1245.
7 Dawson-Hughes B, Dallal GE, Kraal EA, et al. Effect of vitamin D supplementation on wintertime and overall bone loss in healthy postmenopausal women. *Ann Intern Med* 1991; 115: 505–512.
8 Ooms ME, Roos JC, Bezemer PD, et al. Prevention of bone loss by vitamin D supplementation in elderly women: a randomised double-blind trial. *J Endocrinol Metab* 1995; 80: 1052–1058.
9 Dawson-Hughes B, Harris SS, et al. Rates of bone loss in postmenopausal women randomly assigned to one of two dosages of vitamin D. *Am J Clin Nutr* 1995; 61: 1140–1145.
10 Chapuy MC, Arlot ME, Duboeuf F, et al. Vitamin D and calcium to prevent hip fractures in elderly women. *N Engl J Med* 1992; 327: 1637–1642.
11 Dawson-Hughes B, Harris SS, Krall EA, Dallal GE. Effect of calcium and vitamin D supplementation on bone density in men and women 65 years of age or older. *N Engl J Med* 1997; 337: 670–676.
12 Recker RR, Davies KM, Dowd RM, Heaney RP. The effect of low-dose continuous estrogen and progesterone therapy with calcium and vitamin D on bone in elderly women. A randomized, controlled trial. *Ann Intern Med* 1999; 130: 897–904.
13 Lips P, Graafmans WC, Ooms ME, et al. Vitamin D supplementation and fracture incidence in elderly persons. A randomized, placebo-controlled clinical trial. *Ann Intern Med* 1996; 124: 400–406.
14 Vieth R. The role of vitamin D in the prevention of osteoporosis. *Ann Med* 2005; 37: 278–285.
15 Bischoff-Ferrari H, Wong J, Giovannucci E, et al. Fracture prevention with vitamin D supplementation: a meta-analysis of randomized controlled trials. *JAMA* 2005; 293: 2257–2264.
16 Jackson R, LaCroix A, Gass M, et al. Calcium plus vitamin D supplementation and the risk of fractures. *N Engl J Med* 2006; 354: 669–683.
17 Porthouse J, Cockayne S, King C, et al. Randomised controlled trial of calcium and supplementation with cholecalciferol (vitamin D3) for prevention of fractures in primary care. *BMJ* 2005; 330: 1003.
18 Richy F, Schacht E, Bruyere O, et al. Vitamin D analogs versus native vitamin D in preventing bone loss and osteoporosis-related fractures: a comparative meta-analysis. *Calcif Tissue Int* 2005; 76: 176–186.
19 Avenell A, Gillespie W, Gillespie L, O'Connell D. Vitamin D and vitamin D analogues for preventing fractures associated with involutional and postmenopausal osteoporosis. Cochrane database, issue 3, 2005. London: Macmillan.
20 Janssen H, Samson M, Verhaar H. Vitamin D deficiency, muscle function, and falls in elderly people. *Am J Clin Nutr* 2002; 75: 611–615.
21 Bischoff-Ferrari H, Dietrich T, Orav E, et al. Higher 25-hydroxyvitamin D concentrations are associated with better lower extremity function in both active and inactive persons aged 60 years or more. *Am J Clin Nutr* 2004; 80: 752–758.
22 Bischoff-Ferrari H, Dawson-Hughes B, Willett W, et al. Effect of vitamin D on falls: a meta-analysis. *JAMA* 2004; 291: 1999–2006.
23 Bischoff-Ferrari H, Orav EJ, Dawson-Hughes B. Effect of cholecalciferol plus calcium on falling in ambulatory older men and women. *Arch Intern Med* 2006; 166: 424–430.

24 Guyton K, Kensler T, Posner G. Cancer chemo-prevention using natural vitamin D and synthetic analogs. *Ann Rev Pharmacol Toxicol* 2001; 41: 421–442.

25 Garland C, Garland F, Gorham E, *et al*. The role of vitamin D in cancer prevention. *Am J Pub Health* 2006; 96: 252–261.

26 Zitterman A. Vitamin D in preventive medicine. Are we ignoring the evidence? *Br J Nutr* 2003; 89: 552–572.

27 Hartman T, Albert P, Snyder K, *et al*. The association of calcium and vitamin D with risk of colorectal adenomas. *J Nutr* 2005; 135: 252–259.

28 Wactawski-Wende J, Kotchen J, Anderson J, *et al*. Calcium plus vitamin D supplementation and the risk of colorectal cancer. *N Engl J Med* 2006; 354: 684–696.

29 Tuohimaa P, Lyakhovich A, Aksenov N, *et al*. Vitamin D and prostate cancer. *J Steroid Biochem Mol Biol* 2001; 76: 125–134.

30 Giovannucci E, Liu Y, Rimm E, *et al*. Prospective study of predictors of vitamin D status and cancer incidence and mortality in men. *J Natl Cancer Inst* 2006; 98: 451–459.

31 Zitterman A. Vitamin D and disease prevention with special reference to cardiovascular disease. *Prog Biophys Mol Biol* 2006; 92: 39–48.

Vitamin E

Description

Vitamin E is a fat-soluble vitamin.

Nomenclature

Vitamin E is a generic term used to describe all tocopherol and tocotrienol derivatives that exhibit the biological activity of alpha-tocopherol.

Units

To determine the number of milligrams of alpha-tocopherol in a supplement expressed in International Units, use the following conversion factors. If the form of vitamin E in the supplement is natural, i.e. *d*-alpha-tocopherol or RRR-alpha-tocopherol, multiply International Units by 0.67. Thus, 100 IU of natural vitamin E = 66.7 mg alpha-tocopherol (100 × 0.67). If the form of vitamin E in the supplement is synthetic, i.e. *d,l*-alpha-tocopherol or *all-rac*-alpha-tocopherol), multiply IUs by 0.45. Thus, 100 IU of synthetic vitamin E = 45 mg alpha-tocopherol (30 × 0.45).

Human requirements

See Table 1 for Dietary Reference Values for vitamin E.

There is an increased requirement for vitamin E in diets high in polyunsaturated fatty acids (PUFAs), but many items high in PUFA (e.g. vegetable oils and fish oils) are also high in vitamin E (see Table 2). In general, the requirement for vitamin E appears to be 0.4 mg/g of linoleic acid; 3–4 mg/g of eicosapentaenoic and docosahexaenoic acid combined.

Dietary intake

In the UK, the average adult daily diet provides 8.3 mg.

Action

Vitamin E is an antioxidant, protecting PUFAs in membranes and other critical cellular structures from free radicals and products of oxidation. It works in conjunction with dietary selenium (a cofactor for glutathione peroxidase), and also with vitamin C and other enzymes, including superoxide dismutase and catalase.

Dietary sources

See Table 2 for dietary sources of vitamin E.

Metabolism

Absorption

Absorption of vitamin E is relatively inefficient (20–80%); the efficiency of absorption falls as the dose increases. Normal bile and pancreatic secretion are essential for maximal absorption. Absorption is maximal in the median part of the intestine; it is not absorbed in the large intestine to any great extent.

Distribution

Vitamin E is taken up principally via the lymphatic system and is transported in the blood bound to lipoproteins. More than 90% is carried by the LDL fraction. There is some evidence that a greater proportion is transported by the HDL fraction in females than in males.

Table 1   Dietary Reference Values for vitamin E (mg/day)

| Age | UK Safe Intake | EVM | USA | | | FAO/WHO RNI |
			EAR	RDA	TUL	EU RDA = 10 mg
0–6 months	0.4 mg/g PUFA[1]		–	4[2]	–	2.7
7–12 months	0.4 mg/g PUFA[1]		–	6[2]	–	2.7
1–3 years	0.4 mg/g PUFA[1]		5	6	200	5.0
4–8 years	–		6	7	300	5.0[6]
9–13 years	–		9	11	600	–
10–65+ years	–				–	7.5[7]/10.0[8]
14–70+ years	–		12	15	1000[3]	
Males						
11–50+ years	> 4		–	727	–	–
Females						
11–50+ years	> 3		–	–	–	–
Pregnancy	–		16	19	800[4]/1000[5]	
Lactation	–		16	19	800[3]/1000[4]	

[1] PUFA = polyunsaturated fatty acid.   [2] Adequate Intakes (AI).   [3] 14–18 years, 800 mg.   [4] Up to 18 years.   [5] 19–50 years.
[6] 7–9 years, 7.0 mg.   [7] Women   [8] Men.
EVM = Likely safe daily intake from supplements alone.
TUL = Tolerable Upper Intake Level from diet and supplements.

Vitamin E is stored in all fatty tissues, in particular adipose tissue, liver and muscle.

Elimination

The major route of elimination is the faeces; usually < 1% of orally administered vitamin E is excreted in the urine. Vitamin E appears in breast milk.

Bioavailability

Absorption is enhanced by dietary fat; medium-chain triglycerides enhance absorption whereas polyunsaturated fats are inhibitory.

Vitamin E is not very stable; significant losses from food may occur during storage and cooking. Losses also occur during food processing, particularly if there is significant exposure to heat and oxygen. There can be appreciable losses of vitamin E from vegetable oils during cooking.

Water-miscible preparations are superior to fat-soluble preparations in oral treatment of patients with fat malabsorption syndromes. The bioavailability of natural vitamin E is greater than that of synthetic vitamin E. However, several studies indicate that these differences may be even greater than originally thought.[1–4]

Deficiency

Deficiency of vitamin E is not generally recognised as a clearly definable syndrome. In premature infants, deficiency is associated with haemolytic anaemia, thrombocytosis, increased platelet aggregation, intraventricular haemorrhage and increased risk of retinopathy (but prophylaxis is controversial – see Precautions/contraindications).

The only children and adults who show clinical signs of vitamin E deficiency are those with severe malabsorption (i.e. in abetalipopro-

Table 2 Dietary sources of vitamin E

Food portion	Vitamin E content (mg)	Food portion	Vitamin E content (mg)
Breakfast cereals		Kidney (75 g)	0.3
1 bowl All-Bran (45 g)	1.0	Sardines (70 g)	0.3
1 bowl muesli (95 g)	**3.0**	*Tinned salmon (100 g)*	*1.5*
2 pieces Shredded Wheat	0.5	Tinned pilchards (100 g)	0.7
1 bowl Start (35 g)	**6.2**	Tinned tuna (100 g)	0.5
2 Weetabix	0.5	2 fillets herring, cooked (110 g)	0.3
Cereal products		2 fillets kipper, cooked (130 g)	0.4
Brown rice, boiled (160 g)	0.5	**Vegetables**	
Brown pasta	0	Broccoli, boiled (100 g)	1.3
Wholemeal bread, 2 slices	*1.5*	Brussels sprouts, boiled (100 g)	0.9
2 heaped tablespoons wheatgerm	**3.6**	**Sweet potatoes, boiled (150 g)**	**6.5**
Milk and dairy products		2 tomatoes	1.8
½ pint whole milk	0.08	1 small can baked beans (200 g)	0.75
½ pint soya milk	1.7	*Chickpeas, cooked (105 g)*	*1.6*
Hard cheese, 50 g	0.25	Red kidney beans, cooked (105 g)	0.2
1 egg, size 2 (60 g)	0.6	**Fruit**	
Fats and oils		1 apple	0.4
Butter, on 1 slice bread (10 g)	0.2	**½ avocado pear**	**3.0**
Margarine, on 1 slice bread (10 g)	0.8	1 banana	0.3
Low-fat spread, on 1 slice bread (10 g)	0.6	*Blackberries, stewed (100 g)*	*2.0*
2 tablespoons ghee (30 g)	1.0	1 orange	0.3
1 tablespoon olive oil	1.0	3 plums	0.6
1 tablespoon sunflower seed oil	**10**	**Nuts**	
1 tablespoon wheatgerm oil	**27**	**20 almonds**	**4.8**
2 teaspoons cod liver oil	*2.0*	*10 Brazil nuts*	*2.5*
Meat and fish		**30 hazelnuts**	**6.2**
Liver, lambs, cooked (90 g)	0.3	**30 peanuts**	**3.3**
Liver, calves, cooked (90 g)	0.4	**1 tablespoon sunflower seeds**	**7.5**
Liver, ox, cooked (90 g)	0.3	Peanut butter, on 1 slice bread (10 g)	0.5

Excellent sources (> 3.0 mg/portion) (**bold**); good sources
(> 1.5 mg/portion) (*italics*).

teinaemia, chronic cholestasis, biliary atresia and cystic fibrosis), or those with familial isolated vitamin E deficiency (rare inborn error of vitamin E metabolism). Clinical signs of deficiency include axonal dystrophy, reduced red blood cell half-life and neuromuscular disturbances.

Possible uses

A large number of claims for vitamin E have been made, but they are generally difficult to evaluate because they are often anecdotal or deduced from poorly designed trials.

Cancer

Vitamin E has been suggested to be protective against cancer, and several epidemiological studies have found either low dietary intakes of vitamin E and/or lower serum levels of vitamin E in patients who have cancer than in people without cancer. However, not all studies have shown protective effects.

The prospective Iowa Women's Health Study[5] showed that a reduced risk of colon cancer was associated with high intakes of supplemental vitamin E in women under 65 years of age. Further data from this study showed that higher intakes of vitamin E are linked to lower risk of gastric, oesophageal, oral and pharyngeal cancers.[6] High dietary intake of vitamin E has been associated with reduced risk of breast cancer,[7] but another study showed no protective effect.[8] There is some evidence that high plasma vitamin E levels protect against cervical cancer,[9] lung cancer,[10] and prostate cancer.[11]

A large Finnish study involving 29 133 male smokers showed that vitamin E supplementation (50 mg daily) reduced the incidence of prostate cancer by 32% and the risk of prostate cancer deaths by 41% compared with those who took no vitamin E.[12] The study also detected a somewhat lower incidence of colorectal cancer in the vitamin E arm compared with the no vitamin E arm, but this was not statistically significant.[13] Further data from this study showed that neither of the treatments used (vitamin E or beta-carotene) had a statistically significant effect on the incidence and mortality rate of pancreatic cancer and incidence of lung and urinary tract cancers.[14]

More recent trials have shown no significant benefit of vitamin E supplementation in cancer. A randomised, double-blind, placebo-controlled international trial (the initial Heart Outcomes Prevention Evaluation [HOPE] trial and the ongoing HOPE trial) investigated the effect of vitamin E (400 units daily) on cardiovascular events and primary prevention of cancer with a median follow-up of 7 years. There were no significant differences for cancer incidence and cancer deaths.[15] In the Women's Health Study, which tested the effect of vitamin E 600 units on alternate days on cardiovascular events and cancer, there were no significant effects on total cancer, breast cancer, lung cancer, colon cancer or cancer deaths.[16]

A 2003 systematic review concluded that there is insufficient evidence to recommend for or against the use of routine vitamin E supplementation for the prevention of cancers other than lung cancer (i.e. oesophageal, stomach, colorectal, urological and prostate) in the general population. The reviewers also concluded that there is good evidence to recommend against the use of routine vitamin E supplementation for the prevention of lung cancer.[17]

Cardiovascular disease

Epidemiological studies have shown that low dietary intakes of vitamin E are associated with an increased risk of CVD in both men[18] and women.[19] Plasma vitamin E levels have also been found to be low in patients with variant angina.[20]

Several randomised, placebo-controlled trials have looked at the effects of vitamin E supplementation in CVD. The Cambridge Heart Antioxidant Study (CHAOS),[21] which involved a total of 2002 subjects with angiographically proven CVD, showed that those who received vitamin E (400 or 800 units daily) had a 47% reduction in death from cardiovascular death and non-fatal myocardial infarction. This effect was due to a significant reduction (77%) in the risk of non-fatal myocardial infarction.

However, there was no effect on death from CVD alone. A non-significant increase in death from CVD was found in the supplemented group. However, a subsequent analysis of the deaths[22] showed that, of the 59 deaths due to ischaemic heart disease, six were in the group of patients that complied with vitamin E supplementation, 21 were in the non compliant group and 32 in the placebo group. This subsequent analysis has reduced concern about the possible adverse effects of vitamin E in this group of patients with established CVD.

An Italian trial – the Gruppo Italiano per lo Studio Della Sopravvivenza nell'Infarto Miocardio (GISSI)[23] – involved 11 324 patients who had survived a myocardial infarction within the 3-month period before enrolment. The four arms of the study included vitamin E, n-3 PUFA, a mixture of the two, or placebo, and the primary end points were death, non-fatal myocardial infarction and stroke. Vitamin E reduced the risk for the primary end points by 11%, and the n-3 PUFA by 15%, with only the latter reaching statistical significance. Possible explanations for the differences in the results between CHAOS and GISSI have been suggested, and include the fact that 50% of the GISSI subjects were on lipid-lowering drugs and that they presumably ate a Mediterranean diet with a high intake of fruit and vegetables.

The Alpha-Tocopherol, Beta-Carotene Cancer Prevention (ATBC) Study, involving 27 271 men, was designed to investigate the influence of antioxidant supplements on cancer in Finnish smokers. However, an analysis of heart disease[24] in this trial showed that vitamin E (50 mg) reduced the risk of primary major coronary events by 4% and the incidence of fatal CHD by 8%. Neither of these benefits was found to be statistically significant, but the trial used a small dose of a synthetic vitamin E supplement. A further analysis of the prevention of recurrence of angina for subjects in the ATBC trial[25] showed no significant protective effect of vitamin E.

The Heart Outcomes Prevention Evaluation (HOPE) study[26] enrolled a total of 2545 women and 6996 men aged 55 years or older who were at high risk of cardiovascular events, either because they had CVD or diabetes in addition to one other risk factor. They were assigned to natural vitamin E (400 units daily), an ACE inhibitor or placebo for a mean of 4.5 years. In comparison with placebo, there were no significant differences in the number of deaths from cardiovascular causes, myocardial infarction and stroke with vitamin E. Further analysis of the HOPE study in people with mild-to-moderate renal insufficiency found that vitamin E supplementation had no apparent effect on cardiovascular outcomes.[27] Extension of the HOPE trial by a further 4 years (HOPE-TOO) indicated that there were no differences in cardiovascular events but higher rates of heart failure and hospitalisations for heart failure.[15] The Women's Health Study[16] also concluded that 600 units vitamin E every other day over an average of 10.1 years provided no overall benefit for major cardiovascular events, but it reduced cardiovascular mortality in healthy women.

Systematic reviews[17,28,29] and meta-analyses[30] have concluded that there is no benefit of vitamin E in the prevention of cardiovascular events. A further meta-analysis found that high-dose vitamin E supplements (≥ 400 units daily) may increase all-cause mortality and should be avoided.[31]

Cataract

Epidemiological evidence suggests an association between cataract incidence and antioxidant status. Subjects with a low to moderate intake of vitamin E from foods had a higher risk of cataract relative to subjects with higher intakes,[32] and low serum levels of vitamin E and beta-carotene were related to increased risk of cataract in a Finnish study,[33] a French study,[34] and a US study.[35] However, an analysis of the ATBC Study showed that vitamin E (50 mg daily) had no effect on cataract prevalence in middle-aged smoking men.[36] Another study in 750 elderly people with cataracts[37] showed that those who took vitamin E supplements halved the risk of their cataracts progressing over a period of 4.5 years. A further trial in 1193 people with early or no cataract found that vitamin E 500 units daily given for 4 years did not reduce the incidence or progression of nuclear, cortical or posterior subcapsular cataracts.[38]

Diabetes

In a double-blind, placebo-controlled crossover study, 25 elderly patients with type 2 diabetes were randomised to receive 900 mg vitamin E or placebo daily for 3 months. Vitamin E supplementation was associated with a significant reduction in plasma glucose, haemoglobin A_{1c}, triglycerides, free fatty acids, total and LDL cholesterol and apoprotein B levels. The authors concluded that daily vitamin E supplementation produces a small but significant improvement in metabolic control in type 2 diabetes, but that more studies are needed to draw conclusions about the safety of long-term supplementation.[39]

Vitamin E could help to decrease the development of vascular disease in diabetes. Vitamin E supplementation (1200 units for 3 months) in 75 subjects who were diabetic or diabetic with vascular disease reduced the oxidation of LDL cholesterol, and reduced free radical levels and other markers of inflammation.[40] However in this study, the diabetics with or without vascular disease were not distinguishable by any of the markers of inflammation. Much larger, longer-term studies are needed to show that vitamin E has an anti-inflammatory effect in patients with vascular disease.

Neuropsychiatric disorders

Vitamin E supplementation has been associated with some success in tardive dyskinesia.[41,42]

In a double-blind, placebo-controlled study, 341 patients with Alzheimer's disease were randomised to receive 2000 units alpha-tocopherol, 10 mg selegiline, selegiline plus alpha-tocopherol or placebo. There was no significant difference in outcomes between the groups, but after adjustment for confounding factors, there were significant improvements in outcome with all three treatment groups compared with placebo. Vitamin E led to the greatest improvement, followed by selegiline, followed by the combination.[43]

Miscellaneous

Some studies have shown that vitamin E reduces oxidative damage in exercise,[44] improves lung function,[45] and improves immune function in the elderly.[46]

Vitamin E has been suggested to be of benefit in a vast range of conditions including arthritis, asthma, infertility and Parkinson's disease. Preliminary trials have shown some positive benefits, but larger trials are required to confirm these findings. There is some evidence that vitamin E (together with vitamin C) may raise the tolerance to UV rays and therefore reduce the risk of sunburn.

> ### Conclusion
> Several epidemiological studies have shown a link between low vitamin E intakes and CHD. There is some evidence that supplements (>100 units daily) reduce the risk of CHD, but some studies do not demonstrate a benefit. Evidence therefore remains promising but inconclusive. There is little evidence of benefit with vitamin E supplements in cancer prevention. There is preliminary evidence that vitamin E supplements improve immune function and lung function, and reduce oxidative damage in exercise. They may also improve glucose utilisation in diabetes, reduce the risk of cataract, delay the progress of Alzheimer's disease, and improve symptomology in tardive dyskinesia. However, further research is required before vitamin E can be recommended as a supplement for these purposes.

Precautions/contraindications

Vitamin E supplements should be avoided: by patients taking oral anticoagulants (increased bleeding tendency); in iron-deficiency anaemia (vitamin E may impair haematological response to iron) and hyperthyroidism.

Pregnancy and breast-feeding

No problems reported at normal intakes.

Adverse effects

Vitamin E is relatively non-toxic (fractional absorption declines rapidly with increasing intake, thereby preventing the accumulation of toxic concentrations of vitamin E in the tissues). Most adults can tolerate 100–800 mg daily and even doses of 3200 mg daily do not appear to lead to consistent adverse effects.

Large doses (>1000 mg daily for prolonged periods) have occasionally been associated with the following side-effects: increased bleeding tendency in vitamin K-deficient patients; altered endocrine function (thyroid, adrenal and pituitary); rarely, blurred vision, diarrhoea, dizziness, fatigue and weakness, gynaecomastia, headache and nausea.

However, a recent meta-analysis found that high-dose vitamin E supplements ($\geq$ 400 units daily) may increase all-cause mortality and concluded that they should be avoided.[31]

Interactions

Drugs

Anticoagulants: large doses of vitamin E may increase the anticoagulant effect.

Anticonvulsants (phenobarbitone, phenytoin, carbamazepine): may reduce plasma levels of vitamin E.

Colestyramine or colestipol: may reduce intestinal absorption of vitamin E.

Digoxin: requirement for digoxin may be reduced with vitamin E (monitoring recommended).

Insulin: requirement for insulin may be reduced by vitamin E (monitoring recommended).

Liquid paraffin: may reduce intestinal absorption of vitamin E (avoid long-term use of liquid paraffin).
Oral contraceptives: may reduce plasma vitamin E levels.
Sucralfate: may reduce intestinal absorption of vitamin E.

Nutrients

Copper: large doses of copper may increase requirement for vitamin E.
Iron: large doses of iron may increase requirements for vitamin E; vitamin E may impair the haematological response in iron-deficiency anaemia.
Polyunsaturated fatty acids: the dietary requirement for vitamin E increases when the intake of PUFA increases.
Vitamin A: vitamin E spares vitamin A and protects against some signs of vitamin A toxicity; very high levels of vitamin A may increase requirement of vitamin E; excessive doses of vitamin E may deplete vitamin A.
Vitamin C: vitamin C can spare vitamin E; vitamin E can spare vitamin C.
Vitamin K: large doses of vitamin E (1200 mg daily) increase the vitamin K requirement in patients taking anticoagulants.
Zinc: zinc deficiency may result in reduced plasma vitamin E levels.

Dose

Vitamin E is available in the form of tablets and capsules and is an ingredient of multivitamin preparations. Dietary supplements provide 10–1000 mg per daily dose.

Doses for use as an over-the-counter supplement above the RDA have not been established to be of value. There is no evidence to recommend doses higher than 400 units daily.

References

1   Ferslew KE, Acuff RV, Daigneault EA, *et al*. Pharmacokinetics and bioavailability of the RRR and all racemic stereoisomers of alpha-tocopherol in humans after single oral administration. *J Clin Pharmacol* 1993; 33: 84–88.

2   Acuff RV, Thedford SS, Hidiroglou NN, *et al*. Relative bioavailability of RRR- and all-rac-alpha-tocopherol acetate in humans: studies using deuterated compounds. *Am J Clin Nutr* 1994; 60: 397–402.

3   Kiyose C, Muramtsu R, Kameyana Y, *et al*. Biodiscrimination of alpha-tocopherol stereoisomers in humans after oral adminstration. *Am J Clin Nutr* 1997; 65: 785–789.

4   Burton GW, Traber MG, Acuff RV, *et al*. Human plasma and tissue alpha-tocopherol concentrations in response to supplementation with deuterated natural and synthetic vitamin E. *Am J Clin Nutr* 1998; 67: 669–684.

5   Bostick RM, Potter JD, McKenzie DR, *et al*. Reduced risk of colon cancer with high intake of vitamin E: The Iowa Women's Health Study. *Cancer Res* 1993; 53: 4230–4237.

6   Zheng W, Sellers TA, Doyle TJ, *et al*. Retinol, antioxidant vitamins and cancers of the upper digestive tract in a prospective cohort study of postmenopausal women. *Am J Epidemiol* 1995; 142: 955–960.

7   London SJ, Stein EA, Henderson IC, *et al*. Carotenoids, retinol and vitamin E and risk of proliferative benign breast disease and breast cancer. *Cancer Causes Control* 1992; 3: 503–512.

8   Hunter DJ, Manson JE, Colditz GA, *et al*. A prospective study of the intake of vitamins C, E and A and the risk of breast cancer. *N Engl J Med* 1993; 329: 234–240.

9   Palan PR, Mikhail MS, Basu J, Romney SL. Plasma levels of antioxidant beta-carotene and alpha-tocopherol in uterine cervix dysplasias and cancer. *Nutr Cancer* 1991; 15: 13–20.

10 Comstock GW, Helzlouser KJ, Bush TL. Prediagnostic serum levels of carotenoids and vitamin E as related to subsequent cancer in Washington County, Maryland. *Am J Clin Nutr* 1991; 53 (Suppl. 1): S260–264.

11 Eichholzer M, Stahelin HB, Ludin E, Bernasconi F. Smoking, plasma vitamins C, E, retinol and carotene and fatal prostate cancer: seventeen year follow up of the prospective Basel study. *Prostate* 1999; 38: 189–198.

12 Heinonen OP, Albanes D, Virtamo J, *et al*. Prostate cancer and supplementation with alpha-tocopherol and beta-carotene; incidence and mortality in a controlled trial. *J Natl Cancer Inst* 1998; 90: 440–446.

13 Rautalahti MT, Virtamo J, Taylor PR, *et al*. The effects of supplementation with alpha-tocopherol and beta-carotene on the incidence and mortality of carcinoma of the pancreas in a randomized controlled trial. *Cancer* 1999; 86: 37–42.

14 Virtamo J, Edwards BK, Virtanen M, *et al*. Effects of supplemental alpha-tocopherol and beta-carotene

on urinary tract cancer: incidence and mortality in a controlled trial (Finland). *Cancer Causes Control* 2000; 11: 933–939.

15 Lonn E, Bosch J, Yusuf S, *et al*. Effects of long-term vitamin E supplementation on cardiovascular events and cancer: a randomized controlled trial. *JAMA* 2005; 293: 1338–1347.

16 Lee IM, Cook NR, Gaziano JM, *et al*. Vitamin E in the primary prevention of cardiovascular disease and cancer: the Women's Health Study: a randomized controlled trial. *JAMA* 2005; 294: 56–65.

17 Alkhenizan A, Palda VA, and the Canadian Task Force on Preventive Health Care. The role of vitamin E supplements in the prevention of cardiovascular disease and cancer: systematic review and recommendations. London, Ontario: Canadian Task Force on Preventive Health care (CTFPHC), 2003:36.

18 Rimm BE. Vitamin E consumption and the risk of coronary heart disease in men. *N Engl J Med* 1993; 328: 1450–1456.

19 Kushi LH, Fee RM, Sellers TA, *et al*. Intake of vitamins A, C and E and postmenopausal breast cancer. The Iowa Women's Health Study. *Am J Epidemiol* 1996; 144: 165–174.

20 Miwa K, Miyagi Y, Igawa A, *et al*. Vitamin E deficiency in variant angina. *Circulation* 1996; 94: 14–18.

21 Stephens NG, Parsons A, Schofield PM, *et al*. Randomised controlled trial of vitamin E in patients with coronary disease: Cambridge heart antioxidant study (CHAOS). *Lancet* 1996; 347: 781–786.

22 Mitchinson MJ, Stephens NG, Parsons A, *et al*. Mortality in the CHAOS trial. *Lancet* 1999; 353: 381–382.

23 Marchioli R. GISSI-Prevenzione Investigators. Dietary supplementation with n-3 polyunsaturated fatty acids and vitamin E after myocardial infarction: results of the GISSI-Prevenzione trial. *Lancet* 1999; 354: 447–455.

24 Virtamo J, Rapola JM, Ripatti S, *et al*. Effects of vitamin E and beta carotene on the incidence of primary non-fatal myocardial infarction and fatal coronary heart disease. *Arch Intern Med* 1998; 158: 668–675.

25 Rapola JM, Virtamo J, Ripatti S, *et al*. Effects of alpha tocopherol and beta carotene supplements on symptoms, progression and prognosis of angina pectoris. *Heart* 1998; 79: 454–458.

26 The Heart Outcomes Prevention Evaluation Study Investigators. Vitamin E supplementation and cardiovascular events in high risk patients. *N Engl J Med* 2000; 342: 145–153.

27 Mann JF, Lonn EM, Yi Q, *et al*. Effects of vitamin E on cardiovascular outcomes in people with mild-to-moderate renal insufficiency: results of the HOPE study. *Kidney Int* 2004; 65: 1375–1380.

28 Shekelle PG, Morton SC, Jungvig LK, *et al*. Effect of supplemental vitamin E for the prevention and treatment of cardiovascular disease. *J Gen Intern Med* 2004; 19: 380–389.

29 Eidelman RS, Hollar D, Hebert PR, *et al*. Randomized trials of vitamin E in the treatment and prevention of cardiovascular disease. *Arch Intern Med* 2004; 164: 1552–1556.

30 Vivekananthan DP, Penn MS, Sapp SK, *et al*. Use of antioxidant vitamins for the prevention of cardiovascular disease: meta-analysis of randomised trials. *Lancet* 2003; 361: 2017–2023.

31 Miller ER III, Pastor-Barriuoso R, Dalal D, *et al*. Meta-analysis: high-dosage vitamin E supplementation may increase all-cause mortality. *Ann Intern Med* 2005; 142: 37–46.

32 Jacques PF, Chylack LT. Epidemiologic evidence of a role for the antioxidant vitamins and carotenoids in cataract prevention. *Am J Clin Nutr* 1991; 53: S352–355.

33 Knekt P, Heliovaara M, Rissanen A, *et al*. Serum antioxidant vitamins and risk of cataract. *BMJ* 1992; 305: 1392–1394.

34 Delcourt C, Cristol JP, Tessier F, *et al*. Age-related macular degeneration and antioxidant status in the POLA study. POLA Study Group. Pathologies Oculaires Liees a l'Age. *Arch Ophthalmol* 1999; 117: 1384–1390.

35 Lyle BJ, Mares-Perlman JA, Klein BE, *et al*. Serum carotenoids and tocopherols and incidence of age-related cataract. *Am J Clin Nutr* 1999; 69: 272–277.

36 Teikari JM, Virtamo J, Rautalahti M, *et al*. Long-term supplementation with alpha-tocopherol and beta-carotene and age-related cataract. *Acta Ophthalmol Scand* 1997; 75: 634–640.

37 Leske MC, Chylack LT, He Q, *et al*. Antioxidant vitamins and nuclear opacities: the longitudinal study of cataract. *Ophthalmology* 1998; 105: 831–836.

38 McNeill JJ, Robman L, Tikellis G, *et al*. Vitamin E supplementation and cataract: randomized controlled trial. *Ophthalmology* 2004; 111: 75–84.

39 Paolisso G, D'Amore A, Galzerano D, *et al*. Daily vitamin E supplements improve metabolic control but not insulin secretion in elderly type II diabetic patients. *Diabetes Care* 1993; 16: 1433–1437.

40 Devaraj S, Jialal I. Low-density lipoprotein post-secretory modification, monocyte function, and circulating adhesion molecules in type 2 diabetic patients with and without macrovascular complications. *Circulation* 2000; 102: 191–196.

41 Lohr JB, Caliguiri MP. A double–blind, placebo-controlled study of vitamin E treatment of tardive dyskinesia. *J Clin Psychiatr* 1996; 57: 167–173.

42 Adler LA, Edson R, Lavori P, *et al*. Long-term treatment effects of vitamin E treatment of tardive dyskinesia. *Biol Psychiatr* 1998; 43: 868–872.

43 Sano M, Ernesto C, Thomas RG, *et al*. A controlled trial of selegiline, alpha-tocopherol, or both, as treatment for Alzheiimer's disease. The Alzheimer's Disease Co-operative Study. *N Engl J Med* 1997; 336: 1216–1222.

44 Meydani M, Evans WJ, Handelman G, *et al*. Protective effect of vitamin E on exercise-induced oxidative damage in young and older adults. *Am J Physiol* 1993; 264 (5 Pt 2): R992–998.

45 Dow L, Tracey M, Villar A, *et al*. Does dietary intake of vitamin C and E influence lung function in older people? *Am J Respir Crit Care Med* 1996; 154: 1401–1404.

46 Meydani SM, Han SN, Wu D. Vitamin E and immune response in the aged: molecular mechanisms and clinical implications. *Immunol Rev* 2005; 205: 268–284.

Vitamin K

Description

Vitamin K is a fat-soluble vitamin.

Nomenclature

Vitamin K is a generic term for 2-methyl-1,4-naphthaquinone and all derivatives that exhibit qualitatively the biological activity of phytomenadione. The form of vitamin K present in foods is phytomenadione (vitamin K_1). The substances synthesised by bacteria are known as menaquinones (vitamin K_2). The parent compound of the vitamin K series is known as menadione (vitamin K_3); it is not a natural substance and is not used in humans. Menadiol sodium phosphate is a water-soluble derivative of menadione.

Human requirements

See Table 1 for Dietary Reference Values for vitamin K.

Action

Vitamin K is an essential cofactor for the hepatic synthesis of proteins involved in the regulation of blood clotting. These are prothrombin (factor II), factors VII, IX, X and proteins C, S and Z. Vitamin K is responsible for the carboxylation of the bone protein, osteocalcin, to its active form. Osteocalcin regulates the function of calcium in bone turnover and mineralisation. Vitamin K is also required for the biosynthesis of some other proteins found in plasma and the kidney.

Dietary sources

See Table 2 for dietary sources of vitamin K.

Metabolism

Absorption

Vitamin K is absorbed into the lymphatic system, predominantly in the upper part of the small intestine (jejunum and ileum), by a process that requires bile salts and pancreatic juice. The absorption of the different forms of vitamin K differs. Vitamin K_1 (phytomenadione) is absorbed by an active energy-dependent process from the proximal portion of the small intestine; menadione is absorbed by a passive non-carrier-mediated process from both the small and large intestines.

There is evidence that bacterially synthesised vitamin K can be a source of the vitamin for humans, although the availability of a sufficient concentration of bile salts for absorption is questionable (plasma levels of menaquinones suggest that some absorption occurs).

Distribution

Vitamin K is transported in the plasma and metabolised in the liver. Vitamin K_1 is concentrated and retained in the liver. Menadione is poorly retained by the liver but widely distributed in all other tissues.

Elimination

Vitamin K is eliminated partly in the bile (30–40%) and partly in the urine (15%).

Bioavailability

The effect of cooking and food processing on vitamin K has not been carefully studied, but it appears to be relatively stable.

Table 1   Dietary Reference Values for vitamin K (μg/day)

Age	UK Safe Intake	EVM	US RDA	FAO/WHO RNI
0–6 months	10		2.0[1]	5
7–12 months	10		2.5[1]	10
1–3 years	–		30[1]	15
4–6 years	–		–	20
4–8 years	–		55[1]	–
7–9 years	–		–	25
9–13 years	–		60	–
10–18 years	–		–	35–55
14–18 years	–		75	–
Males				
19–70+ years	1 μg/kg body weight	1000	120	65
Females				
19–70+ years	1 μg/kg/body weight	1000	90	55
Pregnancy	1 μg/kg/body weight		90	–
Lactation	1 μg/kg/body weight		90	–

Some of the requirement for vitamin K is met by synthesis in the intestine.

[1] Adequate intakes (AI).

EVM = Likely safe daily intake from supplements alone.

TUL = Tolerable Upper Intake Level from diet and supplements.

Table 2   Dietary sources of vitamin K

Food portion	Vitamin K content (μg)
Broccoli, boiled (100 g)	175
Brussels sprouts, boiled (100 g)	100
Cabbage, boiled (100 g)	125
Cauliflower, boiled (100 g)	150
Kale, boiled (100 g)	700
Lettuce (30 g)	45
Spinach, boiled (100 g)	400
Soya beans, cooked (100 g)	190
Meat, average, cooked (100 g)	50
Cheese (100 g)	50
Bread and cereals (100 g)	< 10
Fruit (100 g)	< 10

Excellent sources (> 100 μg/portion) (**bold**).

Deficiency

Vitamin K deficiency is rare and usually only occurs in people who have malabsorption problems or liver disease. However, it can occur in newborn babies, and all newborns should be given vitamin K. Deficiency leads to a prolonged prothrombin time, which can be corrected by vitamin K supplementation.

Possible uses

Osteoporosis

Vitamin K is not in common use as a dietary supplement, and few products contain it. However, there is increasing evidence that vitamin K deficiency may contribute to osteoporosis by reducing the carboxylation of osteocalcin in bone. Low serum levels of vitamin K and high levels of under-carboxylated osteocalcin have been reported in both post-menopausal women and individuals who have sustained hip fractures,[1–3] and low intakes of vitamin K may increase the risk of hip fracture.[4] In addition, some studies have shown that patients taking oral anticoagulants (which are vitamin K antagonists) are at increased risk of osteoporosis.

Intervention trials have shown positive effects on bone and risk of fracture. A study in which vitamin K_2 45 mg daily was given by mouth to 120 subjects with osteoporosis was found to reduce the risk of fractures and to sustain lumbar BMD.[5] Combined administration of vitamin K_2 (45 mg daily) and vitamin D_3 (1-alpha-hydroxyvitamin D_3 0.75 μg daily) increased the BMD of the lumbar spine in post-menopausal women with osteoporosis compared with calcium.[6] Combined therapy with vitamin K_2 and vitamin D_3 has been found to increase BMD more than vitamin K_2 alone.[7] Vitamin K_1 1 mg daily (co-administered with calcium, magnesium, zinc and vitamin D) reduced bone loss at the femoral neck in post-menopausal women between 50 and 60 years of age to a greater extent than vitamin D and the minerals alone.[8]

In a Dutch study in post-menopausal women, 80 μg of vitamin K_1 daily for 1 year increased carboxylated osteocalcin to pre-menopausal levels.[9] In another study, vitamin K_2 (45 mg daily) in elderly women with osteoporosis reduced serum under-carboxylated osteocalcin levels within 2 weeks, without any significant change in intact osteocalcin, suggesting that under-carboxylated osteocalcin is changed to carboxylated osteocalcin with potentially beneficial effects on bone metabolism.[10]

Vitamin K_2 has also been found to be protective in glucocorticoid-induced bone loss. In one study involving 60 patients, vitamin K_2 alone (45 mg daily), vitamin K_2 plus vitamin D_3 (alfacalcidol 0.5 μg daily) and vitamin D_3 alone prevented BMD loss at the lumbar spine caused by prednisolone.[11] Results from a further study suggested that vitamin K_2 (15 mg daily) could help to prevent glucocorticoid-induced bone loss.[12]

Precautions/contraindications

None reported (except Interactions – see below).

Pregnancy and breast-feeding

No problems reported.

Adverse effects

Oral ingestion of natural forms of vitamin K is not associated with toxicity. A rare hypersensitivity reaction (occasionally results in death) has been reported after intravenous administration of phytomenadione (especially if rapid).

Interactions

Drugs

Antibiotics: may increase requirement for vitamin K.

Anticoagulants: anticoagulant effect reduced by vitamin K (vitamin K is present in several tube feeds); dosage adjustment of anticoagulant may be necessary, especially when vitamin K has been used to antagonise excessive effects of anticoagulants (see the *British National Formulary*).

Colestyramine or colestipol: may reduce intestinal absorption of vitamin K.

Liquid paraffin: may reduce intestinal absorption of vitamin K (avoid long-term use of liquid paraffin).

Sucralfate: may reduce intestinal absorption of vitamin K.

Nutrients

Vitamin A: under conditions of hypervitaminosis A, hypothrombinaemia may occur; it can be corrected by administering vitamin K.

Vitamin E: large doses of vitamin E (1200 mg daily) increase the vitamin K requirement in patients taking anticoagulants, but no confirmed effect in individuals not taking anticoagulants.

Dose

Vitamin K is not generally available in isolation as a supplement. It is an ingredient in some multivitamin preparations. No dose has been established.

Upper safety levels

The UK Expert Group on Vitamins and Minerals (EVM) has identified a safe upper level of vitamin K for adults from supplements alone of 1000 μg daily.

References

1 Binkle NC, Suttie JW. Vitamin K nutrition and osteoporosis. *J Nutr* 1995; 125: 1812–1821.
2 Kanai T, Takagi T, Masuhiro K, *et al*. Serum vitamin K level and bone mineral density in post-menopausal women. *Int J Gynaecol Obstet* 1997; 56: 25–30.
3 Vermeer C, Gijsbers BL, Cracium AM, *et al*. Effects of vitamin K on bone mass and bone metabolism. *J Nutr* 1996; 126 (Suppl. 4): S1187–1191.
4 Feskanich D, Weber P, Willett WC, *et al*. Vitamin K intake and hip fractures in women: a prospective study. *Am J Clin Nutr* 1999; 69: 74–79.
5 Shikari M, Shikari Y, Aoki C, Miura M. Vitamin K2 (menatetrone) effectively prevents fractures and sustains lumbar bone mineral density in osteoporosis. *J Bone Miner Res* 2000; 15: 515–521.
6 Iwamoto J, Takeda T, Ichimura S. Effect of combined administration of vitamin D3 and vitamin K2 on bone mineral density of the lumbar spine in postmenopausal women with osteoporosis. *J Orthop Sci* 2000; 5: 546–551.
7 Braam LA, Knapen MH, Geusens P, *et al*. Vitamin K1 supplementation retards bone loss in postmenopausal women between 50 and 60 years of age. *Calcif Tissue Int* 2003; 73: 21–26.
8 Schaafsma A, Muskiet FA, Storm H, *et al*. Vitamin D(3) and vitamin K(1) supplementation of Dutch postmenopausal women with normal and low bone mineral densities: effects of serum 25-hydroxyvitamin D and carboxylated osteocalcin. *Eur J Clin Nutr* 2000; 54: 626–631.
9 Miki T, Nakatsuka K, Naha H, *et al*. Vitamin K(2) (menaquinone 4) reduces serum undercarboxylated osteocalcin level as early as 2 weeks in elderly women with established osteoporosis. *J Bone Miner Metab* 2003; 21: 161–165.
10 Ushiroyama T, Ikeda A, Ueki M. Effect of continuous combined therapy with vitamin K(2) and vitamin D(3) on bone mineral density and coagulofibrinolysis function in postmenopausal women. *Maturitas* 2002; 41: 211–221.
11 Yonemura K, Fukasawa H, Fujigaki Y, Hishida A. Protective effect of vitamin K2 and D3 on prednisolone-induced loss of bone mineral density in the lumbar spine. *Am J Kidney Dis* 2004; 43: 53–60.
12 Sasaki N, Kusano E, Takahashi H, *et al*. Vitamin K2 inhibits glucocorticoid-induced bone loss partly by preventing the reduction of osteoprotegerin (OPG). *J Bone Miner Metab* 2005; 23: 41–47.

Zinc

Description

Zinc is an essential trace mineral.

Human requirements

See Table 1 for Dietary Reference Values for zinc.

Dietary intake

In the UK, the average adult daily diet provides: for men, 10.2 mg; for women, 7.4 mg.

Action

The human body contains approximately 2 g of zinc, making this trace element the most abundant in the body after iron.[1] Zinc is an essential component of over 200 enzymes. It plays an important role in the metabolism of proteins, carbohydrates, lipids and nucleic acids. It is a cofactor in a range of biochemical processes, including the synthesis of DNA, RNA and protein.[2] Zinc is also required for the hepatic synthesis of retinol-binding protein, the protein involved in transporting vitamin A. Without adequate zinc, symptoms of vitamin A deficiency can appear even if supplements of vitamin A are taken.[3]

Zinc is also crucial for maintaining the structure and integrity of cell membranes. Reduction in the concentration of zinc in biomembranes results in increased susceptibility to oxidative damage and alteration in specific transport systems and receptor sites, and may underlie some of the disorders associated with zinc deficiency.[4] Accumulation of zinc in cell membranes can block receptor sites for histamine release, leading to reduction in release of histamine from mast cells.[5]

Another important structural role for zinc is the so-called zinc-finger motif in proteins.[6] Zinc fingers enable polypeptides that are too small to fold by themselves to fold stably when stabilised by bound zinc. Zinc finger proteins regulate gene expression[7] by acting as transcription factors (binding to DNA and influencing the transcription of specific genes). These proteins are involved in the metabolism of reproductive hormones (e.g. androgens, oestrogens and progesterone). Prostaglandins and nuclear receptors for steroids are also zinc finger proteins. Zinc has regulatory roles in cell signalling and influences nerve impulse transmission. It also has a role in apoptosis (gene-directed cell death), a critical cellular regulatory process with implications for growth and development, as well as a number of chronic diseases.[8]

Zinc plays a role in immune function, which explains why it has been investigated for possible benefit in infections, such as colds. It is involved in the function of cells contributing to non-specific immunity, such as neutrophils and natural killer cells. Zinc also plays a role in T-lymphocyte function and the development of acquired immunity.[9]

Zinc is essential for reproduction. It is necessary for the metabolism of reproductive hormones, ovulation, testicular function, the formation and maturation of sperm, fertilisation and the health of the mother and foetus during pregnancy.[10] Deficiency of zinc during early development can be teratogenic. In men, the prostate gland has the highest concentration of zinc of any organ in the body.

359

Table 1 Dietary Reference Values for zinc (mg/day)

EU RDA = 15 mg

Age	UK				USA		FAO/WHO RNI[5]
	LNRI	EAR	RNI	EVM	RDA	TUL	
0–3 months	2.6	3.3	4.0		2.0[1]	0	1.1–6.6
4–6 months	2.6	3.3	4.0		2.0[1]	0	1.1–6.6
7–12 months	3.0	3.8	5.0		3.0	5.0	2.5–8.4
1–3 years	3.0	3.8	5.0		3.0	7.0	2.4–8.3
4–6 years	4.0	5.0	6.5		–	–	2.9–9.6
4–8 years	–	–	–		5.0	12.0	–
7–10 years	4.0	5.4	7.0		–	–	3.3–11.2[a]
Males							
11–14 years	5.3	7.0	9.0		–	–	5.1–17.1[b]
14–18 years	–	–	–		11.0	34.0	5.1–17.1
15–18 years	5.5	7.3	9.5		–	–	–
19–50+ years	5.5	7.3	9.5	25	11.0	40.0	–
19–65+ years	–	–	–		–	–	4.2–14.0
Females							
11–14 years	5.3	7.0	9.0		–	–	4.3–14.4[b]
14–18 years	–	–	–		9.0	34.0	4.3–14.4
15– 18 years	4.0	5.5	7.0		–	–	–
19–50+ years	4.0	5.5	7.0	25	8.0	40.0	–
19–65+ years	–	–	–		–	–	3.0–9.8
Pregnancy	*	*	*		11.0[2]	40.0[3]	–
Lactation	–	–	–		12.0[4]	40.0[3]	–
0–4 months			+6.0		–	–	–
4+ months			+2.5		–	–	–

* No increment.
[a] 7–9 years.　[b] 10–14 years.
[1] Adequate Intakes (AIs).　[2] aged <18 years, 13 mg daily.　[3] aged <18 years, 34 mg daily.
[4] aged <18 years, 14 mg daily.　[5] Recommended intake varies from diet of high to low zinc bioavailability.
EVM = Likely safe daily intake from supplements alone.
TUL = Tolerable Upper Intake Level from diet and supplements.

Other roles for zinc include wound healing, behaviour and learning, taste and smell, blood clotting, thyroid hormone function and insulin action. Present in high concentrations in the eye, particularly in the retina and choroid, zinc plays a role in the maintenance of vision.[11]

Zinc also acts as an antioxidant, restricting endogenous free radical production and acting as a structural component of the extracellular antioxidant enzyme, superoxide dismutase. It also helps to protect against depletion of vitamin E and maintains tissue concentrations of metallothionein – a possible scavenger of free radicals.[11]

Dietary sources

See Table 2 for dietary sources of zinc.

Table 2 Dietary sources of zinc

Food portion	Zinc content (mg)	Food portion	Zinc content (mg)
Breakfast cereals		1 beef steak (155 g)	7.0
1 bowl All-Bran (45 g)	**3.0**	**Minced beef, lean, stewed (100 g)**	**6.0**
1 bowl Bran Flakes (45 g)	*1.5*	*1 chicken leg (190 g)*	*2.0*
1 bowl Corn Flakes (30 g)	0.1	**Liver, lambs, cooked (90 g)**	**4.0**
1 bowl muesli (95 g)	*2.0*	**Kidney, lambs, cooked (75 g)**	**3.0**
2 pieces Shredded Wheat	1.0	*Fish*	
2 Weetabix	1.0	*Pilchards, canned (105 g)*	*1.5*
Cereal products		*Sardines, canned (70 g)*	*2.0*
Bread, brown, 2 slices	0.7	**Crab (100 g)**	**5.5**
white, 2 slices	0.4	**1 dozen oysters**	**78.7**
wholemeal, 2 slices	1.3	*Vegetables*	
1 chapati	0.7	Green vegetables, average, boiled (100 g)	0.4
Pasta, brown, boiled (150 g)	*1.5*	Potatoes, boiled (150 g)	0.5
white, boiled (150 g)	0.7	1 small can baked beans (200 g)	1.0
Rice, brown, boiled (165 g)	1.0	Lentils, kidney beans or other pulses (105 g)	1.0
white, boiled (165 g)	1.0	*Dahl, chickpea (155 g)*	*1.5*
Milk and dairy products		*lentil (155 g)*	*1.5*
½ pint milk, whole, semi-skimmed or skimmed	1.0	Soya beans, cooked (100 g)	1.0
1 pot yoghurt (150 g)	1.0		
Cheese, Brie (50 g)	1.0	*Fruit*	
Camembert (50 g)	1.3	8 dried apricots	0.2
Cheddar (50 g)	1.1	4 figs	0.3
Cheddar, reduced fat (50 g)	1.4	Half an avocado pear	0.3
Cottage cheese (100 g)	0.5	1 banana	0.2
Cream cheese (30 g)	0.2	Blackberries (100 g)	0.2
Edam (50 g)	1.1	Blackcurrants (100 g)	0.3
Feta (50 g)	0.4	*Nuts*	
Fromage frais (100 g)	0.3	20 almonds	0.6
White cheese (50 g)	*1.5*	10 Brazil nuts	1.0
1 egg, size 2 (60 g)	0.8	30 hazelnuts	0.7
Meat and fish		1 small bag peanuts (25 g)	1.0
Red meat, roast (85 g)	**4.0**		

Excellent sources (**bold**); good sources (*italics*)

Metabolism

Absorption
Absorption occurs throughout the length of the small intestine, mostly in the jejunum, both by a carrier-mediated process and by diffusion.

Distribution
Zinc is transported in association with albumin, amino acids and a 2-macroglobulin. Zinc is principally an intracellular ion and approximately 95% is found within the cells. Approximately 57% of the body pool is stored in skeletal muscle, 29% in bone and 6% in the skin, but zinc is found in all body tissues and fluids, including the liver, kidneys, pancreas, prostate gland and retina.[2]

Elimination
Elimination of zinc is mainly in the faeces; smaller amounts are excreted in the urine and via the skin.

Bioavailability

Absorption of zinc is enhanced by certain amino acids such as cysteine and histidine; meat, dairy produce and fish contain these amino acids and therefore their zinc is efficiently absorbed. Zinc from wholegrain cereals, including bran products, and also soy protein, is less available, partly because of the presence of phytate. The effect of non-starch polysaccharides (dietary fibre), tannic acid and caffeine is equivocal. High calcium intake may reduce absorption, but this is likely only at higher than recommended intakes of calcium (e.g. >1500 mg daily).

Deficiency

Clinical manifestations of severe zinc deficiency include alopecia, diarrhoea, dermatitis, psychiatric disorders, weight loss, intercurrent infection (due to impaired immune function), hypogonadism in males, and poor ulcer healing. Signs of mild to moderate deficiency include growth retardation, male hypogonadism, poor appetite, rough skin, mental lethargy, delayed wound healing and impaired taste acuity.

Maternal zinc deficiency before and during pregnancy may lead to intrauterine growth retardation and congenital abnormalities in the foetus.

Possible uses

Anorexia nervosa

It has been suggested that zinc deficiency is involved in the aetiology of anorexia nervosa. Teenage girls who are restricting their food intake during the period of rapid growth may develop a state of zinc deficiency and anorexia nervosa. A daily supplement of 45 mg of zinc, as zinc sulphate, has been reported to result in weight gain in 17 young female patients with long-standing anorexia nervosa.[12] The weight gain continued over a 4-year follow-up period. Compared with placebo, a daily dose of 100 mg of zinc gluconate doubled the rate of increase in body mass index in 35 female patients with anorexia.[13]

Wound healing

Zinc is essential in wound healing and zinc supplementation is valuable in cases of wounds where there is zinc deficiency or malnutrition. According to one review, zinc administered orally or topically to wounds can promote healing and reduce infection.[14] In patients with low serum zinc levels, topical zinc oxide has been shown to promote cleansing and re-epithelialisation of leg ulcers, reducing deterioration of ulcers and the risk of infection.[15] A Cochrane review assessed six placebo-controlled trials of zinc supplementation in arterial and venous leg ulcers and found no overall benefit on the number of ulcers healed.[16] However, in people with low serum zinc levels, there is some evidence that oral zinc might improve healing of leg ulcers.

Common cold

The use of zinc lozenges within 24 h of the onset of cold symptoms and continued every 2–3 h while awake has been advocated for reducing the duration of the common cold. One proposed mechanism is that zinc may bind with proteins of critical nerve endings in the respiratory tract and surface proteins of the rhinovirus, thereby interrupting virus infection.[17] However, results from RCTs in humans are conflicting. A meta-analysis of six RCTs reported no statistical benefit of using zinc lozenges to reduce cold duration.[18] Two additional analyses of RCTs of zinc for the common cold found that evidence is inconclusive.[19,20] A total of 10 RCTs have now been conducted to evaluate the use of zinc lozenges on the duration of colds. Of these, five showed a positive effect and five reported no effect.

Researchers have suggested that discrepancies may be caused by inadequate placebo control and differences in lozenge formulation, administration and dosage. The amount of available ionised zinc may influence the effectiveness of zinc and this varies with different lozenge formulations. The addition of flavouring agents such as citric acid, mannitol or sorbitol to zinc gluconate lozenge preparations decreases the effect of zinc ionisation, and hence its release, while the addition of glycine to zinc gluconate lozenges does not.[21] Positive results in the common cold are generally associated with zinc gluconate or zinc acetate, while other forms are less effective.

Some researchers question the clinical relevance of oral zinc levels because the rhinovirus replicates in the nasal mucosa. Zinc nasal preparations have also been investigated for the common cold. One study showed that a nasal gel formulation reduced cold duration compared with placebo when used within 24 h of onset of symptoms,[22] while others showed no effect of a nasal spray on duration of cold symptoms.[23,24]

Taking lozenges every 2–3 h while awake may result in daily zinc intakes above the safe upper level of 25 mg daily. Short-term use of zinc lozenges (up to 5 days) has not resulted in serious side-effects, although some individuals experience gastrointestinal irritation. Use of zinc at above the upper limit for prolonged periods (e.g. 6–8 weeks) is not recommended and may lead to copper deficiency.

Male fertility

Zinc is necessary for growth, sexual maturation and reproduction. Infertile men have been reported to have reduced seminal and serum zinc levels compared with fertile men.[25–27] However, other research has shown no statistically significant relationship between zinc in serum or seminal plasma and semen quality or IgA or IgG antisperm antibody. In the same study, zinc levels had no influence on sperm capacity to penetrate cervical mucus *in vitro* or *in vivo* and had no effect on subsequent fertility.[28]

Age-related macular degeneration (ARMD)

Several studies have investigated the effects of zinc and antioxidant vitamins on the progression of age-related macular degeneration (ARMD). The highest profile study is the Age-Related Eye Disease Study (AREDS) in which high-dose zinc supplements (80 mg daily, which is about 10 times the Reference Nutrient Intake), together with antioxidants, were shown to reduce the risk of progression to advanced ARMD among patients who already had extensive drusen.[29] A Cochrane review looked at the overall evidence to date, including AREDS, and concluded that current data are insufficient

to state that antioxidant vitamin and mineral supplementation should be taken during early signs of the disease and that more research is needed.[30]

Miscellaneous

There is limited evidence that zinc may play a role in the treatment of benign prostatic hyperplasia (BPH), exercise performance,[31] and immune function in the elderly.[32] In AIDS patients receiving azidothymidine (AZT) supplemented with zinc for 30 days, body weight was stabilised and the frequency of opportunistic infections reduced in the following 2 years.[33] However, further controlled trials are needed. The role of zinc supplements in acne, white spots on the finger nails and treatment of brittle nails is controversial.

Conclusion

Results from studies investigating the effect of zinc supplements on the common cold are conflicting. There is limited evidence for a benefit of zinc in male infertility and immune function. Further controlled trials are needed.

Adverse effects

Signs of acute toxicity (doses >200 mg daily) include gastrointestinal pain, nausea, vomiting and diarrhoea. Prolonged exposure to doses >50 mg daily may induce copper deficiency (marked by low serum copper and caeruloplasmin levels, microcytic anaemia and neutropenia), and iron deficiency. Doses >150 mg daily may reduce serum HDL levels, depress immune function and cause gastric erosion.

Interactions

Drugs

Ciprofloxacin: reduced absorption of ciprofloxacin.
Oral contraceptives: may reduce plasma zinc levels.
Penicillamine: reduced absorption of penicillamine.

Tetracyclines: reduced absorption of zinc and vice versa.

Nutrients

Copper: large doses of zinc may reduce absorption of copper.

Folic acid: may reduce zinc absorption (raises concern about pregnant women who are advised to take folic acid to reduce the risk of birth defects).

Iron: reduces absorption of oral iron and vice versa (raises concern about pregnant women who are often given iron; this may reduce zinc status and increase the risk of intrauterine growth retardation and congenital abnormalities in the foetus).

Dose

Zinc is available in the form of tablets and capsules and as an ingredient in multivitamin preparations.

The dose beyond the RDA is not established. Dietary supplements contain 5–50 mg (elemental zinc) per daily dose.

The zinc content of some commonly used zinc salts is as follows: zinc amino acid chelate (100 mg/g); zinc gluconate (130 mg/g); zinc orotate (170 mg/g); zinc sulphate (227 mg/g).

Upper safety limits

The UK Expert Groups on Vitamins and Minerals (EVM) has identified a safe upper limit of zinc for adults from supplements alone of 25 mg daily.

References

1 Grahn BH, Paterson PG, Gottschall-Pass KT, Zhang Z. Zinc and the eye. *J Am Coll Nutr* 2001; 20: 106–118.

2 King JC, Keen CL. Zinc. In: Shils ME, Olson JA, Shike M, Ross AC, eds. *Modern Nutrition in Health and Disease*, 9th edn. Philadelphia: Lippincott Williams & Wilkins, 1998: 223–239.

3 Christian P, Khatry SK, Yamini S, *et al*. Zinc supplementation might potentiate the effect of vitamin A in restoring night vision in pregnant Nepalese women. *Am J Clin Nutr* 2001; 73: 1045–1051.

4 Bettger WJ, Fish TJ, O'Dell BL. Effects of copper and zinc status of rats on erythrocyte stability and superoxide dismutase activity. *Proc Soc Exp Biol Med* 1978; 158: 279–282.

5 Kazimierczak W, Adamas B, Maslinski C. The action of the complexes of lidocaine with zinc on histamine release from isolated rat mast cells. *Biochem Pharmacol* 1978; 27: 243–249.

6 Klug A, Rhodes D. 'Zinc fingers': a novel protein motif for nucleic acid recognition. *Trends Biochem Sci* 1987; 12: 464–469.

7 Cousins RJ, Blanchard RK, Moore RB, *et al*. Regulation of zinc metabolism and genomic outcomes. *J Nutr* 2003; 133 (5 Suppl. 1): S1521–1526.

8 Thompson CB. Apoptosis in the pathogenesis and treatment of disease. *Science* 1995; 267: 1456–1462.

9 Shankar AH, Prasad AS. Zinc and immune function: the biological basis of altered resistance to infection. *Am J Clin Nutr* 1998; 68: S447–463.

10 Barceloux DG. Zinc. *J Toxicol Clin Toxicol* 1999; 37: 279–292.

11 Powell SR. The antioxidant properties of zinc. *J Nutr* 2000; 130: S1447–1454.

12 Safai-Kutti S. Oral zinc supplementation in anorexia nervosa. *Acta Psychiatr Scand Suppl* 1990; 361: 14–17.

13 Birmingham CL, Goldner EM, Bakan R. Controlled trial of zinc supplementation in anorexia nervosa. *Int J Eat Disord* 1994; 15: 251–255.

14 Landsdown AB. Zinc in the healing wound. *Lancet* 1996; 346; 706–707.

15 Agren MS. Studies in zinc wound healing. *Acta Derm Venereol* 1990; 154 (Suppl.): 1–36.

16 Wilkinson EA, Hawke CI. Oral zinc for arterial and venous leg ulcers. Cochrane database, issue 4, 1998. London: Macmillan.

17 Novick SG, Godfrey JC, Pollack RL, Wilder HR. Zinc-induced suppression of inflammation in the respiratory tract, caused by infection with human rhinovirus and other irritants. *Med Hypotheses* 1997; 49: 347–357.

18 Jackson JL, Peterson C, Lesho E. A meta-analysis of zinc salt lozenges and the common cold. *Arch Intern Med* 1997; 157: 2373–2376.

19 Jackson JL, Lesho E, Peterson C. Zinc and common cold: a meta-analysis revisited. *J Nutr* 2000; 130: S1512–1515.

20 Marshall I. Zinc and the common cold. Cochrane database, issue 2, 2000. London: Macmillan.

21 Eby GA. Zinc ion availability – the determinant of efficacy in zinc lozenge treatment of common colds. *J Antimicrob Chemother* 1997; 40: 483–493.

22 Hirt M, Nobel S, Barron E. Zinc nasal gel for the treatment of common cold symptoms: a

double-blind, placebo-controlled trial. *Ear Nose Throat J* 2000; 79: 778–80, 782.

23 Belongia EA, Berg R, Liu K. A randomized trial of zinc nasal spray for the treatment of upper respiratory illness in adults. *Am J Med* 2001; 111: 103–108.

24 Turner RB. Ineffectiveness of intranasal zinc gluconate for prevention of experimental rhinovirus colds. *Clin Infect Dis* 2001; 33: 1865–1870.

25 Mohan H, Verma J, Singh I. Inter-relationship of zinc levels in serum and semen in oligospermic infertile patients and fertile males. *Indian J Pathol Microbiol* 1997; 40: 451–455.

26 Kvist U, Bjornadahl L, Kjellberg S. Sperm nuclear zinc, chromatin stability and male fertility. *Scanning Microsc* 1987; 1: 1241–1247.

27 Chia SE, Ong CN, Chua LH, Ho LM, Tay SK. Comparisons of zinc concentrations in blood and seminal plasma and the various sperm parameters between fertile and infertile men. *J Androl* 2000: 21: 53–57.

28 Eggert-Kruse W, Zwick EM, Batschulat K, *et al*. Are zinc levels in seminal plasma associated with seminal leukocytes and other determinants of semen quality? *Fertil Steril* 2002; 77: 260–269.

29 Age Related Eye Disease Study Research Group. A randomized, placebo-controlled, clinical trial of high-dose supplementation with vitamins C and E, beta carotene, and zinc for age-related macular degeneration and vision loss: AREDS report no.8. *Arch Ophthalmol* 2001; 119: 1417–1436.

30 Evans JR. Antioxidant vitamin and mineral supplements for age-related macular degeneration. Cochrane database, issue 2, 2006. London: Macmillan.

31 Krotiewski M, Gudmundson M, Backsrtrom P, *et al*. Zinc and muscle strength and endurance. *Acta Physiol Scand* 1982; 116: 309–311.

32 Bodgen JD, Oleske JM, Lavenhar MA, *et al*. Effects of one year supplementation with zinc and other micronutrients on cellular immunity in the elderly. *J Am Coll Nutr* 1990; 9: 214–215.

33 Mocchegiani E. Benefit of oral zinc supplementation as an adjunct to zidovudine (AZT) therapy against opportunistic infections in AIDS. *Int J Immunopharmacol* 1995; 17: 719–727.

Appendix 1

Guidance on safe upper levels of vitamins and minerals

Vitamin/mineral	EU RDA	EVM UK	TUL USA	SCF EU
Vitamin A (retinol equivalent μg)	800	1500[1]	3000	3600
Vitamin B$_1$ (thiamine) mg	1.4	100[1]	–	
Vitamin B$_2$ (riboflavin) mg	1.6	100[1]	–	–
Vitamin B$_6$ (pyridoxine) mg	2	10[2]	100	25
Vitamin B$_{12}$ (cobalamin) μg	1	1000[1]	–	–
Vitamin C (ascorbic acid) mg	60	1000[1]	2000	–
Vitamin D (cholecalciferol) μg	5	25[1]	50	50
Vitamin E (tocopherol) mg	10	727[2]	1000	300
Niacin mg	18		30	
Nicotinamide mg	–	500[1]		900
Nicotinic acid mg	–	17[1]		10
Biotin μg	150	970[1]	–	–
Folic acid μg	200	1000[1]	1000	1000
Pantothenic acid mg	6	200[1]	–	–
Calcium mg	800	1500[1]	2500	2500
Iodine μg	150	500[1]	1100	600
Iron mg	14	17[1]	45	
Magnesium mg	300	400[1]	350	250
Phosphorus mg	800	250[1]	4000	
Zinc mg	15	25[2]	40	25
Vitamin K mg	–	1[1]	–	–
Beta-carotene mg		7[2]	–	20
Chromium μg	–	–	–	
Copper mg	5[2]	10	5	
Manganese mg		4[1]	11	–
Molybdenum μg		–	2000	600
Selenium μg	–	200[2]	400	300
Boron mg	–	5.9[2]	20	
Nickel mg	–		1	
Vanadium mg	–		1.8	–

EU RDA: the Recommended Daily Allowance considered sufficient to prevent deficiency in most individuals in the population.

EVM: draft figures (2002) produced by the Food Standards Agency (FSA) Expert Vitamin and Mineral (EVM) group.

[1] Likely safe total daily intake from supplements alone.

[2] Safe upper level from supplements alone.

TUL: Tolerable Upper Intake Levels defined by the Food and Nutrition Board of the US National Academy of Sciences as the highest total level of a nutrient (diet plus supplements) that could be consumed safely on a daily basis, which is unlikely to cause adverse health effects to almost all individuals in the general population. As intakes rise above the TUL, the risk of adverse effects increases. The TUL describes long-term intakes, so an isolated dose above the TUL need not necessarily cause adverse effects. The TUL defines safety limits and is not a recommended intake for most people most of the time.

SCF: Tolerable Upper Intake Levels defined by the European Commission's Scientific Committee on Food (SCF) as the maximum level of chronic daily intake of a nutrient (from all sources) judged to be unlikely to pose a risk of adverse effects to humans. http://ec.europa.eu/comm./food/fs/sc/scf/out80_en.html

Note: dashes (–) indicate that the nutrient has been considered but no level set. Where the column is blank, the nutrient has not been considered.

Appendix 2

Drug and supplement interactions

Drug	Food/nutrient	Effect	Intervention
Drugs acting on the gastrointestinal system			
Antacids	Iron	Aluminium-, magnesium- and calcium-containing antacids and sodium bicarbonate reduce absorption of iron	Separate administration of antacids and iron by at least 2 h
Sulfasalazine	Folic acid	Sulfasalazine can reduce absorption of folic acid	Monitor and give a supplement if necessary
Stimulant laxatives	Potassium	Prolonged use of stimulant laxatives can precipitate hypokalaemia	Avoid prolonged use of laxatives
Liquid paraffin	Fat-soluble vitamins	Liquid paraffin reduces absorption of vitamins A, D, E and K	Avoid prolonged use of liquid paraffin
Drugs acting in the treatment of diseases of the cardiovascular system			
Thiazide diuretics	Calcium/vitamin D	Excessive serum calcium levels can develop in patients given thiazides with supplements of calcium and/or vitamin D	Concurrent use of thiazides with calcium and/or vitamin D need not be avoided but serum calcium levels should be monitored
ACE inhibitors	Potassium	Concurrent use of ACE inhibitors with potassium may induce severe hyperkalaemia	Avoid
Potassium-sparing diuretics	Potassium	Concurrent use of potassium-sparing diuretics and either potassium supplements or potassium-containing salt substitutes may induce severe hyperkalaemia	Avoid concurrent use of potassium-sparing diuretics and potassium supplements unless potassium levels are monitored; warn patients about risks of salt substitutes
Calcium-channel blockers	Calcium	Therapeutic effects of verapamil can be antagonised by calcium	Calcium supplements should be used with caution in patients taking verapamil
Hydralazine	Vitamin B_6	Long-term administration of hydralazine may lead to pyridoxine deficiency	Vitamin B_6 supplement may be needed if symptoms of peripheral neuritis develop

Drug	Food/nutrient	Effect	Intervention
Anticoagulants	Vitamin E	Effects of warfarin may be increased by large doses of vitamin E (>100 units daily)	Avoid high-dose vitamin E supplements
	Vitamin K	Effects of anticoagulants can be reduced or abolished by large intakes of vitamin K	Avoid excessive intake of vitamin K (e.g. check labels of enteral feeds)
	Bromelain Chondroitin Fish oils Garlic Ginkgo biloba Ginseng Grape seed extract Green tea S-adenosyl methionine	Effects of anticoagulants may be increased by these supplements	Care with these supplements in people taking anticoagulants, aspirin and anti-platelet drugs. Avoid if possible, otherwise monitor carefully
Colestyramine Colestipol	Fat-soluble vitamins	Prolonged use of these drugs may result in deficiency of fat-soluble vitamins	Supplements of vitamins A, D, E and K may be needed if these drugs are administered for prolonged periods

Drugs acting on the central nervous system

Drug	Food/nutrient	Effect	Intervention
Phenothiazines	Evening primrose oil	Evening primrose oil supplements may increase the risk of epileptic side-effects	Avoid evening primrose oil supplements
Monoamine oxidase inhibitors	Brewer's yeast	Brewer's yeast may provoke a hypertensive crisis	Avoid brewer's yeast supplements
Anti-epileptics*	Folic acid	Anti-epileptics may cause folate deficiency, but use of folic acid supplements may lead to a fall in serum anticonvulsant levels and reduced seizure control	Folic acid supplements should be given only to those folate-deficient patients on anti-epileptics who can be monitored
	Vitamin B_6	Large doses of vitamin B_6 may reduce serum levels of phenytoin and phenobarbitone	Avoid large doses of vitamin B_6 from supplements (>10 mg daily)
	Vitamin D	Anti-epileptics may disturb metabolism of vitamin D leading to osteomalacia	Susceptible individuals should take 10 μg vitamin D daily
	Vitamin K	Anti-epileptics have been associated with foetal haemorrhage. This is because the drug crosses the placenta and decreases vitamin K status, resulting in bleeding in the infant	Vitamin K should be provided to the newborn infant
Levodopa	Iron	Iron reduces the absorption of levodopa	Separate doses of iron and levodopa by at least 2 h
	Vitamin B_6	Effects of levodopa are reduced or abolished by vitamin B_6 supplements (>5 mg daily), but dietary vitamin B_6 has no effect	Avoid all supplements containing any vitamin B_6. Suggest co-careldopa or co-beneldopa as an alternative to levodopa

Drug	Food/nutrient	Effect	Intervention
Drugs used in the treatment of infections			
Tetracyclines	Iron	Absorption of tetracyclines is reduced by iron and vice versa	Separate doses of iron and tetracyclines by at least 2 h
	Calcium/magnesium/zinc	Absorption of tetracyclines may be reduced by mineral supplements and vice versa	Separate doses of mineral supplements and tetracyclines by at least 2 h
Trimethoprim	Folic acid	Folate deficiency in susceptible individuals	Folic acid supplement may be needed if drug used for prolonged periods
4-quinolones	Iron/zinc	Absorption of 4-quinolones may be reduced by mineral supplements and vice versa	Separate doses of mineral supplements and 4-quinolones by at least 2 h
Cycloserine	Folic acid	Folate deficiency in susceptible individuals	Monitor folate status and give supplement if necessary
Isoniazid	Vitamin B_6	Long-term administration of isoniazid may lead to pyridoxine deficiency	Vitamin B_6 supplement may be needed if symptoms of peripheral neuritis develop
Rifampicin	Vitamin D	Rifampicin may disturb metabolism of vitamin D leading to osteomalacia in susceptible individuals	Monitor serum vitamin D levels
Drugs used in the treatment of disorders of the endocrine system			
Oral hypoglycaemics and insulin	Aloe vera	These supplements could theoretically potentiate the effects of oral hypoglycaemics and insulin	Care in people on medication for diabetes
	Alpha-lipoic acid Chromium		
	Glucosamine	Glucosamine might reduce the effects of oral hypoglycaemics and insulin	Care in people on medication for diabetes
Oestrogens (including HRT and oral contraceptives)	Vitamin C	Concurrent administration of oestrogens and large doses of vitamin C (1 g daily) increases serum levels of oestrogens	Avoid high-dose vitamin C supplements
	DHEA	May potentiate hormonal effects	Care in people using HRT
	Isoflavones	May potentiate hormonal effects	Care in people using HRT
Bisphosphonates	Calcium	May lead to reduced absorption of bisphosphonate	Take 2 h apart
Thyroid medication	Kelp/iodine	May lead to poor control of thyroid condition	Avoid without a doctor's advice.
Drugs used in the treatment of musculo-skeletal and joint diseases			
Penicillamine	Iron/zinc	Absorption of penicillamine reduced by mineral supplements and vice versa	Separate doses of mineral supplements and penicillamine by at least 2 h

*This interaction applies to the older anti-epileptic drugs (e.g. phenytoin, primidine, phenobarbitone, valproate and carbamazepine). There is little information on newer anti-epileptic drugs except with the possibility of lamotrigine, which may have anti-epileptic properties. (Gilman JT. Lamotrigine: an antiepileptic agent for the treatment of partial seizures. *Ann Pharmacother* 1995; 29: 144–151.)

Appendix 3

Additional resources

Government web sites related to dietary supplements

United Kingdom

UK Food Standards Agency Expert Group on Vitamins and Minerals (EVM)
A group of independent experts established to consider the safety of vitamins and minerals sold under food law. Produced a report, *Safe Upper Levels for Vitamins and Minerals*, in May 2003.
http://www.food.gov.uk

Medicines and Healthcare products Regulatory Agency (MHRA)
The UK body that licenses medicines. Provides information on legislation relating to herbals and supplements.
http://www.mhra.gov.uk

Europe

European Union Food Safety web site
Gives details of all EU regulation on food supplements.
http://www.europa.eu/pol/food/index_en.htm

European Food Safety Authority (EFSA)
http://ec.europa.eu/comm./food/efsa/efsa_admin_en.htm

USA

US Food and Drug Administration (FDA)
FDA Center for Food Safety and Applied Nutrition
http://vm.cfsan.fda.gov/list.html

FDA press releases and fact sheets
http://vm.cfsan.fda.gov/~lrd/press.html

FDA what's new
http://vm.cfsan.fda.gov/~news/whatsnew.html

Announcements about dietary supplements
Includes details of adverse effects reported to the FDA about individual supplements.
http://vm.cfsan.fda.gov/~dms/supplmnt.html

Overview and history of FDA and the Center for Food Safety and Applied Nutrition
http://vm.cfsan.fda.gov/~lrd/fdahist.html

National Institutes of Health Office of Dietary Supplements
http://dietary-supplements.info.nih.gov

Associations representing industry

Association of the European Self-Medication Industry (AESGP)
European trade association representing the over-the-counter healthcare products industry.
http://www.aesgp.be

Council for Responsible Nutrition (CRN)
Provides member companies with legislative guidance, regulatory interpretation, scientific information on supplement benefits and safety issues and communications expertise.
UK web site: http://www.crn-uk.org
US web site: http://www.crnusa.org

Health Food Manufacturers' Association (HFMA)
A trade association that acts as a voice for the industry; covers food supplements, health foods, herbal remedies, etc.
http://www.hfma.co.uk

International Alliance of Dietary/Food Supplement Associations (IADSA)
Aims to facilitate a sound legislative and political environment to build growth in the international market for dietary supplements based on scientific principles.
http://www.iadsa.org

Proprietary Association of Great Britain (PAGB)
UK trade association representing the consumer healthcare industry.
http://www.pagb.co.uk

Journals and newsletters

American Journal of Clinical Nutrition
Official journal of the American Society for Clinical Nutrition. Published monthly.
http://www.ajcn.org

Focus on Alternative and Complementary Therapies (FACT)
Provides summaries and commentaries on various aspects of complementary medicine, including vitamins, minerals and supplements. Published quarterly.
http://www.pharmpress.com

Journal of Dietary Supplements
A peer-reviewed academic publication, providing the latest information on food supplements. Published quarterly.
The Haworth Press Inc.
http://www.haworthpressinc.com
Tel: +1 800 342 9678

Medicinal Foods News
An online magazine devoted to medical and functional foods.
http://www.medicinalfoodnews.com

Veris Newsletter
Source of information on the role of nutrition in health, with emphasis on antioxidants, botanicals and other ingredients from natural sources.
http://www.cognis.com/veris/verisdefault.htm

On-line research information and comment

Arbor Nutrition Guide
Provides regular updates on nutritional issues, including those with relevance to supplements.
http://arborcom.com (for subscriptions, see http://www.nutritionupdates.org/sub/sub01.php?item=3)

International bibliographic information on dietary supplements (IBIDS)
The aim of this database is to help health professionals, researchers and the general public find scientific literature on dietary supplements.
http://ods.od/nih.gov/Health_Information/IBIDS.aspx

Medline
The US National Library of Medicine's bibliographic database providing extensive coverage of medicine and healthcare from approximately 3900 current biomedical journals, published in about 70 countries.
http://www.ncbi.nlm.nih.gov/pubmed

Medline Dietary Supplements
http://www.nlm.nih.gov/medlineplus/dietarysupplements. html

Medline Vitamins
http://www.nlm.nih.gov/medlineplus/vitamins.html

Other information

Consumer Lab
Tests the content of diet supplements in the USA and provides reports on its work.
http://consumerlab.com

Health Supplement Information Service (HSIS)
Developed by the Proprietary Association of Great Britain (PAGB) to present the facts about health supplements in a straightforward way. Aims to eliminate confusion and provide reliable data about individual nutrients and supplements.
http://www.hsis.org

Joint Health Claims Initiative (JHCI)
Established as a joint venture by consumer organisations, enforcement authorities and industry trade associations to concerns relating to health claims and develop a code of practice to regulate the use of health claims on foods and supplements.
http://www.jhci.org.uk

Quackwatch
A non-profit organisation with the aim of debunking health-related frauds, myths, fads and fallacies. There are sections on dietary supplements.
http://www.quackwatch.com/index.html

Index